Atlas of
INFECTIOUS DISEASES

Volume XI

Pediatric Infectious Diseases

Atlas of
INFECTIOUS DISEASES

Volume XI

PEDIATRIC INFECTIOUS DISEASES

Editor-in-Chief

Gerald L. Mandell, MD

Professor of Medicine
Owen R. Cheatham Professor of the Sciences
Chief, Division of Infectious Diseases
University of Virginia Health Sciences Center
Charlottesville, Virginia

Editor

Catherine M. Wilfert, MD

Professor Emerita
Pediatric Infectious Diseases
Department of Pediatrics
Division of Infectious Diseases and AIDS Clinical Trials Unit
Duke University Medical Center
Durham, North Carolina

With 26 contributors

CHURCHILL LIVINGSTONE

DEVELOPED BY CURRENT MEDICINE, INC.
PHILADELPHIA

CURRENT MEDICINE
400 MARKET STREET, SUITE 700
PHILADELPHIA, PA 19106

Library of Congress Cataloging-in-Publication Data

Pediatric infectious diseases / editor, Catherine M. Wilfert.
p. cm. — (Atlas of infectious diseases; v. 11)
Includes bibliographical references and index.
1. Communicable diseases in children—Atlases. I. Wilfert, Catherine M. II. Series
[DNLM: 1. Communicable Diseases—in infancy & childhood atlases. WC 17 P371 1998]
RJ401.P4 1998
618.92'9-dc21
DNLM/DLC
for Library of Congress 98-25168
CIP

Director of Product Development....................................**Lori J. Bainbridge**
Developmental Editor....................................**Scott Thomas Hurd**
Assistant Editor....................................**Jennifer Wood**
Art Director....................................**Paul Fennessy**
Design and Layout....................................**Erika Mangan**
Illustration Director....................................**Ann Saydlowski**
Illustrator....................................**Nicole Mock, Debra Wertz**
Production Manager....................................**Lori Holland**
Production and Marketing Associate....................................**Amy Watts**
Indexer....................................**Ann Cassar**

ISBN 0-443-06526-8

Printed in Hong Kong by Paramount Printing Group Limited.

10 9 8 7 6 5 4 3 2 1

PREFACE

This volume on pediatric infectious diseases is a selective presentation of an array of infectious diseases as they appear in children. Although some of these infections, such as HHV-6, are almost always limited to children who incur the primary infection. Other infections, such as herpes simplex, may be recurrent and are observed in adults and children. The manifestations of infections often differ in children and these unique presentations and the epidemiology are presented in these pages. The continuing evolution of diseases are affected by human interventions and thus many of these infections, such as measles, rubella, and poliomyelitis, are becoming rare in the developed world because of the advent of successful immunizations. The changing epidemiology and the common disparity observed between resource-poor countries and developed nations is all too clear. HIV infection is a global problem, yet mother to infant transmission can be dramatically reduced by antiretroviral treatment of the pregnant woman. Resource-poor nations have not yet benefited from this knowledge. *Haemophilus influenzae* diseases have almost disappeared in the developed world employing immunization, whereas the morbidity is often not yet even known in less-developed regions.

The compilation of information contained in these pages is due to the industrious and time-consuming efforts of all of the authors. They have done a masterful job in presenting materials that will be helpful in teaching others, in documenting our progress, and in describing how much work remains to be done.

Catherine M. Wilfert

Contributors

Mark J. Abzug, MD
Associate Professor
Department of Pediatrics
University of Colorado School of Medicine
Denver, Colorado

Kenneth A. Alexander, MD, PhD
Assistant Professor
Department of Pediatrics
Division of Pediatric Infectious Diseases
Duke University Medical Center
Durham, North Carolina

Larry J. Anderson, MD
Chief
Respiratory and Enteric Viruses Branch
Division of Viral and Rickettsial Diseases
National Center for Infectious Diseases
Centers for Disease Control and Prevention
Atlanta, Georgia

Ann M. Arvin, MD
Professor
Department of Pediatrics and Microbiology
Stanford University;
Lucile Salter Packard Children's Hospital
Stanford, California

Jane C. Burns, MD
Associate Professor
Department of Pediatrics
University of California, San Diego School of Medicine
La Jolla, California

Mary T. Caserta, MD
Assistant Professor
Department of Pediatrics
University of Rochester;
Attending Physician in Pediatric Infectious Diseases
University of Rochester Medical Center
Rochester, New York

Kenji M. Cunnion, MD, MPH
Fellow
Department of Pediatrics
Duke University Medical Center
Durham, North Carolina

Adnan S. Dajani, MD
Professor
Department of Pediatrics
Wayne State University School of Medicine;
Director of Infectious Diseases
Children's Hospital of Michigan
Detroit, Michigan

Dan Danielsson, MD, PhD
Visiting Professor
Department of Pediatrics
Emory University School of Medicine
Atlanta, Georgia;
Professor
Orebro Medical Center Hospital
Orebro, Switzerland

Gail J. Demmler, MD
Associate Professor
Department of Pediatrics and Pathology
Baylor College of Medicine;
Attending Physician
Director of Diagnostic Virology Laboratory
Texas Children's Hospital
Houston, Texas

Patricia Ferrieri, MD
Professor
Department of Laboratory Medicine, Pathology, and Pediatrics
University of Minnesota Medical School;
Director
Clinical Microbiology Laboratory
University of Minnesota Hospital
Minneapolis, Minnesota

Patricia Flynn, MD
Associate Professor
Department of Pediatrics
University of Tennessee;
Associate Member
St. Jude's Children's Research Hospital
Memphis, Tennessee

Mary P. Glodé, MD
Professor
Department of Pediatrics
University of Colorado;
Vice Chair
Department of Pediatrics
Children's Hospital
Denver, Colorado

Caroline Breese Hall, MD
Professor
Department of Medicine and Pediatrics
University of Rochester;
Attending Physician in Pediatric Infectious Diseases
University of Rochester Medical Center
Rochester, New York

Sheryl Henderson, MD, PhD
Assistant Professor
Department of Pediatrics
Emory University School of Medicine;
Attending Physician in Pediatric Infectious Diseases
Grady Memorial Hospital and Egleston Children's Hospital
Atlanta, Georgia

Richard F. Jacobs, MD, FAAP
Horace C. Cabe Professor
Department of Pediatrics
University of Arkansas for Medical Sciences;
Chief of Pediatric Infectious Diseases
Arkansas Children's Hospital
Little Rock, Arkansas

Mark W. Kline, MD
Professor
Department of Pediatrics
Baylor College of Medicine;
Attending Physician
Texas Children's Hospital
Houston, Texas

Yvonne A. Maldonado, MD
Associate Professor
Department of Pediatrics
Stanford University;
Attending Physician
Lucile Salter Packard Children's Hospital
Stanford, California

André J. Nahimas, MD, PhD
Professor
Department of Pediatrics
Emory University;
Director of Pediatric Infectious Diseases
Grady Memorial Hospital and Egleston Children's Hospital
Atlanta, Georgia

Robert L. Roberts, MD, PhD
Associate Professor
Department of Pediatrics
University of California, Los Angeles
Los Angeles, California

Eric A.F. Simoes, MD, DCh
Associate Professor
Department of Pediatrics
University of Colorado School of Medicine
Denver, Colorado

David H. Spach, MD
Associate Professor of Medicine
Division of Infectious Diseases
University of Washington;
Director
Infectious Diseases Clinic
Harborview Medical Center;
Director
AIDS Medical Education
Northwest AIDS Education and Training Center
Seattle, Washington

James K. Todd, MD
Professor of Pediatrics, Microbiology, and Preventive Medicine
University of Colorado School of Medicine
Denver, Colorado

Thomas J. Török, MD
Medical Officer
Centers for Disease Control and Prevention
Atlanta, Georgia

Elaine Tuomanen, MD
Chair
Department of Infectious Diseases
St. Jude's Children's Research Hospital
Memphis, Tennessee

Sherif R. Zaki, MD, PhD
Adjunct Assistant Professor
Department of Pathology
Emory University;
Chief of Infectious Diseases
Centers for Disease Control and Prevention
Atlanta, Georgia

Contents

CHAPTER 1

Measles, mumps, and rubella

Yvonne A. Maldonado

MEASLES AND RUBELLA are exanthemous and enanthemous illnesses of childhood. Mumps is a generalized viral illness whose major clinical feature is parotitis. In general, all three illnesses are rarely accompanied by serious complications among children living in the United States, and infection is preventable by highly effective vaccines that are administered as a combination (*ie*, measles, mumps, rubella vaccine) in the first year of life. Because the major clinical manifestation of measles and rubella may be an exanthem or enanthem, the differential diagnosis for these two viral infections is extensive. In contrast, mumps is only one of a few infectious agents that cause parotitis; therefore, the differential diagnosis is restricted to a few viral and bacterial pathogens. No effective antiviral therapy exists for any of these illnesses, but in general most children who contract these infections have few to no sequelae. Complications are more common, however, among infants acquiring measles infection, especially those living in developing countries, older children and adults with measles or mumps, and among infants with congenitally acquired rubella. Until recently, all three illnesses were extremely prevalent in the United States and elsewhere; however, development of safe and effective vaccines directed against all three pathogens has decreased the prevalence dramatically in the United States. The major strategy for global elimination of measles, mumps, and rubella, therefore, is strict adherence to immunization of infants against all three pathogens.

MEASLES

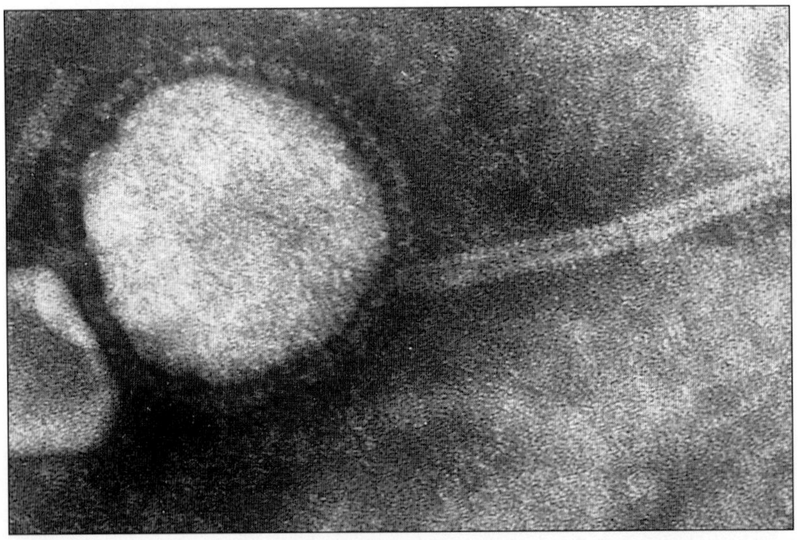

FIGURE 1-1 Measles virus. Measles is an RNA virus and a member of the paramyxovirus family, which includes human pathogens such as mumps, parainfluenza, and respiratory syncytial viruses. Measles virus, however, is in the genus Morbillivirus, which is most related to paramyxoviruses. Paramyxoviruses are animal pathogens that include canine distemper virus and rinderpest, a disease of cattle. Only one measles antigenic type exists [1,2], although there is recent evidence of geographic differences in genetic sequences of wild-type measles viruses [3,4] that have not affected measles immunity [5,6]. Measles virions are spherical, enveloped, and pleomorphic and have a diameter of 100 to 250 nm. (*From* Almeida [7]; with permission.)

Clinical stages of measles infection

Stage	Onset, *d*	Manifestations
1 (incubation)	8–12	None
2 (prodrome)	2–4	Prodrome Fever Catarrhal symptoms Cough Conjunctivitis
3 (enanthem)	4–6	Enanthem Koplik's spots Mild fever and respiratory symptoms
4 (exanthem)	4–8	Exanthem Maculopapular Occasionally confluent Moderate to severe fever and respiratory symptoms

FIGURE 1-2 Clinical stages of measles infection. Typical manifestations of measles infection are divided into three stages. The first is the asymptomatic incubation period, which usually lasts from 8 to 12 days. The second is the prodromal stage, which lasts approximately 2 days and is marked by the beginning symptoms of low-grade fever and the classic triad of cough, coryza, and conjunctivitis. Within 2 to 3 days, the enanthemous stage begins, which consists of a mild erythematous hue in the oral mucosa along with the pathognomonic Koplik's spots. The third stage, exanthemous, is marked by development of a maculopapular rash progressing in a cephalocaudal direction and a worsening of the prodromal symptoms. Fever and respiratory symptoms generally peak within 2 days of development of the exanthem and resolve quickly thereafter, unless there are respiratory complications.

Measles pathogenesis

Transmission
- Respiratory, highly infectious
- Most common in winter and spring
- Prevaccine era epidemics in 2–5-y cycles

Course of infection
- Virus attaches to respiratory epithelium
- Regional lymphatics infected
- Primary viremia
- Replication in reticuloendothelial tissue
- Secondary viremia throughout all organ systems

Immunity
- Develops within 15–17 d after infection; lifelong

FIGURE 1-3 Pathogenesis of measles virus infection. Measles, one of the most contagious pathogens in humans, is transmitted via the respiratory route by aerosolized particles. Individuals are most infectious during the prodromal stage. Once infection occurs, the virus rapidly invades upper respiratory epithelium, spreads to lymphatics, replicates through the reticuloendothelial system, and produces a significant secondary viremia throughout the body that is the source of all the clinical manifestations of measles infection, *eg*, fever, rash, and respiratory symptoms.

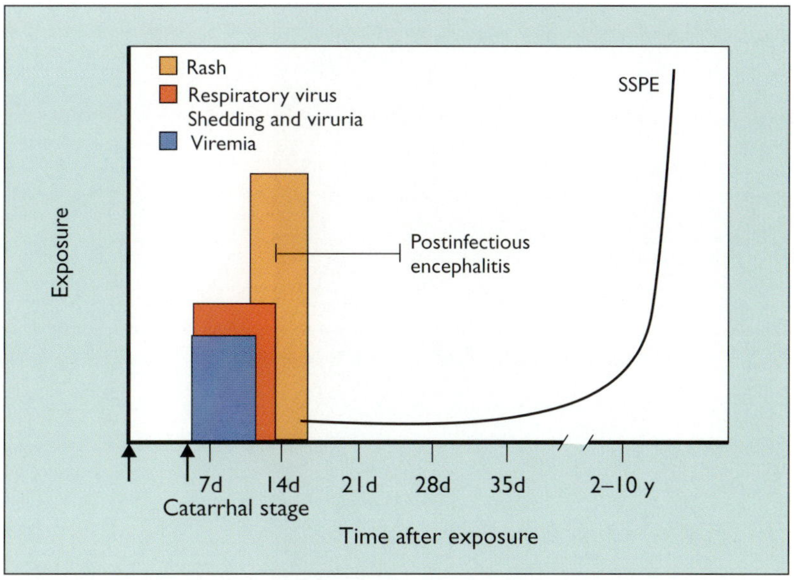

FIGURE 1-4 The pathogenesis of measles infection. This schematic depicts the pathogenesis of measles infection as outlined in Figure 1-3, including the incubation period, course of infection, and complications (*eg*, subacute sclerosing panencephalitis [SSPE]).

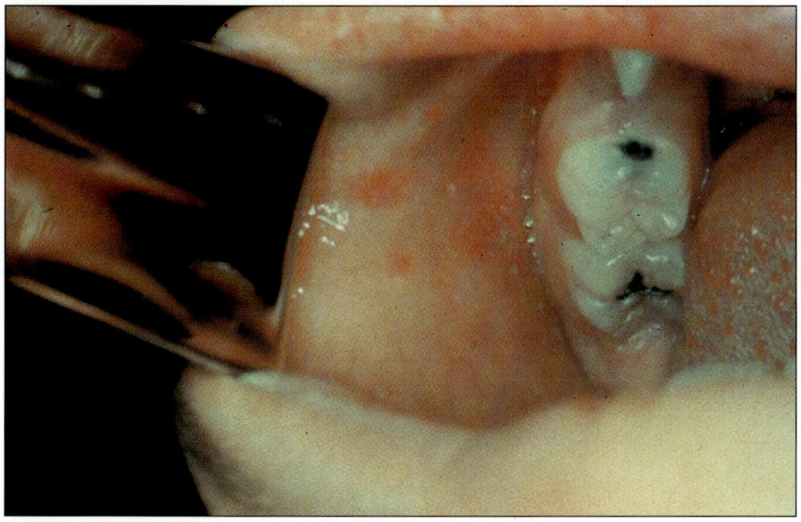

FIGURE 1-5 Koplik's spots. The enanthem of measles infection is manifested primarily by erythematous oral mucosa and by Koplik's spots, which are white, macular, 1-mm lesions that appear on the buccal mucosa usually opposite the premolars. Eventually these lesions may coalesce and spread throughout the buccal mucosa, including the hard and soft palate. Koplik's spots precede the development of the classic measles exanthem by 2 to 3 days and may be fleeting, usually lasting only 12 to 72 hours. (*Courtesy of* Centers for Disease Control and Prevention).

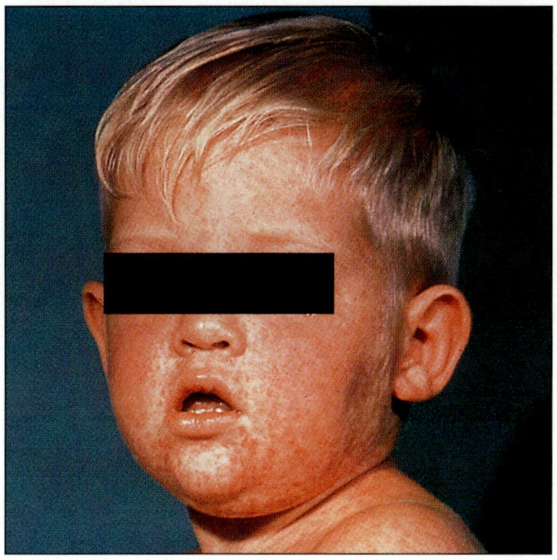

FIGURE 1-6 Early measles exanthem, day 3. This young boy displays the classic form of the early measles exanthemous phase, with conjunctivitis, coryza, and an initially discrete maculopapular rash beginning on the face and spreading to the trunk and extremities. The rash will begin to coalesce in a cephalocaudal direction, as seen in this child. (*Courtesy of* Centers for Disease Control and Prevention).

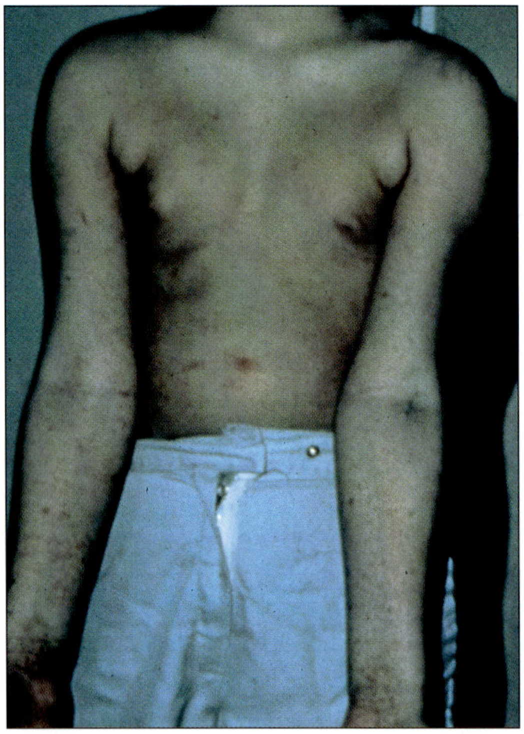

FIGURE 1-7 Atypical measles. Rarely seen now, this form of measles is characteristic of infected individuals who had previously received killed measles vaccines between 1963 and 1968 [8,9]. The incomplete immunity provided by the killed vaccines led to the atypical clinical manifestations of measles. These include sudden onset of high fever, cough, vomiting, pleuritic chest pain, absence of enanthemous phase, and an atypical rash. The rash of atypical measles typically begins distally and proceeds in a centripetal direction, primarily involving the extremities and the lower trunk. Vesicular lesions may also be seen in addition to the maculopapular exanthem.

Complications of typical measles infection

Complication	Rate per 100,000 cases	Cases, %
Otitis Media	8500–15,000	7–9
Pneumonia	3800–7300	1–6
Seizures	500–1000	1–2
Encephalitis	50–400	0.10–0.01
Systemic side effects	0.5–2.0	0.0001*
Deaths	10–10,000	0.001–10

* Prevaccine era.

FIGURE 1-8 Complications of typical measles infection. Because of the extensive viremia and viral replication throughout all organ systems, measles infection is associated with several of complications. Another factor associated with complications of measles is the inherent ability of measles infection to produce transient immunosuppression in the infected individual. Morbidity and mortality rates are represented here for measles cases reported throughout the world; however, the higher rates are noted in lesser developed areas of the world, especially among the malnourished. Even in developed areas of the world, measles deaths may occur in as many as one out of 1000 cases in young children [10]. Secondary bacterial pneumonia accounts for up to 60% of deaths, and diarrhea is also an important cause of death in developing areas of the world [11].

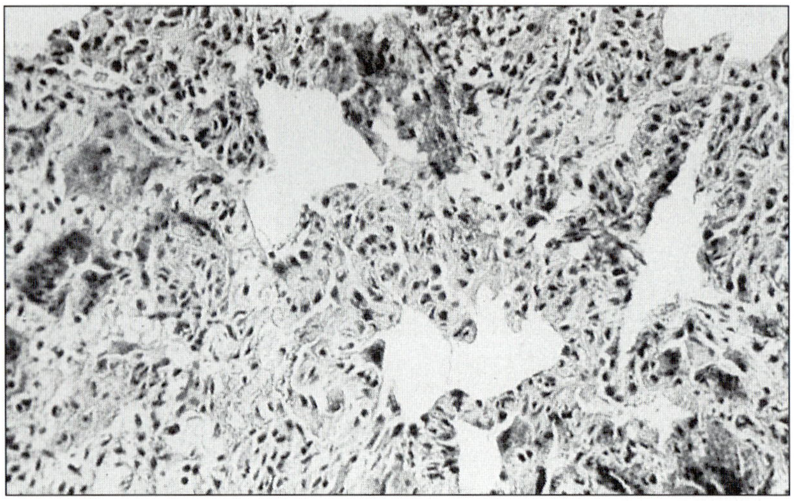

FIGURE 1-9 Histologic features of measles pneumonia. Measles-infected respiratory cells will fuse and form multinucleated giant cells. Among immunocompromised hosts, measles pneumonia may evolve to giant cell pneumonia, which is often fatal.

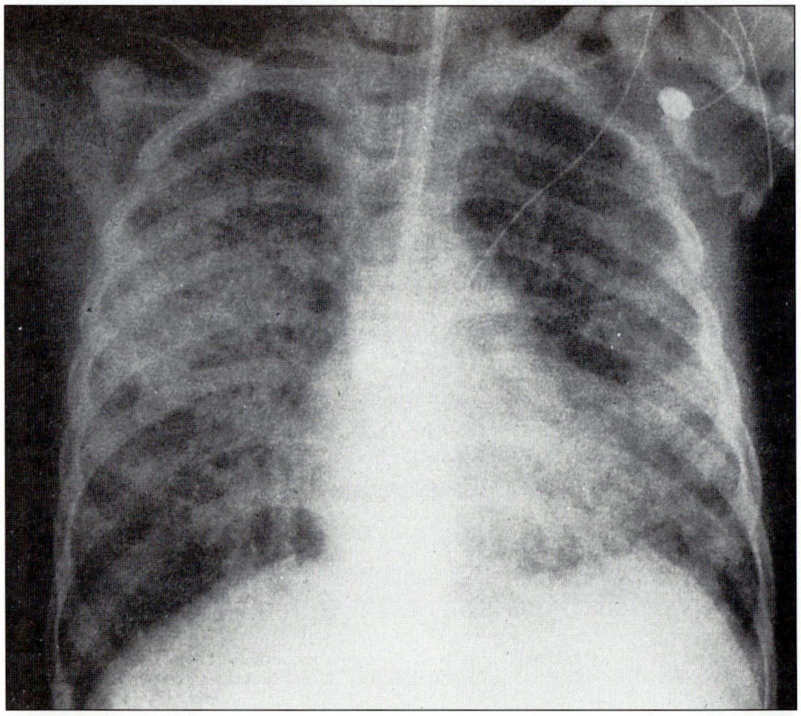

FIGURE 1-10 Giant cell measles pneumonia in the immunosuppressed host. Among malnourished or immunosuppressed individuals, prominent clinical manifestations are giant cell pneumonitis and encephalitis, and the mortality rate may be as high as 70%. Frequently, these infections may present without an exanthemous phase.

Laboratory diagnosis of measles infection

Method	Phase of illness	Sample needed	Interpretation
Antigen detection			
Immunofluorescence	Catarrhal (4 d before to 10 d after rash onset)	Nasopharyngeal Urine	Acute infection
Immunoperoxidase	Catarrhal (4 d before to 10 d after rash onset)	Nasopharyngeal Urine	Acute infection
Tissue culture	Up to 2 d after rash onset	Nasopharyngeal Blood buffy coat Urine	Acute infection
Antibody detection			
Complement fixation	Acute and convalescent	Serum	Evidence of past infection
Radioimmunoassay	Acute and convalescent	Serum	Evidence of past infection
ELISA	Acute and convalescent	Serum	Evidence of past infection
Plaque neutralization	Acute and convalescent	Serum	Evidence of past infection

ELISA—enzyme-linked immunoassay.

Figure 1-11 Laboratory diagnosis of measles infection. Patient samples from a number of sites may be used in direct detection of measles virus during active infection. In general, most detection methods provide identification of virus or viral antigens. Tissue culture is a cumbersome and sometimes inaccurate method and, therefore, is generally not useful in the diagnosis of measles infection. Evidence of current or previous measles infection can be found by measles antibody assays. The most commonly used assay is the enzyme-linked immunoassay (ELISA) [12–14]).

Differential diagnosis of measles infection

Phase of illness	Differential diagnosis	Distinctive clinical features of measles
Prodrome	Respiratory syncytial virus	None
	Influenza	None
	Parainfluenza viruses	None
	Kawasaki disease	Lack of typical Kawasaki enanthem and prolonged fever
Enanthem	Streptococci	Koplik's spots
	Staphylococci	Koplik's spots
	Kawasaki disease	Koplik's spots
Exanthem	Streptococci	Evolution of measles exanthem
	Rubella	Evolution of measles exanthem
	Parvovirus	Evolution of measles exanthem
	Enterovirus	Evolution of measles exanthem
	Epstein–Barr virus	Evolution of measles exanthem; lack of hepatosplenomegaly
	Cytomegalovirus	Evolution of measles exanthem; lack of hepatosplenomegaly
	Mycoplasma pneumoniae	Evolution of measles exanthem
	Erythema multiforme	Constitutional symptoms; evolution of exanthem
	Secondary syphilis	Constitutional symptoms; evolution of exanthem
	Drug rash	Constitutional symptoms; evolution of exanthem
	Connective tissue disease	Constitutional symptoms; evolution of exanthem

Figure 1-12 Differential diagnosis of measles infection. Because of the exanthemous phase of measles infection, the differential diagnosis for typical measles may be broad. During the prodrome, many respiratory viruses can be included in the differential diagnosis. However, once the development of Koplik's spots occurs (if they are detected), the diagnosis of measles is clear. During the exanthem phase of measles infection, most exanthemous illnesses can be included in the differential diagnosis, but most commonly the early measles exanthem is confused with scarlet fever because of the character of the exanthem and the nature of the constitutional symptoms. The evolution of the measles exanthem differentiates this illness from other causes.

Recommendations for measles vaccination

Category	Recommendations
Unvaccinated, no history of measles (12–15 mo of age)	A two-dose schedule (with MMR) is recommended if born after 1956; the first dose is recommended at 12–15 mo of age; the second is recommended at 4–6 y of age
Children 12 mo of age in areas of recurrent measles transmission	Vaccinate; a second dose is indicated at 4–6 y of age (at school entry)
Children 6–11 mo in epidemic situations	Vaccinate (with monovalent measles vaccine or, if not available, MMR); revaccination (with MMR) at 12–15 mo of age is necessary, and a third dose is indicated at 4–6 y
Children 11–12 y who have received one dose of measles vaccine at ≥12 mo of age	Revaccinate (1 dose)
Students in college and other post–high school institutions who have received one dose of measles vaccine at ≥12 mo of age	Revaccinate (1 dose)
History of vaccination before first birthday	Consider susceptible and vaccinate (two doses)
Unknown vaccine, 1963–1967	Consider susceptible and vaccinate (two doses)
Further attenuated or unknown vaccine given with immunoglobulin	Consider susceptible and vaccinate (two doses)
Egg allergy	Vaccinate; no reactive likely
Neomycin allergy, nonanaphylactic	Vaccinate; no reactive likely
Tuberculosis	Vaccinate; vaccine does not exacerbate infection
Measles exposure	Vaccinate or give immunoglobulin, depending on circumstances
HIV infected	Vaccinate (2 doses) unless severely compromised
Immunoglobulin or blood product received	Vaccinate at the appropriate interval (*see* Table 1-18)

MMR—measles-mumps-rubella vaccine.

FIGURE 1-13 Recommendations for measles immunization in the United States. The two-dose schedule of measles administration in childhood is important in maximizing prevention of primary vaccine failure. (*From* the American Academy of Pediatrics [15]; with permission.)

Suggested intervals between immunoglobulin administration and measles vaccination (measles-mumps-rubella vaccine or monovalent measles vaccine)

Indication for immunoglobulin	Route	Dose: Units or mL	Dose: mg IgG/kg	Interval, *mo**
Tetanus (as TIG)	IM	250 U	~10	3
Hepatitis A prophylaxis (as Ig)				
Contact prophylaxis	IM	0.02 mL/kg	3.3	3
International travel	IM	0.06 mL/kg	10	3
Hepatitis B prophylaxis (as HBIG)	IM	0.06 mL/kg	10	3
Rabies prophylaxis (as RIG)	IM	20 IU/kg	22	4
Measles prophylaxis (as Ig)				
Standard	IM	0.25 mL/kg	40	5
Immunocompromised host	IM	0.50 mL/kg	80	6
Varicella prophylaxis (as VZIG)	IM	125 U/10 kg (maximum, 625 U)	20–39	5
Blood transfusion				
Washed erythrocytes	IV	10 mL/kg	Negligible	0
Erythrocytes (adenine-saline added)	IV	10 mL/kg	10	3
Packed erythrocytes	IV	10 mL/kg	20–60	5
Whole blood	IV	10 mL/kg	80–100	6
Plasma or platelet products	IV	10 mL/kg	160	7
Replacement (or therapy) of immune deficiencies (as IVIG)	IV	—	300–400	8
ITP (as IVIG)	IV	—	400	8
RSV–IVIG	IV	—	750	9
ITP	IV	—	1000	10
ITP or Kawasaki disease	IV	—	1600–2000	11

* These intervals should provide sufficient time for decreases in passive antibodies in all children to allow for an adequate response to measles vaccine. Physicians should not assume that children are fully protected against measles during these intervals. Additional doses of Ig or measles vaccine may be indicated after exposure to measles.

HBIG—hepatitis B immunoglobulin; Ig—immunoglobulin; IM—intramuscular; ITP—immune thrombocytopenia purpura; IV—intravenous; IVIG—intravenous immunoglobulin; RIG—rabies immunoglobulin; RSV-IVIG—respiratory syncytial virus intravenous immunoglobulin; TIG—tetanus immunoglobulin; VZIG—varicella-zoster immunoglobulin.

FIGURE 1-14 Intervals for immune globulin administration after measles vaccination. Because measles vaccine uses a live attenuated virus, immunoglobulin preparations may inactivate the vaccine and lead to insufficient or absent immune response. Measles immunization must be given at different intervals after administration of various immunoglobulin preparations, as outlined in the table, in order to allow for an adequate immune response to the measles vaccine. (*From* the American Academy of Pediatrics [15]; with permission.)

Recommendations for control of measles outbreaks

Setting	Control measures
Outbreaks in preschool-age children	Age for vaccination should be lowered to 6 mo in outbreak area if cases are occurring in children <1 y*
Outbreaks in institutions (child care centers, K-12th grades, colleges, and other institutions)	All students, their siblings, and school personnel born after 1956 who do not have documentation of immunity to measles† should have received two doses of measles vaccine
Outbreaks in medical facilities	Revaccination of all medical workers born after 1956 who have direct patient contact and who do not have proof of immunity to measles†; vaccination may also be considered for workers born before 1957

* Children initially vaccinated before the first birthday should be revaccinated at 12–15 mo of age, and a third dose should be administered at 4–6 y of age.

† Proof consists of documentation of physician-diagnosed measles disease, serologic evidence of immunity to measles, or documentation of receipt of two doses of measles vaccine on or after the first birthday.

FIGURE 1-15 Public health considerations and outbreak control. Because of the potential for resurgence of measles in the United States, a variety of vaccination strategies may be employed when measles outbreaks occur. (*From* the American Academy of Pediatrics [15]; with permission.)

MUMPS

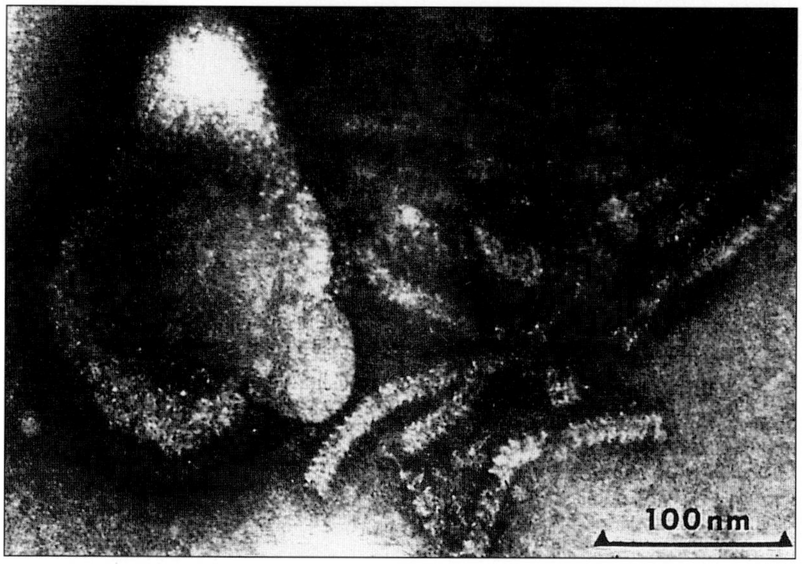

FIGURE 1-16 Mumps virus. Mumps, an RNA virus, was originally classified with the influenza viruses as a member of the myxovirus family. However, it is now classified as a member of the paramyxovirus family, which includes human pathogens such as measles, parainfluenza, and respiratory syncytial viruses. Mumps virus is in the genus Paramyxovirus and is most related to Sendai virus [16,17]. Mumps virions are pleomorphic, enveloped particles with a diameter of 120 to 200 nm. (*From* Wolinsky [18]; with permission.)

Clinical stages of mumps infection

Stage	Onset, *d*	Manifestations
1 (Incubation)	12–25, usually 16–18	None
2 (Prodrome)	1–7, usually 1–2	Prodrome
		Mild fever
		Anorexia
		Malaise
		Myalgia
3 (Parotitis)	1–7, usually 1–2	Unilateral parotitis
	1–3	Bilateral parotitis (70%)
4 (Resolution)	3–5	Systemic symptoms
	7–10	Parotitis

FIGURE 1-17 Clinical stages of mumps infection. Typical characteristics of mumps infection are divided into four stages. The first is the asymptomatic incubation period. The second is the prodromal stage, which lasts approximately 2 days and is marked by the beginning symptoms of low-grade fever and mild constitutional symptoms. Within 1 to 7 days and generally within 1 day, unilateral parotid swelling will become evident; approximately 70% of patients with unilateral parotitis will develop bilateral parotitis within 12 to 24 hours. Resolution of systemic illness occurs within 3 to 5 days and parotitis within 7 to 10 days.

Mumps pathogenesis

Transmission
- Contact with infected respiratory secretions
- Most common in late winter and early spring
- Prevaccine era: 3–4-y cycles

Course of infection
- Virus attaches to respiratory epithelium
- Regional lymphatics infected
- Primary viremia
- Replication throughout all organ systems and glandular epithelium

Immunity
- Long-lasting, possibly lifelong

FIGURE 1-18 Pathogenesis of mumps virus infection. The transmissibility of mumps virus is probably underestimated because 20% to 40% of infections may be asymptomatic. Mumps virus is transmitted by contact with infected respiratory secretions. Individuals are usually infectious during the asymptomatic prodromal period and for up to 1 week after the onset of parotitis. It is clear that mumps infection is not limited to the parotid glands, and that disseminated systemic infection occurs and is the primary source of complications of mumps infection. Immunity is long-lasting, but the onset of immunity after infection is not known.

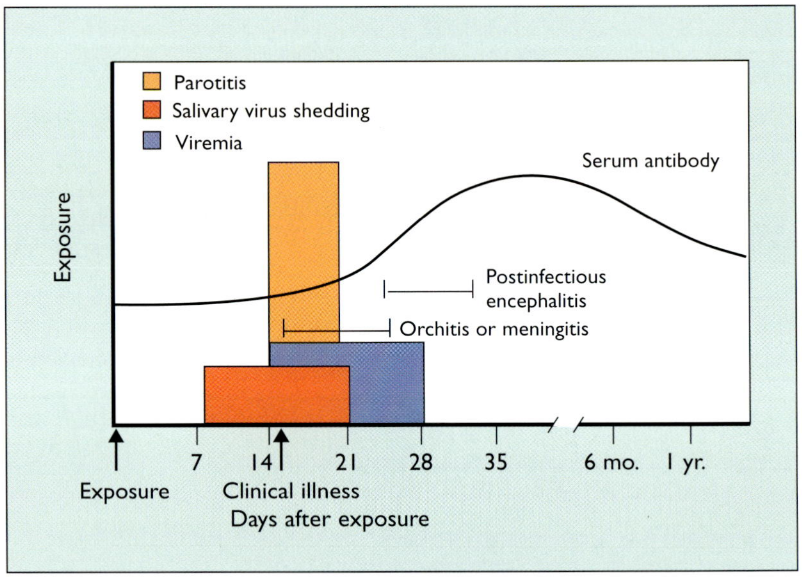

FIGURE 1-19 Pathogenesis of mumps infection as outlined in Figure 1-23.

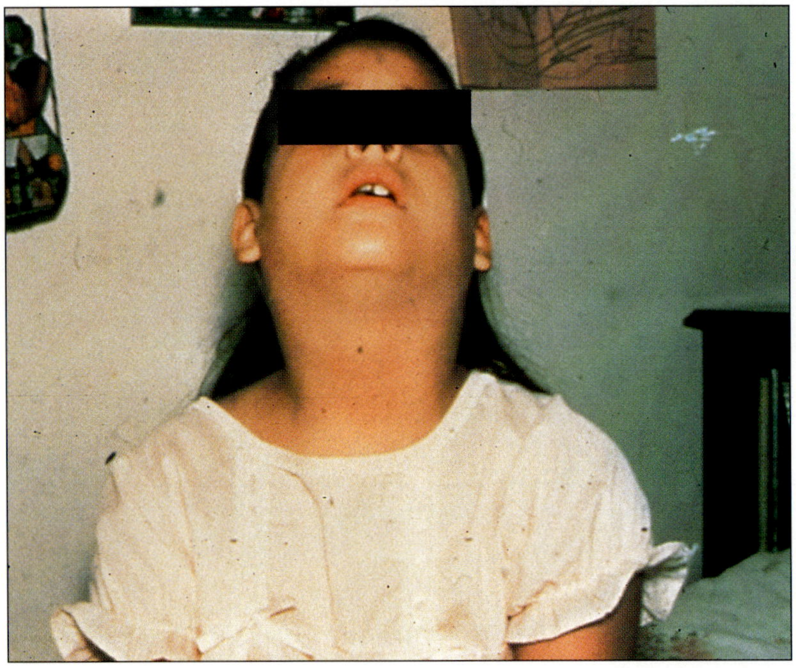

FIGURE 1-20 Bilateral parotitis. This child displays the typical manifestations of bilateral parotitis, which will occur in 70% of patients who develop parotitis during mumps infection. Bilateral involvement typically occurs within 2 to 3 days after onset of unilateral parotitis. Clinical manifestations are similar to those of unilateral parotitis, during which the swollen parotid gland may frequently lift the adjacent ear upward and outward and will obscure the mandibular angle. Within the buccal mucosa, the orifice leading into Stensen's duct may be inflamed and erythematous. The patient may also complain of earache on the affected side and discomfort on ingesting acidic foods or liquids. The parotid gland will reach maximal swelling within 2 days.

Complications of mumps infection

Complication	Cases, %
Orchitis	30–38 (postpubertal males only)
Mastitis	30 (postpubertal females only)
Encephalitis/Meningoencephalitis	1–10
Deafness	Rare
Pancreatitis	Rare
Arthritis	Rare
Deaths	Rare (1.4% of mumps encephalitis)

FIGURE 1-21 Complications of mumps infection. Despite the extensive viremia and viral replication throughout all organ systems, mumps infection is not associated with severe sequelae in most cases. Most complications of acute mumps infection occur among older, postpubertal children and adults. Orchitis is the most common clinical complication of mumps infection. Orchitis is most likely to occur after acute infection among men in the second through fourth decades of life. Testicular pain usually begins within 4 to 8 days after the onset of parotid swelling, is generally unilateral, and may last for 3 to 7 days. Unilateral orchitis occurs in 20% to 30% of male patients who develop mumps after puberty. Of these patients, 25% will develop bilateral orchitis. Half of all male patients with mumps orchitis will develop testicular atrophy, and thus, sterility is likely to occur in less than 1% of patients. Central nervous system involvement is very common, occurring in up to 50% of those with parotitis, but clinical manifestations occur in only 1% to 10% of patients. Symptoms include fever, headache, nuchal rigidity, and mental status changes. Seizures may occur in up to 20% of patients. Most sequelae are self-limited but infrequently may be permanent. Most deaths from mumps occur in adults and are generally secondary to late complications, especially meningoencephalitis.

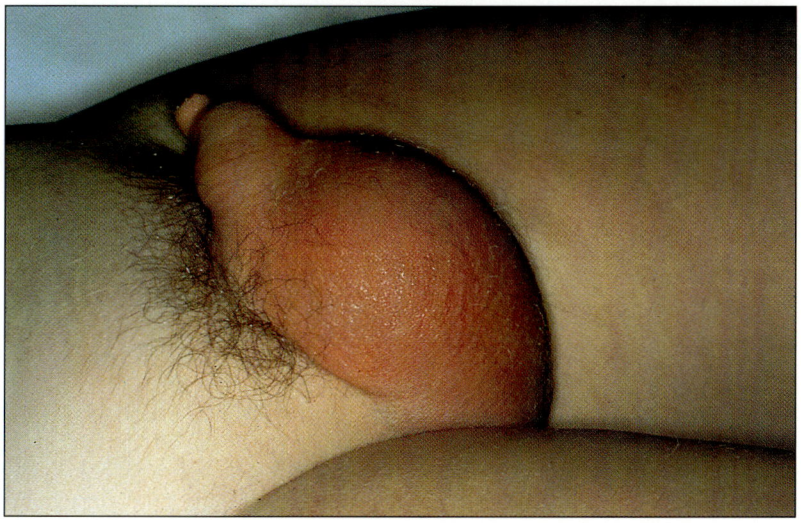

FIGURE 1-22 Mumps orchitis. Note the extensive swelling and erythema.

Recommendations for Mumps Immunization in the United States

Mumps vaccine
- Live virus vaccine prepared in chick embryo cells
- Administered 0.5 mL injected subcutaneously

Indications
- Should be given as a combination vaccine with measles and rubella at 12–15 mo of age with a second dose at 4–6 y of age
- Children who have not received a second dose should be revaccinated by 12 y of age
- Children, adolescents and adults without documentation of receipt of two doses should be vaccinated before travel outside the United States
- Mumps is not routinely indicated for those born before 1957, but is not contraindicated in this group
- Mumps vaccine may be given simultaneously with other vaccines

FIGURE 1-23 Recommendations for mumps immunization in the United States. These recommendations parallel those for measles immunization. (*Adapted from* American Academy of Pediatrics [19]; with permission.)

Rubella

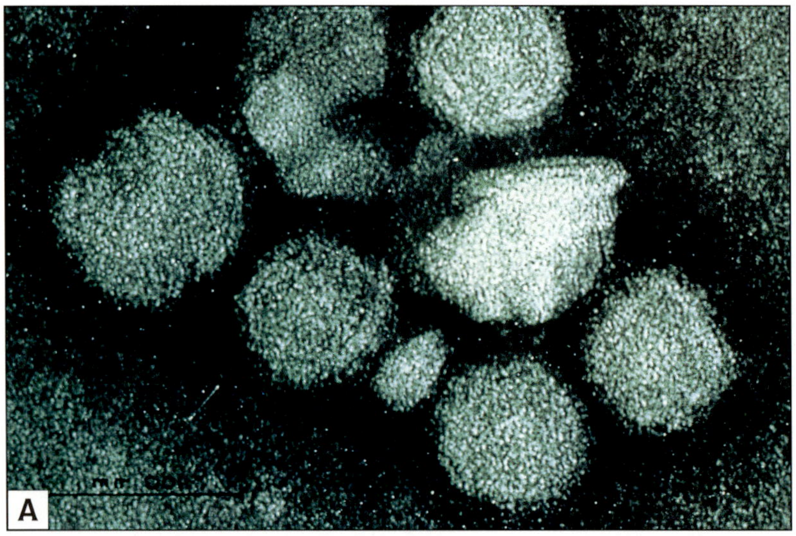

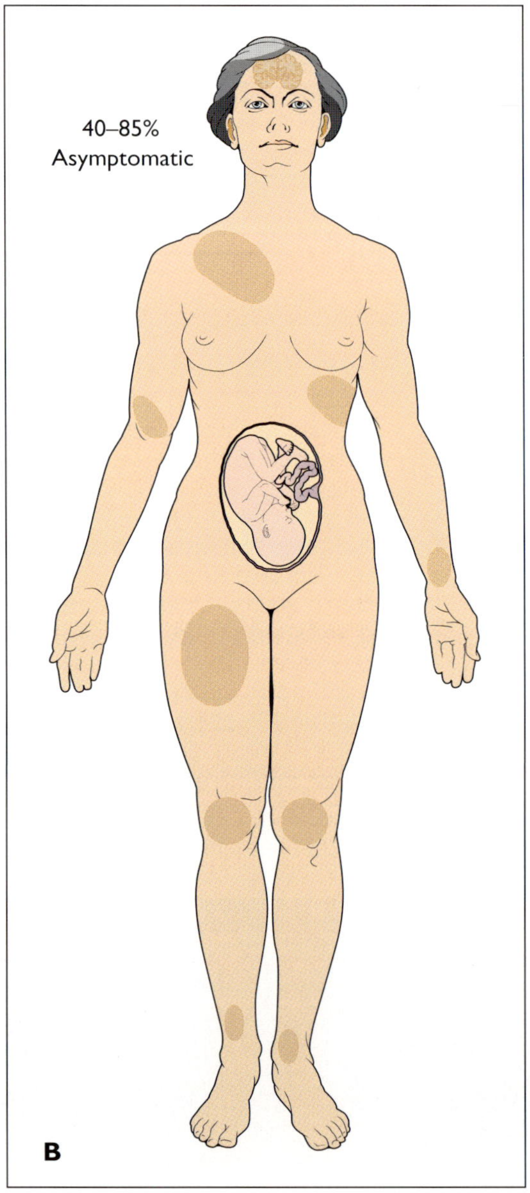

Figure 1-24 Rubella virus. **A**, Rubella virus is a member of the togavirus family and the only member of the genus *Rubivirus*. It has no antigenic relationship to other viruses. Only one rubella antigenic type exists [20]. Rubella virions are pleomorphic, ovoid-shaped, and have a diameter of 120 to 180 nm. **B**, Major organ systems affected by rubella infection.

Clinical stages of acquired rubella infection

Stage	Onset, *d*	Manifestations
1 (Incubation)	14–21	None
2 (Prodrome)	1–5	Prodrome Catarrhal symptoms Lymphadenopathy
3 (Enanthem)	1–2	Enanthem Not Koplik's spots
4 (Exanthem)	0–3	Exanthem Maculopapular Flushed areas Scarlet fever–like rash Mild fever Mild pharyngeal and conjunctival edema

Figure 1-25 Clinical stages of acquired rubella infection. Frequently acquired rubella may be mild enough to go unnoticed or may be completely asymptomatic. The prodrome stage is very mild, but pathognomonic tender extensive enlargement of retroauricular, posterior cervical, and postoccipital lymph nodes occurs during this stage. Lymphadenopathy may persist for a week or longer. Shortly after the prodrome begins, a mild enanthem may appear, characterized by discrete erythematous spots on the soft palate that may coalesce and darken. During the exanthemous phase, the rash begins on the face and spreads rapidly over the entire body within a day. The nature of the rash is variable, and may take on a maculopapular, confluent, or even scarlet fever–like "pinpoint" character. Minimal desquamation will occur by the third day. Splenomegaly may sometimes accompany acquired rubella infection. In older girls or women, polyarthritis with arthralgias may occur and persist for up to 2 weeks without sequelae.

Acquired rubella pathogenesis

Transmission
Direct or droplet contact from infectious nasopharyngeal secretions
Course of infection
Virus attaches to respiratory epithelium
Regional lymphatics infected
Primary viremia
Replication in reticuloendothelial tissue
Secondary viremia throughout all organ systems
Immunity
Develops during clinical manifestations of inaction, usually lifelong but second infections have been serologically documented

FIGURE 1-26 Pathogenesis of acquired rubella infection. Rubella is most likely transmitted via the respiratory route by aerosolized particles from infectious nasopharyngeal secretions. Infectivity correlates with nasopharyngeal shedding of rubella virus, which begins within 3 to 8 days after exposure and may continue for up to 2 weeks. Once infection occurs, the virus rapidly invades upper respiratory epithelium, spreads to lymphatics, replicates through the reticuloendothelial system, and 6 to 20 days after exposure produces a significant secondary viremia throughout the body. During this time, rubella virus can be recovered from a variety of sites, including the respiratory tract, blood, urine, lymph nodes, breast milk, and cerebrospinal fluid. Immunity generally develops during the period of clinical illness.

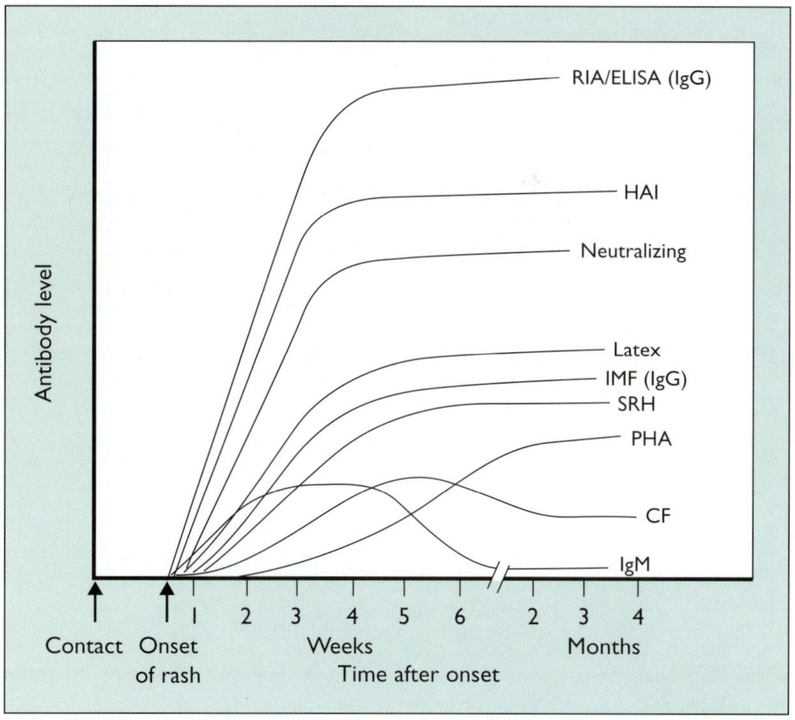

FIGURE 1-27 Antibody response in acute rubella infection. A variety of antibody types are produced in response to acute rubella infection. Development of neutralizing and hemagglutination-inhibition (HAI) antibodies correlates with onset of the rubella exanthem. These antibodies persist for life. CF—complement fixation; RIA/ELISA—radioimmunoassay/enzyme-linked immunosorbent assay; IMF—intermaxillary fixation; PHA—passive hemagglutinating; SRH—somatotropin-releasing hormone. (*Adapted from* Best and O'Shea [21]; with permission.)

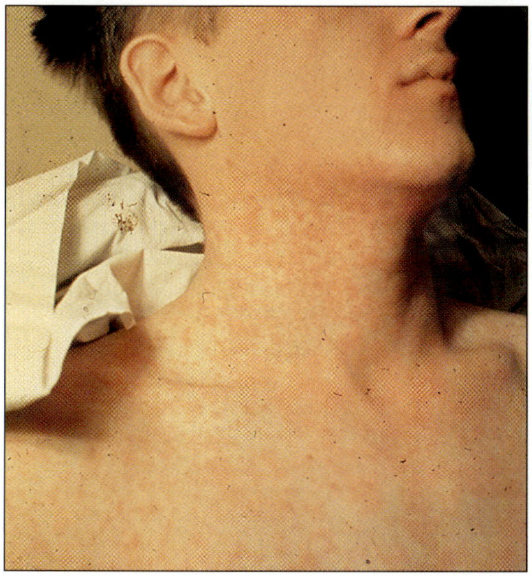

FIGURE 1-28 Rash of acquired rubella. The rash of acquired rubella is usually maculopapular, which may eventually coalesce. The rash is usually mild.

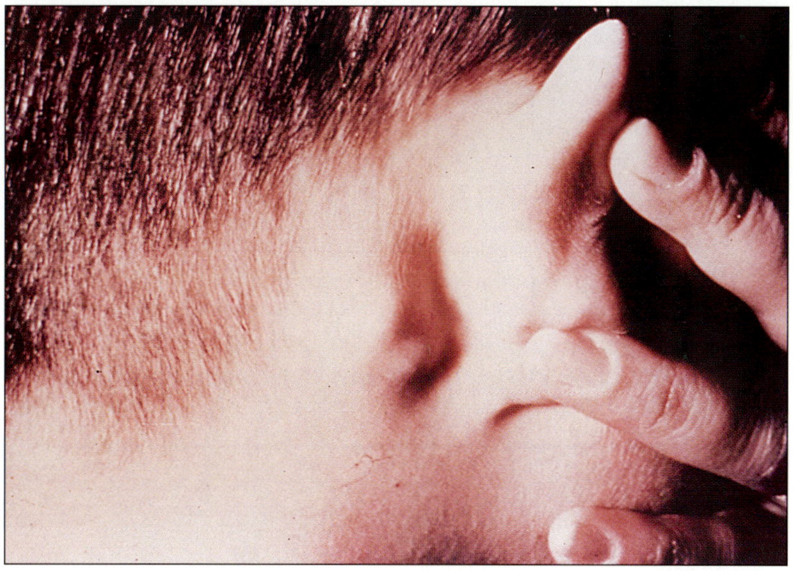

FIGURE 1-29 Posterior auricular adenopathy associated with acquired rubella. Posterior auricular adenopathy is associated most frequently with acquired rubella infection.

Differential diagnosis of acquired rubella infection

Phase of illness	Differential diagnosis	Distinctive clinical features of rubella
Prodrome	Respiratory syncytial virus	None
	Influenza	None
	Parainfluenza viruses	None
	Kawasaki disease	Lack of typical Kawasaki enanthem and prolonged fever
Enanthem	Streptococci	Usually milder
	Staphylococci	Usually milder
	Kawasaki disease	Usually milder
	Measles	No Koplik's spots
Exanthem	Streptococci	Milder, transient exanthem
	Measles	Milder, transient exanthem
	Parvovirus	No associated anemia or distinct exanthem
	Enterovirus	None
	Epstein–Barr virus	Milder, transient exanthem; no hepatomegaly
	Cytomegalovirus	Milder, transient exanthem; no hepatomegaly
	Mycoplasma pneumoniae	Milder respiratory symptoms

Figure 1-30 Differential diagnosis of acquired rubella infection. Because of the exanthemous phase of rubella infection, the differential diagnosis may be broad. During the prodrome, many respiratory viruses can be included in the differential diagnosis. However, the catarrhal symptoms of acquired rubella are minimal or absent compared with most respiratory pathogens. Also, the pathognomonic lymphadenopathy associated with acquired rubella may distinguish this from other infections. During the exanthem phase of acquired rubella infection, most exanthemous illnesses can initially be included in the differential diagnosis, but most can be excluded because of the transient mild nature of the rubella rash. Only the rash of scarlet fever may be most likely to be confused with that of acquired rubella infection. In older girls and women, the presence of joint signs and symptoms may aid in the diagnosis of acquired rubella.

Congenital rubella pathogenesis

Transmission
- Maternal–fetal transmission of virus via the placenta

Course of infection
- Maternal infection during pregnancy
- Placental infection
- Disseminated, persistent fetal infection
- Replication in all fetal organ systems
- Generalized virus-induced vasculitis producing disseminated necrosis and subsequent parenchymal hypoplasia
- Development of mitotic arrest and chromosomal defects
- Degree of pathology significantly higher in first-trimester infections

Immunity
- Fetal immunity during congenital infection distinct from that produced by acute postnatal infection; cell-mediated immune responses are depressed after congenital infection

Figure 1-31 Pathogenesis of congenital rubella infection. In contrast to postnatal or acquired rubella infection, congenital rubella infection may produce a wide spectrum of persistent, progressive, and serious sequelae. The major factor affecting this increased susceptibility to serious sequelae is the ability of rubella virus to infect all fetal tissue and cause mitotic arrest, chromosomal damage, angiopathic necrosis, and focal inflammation, all of which lead to generalized parenchymal hypoplasia and disrupted organogenesis. The nature of the congenital defects associated with rubella infection varies depending on the trimester of infection (*see* Fig. 1-33). The most serious sequelae are observed when infection occurs in the first trimester. Infection during this period is also associated with increased risk of miscarriage, abortion, or stillbirth. However, virtually no defects will be identified in congenital infection occurring after 16 weeks gestation.

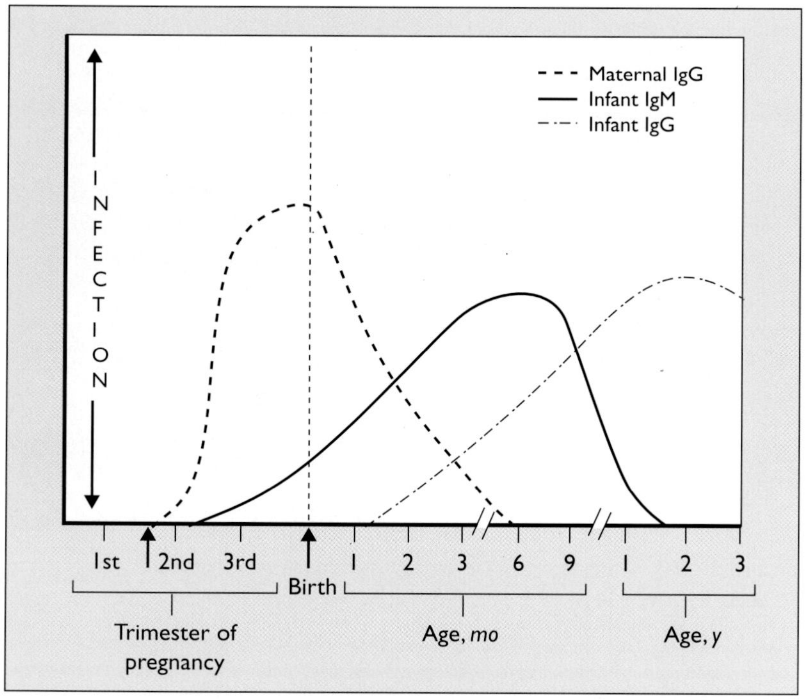

FIGURE 1-32 Immune response in congenitally acquired rubella. The immune response to congenital rubella infection is quite distinct from that observed in postnatal infection. Fetal IgM antibodies may be detected as early as 20 weeks gestation, IgM and IgG levels will rise over the first few months of life, and IgM levels may persist for up to 6 months of age. (*Adapted from* Best and O'Shea [21]; with permission.)

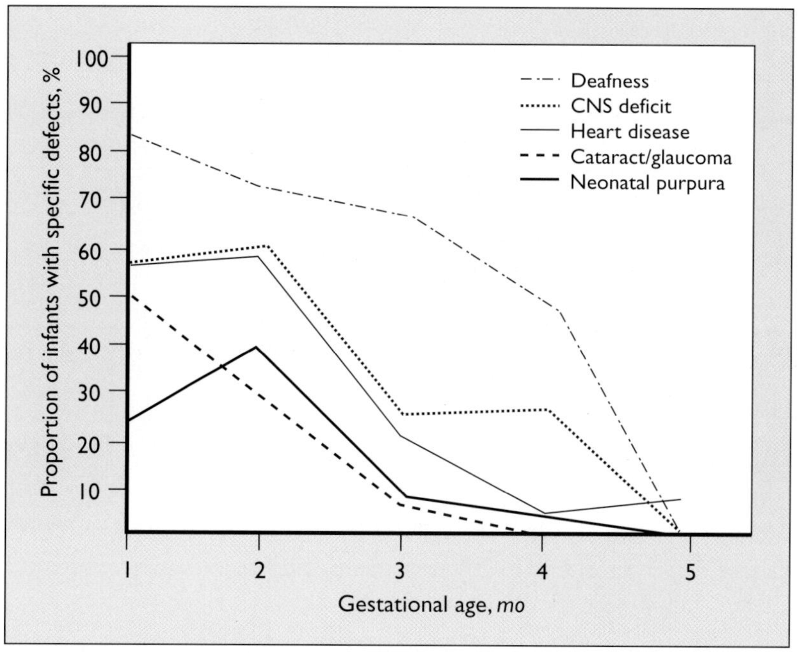

FIGURE 1-33 Sequelae of congenital rubella infection in relation to gestational age at the time of infection [12,27]. CNS–central nervous system. (*Adapted from* Best and O'Shea [21]; with permission.)

Clinical features associated with congenital rubella syndrome

Category	Common	Uncommon
Present at birth		
Transient	Low birth weight Thrombocytopenic purpura Hepatomegaly Splenomegaly Bone lesions	Cloudy corneas Hepatitis Generalized lymphadenopathy Hemolytic anemia Pneumonitis
Permanent	Sensorineural deafness Peripheral pulmonary stenosis Pulmonary valvular stenosis Patent ductus arteriosus Ventricular septal defect Retinopathy Cataract Microphthalmia Psychomotor retardation Cryptorchidism Inguinal hernia Diabetes mellitus	Severe myopia Thyroid disorders Dermatoglyphic abnormalities Glaucoma Myocardial abnormalities
Delayed	Sensorineural deafness Peripheral pulmonary artery stenosis Mental retardation Central language defects Diabetes mellitus Immune complex disease Hypogammaglobulinemia	Severe myopia Thyroiditis Hypothyroidism Growth hormone deficiency Chronic rash Pneumonitis Progressive panencephalitis

FIGURE 1-34 Complications of congenital rubella infection [22–24]. Because of the extensive viremia and viral replication throughout all fetal organ systems, congenital rubella infection is associated with protean sequelae and complications. However, the most common complications of congenital rubella infection are intrauterine growth retardation, cataracts, cardiac defects (myocarditis, patent ductus arteriosus, pulmonary artery stenosis), "blueberry muffin" skin lesions, and deafness. Persistent and late sequelae are not as common but may be progressive. Up to 20% of first trimester infection will end in early miscarriage. Among live births, congenital defects may occur in over 80% of infants infected in the first trimester but in virtually no infants infected after the first 16 weeks of gestation. (*Adapted from* Banatvala and Best [25]; with permission.)

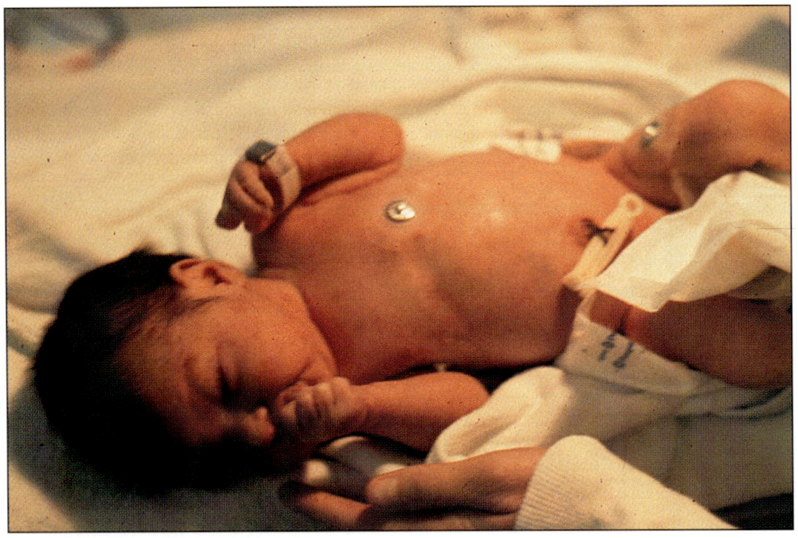

FIGURE 1-35 Infant with "blueberry muffin" lesions and congenital rubella syndrome.

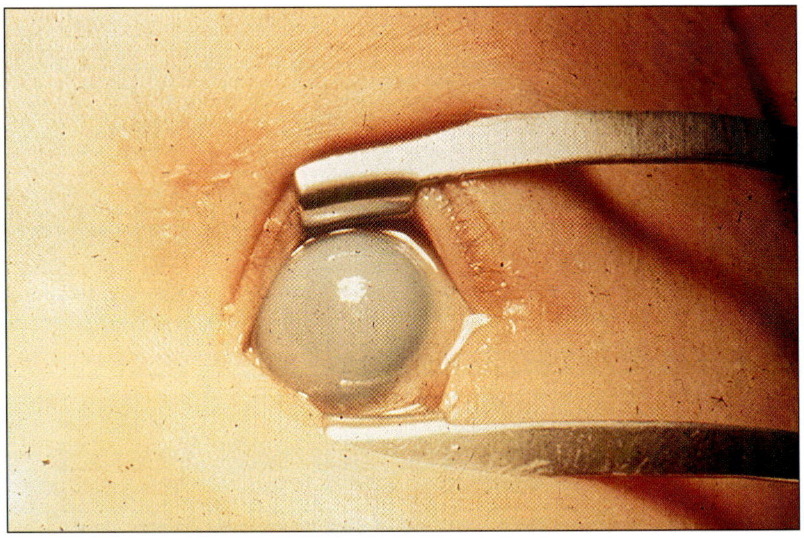

FIGURE 1-36 Cataracts in an infant with congenital rubella syndrome.

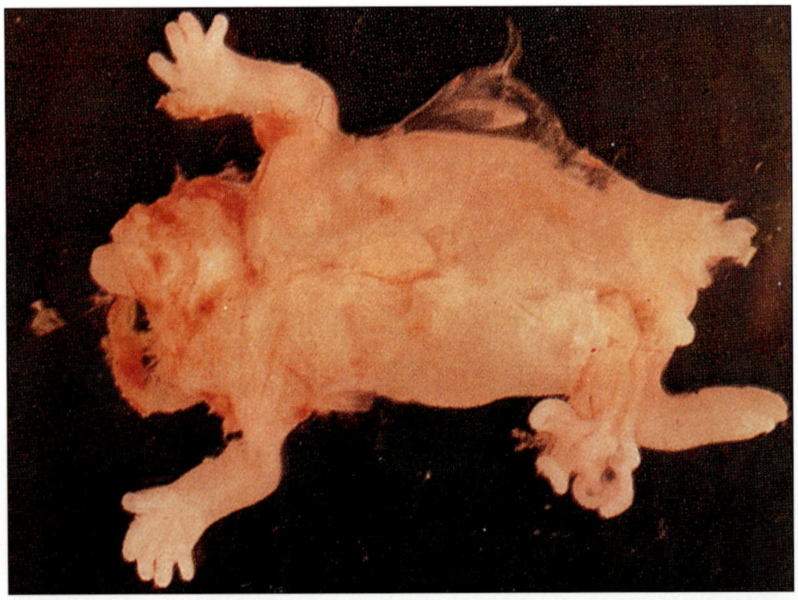

FIGURE 1-37 Embryopathy associated with congenital rubella syndrome.

Differential diagnosis of congenital rubella infection

Differential diagnosis	Distinctive clinical features of rubella
Other congenital and perinatal infections	
Toxoplasmosis	Cataracts, cardiac defects
Cytomegalovirus	Cataracts, cardiac defects
Herpes simplex	Absence of skin, eye, mucous membrane vesicles or lesions
HIV	Congenital HIV is infection generally asymptomatic in the neonatal period
Syphilis	Cataracts, cardiac, auditory, and neurologic defects
Enterovirus	Cataracts, cardiac, auditory, and neurologic defects
Drug-induced hearing loss	Other sequelae of congenital rubella
Noninfectious congenital defects	Dependent on the nature of the congenital syndrome or spectrum of noninfectious defects
Cerebral palsy	Other sequelae of congenital rubella

FIGURE 1-38 Differential diagnosis of congenital rubella infection. The clinical manifestations of congenital rubella syndrome may be varied; thus there is a wide differential diagnosis. However, the majority of other diagnoses may be excluded based on specific sequelae associated with congenital rubella. In addition, certain diagnoses, such as herpes simplex virus infection, have characteristic clinical findings that are usually quite distinct from those of congenital rubella syndrome. In addition, laboratory testing is important in distinguishing congenital rubella syndrome from other diagnoses.

Laboratory diagnosis of congenital rubella infection

Method	Sample timing	Sample needed
Virus detection		Fetal tissue (postmortem)
Tissue culture isolation	Prenatal period	Amniotic fluid (amniocentesis, chorionic villus sampling)
	Neonatal period	Nasopharyngeal, feces, urine
	Postnatal period	Throat, cerebrospinal fluid
Antibody detection		
Complement fixation	Acute and convalescent	Serum
Radioimmunoassay	Acute and convalescent	Serum
Hemagglutination-inhibition		
Enzyme-linked immunoassay	Acute and convalescent	Serum
Plaque neutralization	Acute and convalescent	Serum

Figure 1-39 Laboratory diagnosis of congenital rubella infection. Because clinical manifestations of congenital rubella infection may be nonspecific, the diagnosis of congenital rubella syndrome requires virologic or serologic confirmation. Patient samples from a number of sites may be used in direct detection of rubella virus during active infection, which in congenital rubella syndrome may persist for years [26]. Tissue culture is easily accomplished from several clinical samples but is expensive, time consuming, and becoming less available. Serologic testing is therefore the current mainstay of establishing the diagnosis of congenital rubella infection; however, interpretation of assays is difficult and should be carefully done. Assays include the rubella IgM and IgG antibody assays, of which the most commonly used is the enzyme-linked immunoassay [22,27]. However, false-positive IgM results from cord blood or neonatal serum may occur, and false-negative reactions may result if congenital infection occurred late in pregnancy. Serial measurements of IgG are therefore recommended and samples drawn in the first year of life should be run in parallel. Persistence of hemagglutination-inhibition antibodies is considered diagnostic of congenital infection.

Indications and contraindications for rubella vaccination

Indications	Contraindications
Children ≥12 mo (with measles and mumps vaccines administered as MMR) in a two-dose schedule as indicated for measles and mumps immunization	Pregnancy Immunodeficiency or immune-compromised condition (except HIV infection)
Susceptible individuals in the following groups: Prepubertal girls and boys Adults, especially premarital or postpartum women College students Child care personnel Health care personnel Military personnel	Recipient of immunoglobulin or blood in past 3 mo*

* Rubella vaccine may be given postpartum concurrently of after the administration of anti-Rho (D) immunoglobulin or blood products. If rubella vaccine is given as MMR, longer intervals may be necessary (*see* Fig. 1-17).

MMR—measles-mumps-rubella vaccine.

Figure 1-40 Indications and contraindications for rubella vaccination in the United States. (*Adapted from* American Academy of Pediatrics [28]; with permission.)

Use of immunoglobulin after exposure to rubella

Postexposure prophylaxis in early pregnancy: not recommended unless termination of pregnancy is not an option
Dose: 0.55 mL/kg

Figure 1-41 Uses of immune globulin after exposure to rubella during pregnancy [29]. The use of immune globulin in this situation is generally not recommended. The dose recommended in limited situations has been found to prevent or modify infection. One study found a decrease in clinically apparent infection from 87% among control compared with 18% among immune globulin recipients, but 44% of recipients were found to be infected based on laboratory diagnosis. In addition, infants have been born with congenital rubella syndrome even after their mothers received postexposure prophylaxis during pregnancy. (*Adapted from* American Academy of Pediatrics [29]; with permission.)

References

1. Sheshberadaran H, Chen SN, Norrby E: Monoclonal antibodies against five structural proteins of measles virus: I. Characterization of antigenic determinants on nine strains of measles virus. *Virology* 1983, 128:341–353.
2. Tamin A, Rota PA, Wang ZD, *et al.*: Antigenic analysis of current wild type and vaccine strains of measles virus. *J Infect Dis* 1994, 170:795–801.
3. Rota JS, Hummel KB, Rota PA, Bellini WJ: Genetic variability of the glycoprotein genes of current wild-type measles isolates. *Virology* 1992, 188:135–142.
4. Birrer MJ, Udem S, Nathanson S, Bloom BT: Antigenic variants of measles virus. *Nature* 1981, 293:67–69.
5. Kingsbury DW, Bratt MA, Choppin PE, *et al.*: Paramyxoviridae. *Intervirology* 1978, 10:137–152.
6. Bellini WJ, Rota JS, Rota PA: Virology of measles virus. *J Infect Dis* 1994, 170(suppl 1):S15–S23.
7. Almeida J: Measles. In *Color Atlas of Infectious Diseases*. Chicago: Year Book Medical Publishers; 1974:243.
8. Martin DB, Weiner LB, Neiburg PI, Blair DC: Atypical measles in adolescents and young adults. *Ann Intern Med* 1979, 90:877–881.
9. Laptook A, Wind W, Nussbaum M, Shenker IR: Pulmonary lesions in atypical measles. *Pediatrics* 1978, 62:42–46.
10. Mason WH, Ross LA, Lanson J, Wright HT Jr: Epidemic measles in the post-vaccine era: evaluation of epidemiology, clinical presentation and complications during and urban outbreak. *Pediatr Infect Dis J* 1993, 11:42–48.
11. Centers for Disease Control and Prevention: Progress toward global measles control and elimination, 1990–1996. *MMWR Morb Mortal Wkly Rep* 1997, 46:893–897.
12. Forghani B, Schmidt NJ: Antigen requirements, sensitivity and specificity of enzyme immunoassays for measles and rubella viral antibodies. *J Clin Microbiol* 1979, 9:657–664.
13. Kramer SM, Cremer NE: Detection of IgG antibodies to measles virus using monoclonal antibodies for antigen capture in enzyme immunoassay. *J Virol Methods* 1984, 8:255–263.
14. Salonen J, Vainionpaa R, Halonen P: Assay of measles virus IgM and IgG class antibodies by use of peroxidase labelled viral antigens. *Arch Virol* 1986, 91:93–106.
15. American Academy of Pediatrics: Measles. In *1997 Red Book: Report of the Committee on Infectious Diseases*, ed 24. Edited by Peter G. Elk Grove Village, IL: American Academy of Pediatrics; 1997:349.
16. Julkunen J: Serological diagnosis of parainfluenza virus infections by enzyme immunoassay with special emphasis on purity of viral antigens. *J Med Virol* 1984, 14:177–187.
17. Orvell CR, Rydbeck R, Love A: Immunological relationships between mumps virus and parainfluenza viruses studied with monoclonal antibodies. *J Gen Virol* 1986, 67:1929–1939.
18. Wolinsky JS: Mumps virus. In *Fields' Virology*, ed 3. Edited by Fields BN, Knipe DM, Howley PM. Lippincott-Raven; 1996.
19. American Academy of Pediatrics: Mumps. In *1997 Red Book: Report of the Committee on Infectious Diseases*, ed 24. Edited by Peter G. Elk Grove Village, IL: American Academy of Pediatrics; 1997:366–369.
20. Horzinek MC: *Non-Arthropod Borne Togaviruses*. London: Academic Press; 1981.
21. Best JM, O'Shea S: Rubella virus. In *Diagnostic Procedures for Viral, Rickettsial, and Chlamydial Infection*, ed 6. Edited by Lennette EH, Schmmidt NJ. Washington, DC: American Public Health Association; 1989:731–795.
22. Maldonado YA: Rubeola virus (measles and subacute sclerosing panencephalitis). In: *Principles and Practice of Infectious Diseases*. Edited by Long SE, Pickering LK, Prober CG. New York: Churchill Livingstone; 1997.
23. Dudgeon JA: Congenital rubella. *J Pediatr* 1975, 87:1078–1086.
24. Chiriboga-Klein S, Oberfield SE, Casullo AM, *et al.*: Growth in congenital rubella syndrome and correlation with clinical manifestations. *J Pediatr* 1989, 115:251–255.
25. Banatvala JE, Best JM: Rubella. In *Diagnostic Procedures for Viral, Rickettsial, and Chlamydial Infections*, ed 6. Washington, DC: American Public Health Association; 1989:731–795.
26. Shwemon Da, Cherry JD, Kirby DE: Shedding of rubella virus in a 4-1/2 year old boy with congenital rubella. *Pediatr Infect Dis J* 1982, 1:342–343.
27. Levin JM, Oxman MN, Moor MG, *et al.*: Diagnosis of congenital rubella in utero. *N Engl J Med* 1974, 290:1187–1188.
28. American Academy of Pediatrics: Mumps. In *1997 Red Book: Report of the Committee on Infectious Diseases*, ed 24. Edited by Peter G. Elk Grove Village, IL: American Academy of Pediatrics; 1997:460.
29. American Academy of Pediatrics: Mumps. In *1997 Red Book: Report of the Committee on Infectious Diseases*, ed 24. Edited by Peter G. Elk Grove Village, IL: American Academy of Pediatrics; 1997:458.

Chapter 2

Human Herpesvirus 6 and 7

Caroline Breese Hall
Mary T. Caserta

THE FAMILY OF HUMAN HERPESVIRUSES has recently become more prolific with progeny of importance for pediatrics. Human herpesvirus 6 (HHV6) was discovered by the advent of retroviral technology in the peripheral blood lymphocytes of adults with lymphoproliferative diseases and HIV infection [1]. Its role in pediatric infectious diseases was first illuminated 2 years later when the virus was identified in the lymphocytes of four infants with roseola. HHV6 thus assumed the provocative position of a pathogen that potentially could span the ages from infancy to adulthood. Its role as the major cause of the ubiquitous childhood exanthem, roseola, has now been well established. However, the relationship of primary infection in infancy to its association with immunocompromised diseases later in life is unexplained, and its ability to become latent and to reactivate itself are subjects of much current interest and investigation.

Three years after the recognition of HHV6, human herpesvirus 7 (HHV7) was discovered in 1989 in the peripheral blood lymphocytes of a healthy adult [2]. The knowledge of this new virus is limited, especially its role in clinical disease. Currently, it appears that HHV7 may cause a relatively small proportion of the cases of roseola, but symptomatic primary illness may be relatively infrequent, particularly in comparison with HHV6. HHV7, however, shares the familial characteristic of its ability to persist after initial infection with asymptomatic shedding, especially from the saliva.

CHARACTERISTICS OF THE VIRUS

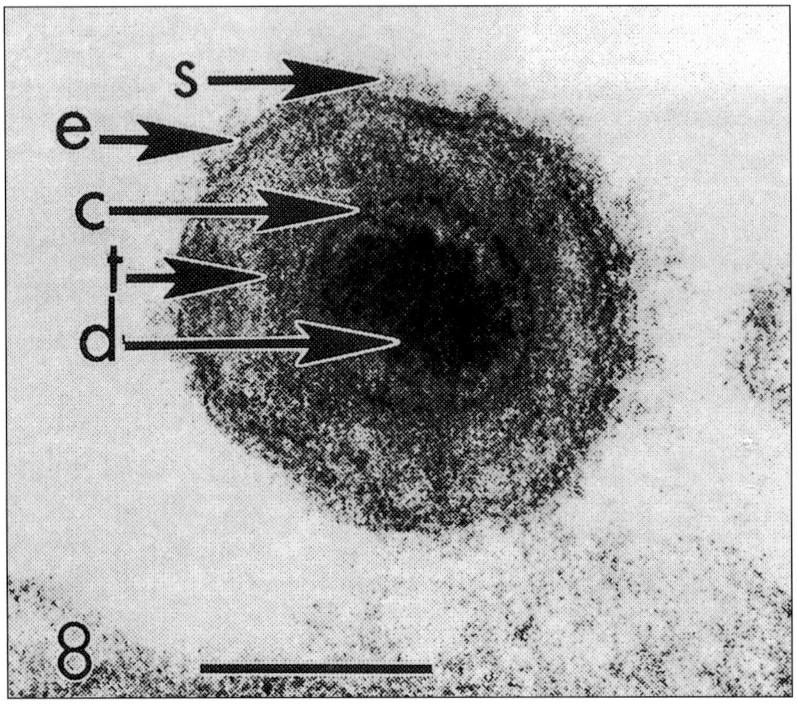

FIGURE 2-1 The ultrastructure of human herpesvirus 6. Depicted in this electron micrograph of an extracellular human herpesvirus 6 virion is the characteristic structure of the herpesvirus family. The virus is enveloped (*e*) with an approximate diameter of 160 to 200 nm with a DNA core (*d*)—a linear, double-stranded DNA genome of 160 to 170 kb—surrounded by a nucleocapsid (*c*) of icosahedral symmetry containing 162 capsomeres. Internal to the envelope, studded with surface spikes (*s*), lies the tegument (*t*). (*From* Kramarsky and Sander [3]; with permission.)

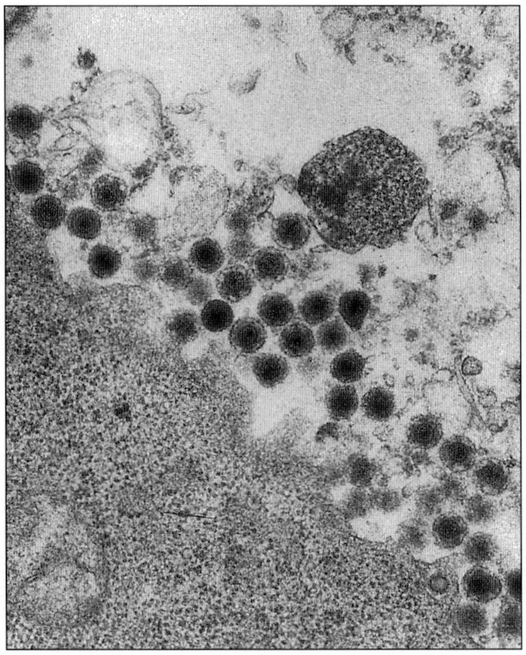

FIGURE 2-2 An electron micrograph of the replication of human herpesvirus 6 in HSB-2 cells (human T-cell line). Human herpesvirus 6 replicates in the nucleus of the infected cell, producing nucleocapsids that become coated with the tegument and subsequently with the lipid envelope and surface spikes. The extracellular virions, as shown in this electron micrograph, are released by exocytosis. (*From* Ablashi and Hung [4]; with permission.)

Characteristics of Human Herpesvirus 6

Characteristics of human herpesvirus 6
Uniformity of shape and size
Enveloped particles 200 nm in diameter
Icosahedral symmetry of core, 162 capsomeres
Viral particles develop in nucleus and are released by exocytosis and eventual cell death
Large double-stranded DNA genome (160 kb)
Low guanine cytosine content (42%) compared with other herpesviruses
Unique sequence flanked by 10-kb direct-repeat elements
Genome contains areas of cross-hybridizing with cytomegalovirus, Marek's disease virus, and human herpesvirus 7
Infects mostly CD4+ lymphocytes; other T, B, and NK cells; megakaryocytes; glial cells; and colorectal cell lines
Animal hosts: specimens from roseola patients tried unsuccessfully in nonprimates by Breese [15]; Kempe *et al.* [10] produced febrile illness in rhesus monkeys; recent attempts to repeat results in rhesus monkeys not successful

Figure 2-3 The distinctive virologic characteristics of human herpesvirus 6. Human herpesvirus 6 shares features similar to other human herpesviruses as well as possessing distinctive characteristics.

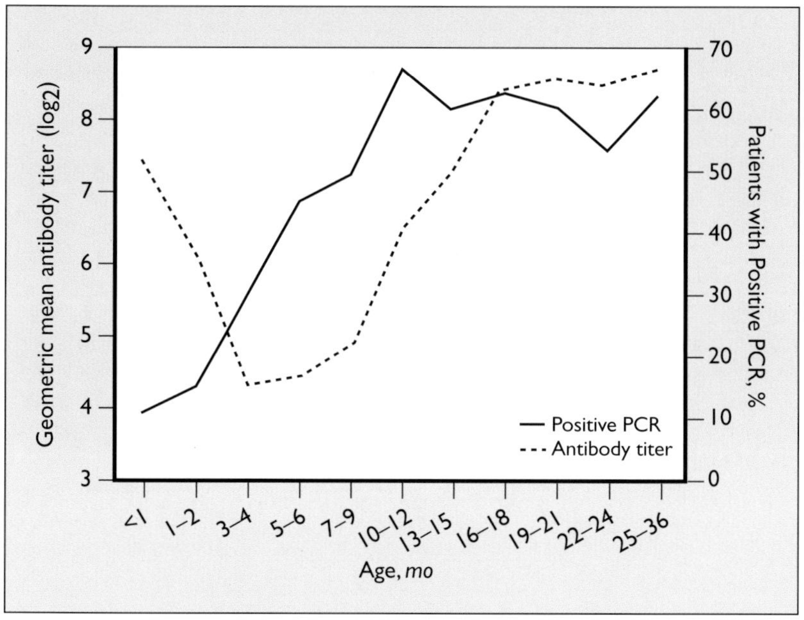

Figure 2-4 Acquisition of human herpesvirus (HHV6) in young children. This figure indicates the ubiquitous and early occurrence of HHV6 infection as determined by the acquisition of specific antibody. Essentially all newborn cord-bloods possess specific antibody, indicating universal acquisition of HHV6 by their mothers. The loss of passive antibody is followed at 3 to 5 months by the rapid climb in antibody titer, resulting from acquisition of primary HHV6 infection by infants. The peak is reached at approximately 1 year of age. The presence of HHV6 DNA (as indicated by the positive polymerase chain reaction [PCR] assay in the peripheral blood mononuclear cells of the infants) also indicates the rapid acquisition of infection once passive antibody has diminished. The continued presence of HHV6 DNA in 50% to 70% of infants beyond 7 months of age indicates the frequent persistence of the HHV6 genome and the possible latency of HHV6 after primary infection. (*Adapted from* Hall *et al.* [5]; with permission.)

Children aged 0 to 45 months with human herpesvirus 6 antibody, DNA, or both in their blood mononuclear cells

		Human herpesvirus 6					
			PCR positive			Antibody positive	
Age, *mo*	Patients, *n*	Patients tested, *n*	Patients, *n*	%	Patients tested, *n*	Patients, *n*	%
0–5	53	53	12	23	48	28	58
6–11	76	74	35	47	73	40	55
0–11	129	127	47	37	121	68	56
12–23	118	116	72	62	107	85	79
0–23	247	243	119	49	228	153	67
24–44	48	48	18	38	43	38	88
0–44	295	291	137	47	271	191	70

PCR—polymerase chain reaction

Figure 2-5 Age of acquisition of human herpesvirus 6 (HHV6) infection according to antibody and presence of HHV6 DNA. This table shows the cumulative percent of children who have acquired HHV6 according to age as detected by the persistence of the HHV6 genome in the peripheral blood lymphocytes and by the presence of specific antibody in a population of 295 normal children from birth to 45 months of age. Note the peak age for detection of HHV6 DNA is from 12 to 23 months, which probably reflects persistence or latency of virus shortly after primary infection in a large proportion of children. The proportion of children with detectable DNA declines with age, suggesting either clearance of the virus or persistence or latency at a separate site or at levels too low to be detected. In contrast, the serologic results represent the cumulative prevalence of infection with HHV6 and show high levels of acquisition by 23 months of age. (*Adapted from* Lanphear *et al.* [6]; with permission.)

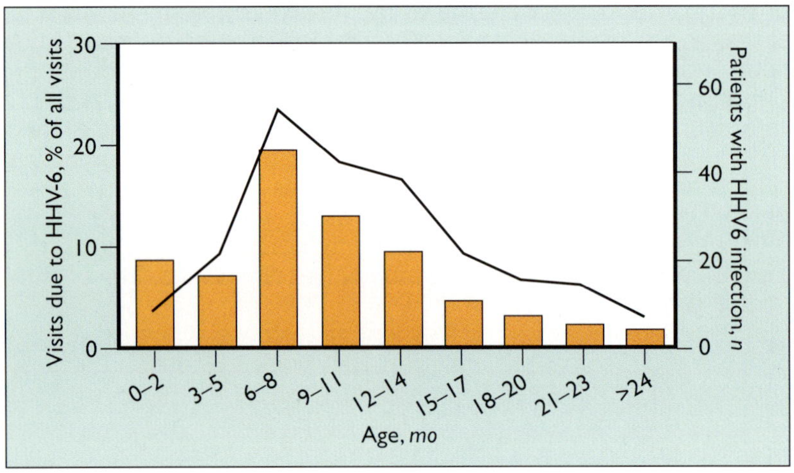

Figure 2-6 The clinical impact of human herpesvirus (HHV6). This graph depicts the number of children presenting to the emergency department with illness from primary HHV6 infection (*bar*) and visits due to primary HHV6 infection as a percentage of all emergency department visits (*curve*) for children presenting with acute febrile illnesses according to their age. Children with primary HHV6 infection were diagnosed by isolation of the virus from their peripheral blood mononuclear cells and with seroconversion. The importance of HHV6 infection as a cause of morbidity and acute medical visits for infants in the first year of life, especially the second 6 months of life, is underscored by the graph. Approximately 20% of the acute visits for children 6 to 8 months of age were due to primary HHV6 infection. (*Adapted from* Hall *et al.* [5]; with permission.)

Sites detected by polymerase chain reaction of human herpesvirus DNA persistence in adults
Peripheral blood mononuclear cells
Saliva, throat swabs, pulmonary secretions
Cervical secretions
Lymph nodes, spleen
Liver
Brain, cerebrospinal fluid

Figure 2-7 Sites of human herpesvirus 6 (HHV6) DNA persistence in adults detected by polymerase chain reaction (PCR). HHV6 DNA has been detected by PCR in a variety of sites in normal adults as well as in immunocompromised patients in whom the frequency of detection and viral load may be greater. Horizontal transmission to susceptible infants is suggested from the persistence and frequency of HHV6 DNA in secretions of close contacts and, as illustrated in Figure 2-6, in the rapid and constant acquisition of infection by infants concurrent with the decline of maternal antibody. Perinatal transmission has been suggested by the detection of HHV6 DNA in 10% to 20% of cervical secretions and by the detection of HHV6 DNA in newborn infants [5,7,8]. HHV6 DNA, however, has not been detected in breast milk [9].

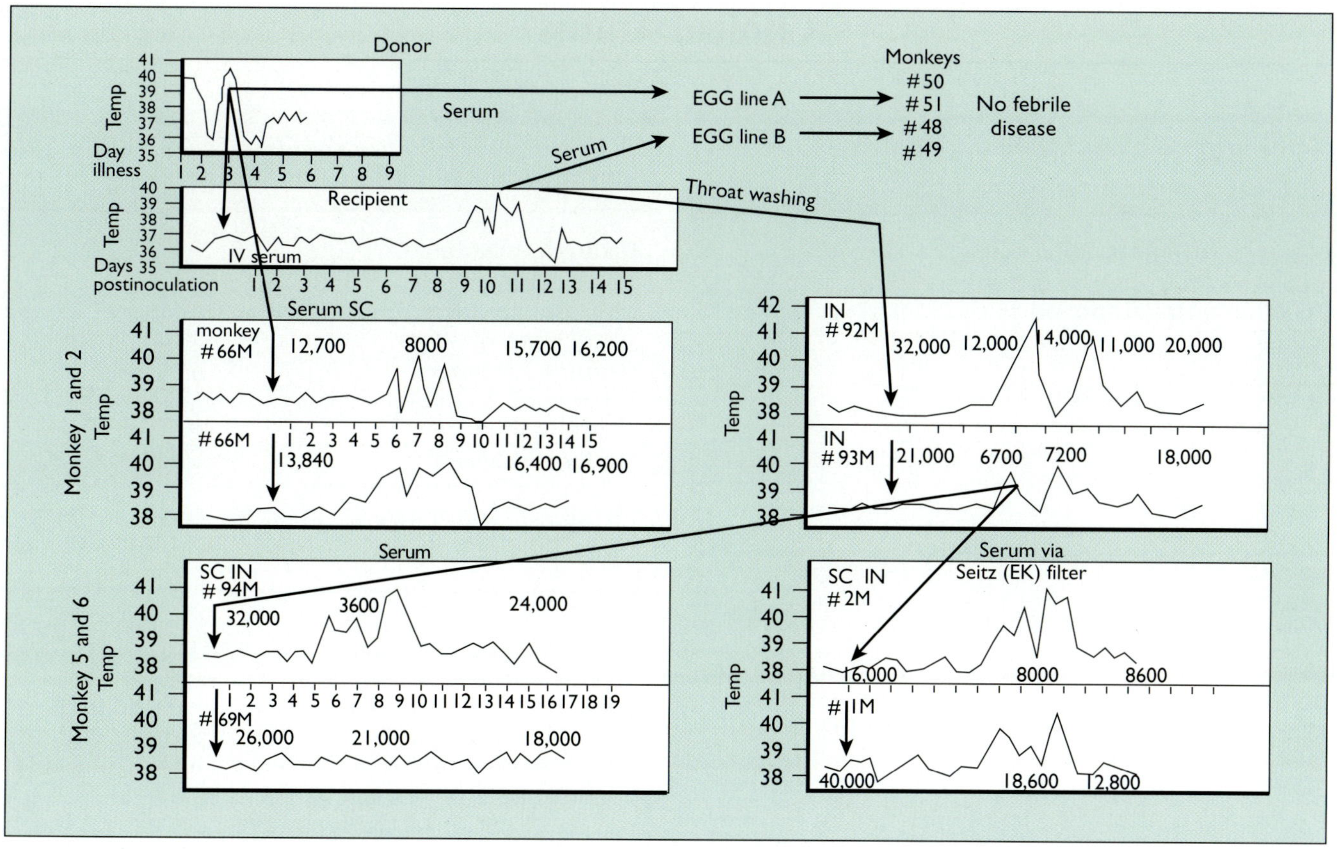

Figure 2-8 Transmission of human herpesvirus 6 infection. Kempe in 1950 demonstrated that roseola was caused by an infectious agent that could be transmitted by the serum of an acutely ill child. Secondly, in the experiments demonstrated in the figure with Rhesus monkeys he showed serum from a child with roseola during the acute febrile stage could be inoculated intravenously or subcutaneously into monkeys resulting in a febrile response and a pattern of illness similar to that of roseola in humans. In addition, throat washings of a child with acute roseola produced a similar febrile illness in monkeys. (*Adapted from* Kempe *et al.* [10]; with permission.)

Immune response

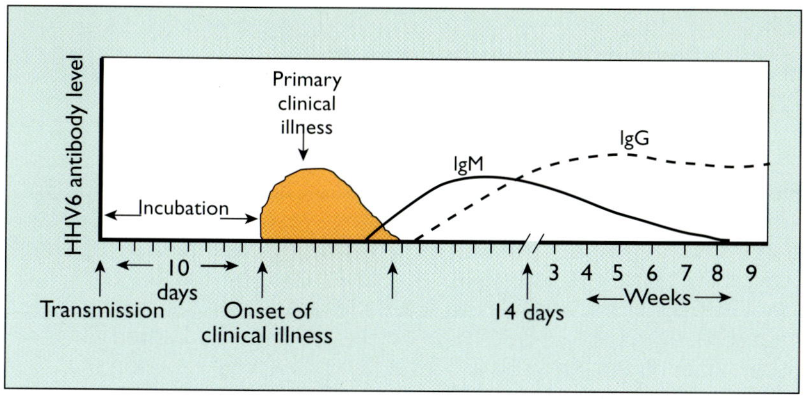

Figure 2-9 Humoral immunity to human herpesvirus 6 (HHV6). The humoral antibody response after primary HHV6 infection appears to consist of both neutralizing immunoglobulin (Ig) M and IgG, but neutralizing IgA antibodies have not been detected. Specific IgM antibodies may be detected approximately 5 to 7 days after the onset of the clinical illness, peak approximately 2 to 3 weeks later, and subsequently diminish, disappearing after approximately 2 months. Detection of IgM antibodies, however, is not always specific for primary infection. HHV6 antibodies of the IgM class may be detected in approximately 5% of normal adults. Specific IgG antibodies generally appear between 2 and 3 weeks from the onset of primary clinical illness, peak within the subsequent 2 to 3 weeks, and may decline in titer subsequently, but remain detectable usually throughout life. The antibody titer also appears to fluctuate, possibly due to reactivation of HHV6 DNA or from infection with other related viruses. (*Adapted from* Suga *et al.* [11]; with permission.)

Clinical strains

Two major strain groups of human herpesvirus 6: variants A and B

Differences in variants may be detected by
- Cellular tropism in vitro, possibly in humans
- Reactivity with monoclonal antibodies
- Restriction fragment length polymorphism analysis

Homology
- Between variants A and B = 95%
- Within same variant group = 99%

Prototypes
- A variants: GS, U1102
- B variants: Z29

Figure 2-10 Strain groups of human herpesvirus 6 (HHV6). Antigenic and genomic analyses of HHV6 isolates have indicated two major strain groups, called HHV6 variant A and HHV6 variant B.

Clinical associations of two major strain groups of human herpesvirus 6: variants A and B

Group A variants
- No clear disease association
- Most isolates from adults with reactivation with immunodeficiency diseases

Group B Variants
- Isolated from children and adults (especially adults with immunodeficiency)
- Hodgkin's disease
- Bone marrow transplant patients
- All isolates from children with primary infection, but four are from Rochester, NY, with A/B genome (some with A phenotype)

Figure 2-11 Clinical disease states associated with each variant group. Group A variants have been associated with a variety of conditions, especially in compromised adults, but no evidence currently exists for variant A strains as the direct cause of these diseases. Group B variants, however, are almost the exclusive cause of primary human herpesvirus 6 infection in infants [12].

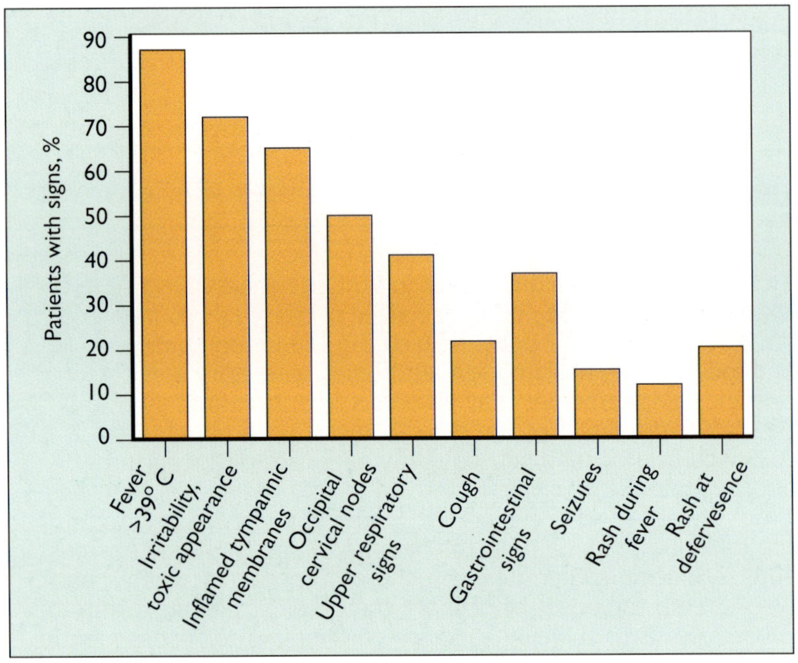

Figure 2-12 Clinical manifestations associated with human herpesvirus 6 (HHV6) primary infection. This graph illustrates the frequency of various signs and symptoms associated with primary infection from a prospective study of over 300 normal children with primary HHV6 infection diagnosed by isolation of the virus from their peripheral blood mononuclear cells and by seroconversion. The clinical presentation of primary HHV6 may be varied, and the signs are often nonspecific. Fever of abrupt onset is the most characteristic finding. Usually the fever is high, averaging 40°C. Second in occurrence are the nonspecific signs, such as irritability, poor feeding, or toxic appearance. Approximately 25% of patients present with manifestations that are primarily gastrointestinal or respiratory. The classical description of roseola, high fever, nonspecific signs, and rash on defervescence occur in the minority of patients, usually less than 20%. (*Adapted from* Hall [13]; with permission.)

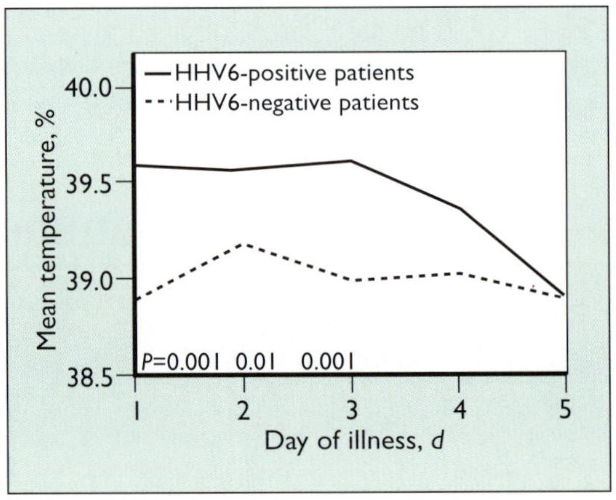

Figure 2-13 The course of fever in human herpesvirus 6 (HHV6) infection. The pattern of fever in children with primary HHV6 infection is compared with children of similar age presenting at the same season for acute medical visits for febrile illnesses not due to HHV6. Over 3000 children with acute febrile illness were evaluated prospectively at the University of Rochester Medical Center. Of these, 335 had primary HHV6 infection proven by isolation of HHV6 from blood and seroconversion. These children were compared with a matched group of children who presented with febrile illnesses from other causes. The children with HHV6 primary infection had significantly higher temperatures that were sustained above 39°C for the first 3 days of illness and then, on average, returned to normal by day 6 or 7 [5,14].

Syndrome of roseola infantum

- Sobriquets: exanthem subitum or sixth disease rose rash of infants
- Incidence highest ages 6–12 mo (average range, 3–36 mo)
- Abrupt onset of high fever for 3–6 d
- Non-specific signs of illness
- Usually does not appear toxic
- Mild palpebral erythema
- Prominent occipital lymphadenopathy
- Rash on defervescence

FIGURE 2-14 Major clinical findings associated with the syndrome of roseola in infants. Roseola infantum is a distinct clinical syndrome of infancy and early adulthood recognized and described by physicians of the early 20th century. The epidemiology and clinical signs and symptoms of roseola are presented in this table.

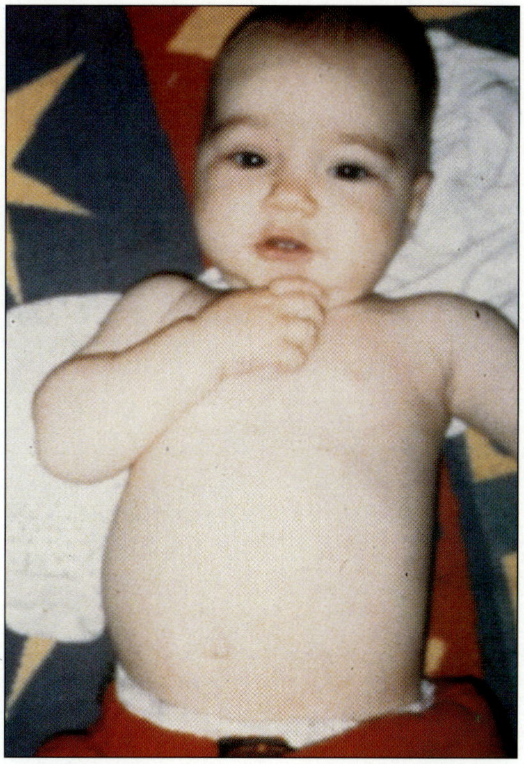

FIGURE 2-15 The rash of roseola. The rash of roseola classically appears at the time of defervescence, although occasionally 1 day before or after. The rash is rose colored, macular, or maculopapular, blanching, and characteristically 2 to 3 mm in diameter. The rash is highly variable in its appearance, location, and duration, and it is not distinctive. Most commonly, the rash is first noted on the trunk with subsequent spread to the neck, face, upper extremities, and lower extremities. Distribution, how-ever, may be much more localized. The rash can be so mild and evanescent (only hours in duration) that it may be missed.

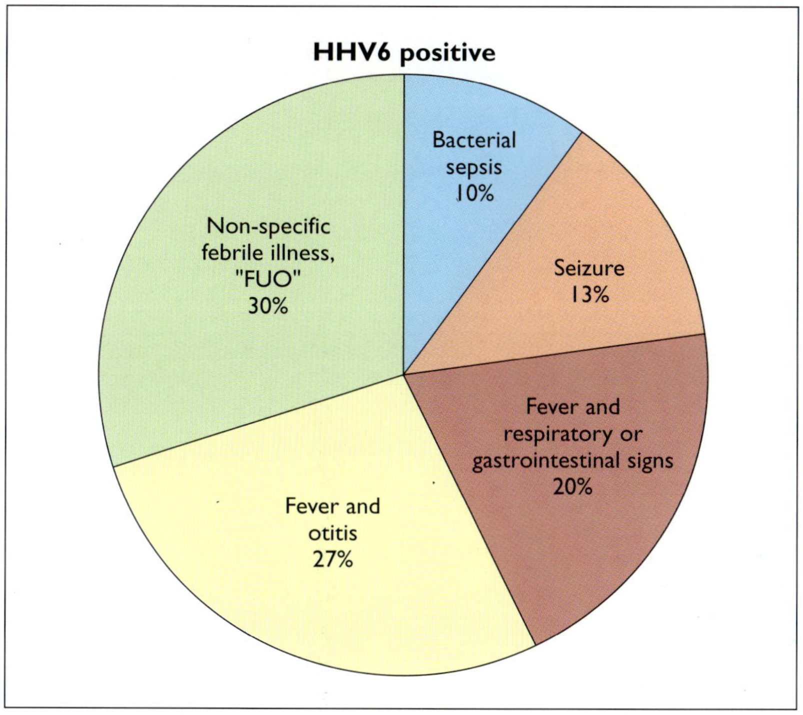

FIGURE 2-16 Initial diagnosis in children subsequently proven to have primary human herpesvirus 6 (HHV6) infection. The difficulty in clinical diagnosis of primary (HHV6) infection is indicated by the data from the prospective study of children presenting with acute febrile illnesses to outpatient facilities and the emergency department at the University of Rochester Medical Center [5]. The most frequent diagnosis at the time of discharge from the acute visit was fever with otitis media. The diagnosis of respiratory or gastrointestinal illness was given to 20% of these children. Ten percent appeared toxic. The appearance of toxicity was great enough to elicit the diagnosis of presumed bacterial sepsis. (*Data from* Hall *et al.* [5].)

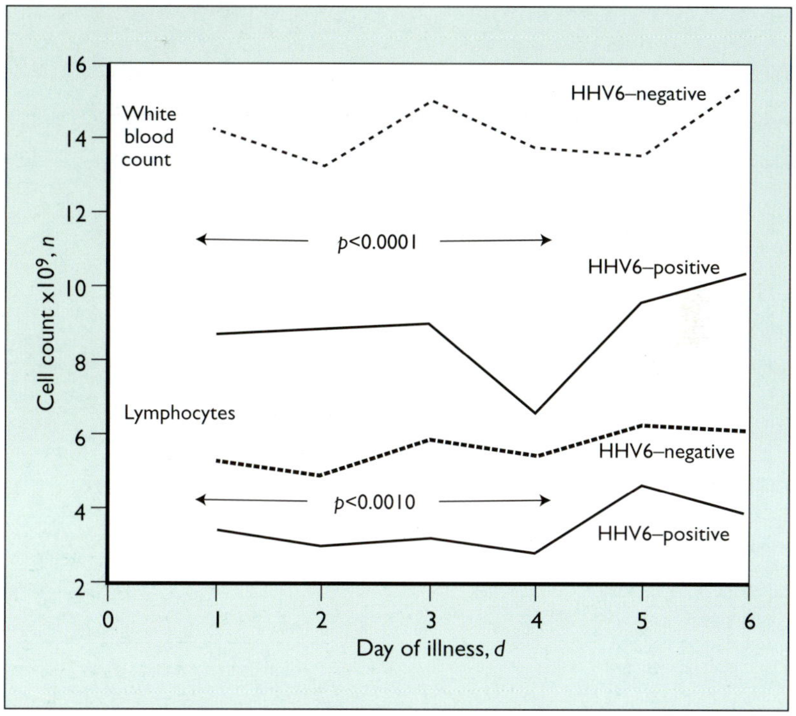

FIGURE 2-17 Laboratory findings associated with primary human herpesvirus 6 (HHV6) infection. Primary HHV6 infection is not distinguished by any specific laboratory findings. However, the total white blood cell count and absolute lymphocyte count are significantly lower in children with primary HHV6 infection than in the matched group of control children from the prospective studies previously described [5,14]. These two points are graphically presented in the figure. Characteristically, the WBC and lymphocytes reach a nadir at approximately 4 days from the onset of clinical illness. This pattern was described 50 years ago as a characteristic finding of children with roseola [15].

Complications and prognosis
Complete recovery (usually)
Asymptomatic persistence of human herpesvirus DNA in peripheral blood mononuclear cells and saliva is common
Most frequent complications involve central nervous system
Febrile seizures
Bulging anterior fontanelle
Encephalopathy
Meningoencephalitis
Transient hemiplegia

FIGURE 2-18 Complications associated with human herpesvirus 6 (HHV6) primary infection and prognosis. Primary HHV6 infection for most children is a benign disease with complete recovery. Silent persistence of the HHV6 genome in the blood and saliva, however, is common. The most common clinical complications associated with the acute febrile disease are those involving the central nervous system, especially febrile seizures, in children 6 months to 2 years of age.

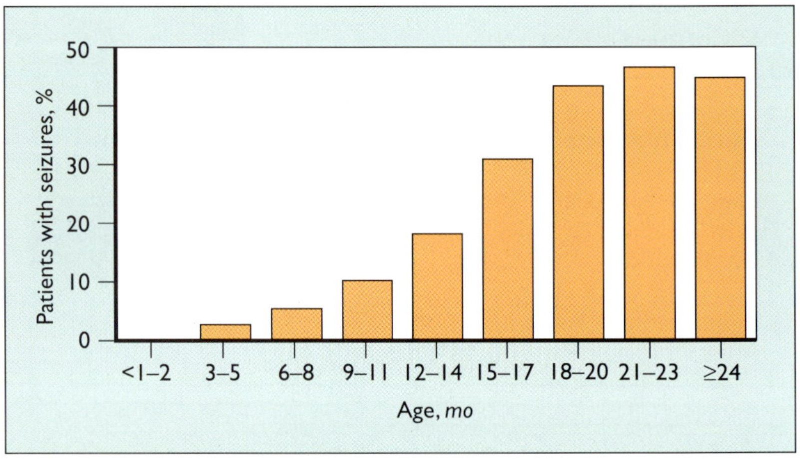

FIGURE 2-19 Incidence of febrile seizures associated with primary human herpesvirus 6 (HHV6) infection. This figure demonstrates the frequency with which the acute febrile phase of HHV6 infection is complicated by seizures. Of the children 18 to 24 months of age evaluated in the emergency department in Rochester, New York, with proven primary HHV6 infection, over 40% had their illness complicated by seizures.

Characteristics of febrile seizures complicating human herpesvirus 6 primary infection
Human herpesvirus 6 is the most frequently identified cause of first febrile seizures evaluated in emergency department
Generalized convulsion accompanies fever in a previously normal infant
Only half of human herpesvirus 6–associated seizures occur on first day of fever
Seizures may be of prolonged duration
Seizures may be recurrent during febrile phase of illness

FIGURE 2-20 Characteristics of febrile seizures complicating human herpesvirus 6 primary infection. Although the seizures complicating human herpesvirus 6 infection are febrile seizures, they may have some differentiating characteristics, suggesting that in some children, the seizures may be more severe.

Human herpesvirus 6 DNA in cerebrospinal fluid
HHV6 DNA in CSF at time of febrile primary infection in ≥25% of patients
HHV6 DNA persists following primary infection in 28%–70% of normal children
HHV6 DNA persistence in CSF is usually asymptomatic
Persistence of HHV6 DNA in CSF is associated with risk of recurrent seizures

FIGURE 2-21 Human herpesvirus 6 (HHV6) DNA in cerebrospinal fluid (CSF). The genome of HHV6 frequently may persist asymptomatically in the CSF of normal children subsequent to primary infection. However, the presence of HHV6 DNA in the CSF has been associated in limited studies with subsequent neurologic complications [16–18].

Clinical and laboratory findings in patients positive and negative for human herpesvirus 6 in cerebrospinal fluid

	Positive ($n = 72$)	Negative control* ($n = 90$)	Negative ($n = 415$)
Age, *mo*			
Average (median)	4.3 (1.5)	4.0 (1.0)	4.3 (1.0)
Range	0.1–20.0	0.1–25.0	0.1–36.0
PBMC			
Culture positive for HHV6, %	7.0 (9.7)	7.0 (7.7)	23.0 (5.5)
HHV6 IgG titer† ($\log_2$)			
Plasma	6.26	6.49	6.24
CSF	2.32	2.32	2.32
CSF WBC count (range)	3 (1–567)	3 (0–1122)	4 (0–3420)
CSF RBC count (range)	2 (0–171,200)	4 (0–377,528)	4 (0–480,000)
Peripheral WBC count†	13.7×10^3	13.4×10^3	
Lymphocytes, %†	45.0	45.0	
Temperature, °C†	38.8	38.8	
Seizures, *n* (%)	13.0 (18.1)	9.0 (10.0)	
Age of children with seizures, *mo*†	11.9	13.2	

*After polymerase chain reaction testing, 90 children negative for HHV6 in CSF were matched to CSF HHV6-positive patients for presence or absence of acute HHV6 infection. HHV6 in PBMC, age, and date or season of evaluation.

†Average value.

IgG—immunoglobulin G; RBC—red blood cell; WBC—white blood cell.

Figure 2-22 Clinical and laboratory findings in patients positive and negative for human herpesvirus 6 (HHV6) in the cerebrospinal fluid (CSF). The table shows the characteristics of children with HHV6 DNA persisting in their CSF in comparison with a control group of children who did not have HHV6 DNA detected in their CSF.

After polymerase chain reaction testing, 90 children negative for HHV6 in the CSF were matched to patients with HHV6 DNA in their CSF for the presence or absence of acute HHV6 infection, HHV6 in their peripheral blood mononuclear cells (PBMC), age, and date or season of evaluation. No statistically significant differences were found between CSF-negative and -positive patients in laboratory or clinical characteristics, such as the degree of fever or the number with seizures at the acute visit. (*From* Caserta *et al.* [17]; with permission.)

Diagnosis

Diagnosis of human herpesvirus 6 infection

- Must differentiate acute primary infection from persistent infection following primary infection, including latent infection and reactivation
- No rapid or clinically feasible assay is currently available for differentiation of above states of viral infection
- Definitive diagnosis of acute primary infection currently requires both isolation of human herpesvirus 6 from peripheral blood mononuclear cells (viremia) and seroconversion of immunoglobulin G human herpesvirus 6 antibody

Figure 2-23 Diagnosis of human herpesvirus 6 infection. Assays for reliable confirmation of acute primary human herpesvirus 6 infection are not commercially available currently.

Diagnostic methods for human herpesvirus 6 infection: isolation of virus

- Primary isolation of HHV6 in cell culture by cocultivation of patients' PBMCs with freshly stimulated cord blood lymphocytes
- Confirmation of isolation of HHV6 in culture by specific antigenic detection with monoclonal antibodies, DNA probes, or specific polymerase chain reaction primers
- Variant differentiation by variant-specific monoclonal antibodies and/or polymerase chain reaction

Figure 2-24 Diagnostic methods for human herpesvirus 6 infection (HHV6): isolation of virus. The isolation of HHV6 from human blood samples is achieved through cocultivation of the patient's peripheral blood mononuclear cells (PBMCs) with stimulated lymphocytes obtained from human umbilical cord blood. The use of stimulated adult donor lymphocytes is not acceptable because of the possibility of reactivation of HHV6 from the donor sample, leading to false-positive culture results.

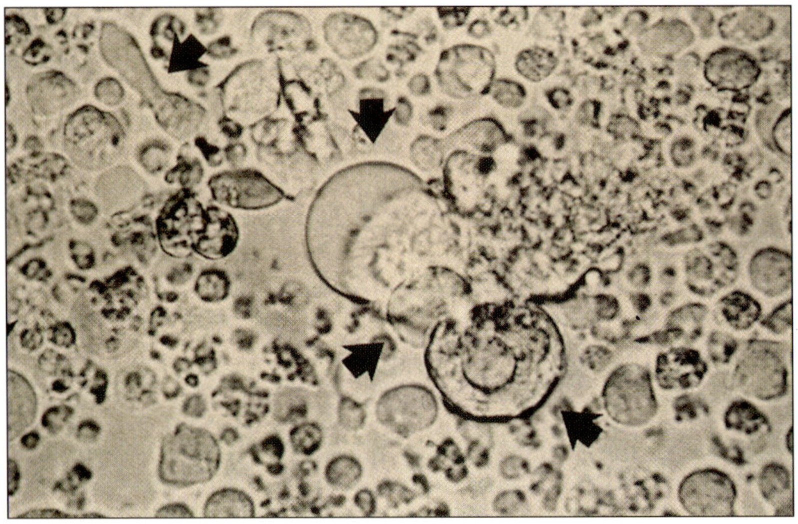

FIGURE 2-25 Isolation of human herpesvirus (HHV6) in cord blood cells. Initial isolation of HHV6 from the peripheral blood lymphocytes of an infant with primary HHV6 infection is depicted in this cord blood cell culture by the ballooning, syncytial appearance. *Arrows* indicate infected cord blood cells. Specific confirmation is subsequently accomplished by monoclonal antibodies, polymerase chain reaction, or both.

Diagnostic methods for human herpesvirus 6 infection: serologic assays
Immunofluorescent assays, indirect and anticomplement
Neutralization assays
Enzyme immunoassays
Competitive radioimmunoassays

FIGURE 2-26 Diagnostic methods for human herpesvirus 6 infection: serologic assays. Several different methods for the detection of a serologic response to human herpesvirus 6 have been described and are outlined in this table.

Diagnostic methods for human herpesvirus 6 infection: problems with serologic assays
Diagnosis of acute infection by seroconversion with acute and convalescent sera is retrospective
Titer of IgG HHV6 antibodies may fluctuate subsequent to primary infection, sometimes with fourfold rise
IgG antibodies are present in essentially all individuals >3 y of age
Differentiation of acute and past infection by detection of specific IgM antibodies is not specific (*ie*, IgM antibodies may be present in sera of normal adults) and by IgM assays of variable intensity
Measurement of cross-reactive antibodies: diminished specificity of assay due to antigenic and genetic similarity of 1) HHV6 to HHV7 and HCMV and 2) between the HHV6 variants

HCMV—human cytomegalovirus; HHV6—human herpesvirus 6; HHV7—human herpesvirus 7; IgG—immunoglobulin G; IgM—immunoglobulin M.

FIGURE 2-27 Diagnostic methods for human herpesvirus 6 infection: problems with serologic assays. The ability to diagnose human herpesvirus 6 infections accurately by serologic methods alone is flawed in several ways as outlined in this table.

Diagnostic methods for human herpesvirus 6 infection: assays for human herpesvirus 6 DNA and human herpesvirus 6 in pathologic specimens
Polymerase chain reaction
Nucleic acid hybridization of Southern blots
In situ hybridization
In situ immunohistochemistry

FIGURE 2-28 Diagnostic methods for human herpesvirus (HHV6): assays for HHV6 DNA and for HHV6 in pathologic specimens. The diagnoses of HHV6 infection requires both methods for detecting the presence of virus or viral DNA and serologic confirmation of infection. This table outlines techniques for the detection of viral DNA proteins in patient samples.

Detection of human herpesvirus 6: DNA in peripheral blood mononuclear cells, secretions, and other body sites

HHV6 DNA detection (as by polymerase chain reaction) indicates present or past infection with HHV6
Quantitative assays may be useful in determining viral load, suggesting change in viral state; examples include:
- Increased viral load with change from latency to reactivation
- Increased viral load associated with immunocompromised state

Figure 2-29 Detection of human herpesvirus 6 (HHV6) DNA in peripheral blood mononuclear cells, secretions, and other body sites. HHV6 causes ubiquitous infection of the human population. HHV6 can remain latent or persistent for many years at various sites, including the peripheral blood mononuclear cells and central nervous system. Laboratory techniques that can distinguish between active replicating virus and latent genome will be very helpful in distinguishing between clinical conditions in which HHV6 is a cause of disease and those in which HHV6 is a mere passenger in pathologic cells.

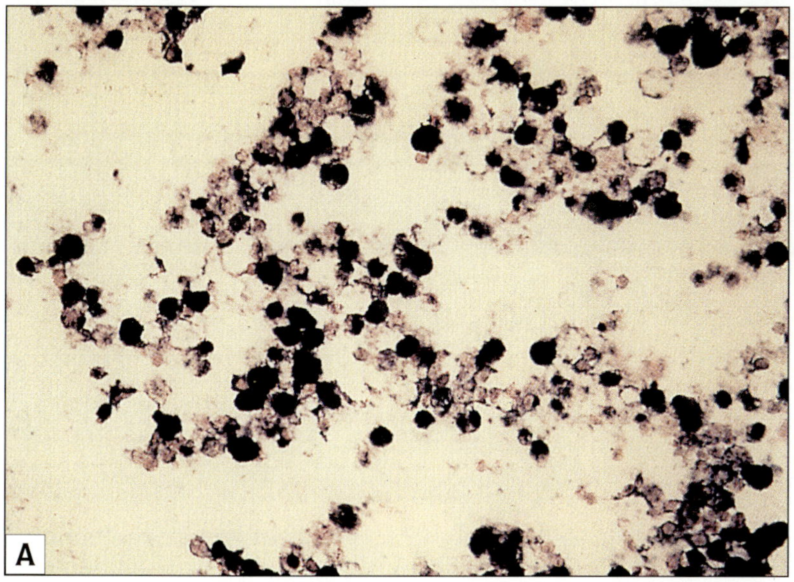

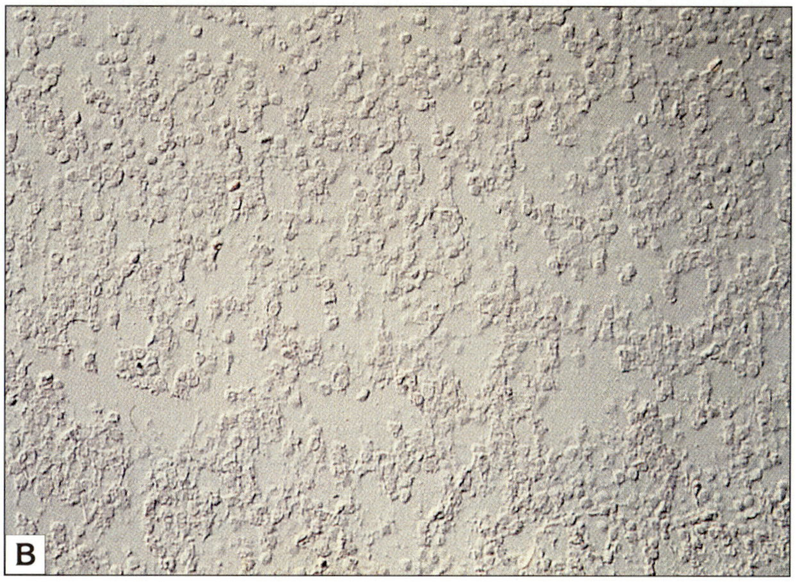

Figure 2-30 Detection of human herpesvirus 6 (HHV6) by in situ hybridization. The HHV6 genome can be detected in the nuclei of infected cells by in situ hybridization techniques as shown in the figures. **A**, HHV6 infected cord blood cells show intense blue nuclear signal using a digoxigenin-labeled DNA probe for the large tegument protein gene of HHV6 whereas, **B**, a 19-week gestation human fetal brain is negative for HHV6 infected cells. (*From* Saito *et al.* [19]; with permission.)

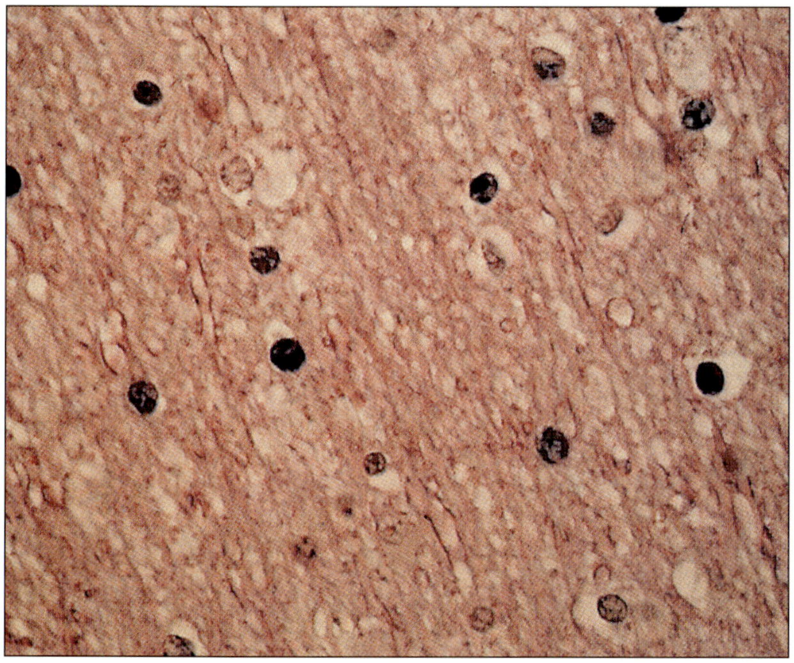

Figure 2-31 Human herpesvirus 6 (HHV6) localization in brain tissue by in situ hybridization. HHV6 DNA has been detected in the brain tissue of both normal and immunocompromised patients by both polymerase chain reaction and in situ hybridization (ISH). The advantage of ISH is the ability to preserve tissue architecture and accurately localize the DNA of interest. This is demonstrated in the ISH figure of subcortical white matter obtained from a child with HIV. Numerous HHV6 containing nuclei are identified primarily in cells with morphologic features of oligodendrocytes (Eosin counterstained, × 380). (*From* Saito *et al.* [19]; with permission.)

Therapy for human herpesvirus 6 infection
Currently no approved therapy
Agents showing in vitro inhibition of HHV6 infection
Ganciclovir
Acyclovir (less inhibitory than ganciclovir)
Foscarnet
Anecdotal clinical experience with foscarnet and ganciclovir in therapy of a few patients with bone marrow transplants

FIGURE 2-32 Therapy for human herpesvirus 6 infection (HHV6). Antiviral therapy for HHV6 infections is not available presently. Drugs demonstrating in vitro activity against HHV6 are outlined in this table. (*Adapted from* Drobyski *et al.* [20].)

HUMAN HERPESVIRUS 7

Characteristics of human herpesvirus 7
Electron micrographs reveal typical herpesvirus virions that have the following characteristics:
Diameter of 180–200 nm
Electron-dense cylindrical core
Nucleocapsid
Tegument
Envelope with spikes

FIGURE 2-33 Characteristics of human herpesvirus 7. This table contains the major ultrastructural characteristics of human herpesvirus 7, which clearly shares the typical features of the herpesvirus family and is similar to human herpesvirus 6.

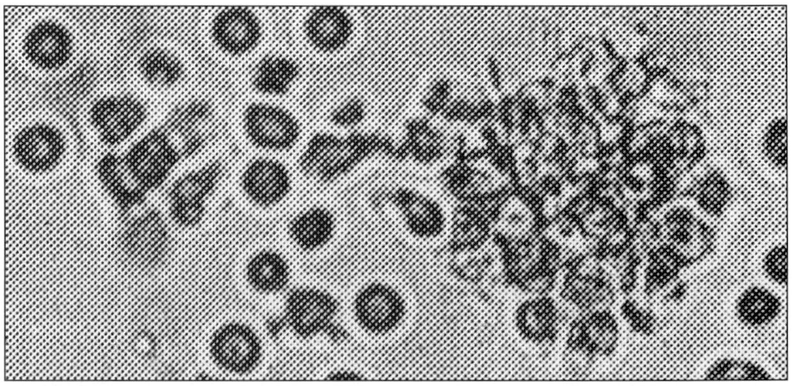

FIGURE 2-34 Ultrastructural characteristics of human herpesvirus 7 (HHV7). This electron micrograph of HHV7 virions illustrates the ultrastructural characteristics of the virus and demonstrates the typical herpesvirus structure. An electron dense core surrounded by the nucleocapsid. This is enclosed by amorphous tegument, which is surrounded by a lipid envelope containing protein spikes. (*From* Frenkel *et al.* [2]; with permission.)

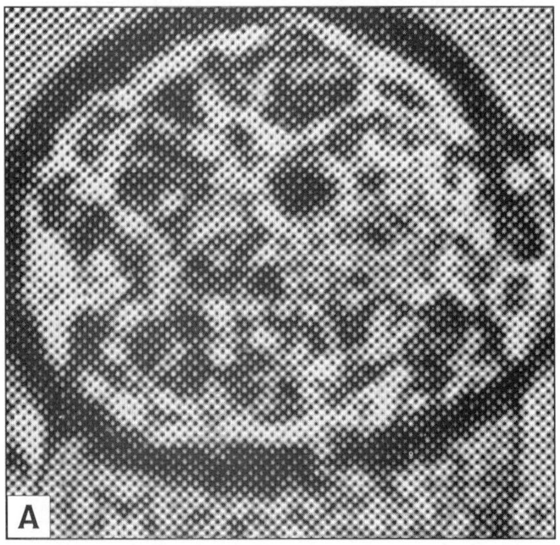

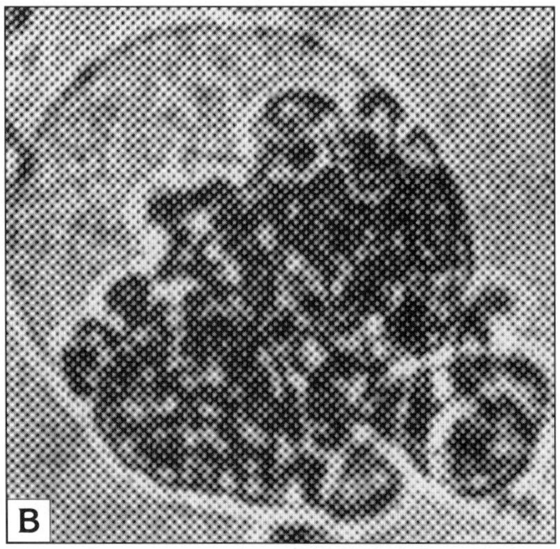

FIGURE 2-35 The propagation of human herpesvirus 7 (HHV7). These photographs were taken through a light microscope 7 days following the infection of stimulated cord blood mononuclear cells with HHV7. HHV7 has been found to infect primarily CD 4+ immature T cells, and the CD 4 molecule is a cellular receptor for the virus. The typical cytopathic effect produced by HHV7 is clearly shown and consists of large refractile ballooning cells (**B** and **C**)

(continued on next page)

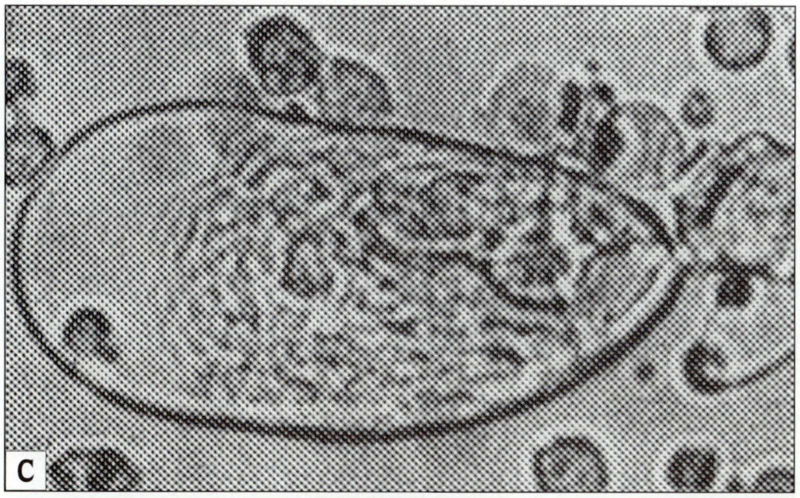

Figure 2-35 *(continued)* with distinct membranes in addition to cells that appear to have undergone fusion (**D**). These cells are in sharp contrast to the appearance of the uninfected control cord blood mononuclear cell culture (**A**) displaying uniform small individual cells. (*From* Frenkel *et al.* [2]; with permission.)

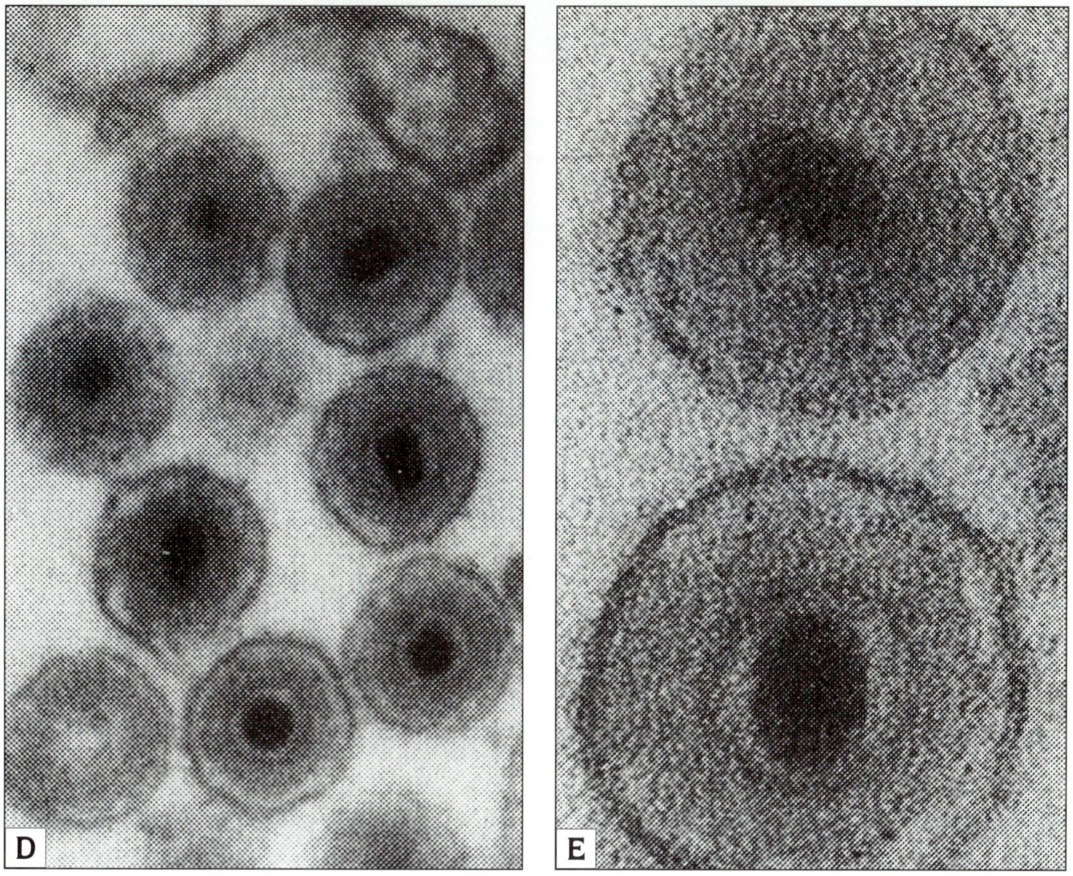

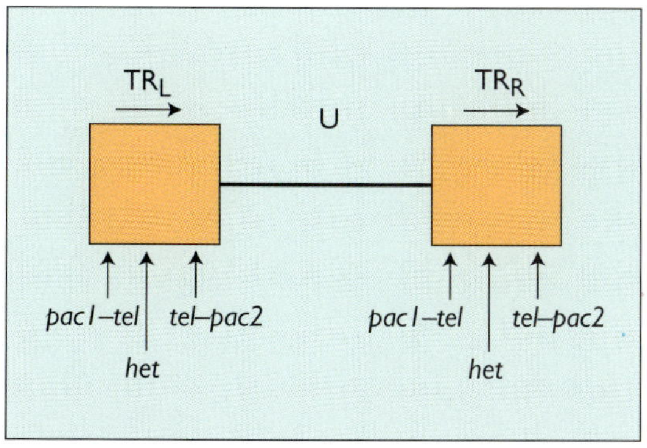

Figure 2-36 Genomic structure of human herpesvirus 7 (HHV7): proposed model of the HHV7 genome. Although the complete structure of HHV7 DNA has not yet been elucidated completely, the genome consists of a single unique component (U), estimated to be 120 kbp, which is bound by two direct terminal repeats, TR_L and TR_R, similar to the structure of human herpesvirus 6 (HHV6). The *pac1* and *pac2* are conserved sequences that function to promote the cleavage and packaging of the viral DNA during replication. The *het* sequences are variable according to the strain of HHV7. Limited regions of the HHV7 genome cross-hybridize significantly with HHV6. (*Adapted from* Frenkel and Roffman [21]; with permission.)

Epidemiology of human herpesvirus 7
Serologic studies show HHV7 is a ubiquitous infection HHV7 is acquired in early childhood, generally after HHV6 Almost all adults are seropositive; thus, all infants have passive HHV7 antibody present at birth
HHV6—human herpesvirus 6; HHV7—human herpesvirus 7.

Figure 2-37 Epidemiology of human herpesvirus 7. This table outlines the epidemiologic characteristics of human herpesvirus 7 as demonstrated in multiple serologic studies.

Children aged 0 to 45 months with human herpesvirus 7 antibody, DNA, or both in their blood mononuclear cells

		Human herpesvirus 7					
		PCR positive			Antibody positive		
Age, *mo*	Patients, *n*	Patients tested, *n*	Patients, *n*	%	Patients tested, *n*	Patients, *n*	%
0–5	53	49	4	8	23	6	29
6–11	76	73	14	19	30	5	17
0–11	129	122	18	15	53	11	21
12–23	118	109	38	35	51	20	39
0–23	247	231	56	24	104	31	30
24–44	48	46	24	52	20	10	50
0–44	295	277	80	29	124	41	33

PCR—polymerase chain reaction

FIGURE 2-38 Acquisition of human herpesvirus 7 (HHV7) infection as determined by the presence of HHV7 antibody, HHV7 DNA, or both in peripheral blood mononuclear cells of children aged 0 to 45 months. In comparison with the acquisition of human herpesvirus 6 infection, which is most common from 6 to 12 months of age, primary HHV7 infection generally occurs later in life with few infants acquiring HHV7 infection before 6 months of age, suggesting that passive antibody is protective. This table summarizes studies of normal children from Rochester, New York, and demonstrates that 17% of children aged 6 to 11 months (when passive antibody should have disappeared) still have antibody to HHV7. Between 24 and 44 months of age, 50% of the children were antibody positive, and a similar percent were demonstrated to possess HHV7 DNA in their peripheral blood mononuclear cells (Hall, Unpublished data).

Persistence of human herpesvirus DNA

- Human herpesvirus 7 DNA detected in saliva of most adults (>75%)
- Frequently persists in peripheral blood mononuclear cells of children after primary infection
- Human herpesvirus 7 DNA detected in other body sites and fluids, including cerebrospinal fluid and urine (<10% of normal adults)

FIGURE 2-39 Sites of asymptomatic persistence of human herpesvirus 7 DNA. Like other herpesviruses, human herpesvirus 7 has been found to persist in normal hosts following primary infection. The precise nature or consequences of persistence or latency have yet to be fully discovered.

The role of human herpesvirus 7 in clinical disease

- HHV7 as a direct cause of clinical diseases currently is not well elucidated
- The frequent persistence of HHV7 DNA in saliva and other body sites leads to its association with a variety of disease states but does not necessarily indicate etiology
- HHV6 and HHV7 commonly persist together, and infection with one may reactivate the other, resulting in difficulty in determining which virus is the cause of the associated clinical manifestations

HHV6—human herpesvirus 6; HHV7—human herpesvirus 7.

FIGURE 2-40 The indeterminate role of human herpesvirus 7 as cause of clinical diseases. Little is known about the pathologic potential of human herpesvirus 7 as outlined in this table.

The role of human herpesvirus 7 in clinical disease in children
HHV7 primary infection appears to cause a small proportion of cases of roseola (exanthem subitum)
HHV7 infection may account for the occasional second or recurrent cases of roseola
Most primary infections with HHV7 appear to be asymptomatic
HHV7—human herpesvirus 7.

FIGURE 2-41 The role of human herpesvirus 7 as the cause of clinical disease in children. Primary infection with human herpesvirus 7 in childhood has been documented and associated with the clinical syndrome described in the table.

Clinical features of primary human herpesvirus 7 infection in 15 Japanese children
Mean age
12.9 mo (range 7–27 mo)
Clinical findings
Fever: in 15 children (100%)
Mean temperature, 38.7°C (range 37.6°–39.8°C)
Mean duration, 2.9 d (range, 1–5 d)
Rash: in 14 children (93%)
Onset of rash, mean of 2.9 d (range, 2–5 d)
Duration of rash, 2.7 d (range, 1–5 d)
Seizure: in 1 child (7%)
Serologic findings
Simultaneous significant rise in human herpesvirus 6 antibody in 8 of 15 patients (53%) with human herpesvirus 7

FIGURE 2-42 The clinical manifestations associated with primary human herpesvirus 7 infection. Suga *et al.* [22] reported the clinical manifestations of primary human herpesvirus 7 infection in 15 Japanese children.

Diagnosis of human herpesvirus 7 infection: difficulties in diagnosing primary infection
Primary infection diagnosis: both isolation of HHV7 from peripheral blood mononuclear cells and serologic conversion in previously seronegative child
Isolation and propagation of HHV7 technically difficult
Serologic assays for HHV6 and HHV7 may detect cross-reactive antibodies
Reactivation of HHV6 by HHV7 infection and possible reactivation of HHV7 by HHV6 infection
HHV6—human herpesvirus 6; HHV7—human herpesvirus 7.

FIGURE 2-43 The difficulties in the diagnosis of primary human herpesvirus 7 infection. The diagnosis of human herpesvirus 7 infection is hampered by the technical challenge of isolating the virus and of its cross-reactivity and interaction with human herpesvirus 6.

Diagnosis of human herpesvirus 7 infection
Isolation of virus
Initial isolation from saliva or peripheral blood mononuclear cells in stimulated T cells (cord blood mononuclear cells)
Propagation in continuous cell lines: generally poor viral replication; Sup-T1 cells (immature T-cell line) commonly used
Seriologic assays
Immunofluorescent assays
Immunoblots
Detection of HHV7 genome
Enzyme immunoassays
Polymerase chain reaction and Southern blot hybridization
In situ hybridization

FIGURE 2-44 The diagnosis of human herpesvirus 7 (HHV7). HHV7 is a difficult virus to isolate and propagate in continuous culture. As with human herpesvirus 6, the diagnosis of HHV7 primary infection requires both viral isolation and seroconversion. The diagnosis of past infection with HHV7 can be ascertained by mononuclear biologic methods for detection of the HHV7 genome as shown in this table.

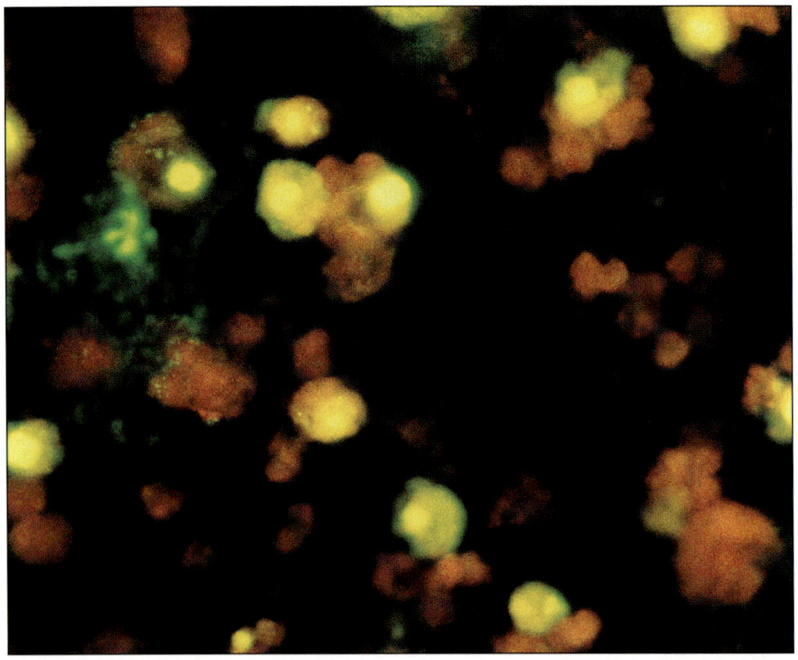

Figure 2-45 Human herpesvirus 7 infected cord blood mononuclear cells. This photograph depicts a positive indirect fluorescent antibody assay for human herpesvirus 7, showing the typical bring apple-green fluorescence primarily in the nuclei of positive cells. The negative cells are stained red and can be seen in the background.

References

1. Salahuddin SZ, Ablashi DV, Markham PD, *et al.*: Isolation of a new virus, HBLV, in patients with lymphoproliferative disorders. *Science* 1986, 234:596–601.
2. Frenkel N, Schirmer EC, Wyatt LS, *et al.*: Isolation of new human herpesvirus from CD4+ T cells. *Proc Natl Acad Sci U S A* 1990, 87:748–752.
3. Kramarsky B, Sander C: Electron microscopy of human herpesvirus-6 (HHV-6). In *Human Herpesvirus-6: Epidemiology, Molecular Biology and Clinical Pathology.* Edited by Ablashi DV, Krueger GRF, Salahuddin SZ. Amsterdam, the Netherlands: Elsevier; 1992:59–66.
4. Ablashi DV, Hung CL: In vitro propagation systems for HHV-6. In *Human Herpesvirus-6: Epidemiology, Molecular Biology and Clinical Pathology.* Edited by Ablashi DV, Krueger GRF, Salahuddin SZ. Amsterdam, the Netherlands: Elsevier; 1992:37–47.
5. Hall CB, Long CE, Schnabel KC, *et al.:* Human herpes virus-6 infection in children: prospective evaluation for complications and reactivation. *N Engl J Med* 1994, 331:432–438.
6. Lanphear BP, Hall CB, Black J: Risk factors for HHV-6 and HHV-7 infections in children. *Pediatr Infect Dis J* 1998, in press.
7. Leach CT, Newton ER, McParlin S, Jenson HB: Human herpesvirus 6 infection on the female genital tract. *J Infect Dis* 1994, 169:1281–1283.
8. Okuno T, Oishi H, Hayashi K, *et al.*: Human herpesvirus 6 and 7 in cervixes of pregnant women. *J Clin Microbiol* 1995, 33:1968–1970.
9. Dunne WM Jr, Jevon M: Examination of human breast milk for evidence of human herpesvirus 6 by polymerase chain reaction. *J Infect Dis* 1993, 168:250.
10. Kempe HC, Shaw EB, Jackson JR, Silver HK: Studies on the etiology of exanthema subitum (Roseola infantum). *J Pediatr* 1950, 37:561–568.
11. Suga S, Yoshikawa T, Asano Y, *et al.*: IgM neutralizing antibody responses to human herpesvirus-6 in patients with exanthem subitum or organ transplantation. *Microbiol Immunol* 1992, 36:495–506.
12. Dewhurst S, McIntyre K, Schnabel K, Hall CB: Human herpesvirus 6 (HHV-6) variant B accounts for the majority of symptomatic primary HHV-6 infections in a population of U.S. infants. *J Clin Microbiol* 1993, 31:416–418.
13. Hall CB: Human herpesviruses 6 (Roseola, Exanthem Subitum). In *Principles and Practice of Pediatric Infectious Diseases.* Edited by Long SS, Prober CG, Pickering LK. New York: Churchill Livingstone, Inc.; 1997:1176–1181.
14. Pruksananonda P, Hall CB, Insel RA, *et al.*: Primary human herpesvirus 6 infection in young children. *N Engl J Med* 1992, 326:1445–1450.
15. Breese BB Jr: Roseola infantum (exanthem subitum). *NY State J Med* 1941, 41:1854–1859.
16. Yamanishi K, Kondo K, Mukai T, *et al.*: Human herpesvirus 6 (HHV-6) infection in the central nervous system. *Acta Paediartica Japonica* 1992, 34:337–343.
17. Caserta MT, Hall CB, Schnabel K, *et al.*: Neuroinvasion and persistence of human herpesvirus-6 in children. *J Infect Dis* 1994, 170:1586–1589.
18. Kondo K, Nagafuji H, Hata A, *et al.*: Association of human herpesvirus 6 infection of the central nervous system with recurrence of febrile convulsions. *J Infect Dis* 1993, 167:1197–1200.
19. Saito Y, Sharer LR, Dewhurst S, *et al.*: Cellular localization of human herpesvirus-6 in the brains of children with AIDS encephalopathy. J Neurovirol 1995, 1:30–39.
20. Drobyski WR, Dunne WM, Burd EM, *et al.*: Human herpesvirus-6 (HHV6) infection in allogeneic bone marrow transplant recipients: evidence of a marrow-suppressive role for HHV-6 in vivo. *J Infect Dis* 1993, 167:735–739.
21. Frenkel N, Roffman E: Human herpesvirus 7. In *Fields Virology*, ed 3. Edited by Fields BN, Knipe DM, Howley PM, *et al.*: Philadelphia: Lippincott-Raven Publishers, 1996:2609–2622.
22. Suga S, Yoshikawa T, Nagai T, Asano Y: Clinical features and virological findings in children with primary human herpesvirus 7 infection. *Pediatrics* 1997, 99:468–469.

Chapter 3

Parvovirus Infections

Larry J. Anderson
Sherif R. Zaki
Thomas J. Török

Taxonomy

The Parvoviridae family

Family Parvoviridae
Subfamily: Parvovirinae
- Genus: *Parvovirus* (pathogens include Aleutian mink disease virus, bovine parvovirus, canine parvovirus, feline panleukopenia virus, porcine minute virus)
- Genus: *Erythrovirus* (pathogens include human parvovirus B19, simian parvovirus)
- Genus: *Dependovirus* (pathogens include adenoassociated viruses 1–5, avian adeno-associated virus)

Subfamily: Densovirinae
- Genus: *Densovirus*
- Genus: *Iteravirus*
- Genus: *Contravirus*

Figure 3-1 The Parvoviridae family. Parvoviruses are small 18- to 26-nm viruses that are stable in the environment, have a single-stranded DNA genome, and require actively dividing cells (the host cell needs to go through the S-phase of cellular replication) to complete the viral replication cycle. The viruses in the subfamily Parvovirinae infect animals whereas those in the subfamily Densovirinae infect arthropods. To date, viruses in the genus *Parvovirus* have been shown to infect only nonprimate animals; those in the genus *Erythrovirus* infect only humans and nonhuman primates, and those in the genus *Dependovirus* infect both humans and various animals. Human parvovirus B19 is the only parvovirus that, to date, has been shown to cause disease in humans [1].

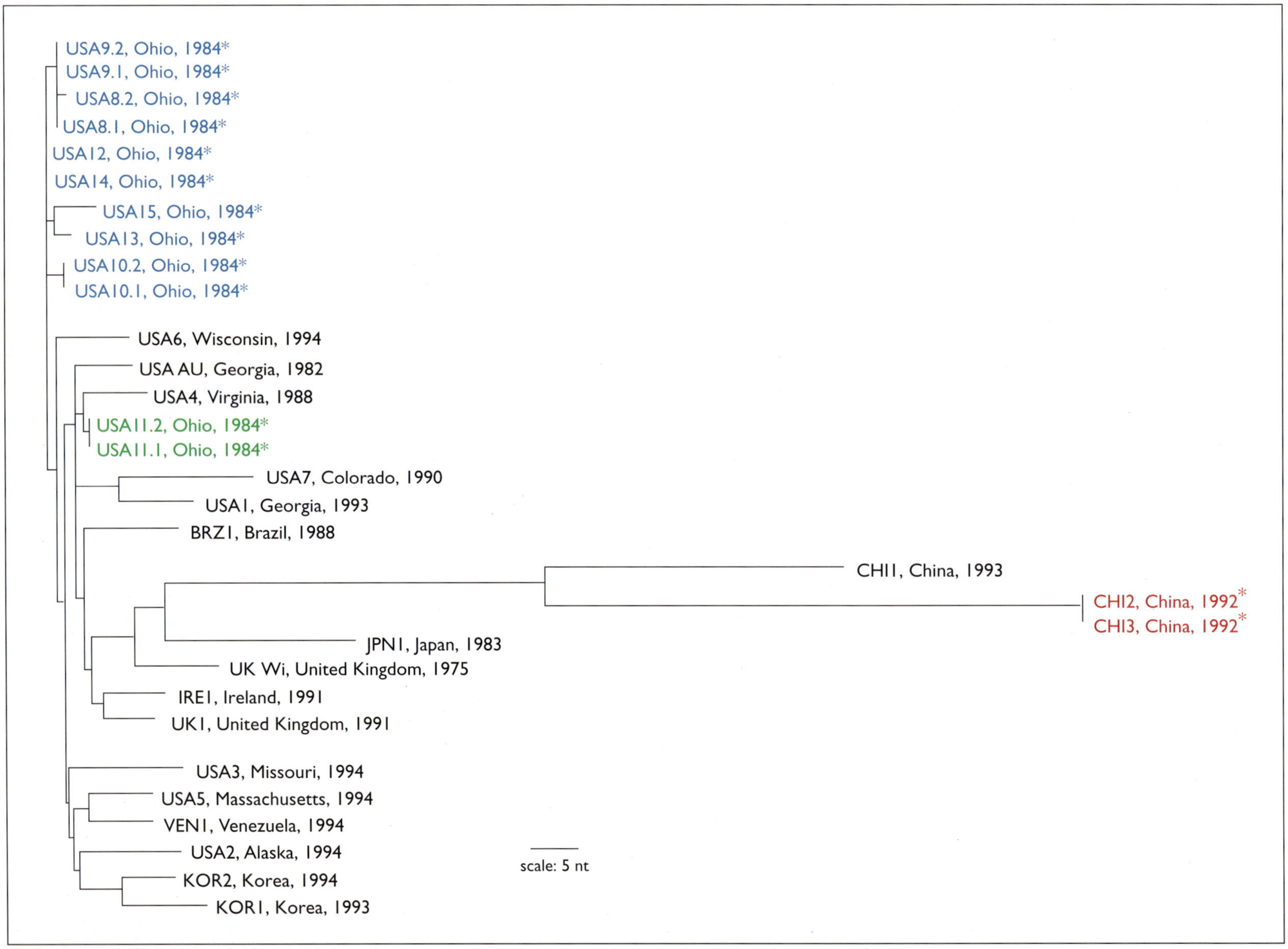

Figure 3-2 Genetic variability in human parvovirus B19 (B19) isolates. Although only one serotype of B19 has been described, the virus does have limited antigenic and genetic variability. This figure illustrates variability over 2343 nucleotides of the *VP1/VP2* gene 1)

(legend continued on next page)

FIGURE 3-2 *(continued)* between sequential isolates from the same patient and same community outbreak (green or blue lettering and labeled USA8.1–USA11.2 [for example, the first isolate for patient 8 is USA8.1 and the second is USA8.2]), and 2) among isolates from other distinct outbreaks in the United States and abroad.

The relative differences between isolates is indicated by distance on the horizontal or X axis. In this study, the maximum divergence between isolates was 4.6% of nucleotides and 1.7% of deduced amino acids. Few changes were seen in viruses isolated over time from the same patient (separated by ~3 wk) (USA8.1–USA11.2) or in viruses isolated from a family cluster (red lettering and labeled CH12 and CH13). Also, note that isolates from seven of eight patients from an outbreak in Ohio in 1984 (blue lettering) had sequences that were more closely related to each other (0 to 8 nucleotide differences) than were isolates from other distinct outbreaks in the United States (15 to 30 nucleotide differences) or isolates from other countries (17 to 108 nucleotide differences). The isolates from the eighth patient (green lettering and labeled USA11.1 and USA11.2) had between 7 and 11 nucleotide differences when compared with isolates from the other seven Ohio patients, suggesting that two distinct strains of B19 were cocirculating during this outbreak. (*Adapted from* Erdman *et al.* [2]; with permission.)

BIOLOGY OF INFECTION

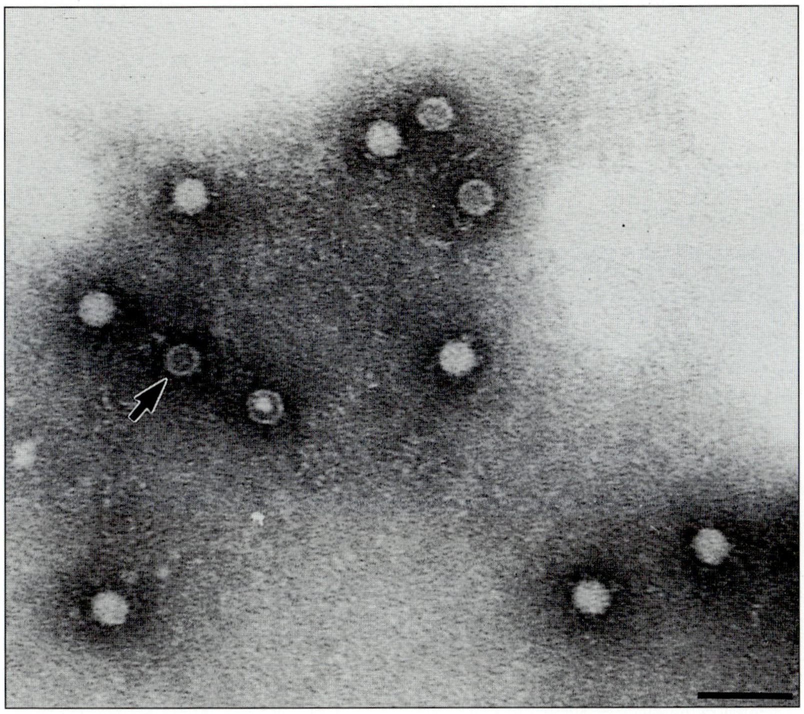

FIGURE 3-3 Electron micrograph of parvovirus particles in serum of a patient with sickle cell disease and transient aplastic crisis. The nonenveloped particles are small (approximately 22 nm) and icosahedral in shape. Occasional empty capsids are seen (*arrow*). The virus has a buoyant density of approximately 1.40 g/mL in cesium chloride. The virion is composed of 60 capsid proteins with 5% being viral protein (VP) 1 (VP1) and 95% being VP2, and a single strand of virion DNA, either with plus or minus sense. In vitro, empty capsids (*ie*, without virion DNA) will form from cloned, expressed VP2 alone or VP2 plus VP1. The two types of empty capsids, VP2 and VP2 plus VP1, have antigenic differences between each other and infectious virions (*ie*, VP2 plus VP1 plus virion DNA). For example, VP2 empty capsids are least effective at inducing neutralizing antibodies, whereas infectious virus is most effective. Radiographic crystallographic studies of B19 empty capsids have resolved its structure to 8.0 Å, a level that provides an overall picture of the virion structure but does not locate the position of individual amino acids. These studies suggest that the internal structure of B19 is similar to that of other parvoviruses, but its surface structure is distinct [3,4]. *Bar* indicates 50 nm.

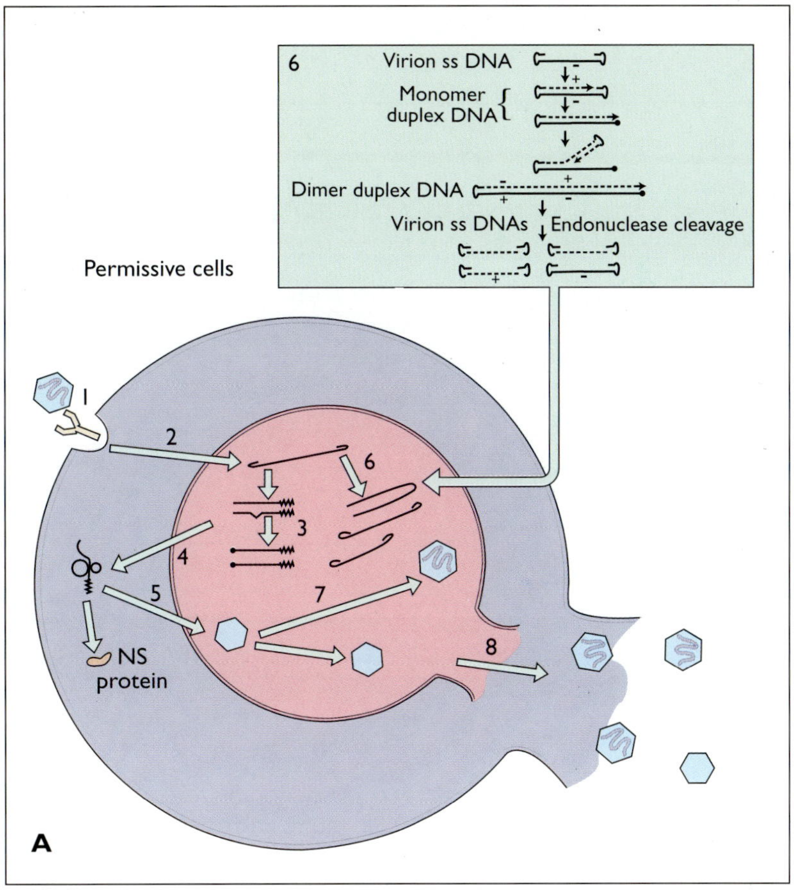

FIGURE 3-4 Infection of permissive and nonpermissive cells by B19. **A**, Permissive cell infection. In permissive cells [5], such as human proerythroblasts (1), B19 attaches to the cell through blood group P antigen (or globoside) [6] and is endocytized; virion DNA migrates to the nucleus (2), where mRNAs are transcribed and processed (3); mRNAs are transported to the cytoplasm, where they attach to ribosomes and translate the corresponding nonstructural (NS) protein, VP1, VP2, 7.5-kD, and 11.0-kD proteins (4); capsids are assembled from VP1 and VP2 (5); dimer duplex intermediates are transcribed and cleaved by cellular endonucleases to form virion single-stranded positive and negative sense DNA (6); capsids incorporate virion positive or negative sense DNA to form infectious virions (7); and the cell lyses and releases infectious virions and empty capsids (8). The cytotoxicity of the NS protein is probably responsible for cell death and lysis.

(continued on next page)

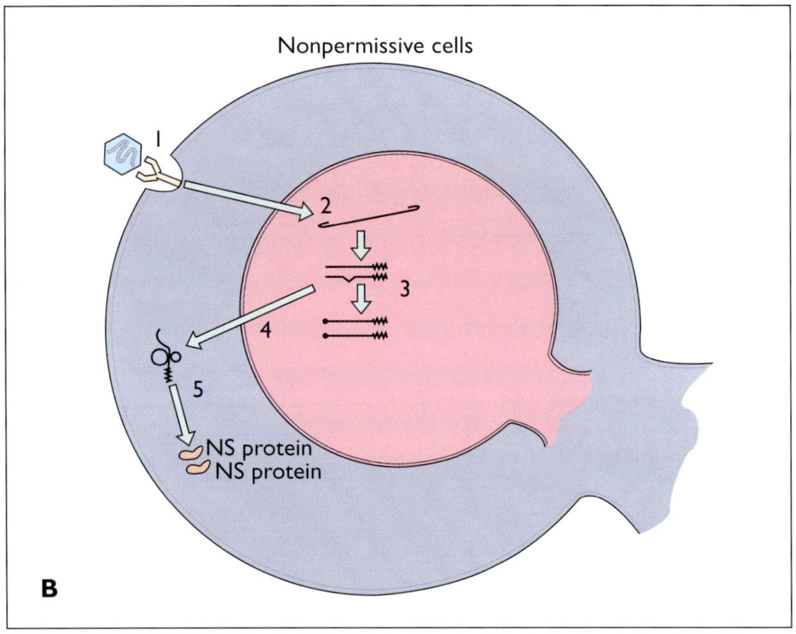

FIGURE 3-4 *(continued)* **B,** Nonpermissive cell infection. When B19 infects nonpermissive cells, presumably it attaches to blood group P antigen and is endocytized (1); virion DNA migrates to the nucleus in a fashion similar to that in permissive cells (2); based on in vitro studies, more NS than VP1 and VP2 mRNAs are transcribed (3); and NS mRNAs are efficiently translated and few or none of the VP1 and VP2 mRNAs are translated (4) [5,7]. The cytotoxicity of the NS protein leads to cell death (5).

B19 can also infect monocytes and macrophages that do not have blood group P antigen, possibly by antibody and virus complexes attaching to Fc receptors on the cell. Infection in monocytes and macrophages does not appear to produce infectious virus; it is not known whether infection results in cell death. ss—single-stranded.

Cell types that can be permissively and nonpermissively infected with B19

Cell type	Documentation	Mechanism of infection	Productive infection
Erythroid precursor cell (pronormoblast)	IFA, EM, I, IH	Blood group P antigen	Yes
Megakaryocytes	IH, IS	Blood group P antigen	Unknown
Granulocyte precursor cells (?)	EM	Unknown	Unknown
Macrophages	IS	Fc receptor (?)	Unknown
Myocytes	EM, IS	Blood group P antigen	Unknown
Endothelial cells	IH	Blood group P antigen	Unknown
Epidermal cells (?)	IH, IS	Unknown	Unknown

EM—electron microscopy; I—infectivity assay; IFA—immunofluorescent assay; IH—immunohistochemical; IS—in situ hybridization.

FIGURE 3-5 Cell types that can be permissively and nonpermissively infected with B19. The primary site of productive B19 infection is proliferating late erythroid progenitor cells, *eg*, the proerythroblast [8]. Other cells, such as megakaryocytes, myocytes, and endothelial cells, also have blood group P antigen and can be infected. Monocytes and macrophages do not have blood group P antigen, but presumably can be infected through virus or antibody complexes attaching to Fc receptors. It is not known whether B19 infection of nonerythroid cells produces infectious virus.

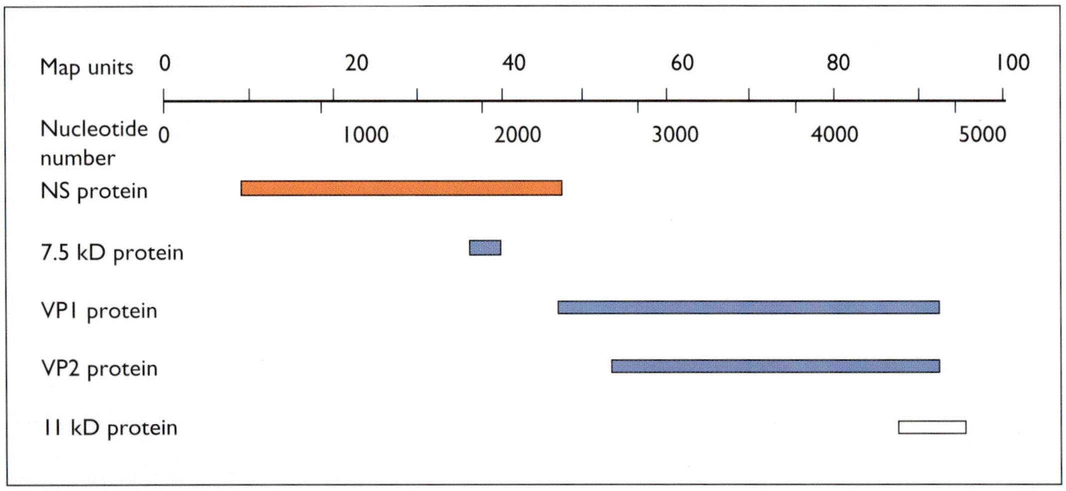

FIGURE 3-6 Organization of the B19 genome. The B19 genome encodes for nine mRNA species that translate five distinct proteins: the nonstructural (NS) protein in open reading frame 1 (*hatched bar*) is involved in virion replication; the two viral capsid proteins, VP1 and VP2, in open reading frame 2 (*closed bar*) form the virion capsid; the function of the 7.5-kD protein in open reading frame 2 is not known; and the function of the 11-kD protein in open reading frame 3 (*open bar*) is not known. The unprocessed NS protein is 671 amino acids and 78 kD; the 7.5-kD protein is 72 amino acids, the VP1 protein is 781 amino acids and 83 kD, the VP2 protein is 554 amino acids and 58 kD, and the 11-kD protein is 94 amino acids [4]. VP1 is identical to VP2 except that it has an additional 227 amino acids at the amino terminus.

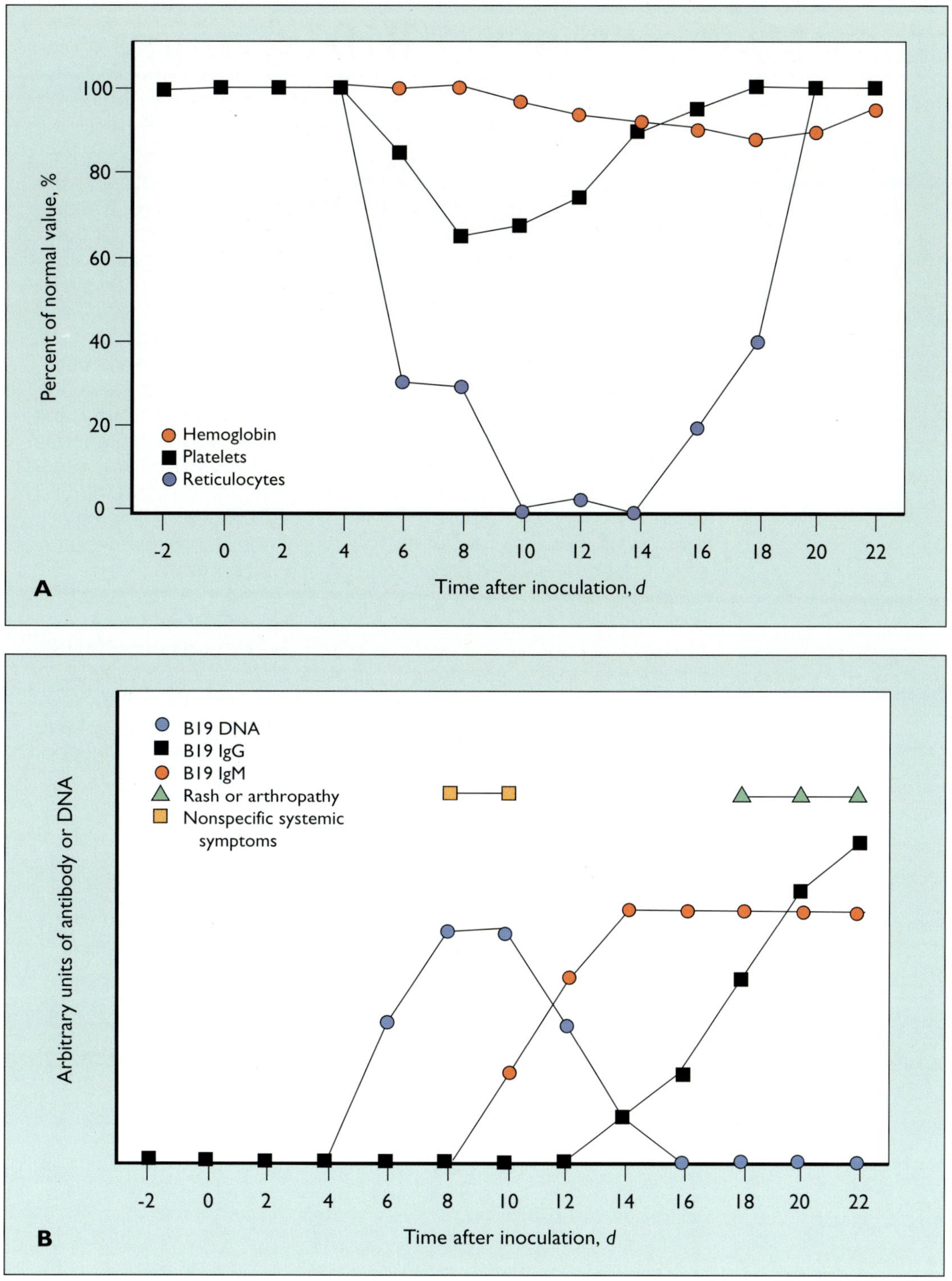

Figure 3-7 Human volunteer study of B19 infection. This study of nine adult volunteers intranasally inoculated with B19 illustrates many of the features of infection in humans [9]. **A,** Composite percentage of normal values of peripheral blood reticulocytes, hemoglobin, and platelets during infection. Four of five B19 IgG antibody–negative volunteers were infected and one of four antibody-positive volunteers became infected. The one antibody-positive, infected volunteer had barely detectable levels of IgG antibody before infection and had a transient viremia and anamnestic antibody response. Viremia developed between 5 and 6 days after inoculation and continued (as measured by DNA hybridization) for 6 to 10 days, with peak titer of virus in serum occurring at 7 to 9 days after infection. Associated with viremia, the antibody-negative volunteers experienced mild systemic symptoms (*ie*, low-grade fever, chills, myalgia, and headache). As expected of a virus that infects erythrocyte precursor cells, a transient erythrocyte aplasia, reticulocytopenia, and a consequent drop in hemoglobin levels were detected several days after the initial viremia and persisted for up to 10 days. Coincident with the viremia was a 30% to 50% drop in numbers of neutrophils, lymphocytes, and platelets. **B,** Composite levels of B19 antibodies or DNA during infection. IgM antibodies developed 10 to 13 days after infection and IgG antibodies a few days later. Only after development of B19 antibodies and clearance of the viremia (as detected by probe hybridization) did the typical symptoms associated with B19 infection (rash and arthritis) appear. Immune complexes were detected after the antibody response and may contribute to the pathogenesis of the rash and arthritis.

Clinical and Pathologic Manifestations of B19 Infection

Clinical manifestations of B19 infection
Common manifestations in the normal host
Asymptomatic infection
Erythema infectiosum (fifth disease)
Arthropathy (acute, self-limited)
Manifestations in the compromised host
Transient aplastic crisis in person with hematologic disorders
Chronic anemia in immunocompromised persons
Fetal anemia with hydrops and death
Uncommon manifestations
Other cutaneous manifestations (*eg*, vesicles, papules, purpura, desquamation)
Chronic arthropathy without joint destruction
Chronic infection in the normal host
Congenital anemia
Hemophagocytic syndrome
Neurologic abnormalities (*eg*, paresthesias, dysesthesias)

Figure 3-8 Clinical manifestations of B19 infection. B19 infection has several distinctive clinical presentations, which vary depending on the age and sex of the patient, and host factors.

In the normal host, the most common manifestations (rash and joint disease) develop after the antibody response occurs and the viremia, as indicated by DNA hybridization, has resolved. These manifestations of infection are not attributable to lytic infection of erythrocyte precursors; they are probably, at least in part, immune mediated and usually require no or only symptomatic therapy.

In patients with underlying hematologic abnormalities or compromised immune systems, or in the pregnant woman, infection can be associated with serious complications. Persons with various hematologic abnormalities (*see* Fig. 3-13) may develop transient aplastic crisis, and patients with compromised immune systems may develop chronic infection and an associated anemia. Maternal infection can lead to fetal infection that usually is associated with no complications but can result in a severe anemia in the fetus, hydrops, and death. B19-associated congenital anomalies, if they occur, are uncommon [10]. Several additional manifestations of infection have been described but are uncommon.

Finally, various diseases have been reported in patients with B19 infection, but an etiologic link between B19 and these diseases has not been established [11]. In some instances, B19 infection is probably present by chance or as an opportunistic infection or based on false-positive IgM antibody or polymerase chain reaction assays. In other instances, the infection may have unmasked the underlying condition. Further studies are needed to clarify which of these many possible associations are real.

Clinical manifestations of B19 infection in persons exposed to children with erythema infectiosum

	Frequency among family contacts, %	
Symptoms	IgM positive (n=36)	IgM negative (n=25)
Rash illness	53*	8
Fever	47	28
Nausea	39*	8
Muscle aches	36*	8
Joint pains	33*	4
Rhinorrhea	31	20
Diarrhea	28*	4
No symptoms	17	72

* Symptoms reported significantly more often (P<0.05) in infected than in uninfected contacts.

Figure 3-9 Clinical manifestations and frequency of signs and symptoms of B19 infection in persons exposed to children with erythema infectiosum. These family contacts were not at increased risk of serious complications of B19 infection. The 36 IgM-positive persons were considered infected and the 25 IgM-negative persons were considered uninfected [12]. Approximately half of infected contacts had no rash illness and 17% reported no symptoms. Higher rates of asymptomatic infection have been reported among B19-infected patients in other settings. In this study, 69% of B19-infected contacts of patients with transient aplastic crisis reported no symptoms with infection. The frequent lack of a typical B19-associated rash probably explains the high prevalence of B19 IgG antibodies but infrequent history of having had erythema infectiosum in adults.

Signs and symptoms reported in children with erythema infectiosum

Signs and symptoms	Sign or symptom occurrence, % (range)
Fever	14–53
Headache	12–53
Sore throat	12–60
Pruritus	0–>50
Upper respiratory tract illness or cough	5–40
Diarrhea	0–40
Nausea or vomiting	0–33
Sore eyes or conjunctivitis	4–27
Arthralgia or arthritis	0–9

Figure 3-10 Signs and symptoms reported in children with erythema infectiosum. Erythema infectiosum is the most commonly recognized manifestation of B19 infection. Onset of illness has been reported to occur between 4 and 20 days after clinically and epidemiologically defined exposure. In the volunteer study described in Figure 3-8, the time from inoculation of the virus to onset of rash and joint symptoms was 17 to 18 days. Erythema infectiosum usually resolves within 2 weeks, but the illness can last for months. Resolution and then recrudescence of rash or other signs and symptoms are common and can be precipitated by a variety of stimuli, including local irritation, bathing, emotional stress, sunlight exposure, and change in ambient temperature. Symptoms reported in children with erythema infectiosum have varied considerably among outbreaks [13]. These differences may be caused by variations in case definitions, patterns of observing or recording clinical signs and symptoms, skin pigmentation, or, possibly, other host or viral factors.

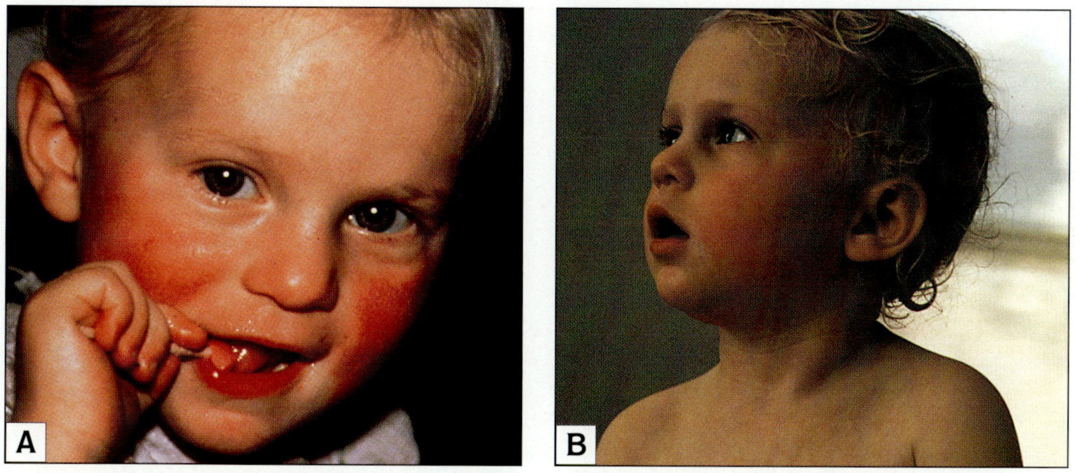

FIGURE 3-11 Children with rash of erythema infectiosum. **A,** Close-up of face. **B,** Head and chest view. The facial rash is characterized by intense erythema of the cheeks with circumoral pallor (slapped-cheek appearance). On the extremities and trunk, the rash is less intensely red, is maculopapular, and has a reticular or lacelike appearance; the palms and soles are usually spared. The rash may be pruritic. Recrudescence of the rash can occur with nonspecific stimuli, such as exposure to heat or cold. Usually, the rash persists for less than 2 weeks. Other cutaneous manifestations of B19 infection are less commonly reported and include vesicles, papules, purpura, and desquamation.

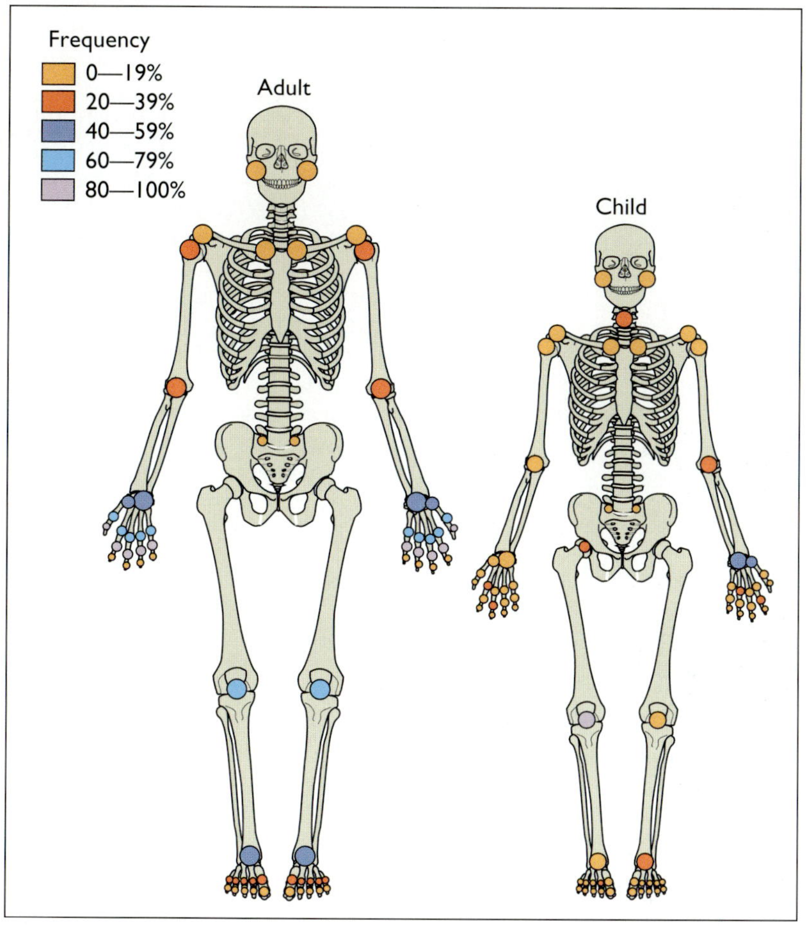

FIGURE 3-12 Human parvovirus B19–associated arthritis and arthralgia. Location and relative frequency of joint disease in adults (*left*) and children (*right*) after B19 infection. Following B19 infection, adults commonly develop a symmetric polyarthropathy affecting primarily the hands and wrists. In the majority of cases, joint manifestations are limited to arthralgias or stiffness that persists for a few days or a few weeks; joint swelling and other signs of joint inflammation are less common. Arthralgia and arthritis are most commonly reported in female adults. In contrast to adults, few children develop joint disease after B19 infection; the distribution of the involved joints is not symmetric and frequently involves four or fewer joints, with the knee being most commonly affected. The joint disease is probably immune mediated because it occurs after the antibody response develops and after viremia (as detected by DNA hybridization) is cleared. The arthropathy can occur with or without a rash. Rheumatoid factor and other autoantibodies may be present transiently. In some cases, arthralgias and arthritis may persist for months and may meet American Rheumatism Association criteria for rheumatoid arthritis, juvenile rheumatoid arthritis, or fibromyalgia. Bone erosions are not evident even with chronic joint disease. The presence of bone erosions should suggest another diagnosis.

Conditions that predispose to serious complications of B19 infections

Hematologic disorders associated with anemia
- Decreased erythrocyte production (*eg,* thalassemia, iron deficiency)
- Increased erythrocyte destruction or loss (*eg,* sickle cell disease, hereditary spherocytosis, malaria, blood loss)

Congenital or acquired immunodeficiency, such as that associated with HIV infection, lymphoproliferative disorders, immunosuppressive therapy for cancer, leukemia, lymphoma, or organ transplantation

Pregnancy

FIGURE 3-13 Conditions that predispose to serious complications of B19 infection. In the normal host, infection produces a self-limited erythrocyte aplasia that is clinically inapparent. Patients with hematologic disorders characterized by decreased erythrocyte production or increased erythrocyte destruction may acutely develop severe acute symptomatic anemia as a result of the erythrocyte aplasia or transient aplastic crisis. Immunocompromised patients may develop chronic B19 infection and anemia. The fetus is at risk of developing both severe anemia and chronic B19 infection.

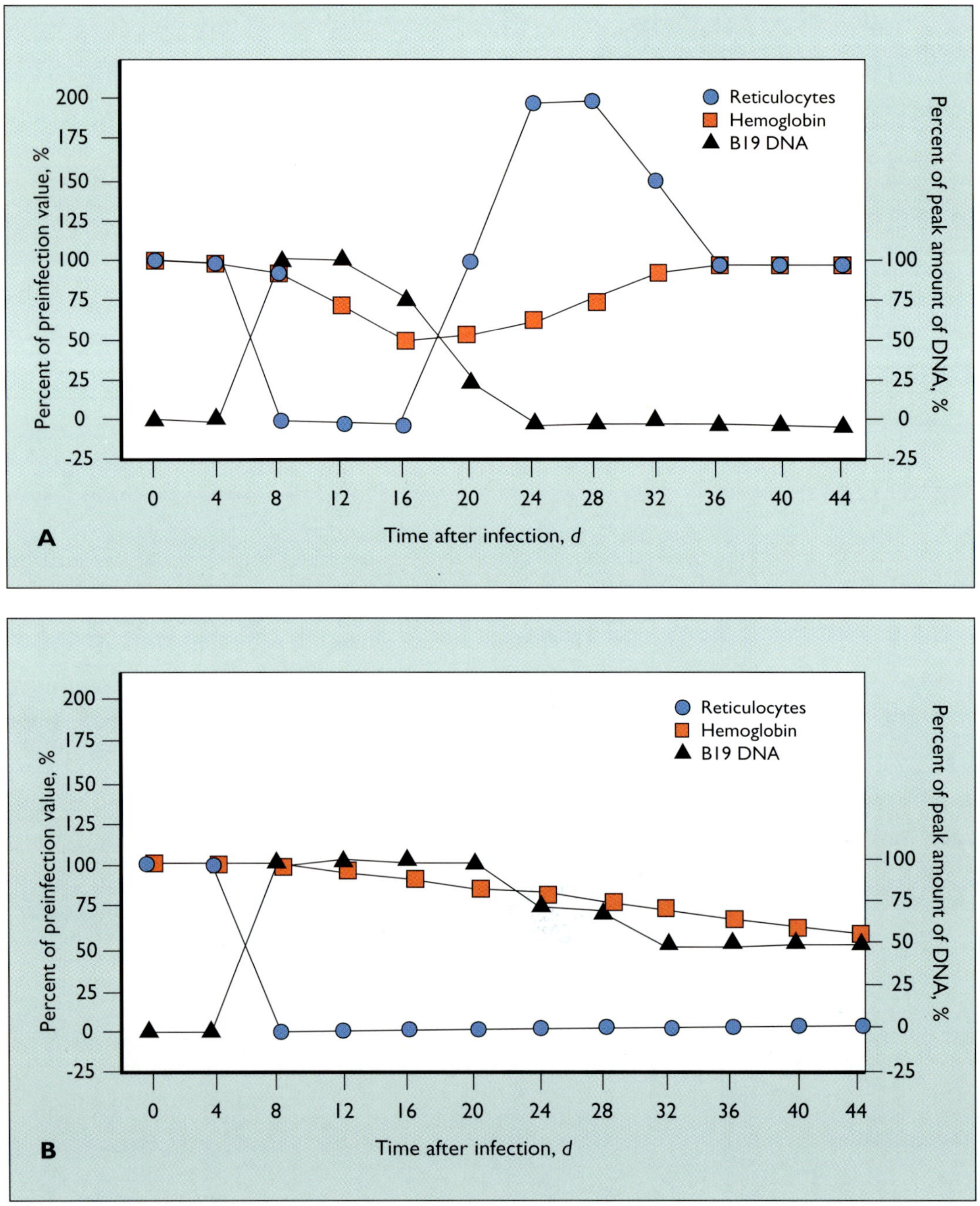

FIGURE 3-14 The pathogenesis of B19-associated anemia in patients with hematologic (*panel A*) versus immunologic (*panel B*) abnormalities. In patients with a hematologic abnormality, the infection of erythrocyte precursors leads to a drop in hemoglobin level that is symptomatic because the level drops precipitously (eg, patients with sickle cell disease (*panel A*)]) or the initial level was sufficiently low that an otherwise inapparent drop causes symptoms (eg, patients with iron-deficient anemia). In patients with transient aplastic crisis, once the immune response cures the infection, erythrocyte production resumes, and the steady-state hemoglobin level is reestablished.

The patient with a compromised immune system that cannot cure the infection has a steady drop in hemoglobin level that eventually leads to a symptomatic anemia (note persistence of B19 DNA and steady drop in hemoglobin levels in the *panel B*) . There are several case reports of patients without a well-documented immune deficiency who developed chronic infection and anemia. Presumably, these patients had a limited immunologic defect that prevented them from controlling B19 infection. Patients can develop chronic infection and anemia with or without circulating B19-specific IgG or IgM antibody, and not all B19-infected patients with the immune deficiencies noted in Figure 3-14 will develop chronic infection and anemia. Patients with chronic B19-associated anemia are likely to respond to immune globulin intravenous treatment as described in Figure 3-39. (*Adapted from* Saarinen *et al.* [14] and Anderson *et al.* [9].)

Symptoms in sickle cell disease patients with transient aplastic crisis

Signs and symptoms	Sign or symptom occurrence, % (range)
Fever	80–100
Headache	35–50
Malaise	40–70
Gastrointestinal symptoms	40–85
Respiratory tract symptoms	0–45
Conjunctivitis or photophobia	0–15
Rash	0–25

FIGURE 3-15 Symptoms in sickle cell disease patients with transient aplastic crisis (TAC). B19 infection can be documented in over 90% of cases of TAC in patients with sickle cell disease [13,15]. Secondary cases of TAC in households usually occur between 6 and 12 days, but sometimes up to 20 days, after the index patient with TAC. The patient often presents 1 to 7 days after onset of the noted symptoms, with reticuloctye counts of 0% to 1% and pallor, and a drop in their baseline hemoglobin levels of up to 50% or more. Hemoglobin levels less than 2.0 gm/dL can occur and patients often require hospitalization and transfusion therapy to maintain hemodynamic stability until their immune response cures the infection and erythrocyte production resumes. Reticulocytosis and recovery usually begin within a week of presentation. Stroke, acute splenic sequestration, acute chest syndrome, and even death may complicate TAC. Erythema infectiosum and joint disease, the usual manifestations of acute B19 infection, are rarely observed in persons with TAC.

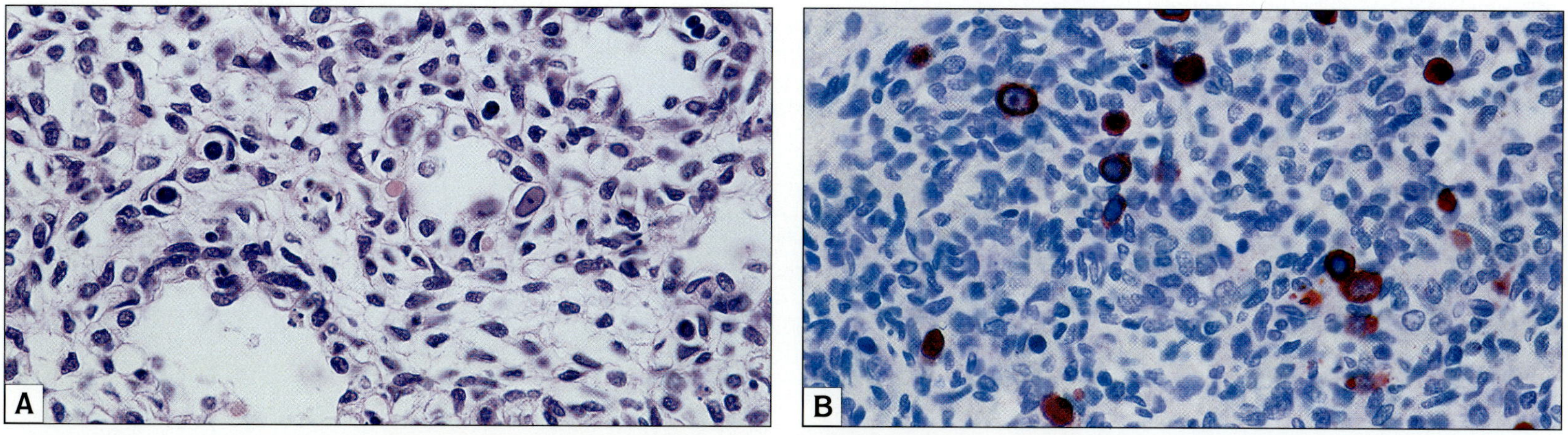

FIGURE 3-23 Histologic findings in the lung of a B19-infected hydropic fetus. **A,** Several erythroid cells containing ground glass inclusions typical of parvovirus B19 are seen. Inclusion-bearing nucleated erythrocytes can frequently be identified in the vascular spaces, even in poorly preserved tissue specimens, making histopathologic examination of the lung a worthwhile endeavor for confirming the diagnosis of intrauterine B19 infection. (Hematoxylin and eosin stain, × 158.) **B,** Confirmation and localization of parvovirus antigens in same patient by using immunohistochemistry. Both nuclear and cytoplasmic immunostaining of erythroid precursors is seen. Although not directly affected by B19 infection, normal lung development may be impaired by large volumes of pleural fluid. (Naphthol fast red with light hematoxylin counterstain, × 158.)

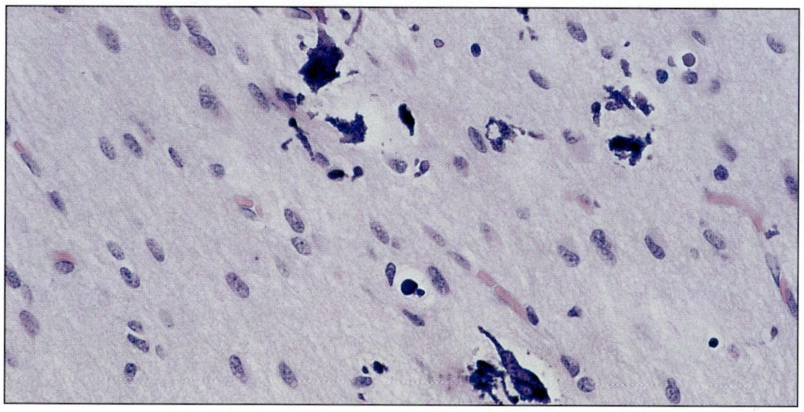

FIGURE 3-24 Histologic findings in the central nervous system of a B19-infected fetus. Neuronal calcifications have been noted in some fetuses following intrauterine B19 infection, and B19 inclusions have been found in erythroid cells in the central nervous system (CNS). Infection of neurons has not been demonstrated, however, suggesting that any B19-associated CNS abnormalities may be caused by hypoxia and not the cytopathic effect of the virus. The fact that experimental and natural intrauterine infection with many animal parvoviruses are associated with CNS malformations has encouraged researchers to look for CNS abnormalities after B19 infection in the human fetus. Although CNS abnormalities have been reported in a few cases of fetal B19 infection, an etiologic link between these abnormalities and the infection has not been established. (Hematoxylin and eosin stain, × 100.)

DIAGNOSIS OF INFECTION

Diagnosis of B19 infection

Acute or active infection
- Indicated by symptoms and documented by detecting B19 antigens, DNA, or virions in serum or tissue specimens; recent infection indicated by presence of B19 IgM antibodies

Chronic infection
- Most often demonstrated by detecting B19 DNA in serum or other specimens over time; can be found with or without presence of IgM or IgG antibodies

Past infection
- Indicated by the presence of B19 IgG antibodies

Site of infection
- Can be demonstrated by identifying infected cells by in situ hybridization, immunohistologic, or immunofluorescence studies or by identifying infection in tissue through detection of replicative forms of DNA and nonstructural protein.

FIGURE 3-25 Diagnosis of B19 infection. The availability of a variety of diagnostic assays or techniques for B19 infection makes it possible to not only diagnose infection but also investigate pathogenesis of disease. The IgM antibody assay has been invaluable in detecting acute infection and linking B19 to erythema infectiosum and arthropathy. The IgG assay has been helpful in determining the prevalence of infection and identifying who is likely to be susceptible to infection. Sensitive DNA detection assays, especially polymerase chain reaction (PCR), have provided some interesting information on chronic infection and possible B19-associated diseases that will require further study. B19 IgM antibody is present at the onset of illness in most patients with erythema infectiosum or B19-associated arthropathy and present somewhat less frequently in patients with transient aplastic crisis (TAC). Patients with TAC who are IgM negative at presentation usually will become IgM positive within a few days. The very sensitive PCR assay has made it possible to usually detect B19 DNA up to a month and sometimes longer after onset of illness. It is not yet clear as to what is the clinical relevance of the low levels of B19 DNA that can be detected in serum or other specimens from patients who do not have an acute B19-associated illness or chronic B19-associated anemia. Histopathologic and other studies to determine site of infection are likely to be especially important to understand the role of chronic B19 infection and disease.

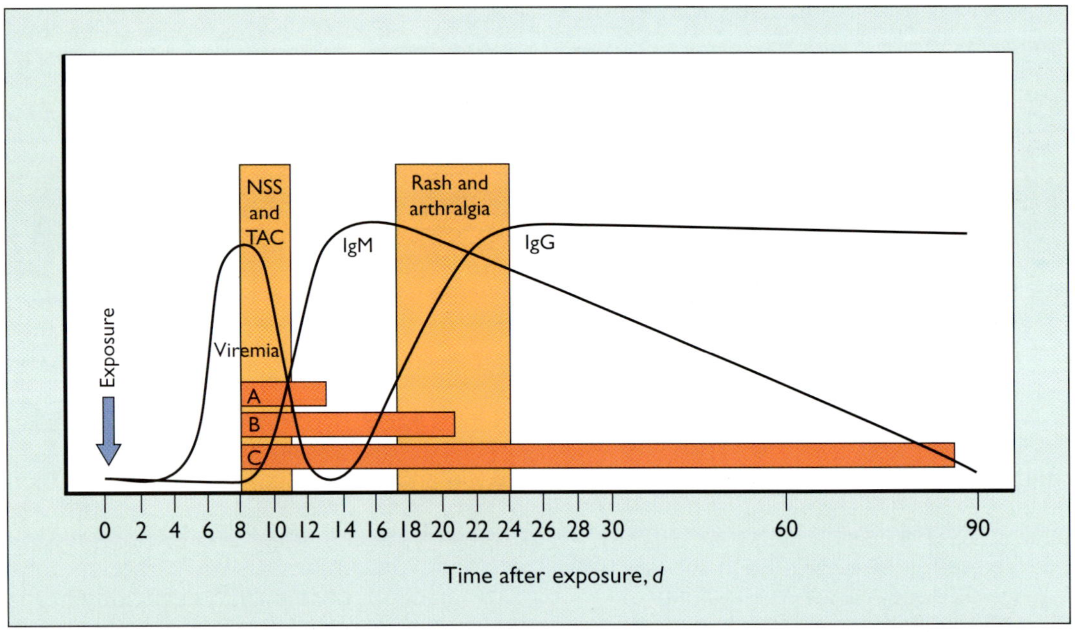

FIGURE 3-26 Time of antibody, antigen, and DNA positivity following B19 infection. B19 infection can be associated with a high-titered viremia (titers as high as 10^{12} particles/mL have been reported) during the acute phase of illness that can be detected by electron microscopy (*bar* A), antigen detection assays (*bar* A), DNA probe hybridizations assays (*bar* B), or polymerase chain reaction (PCR) DNA assays (*bar* C). Patients with transient aplastic crisis (TAC) often present during this acute viremic phase of the infection. With development of an IgM and then IgG antibody response, the titer of virus drops rapidly and virus can be detected for a few days by DNA probe hybridization (*bar* B). Symptoms of erythema infectiosum are usually noted several days after the antibody response is detected and after DNA can no longer be detected by probe hybridization assays. With PCR, B19 DNA can usually be detected for up to a month, sometimes longer. IgM antibodies can usually be detected at the onset of illness and for approximately 2 months thereafter. NSS—nonspecific systemic symptoms.

B19 false-positive IgM antibody assays

Capture IgM assay	Indirect IgM assay* Positive	Indirect IgM assay* Negative	PCR positive for B19 DNA
Positive	2	1	3
Negative	7	9	0

* Sensitivity (compared with the capture antibody assay), 2/3 (67%); specificity (compared with the capture antibody assay), 9/16 (56%).

FIGURE 3-27 Human parvovirus B19 false-positive IgM antibody assays. Some B19 IgM antibody assays, *eg*, some indirect Western blot, immunofluorescent, or enzyme immunoassay, can have low sensitivity and specificity. The capture IgM antibody format in most instances has given the best combination of sensitivity and specificity (*see* Fig. 3-32). These data illustrate the potential problems with indirect IgM antibody assays by comparing results from parallel testing of 19 serum specimens from an outbreak of B19 [17]. Note the discrepancy in results between the indirect and capture antibody assays and that polymerase chain reaction for B19 DNA corroborated all three IgM-positive results by the capture antibody assay, but only two of nine positive results by the indirect assay. Some reports of B19-associated disease are probably based on false-positive IgM antibody results.

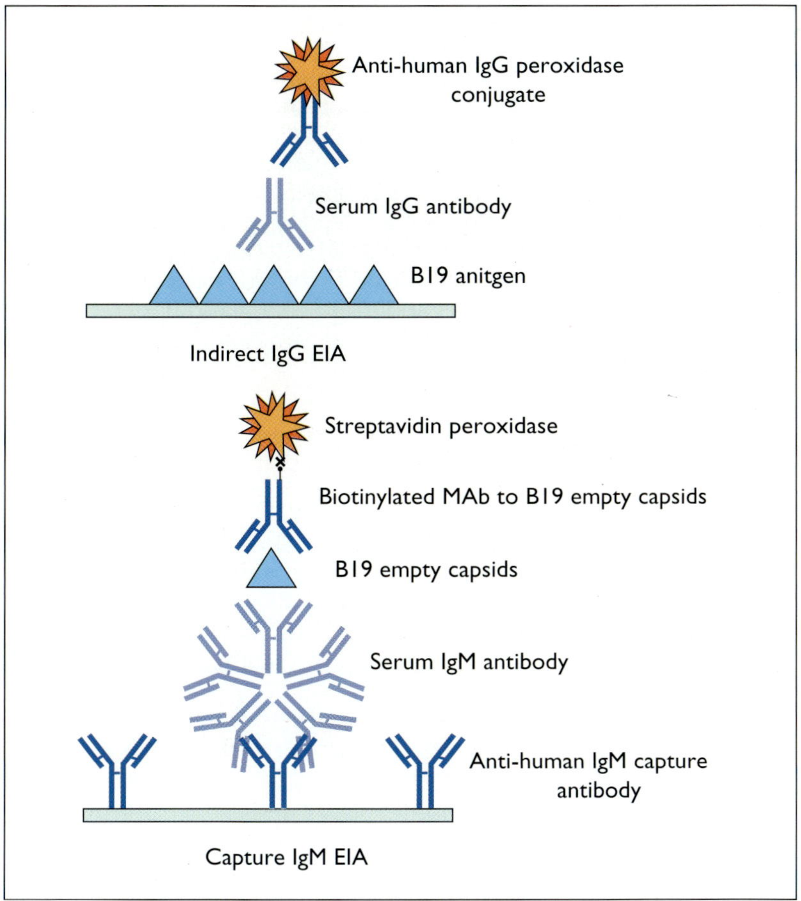

FIGURE 3-28 Human parvovirus B19 IgM antibody capture assay. The antibody capture assay has usually given the best combination of sensitivity and specificity for detecting B19 IgM antibodies. The capture antibody format used with an enzyme immunoassay (EIA) or radioimmunoassay detection system yields essentially identical results. In the capture antibody format, the IgM antibodies are captured by antihuman antibodies attached to the walls of the microtiter plate wells (or other solid phase); the wells are washed, removing IgG antibodies; the captured IgM antibodies are reacted against the B19 antigens; and a biotinylated monoclonal antibody is used to detect B19 antigens that reacted against the captured IgM antibodies. Removal of IgG antibodies before reacting the IgM antibodies against the B19 antigens decreases the chance that B19-specific IgG antibodies will block epitopes on the B19 antigens and give a false-negative result or be captured by IgM rheumatoid factor and give a false-positive result. The capture antibody format also minimizes nonspecific sticking of IgM antibodies.

EPIDEMIOLOGY OF INFECTION

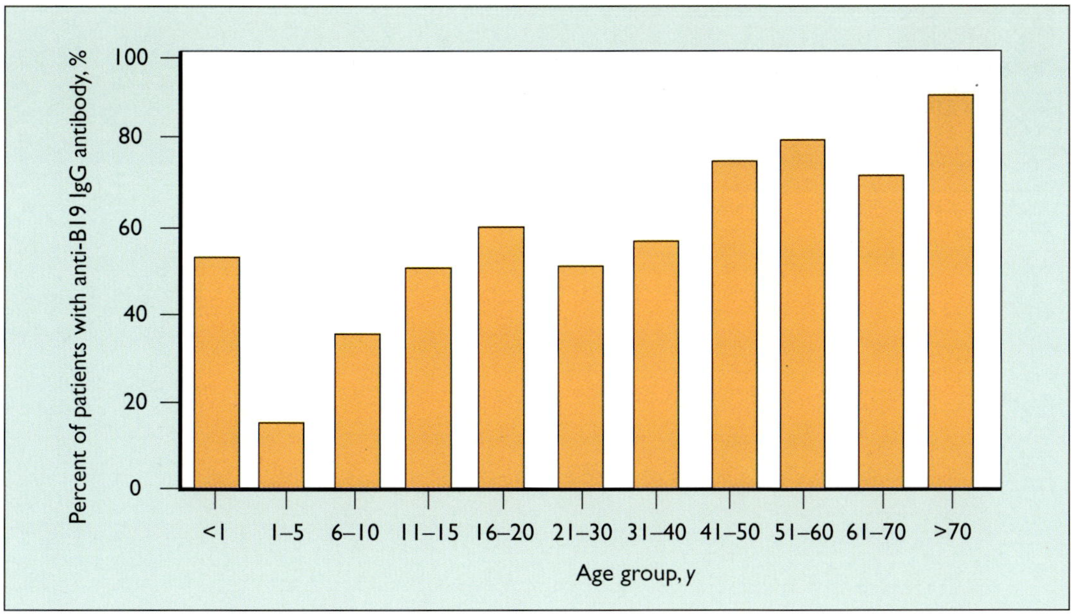

FIGURE 3-29 Human parvovirus B19 IgG positivity by age. Because B19 IgG antibody persists for a long time after infection, it is an indicator of prevalence of infection in a population. The rate of B19 IgG positivity increases most sharply during the early school years, *ie*, from the 1- to 5-year-old age group to the 11- to 15-year-old age group, consistent with the fact that most outbreaks of erythema infectiosum are reported among children during the elementary and middle school years [18]. The rate of IgG positivity gradually rises to reach approximately 80% later in life. The rate of IgG positivity will vary between communities and between years in the same community, depending on timing of recent B19 outbreaks. Rates between 40% and 60% are most commonly reported for adults 20 to 40 years of age.

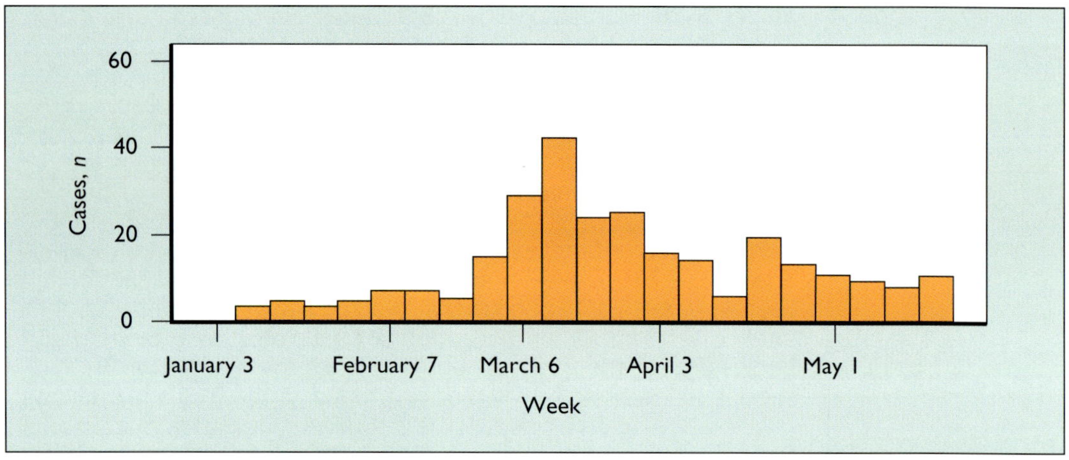

FIGURE 3-30 Community outbreak of erythema infectiosum. Outbreaks of erythema infectiosum in temperate climates are often noted in the late winter and spring months in childcare centers and elementary and middle schools. As illustrated in this epidemic curve of an outbreak of erythema infectiosum in a Connecticut town in 1988, B19 spreads slowly through schools, resulting in outbreaks lasting months and often continuing until schools close for summer vacation [19].

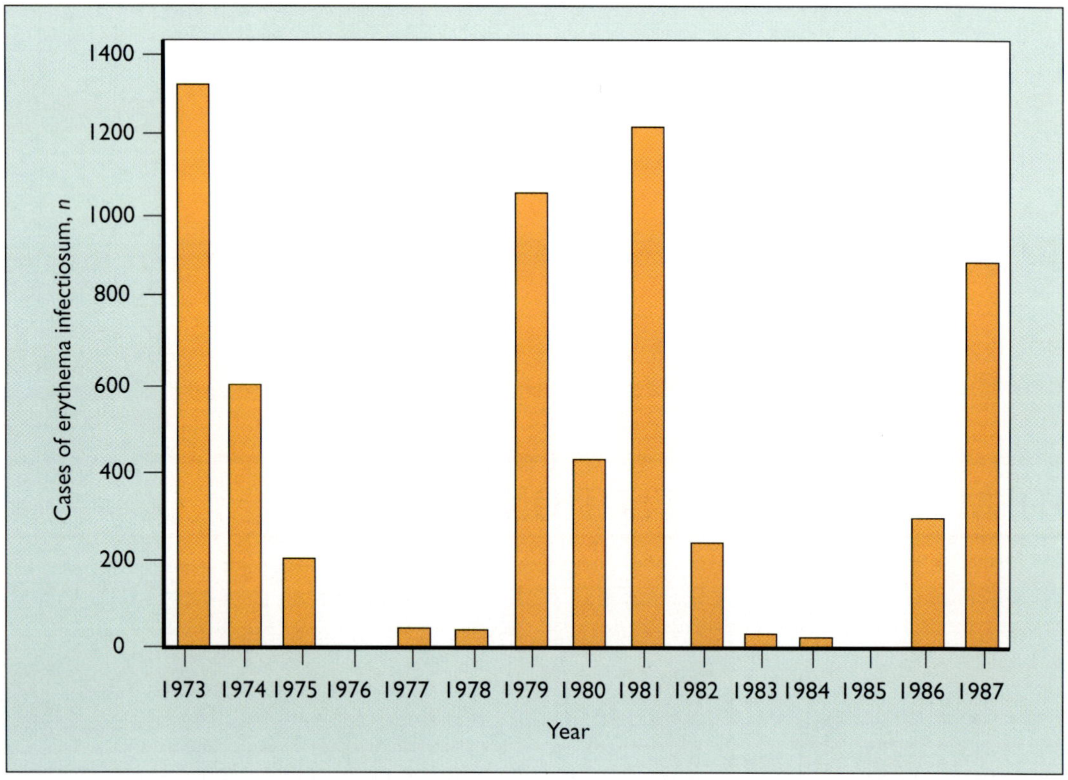

FIGURE 3-31 Cyclical nature of B19 infections in a community. B19 infection is most often recognized as cases of erythema infectiosum during outbreaks in schools. In a given community, high levels of B19 activity will occur for a few years followed by low levels of activity for 3 to 10 years. This graph of erythema infectiosum cases reported by school nurses in Iowa illustrates the cyclical nature of B19 outbreaks [20]. Note that three 2- to 4-year periods of higher numbers of reported cases were interspersed by two 3-year periods of few reported cases.

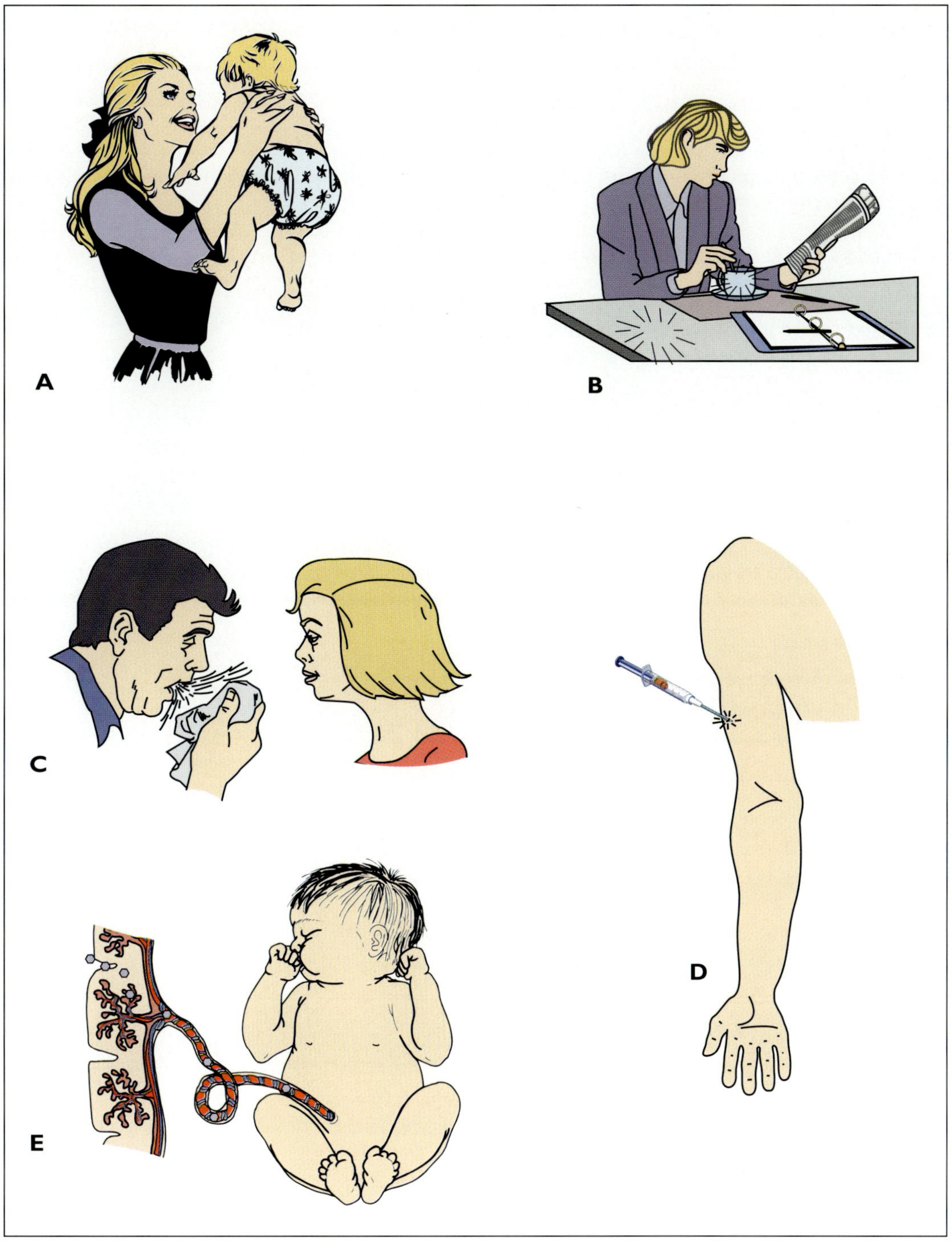

Figure 3-32 Modes of transmission. The fact that B19 spreads efficiently in households but takes months to spread through schools suggests that close contact is important to transmission. **A,** Probably direct person-to-person transmission. After touching an infected person's contaminated hands one can then autoinoculate the virus onto a mucous membrane. B19 has been detected on the hands of a child with erythema infectiosum, as reported by the Centers for Disease Control and Prevention (Unpublished data). **B,** Probably transmission by fomites. After touching an object such as a cup, door knob, or countertop that has been contaminated by a B19-infected person one can then autoinoculate the virus onto a mucous membrane. B19 DNA has been detected on surfaces in a room where a B19-infected abortus was delivered. **C,** Probably large-droplet transmission. This mode of transmission occurs by inhaling large droplets containing infectious virus generated by a cough or sneeze from a B19-infected person. **D,** Percutaneous transmission. B19 has also been transmitted percutaneously through infusion of contaminated blood or blood products such as factor VIII or through contaminated needles (*eg*, tattooing). **E,** Vertical transmission from the mother to her fetus.

Sources of infectious virus

Respiratory tract secretions B19 DNA has been detected by probe hybridization in respiratory tract excretions of person during the acute viremic phase of the illness (*eg*, 2 of 6 respiratory secretion specimens from patients with acute TAC were positive in one study [12]). Blood B19 DNA and infectious virus have been detected in serum frequently by probe hybridization during acute-phase TAC but infrequently during acute-phase erythema infectiosum; the clinical manifestations of EI occur later in the course of infection that those of TAC; titers as high as 10^{12} particles/mL have been found in serum specimens; with PCR, low levels of B19 DNA can be detected for up to a month and sometimes longer after onset of EI [20].	Urine B19 DNA has been found in urine of some patients during the acute viremic phase (*eg*, 2 of 6 urine specimens from patients with acute TAC were positive in one study [12]). Other sources of B19 B19 DNA has also been found in amniotic fluid and a variety of tissues; during the viremic phase of illness, all tissues will contain some virus because of the presence of blood that contains B19.

EI—erythema infectiosum; PCR—polymerase chain reaction; TAC—transient aplastic crisis.

Figure 3-33 Sources of infectious virus. Respiratory secretions are probably the most common source of infectious virus and the principal source of virus for transmission in the community. Blood is an important source of infectious virus for transmission to patients, such as those with hemophilia who receive multiunit blood products during childhood. B19-infected tissue may be a source of virus for nosocomial transmission.

Human parvovirus B19 DNA contamination of blood products

Product	Contaminated, %	Risk of transmission
Start pools	87	Not applicable
Albumin	0–25	Unknown
Clotting factor concentrates	20–100	High
IVIG	20	Unknown but probably low
IMIG	75	Unknown but probably low

IMIG—intramuscular immune globulin; IVIG—intravenous immune globulin.

Figure 3-34 Human parvovirus B19 DNA contamination of blood products. B19 is a common contaminant of multiunit blood products. Because B19 is often associated with mild or no illness, potential blood donors may be unaware of an acute infection. Although B19-viremic blood donors are relatively uncommon (one in 3000 to one in 20,000 by most detection methods), the starting pools for blood products often contain more than 5000 units and, therefore, have a high likelihood of being contaminated. Because the virus is small and able to survive most inactivation procedures, it is difficult to remove from blood products and frequently contaminates the final product, as already noted. B19 DNA was detected in products after various purification and inactivation procedures, including solvent-detergent treatment, affinity or ion exchange chromatography, heating to 80° C for 72 hours, and acid pH (pH 4.5) [22]. Although it is not known how well the presence of B19 DNA correlates with presence of infectious virus, B19 has been transmitted from factor VIII that has been inactivated and purified by a variety of procedures, including heating to 80° C for 72 hours and solvent detergent treatment. Although B19 may be transmitted by intravenous immune globulin or intramuscular immune globulin, the presence of neutralizing antibodies in these preparations probably minimizes the clinical importance of such transmission.

Risk of infection after different types of exposures to B19

Setting	Susceptible persons infected, %
Household	50
Staff working in an elementary or middle school with a B19 outbreak	8–50
Staff working in a child care center with a B19 outbreak	30
No known household or work exposure to B19 but living in a community with a B19 outbreak	6–30
Noscomial	0–42
No known community, household, or work exposure	0.25–1.00

Figure 3-35 Risk of infection after different types of exposures to B19. Investigations of B19 outbreaks have provided an opportunity to determine the rate at which B19 infection occurs after exposure to B19-infected persons in different settings [19,23,24]. In these studies, infected persons were defined as those who were positive for B19 IgM antibodies, and susceptible persons were defined as those who were positive for IgM or negative for IgG antibodies. In one outbreak investigation, the rate of infection among school teachers increased as the number of students in the classroom with erythema infectiosum increased. Nosocomial outbreaks of B19 have been reported, but some suspected nosocomial outbreaks have probably just represented community-acquired infection.

TREATMENT OF INFECTION

Treatment of disease associated with B19 infection

Disease	Treatment
Erythema infectiosum	None or symptomatic
TAC	Transfusion/oxygen therapy (if needed)
Arthritis and arthralgia	Nonsteroidal anti-inflammatory agents
Fetal hydrops	Intrauterine blood transfusions (?)
Chronic infection with anemia	IVIG/transfusions
Chronic infection without anemia	IVIG/transfusions (?)

IVIG—intravenous immune globulin; TAC—transient aplastic crisis.

FIGURE 3-36 Treatment of disease associated with B19 infection. Most B19 infections, including erythema infectiosum, are mild and require no treatment [24]. Infection in patients with a need for increased erythrocyte production to maintain hemodynamic stability can develop a serious, acute, but self-limited anemia (transient aplastic crisis) that should be monitored carefully and may require transfusion therapy. For example, in one study of 62 patients with sickle cell anemia and B19-associated TAC, 87% required blood transfusions, 63% required hospitalization, and one died [25]. B19-associated arthritis and arthralgia is a self-limited illness, but the patient may benefit from symptomatic therapy with nonsteroidal anti-inflammatory agents. Management of the fetus with hydrops is problematic. The severe anemia associated with intrauterine B19 infection has led some investigators to treat the hydropic fetus with intrauterine blood transfusions, and several studies suggest that this treatment may be effective [26]. Intrauterine blood transfusions, however, present a risk to the fetus and the benefit has not yet been clearly demonstrated. Fetal ultrasound is the best method to diagnose the hydropic fetus. Patients with deficient immune systems can develop a chronic severe anemia that may require transfusion therapy and should be treated with intravenous immune globulin. Patients have received intravenous immune globulin at doses of 400 mg/kg for 5 or 10 days or 1 g/kg for 3 days with good results. It is not yet clear whether persons with chronic B19 infection without anemia will benefit from intravenous immune globulin treatment [24].

PREVENTION OF INFECTION

Methods to prevent B19 infection

- Infection control practices
- Avoiding possible exposures, *eg*, staying home from work (?)
- Intravenous immune globulin (?)
- Vaccination (?)

FIGURE 3-37 Methods to prevent B19 infection. The only options presently available to prevent B19 infection are preventing transmission through infection control practices or avoiding exposure [29]. Concern about exposure to B19 has most frequently been raised for pregnant women working with children in schools or childcare centers during outbreaks of erythema infectiosum. It is likely that good hand-washing practices and not sharing food will decrease the risk of acquiring B19 infection in all settings; staying away from potential exposures in the workplace may or may not decrease the risk of acquiring infection because rates of non–work-related, community transmission can be high during some community outbreaks [17] (*see* Fig. 3-44 for estimates of risks of fetal death associated with different types of exposures to B19 infections). Because immune globulin intravenous (IGIV) is an effective treatment for anemia in patients with chronic B19 infection, it has been considered as a possible way to prevent infection during or after B19 exposure. There are, however, no data on IGIV for prevention of B19 infection or disease. A vaccine for B19 is being developed, but its ability to prevent infection or disease has not yet been tested.

$$\text{Rate of fetal death} = \text{Rate of susceptibility} \times \text{Rate of infection after exposure} \times \text{Rate of death after infection}$$

A

FIGURE 3-38 Risk of fetal death associated with different exposures to B19. Exposure or potential exposure to B19 can create considerable concern to the pregnant women. **A**, The risk associated with different exposures can be estimated using an equation. Outbreak investigations and other epidemiologic studies have provided a range of estimated values that can be used in this equation to calculate low and high estimates associated with different types of exposure to B19.

(continued on next page)

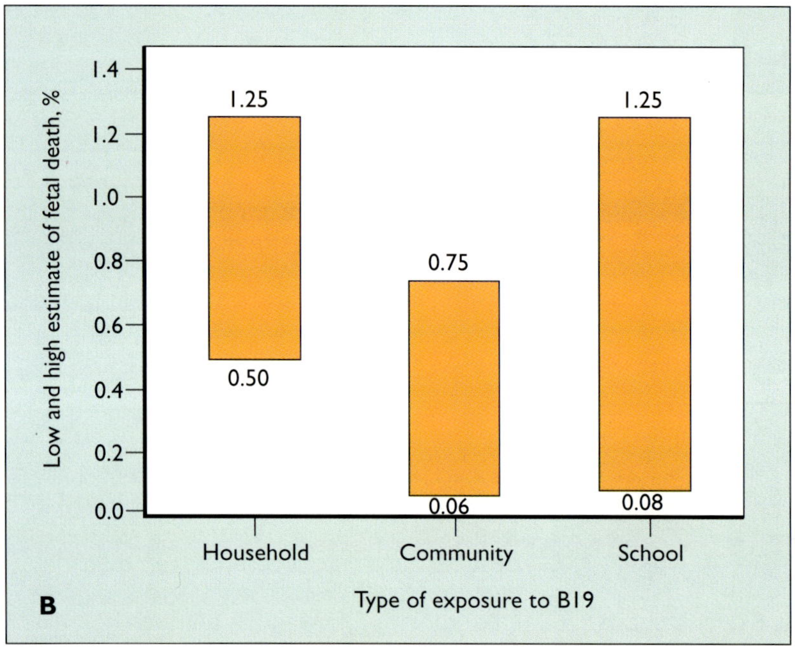

Figure 3-38 *(continued)* **B.** We used a susceptibility (IgG negative) rate of 50% for women in their child-bearing years and the rate of fetal death with maternal infection of 2% to 5%. The estimated rates of infection for different types of exposures is given in Figure 3-39. Note that the highest estimated risk of fetal death is just over 1%, indicating that few exposures during pregnancy will lead to fetal death. The rate of fetal death varies with gestational age of the fetus at time of infection; the greatest risk probably is associated with infection in the first half of the pregnancy.

References

1. Berns KI, Bergion M, Bloom M, *et al.*: Parvoviridae. In *Viral Taxonomy: Classification and Nomenclature of Viruses, Sixth Report of the International Committee on Taxonomy of Viruses.* Edited by Murphy FA, Fauquet CM, Bishop DHL, *et al.* New York: Springer-Verlag; 1995:169–178.
2. Erdman DD, Durigon EL, Wang Q-Y, Anderson LJ: Genetic diversity of human parvovirus B19: sequence analysis of the VP1/VP2 gene from multiple B19 isolates. *J Gen Virol* 1996, 77:2767–2774.
3. Agbandje-McKenna M, Rossman MG: The structure of human parvovirus B19. In *Mongraphs in Virology: Human Parvovirus B19.* Edited by Anderson LJ, Young NS. New York: Karger; 1997:3–15
4. Astell CR, Luo W, Brunstein J, St. Amand J: B19 parvovirus: biochemical and molecular features. In *Monographs in Virology: Human Parvovirus B19.* Edited by Anderson LJ, Young NS. New York: Karger; 1997:16–41.
5. Young NS: Parvoviruses. In *Fields Virology.* Edited by Fields BN, Knipe DM, Howley PM, III. Philadelphia: Lippincott-Raven Publishers; 1996:2199–2220.
6. Brown KE, Anderson SM, Young NS: Erthrocyte P antigen: cellular receptor for B19 parvovirus. *Science* 1993, 262:114–117.
7. Pallier C, Greco A, Junter JL, *et al.*: The 3′ untranslated region of the B19 parvovirus capsid protein mRNAs inhibits its own mRNA translation in nonpermissive cells. *J Virol* 1997, 71:9482–9489.
8. Morey AL, Fleming KA: Immunophenotyping of fetal haemopoietic cells permissive for human parvovirus B19 replication in vitro. *Br J Haematol* 1992, 82:302–309.
9. Anderson MJ, Higgins PG, Davis LR, *et al.*: Experimental parvoviral infection in humans. *J Infect Dis* 1985, 152:257–265.
10. Török TJ: Human parvovirus B19. In *Infectious Diseases of the Fetus and Newborn Infant.* Edited by Remington JS, Klein JO, IV. Philadelphia: WB Saunders; 1995:668–702.
11. Török TJ: Unusual clinical manifestations reported in patients with parvovirus B19 infection. In *Monographs in Virology: Human Parvovirus B19.* Edited by Anderson LJ, Young NS. New York: Karger; 1997:61–92.
12. Chorba T, Coccia P, Holman RC, *et al.*: The role of parvovirus B19 in aplastic crisis and erythema infectiosum (fifth disease). *J Infect Dis* 1986, 154:383–393.
13. Anderson LJ. Role of parvovirus B19 in human disease. *Pediatr Infect Dis J* 1987, 6:711–718.
14. Saarinen UA, Chorba TL, Tattersall P, *et al.*: Human parvovirus B19-induced epidemic red cell aplasia in patients with hereditary hemolytic anemia. *Blood* 1986, 67:1411–1417.
15. Smith JC, Megason GC, Iyer RV, *et al.*: Clinical characteristics of children with hereditary hemolytic anemias and aplastic crisis: a 7-year review. *South Med J* 1994, 87:702–708.
16. Owren PA: Congenital hemolytic jaundice: the pathogenesis of the "hemolytic crisis." *Blood* 1948, 3:231–248.
17. Dowell SF, Török TJ, Thorp JA, *et al.*: Parvovirus B19 infection in hospital workers: community or hospital acquisition? *J Infect Dis* 1995, 172:1076–1079.
18. Cohen BJ, Buckley MM: The prevalence of antibody to human parvovirus B19 in England and Wales. *J Med Microbiol* 1988, 25:151–153.
19. Gillespie SM, Cartter ML, Asch S, *et al.*: Occupational risk of human parvovirus B19 infection for school and day-care personnel during an outbreak of erythema infectiosum. *JAMA* 1990, 263:2061–2065.
20. Naides SJ: Erythema infectiosum (fifth disease) occurrence in Iowa. *Am J Public Health* 1988, 78:1230–1231.
21. Erdman DD, Usher J, Tsou C, *et al.*: Human parvovirus B19 specific IgG, IgA, and IgM antibodies and DNA in serum specimens from persons with erythema infectiosum. *J Med Virol* 1991, 35:110–115.
22. Saldanha J, Minor P: Detection of human parvovirus B19 DNA in plasma pools and blood products derived from these pools: implications for efficiency and consistency of removal of B19 DNA during manufacture. *Br J Haematol* 1996, 93:714–719.
23. Erdman DD, Anderson BC, Török TJ, *et al.*: Possible transmission of parvovirus B19 from intravenous immune globulin. *J Med Virol* 1997, 53:233–236.
24. Anderson LJ: Treatment and prevention human parvovirus B19 disease. In *Monographs in Virology: Human Parvovirus B19.* Edited by Anderson LJ, Young NS. New York: Karger; 1997:137–148.
25. Goldstein AR, Anderson MJ, Serjeant GR: Parvovirus associated aplastic crisis in homozygous sickle cell disease. *Arch Dis Child* 1987, 62:585–588.
26. Fairley CK, Smoleniec JS, Caul OE, Miller E: Observational study of effect of intrauterine transfusions on outcome of fetal hydrops after parvovirus B19. *Lancet* 1995, 346:1335–1337.

CHAPTER 4

Herpes Simplex Virus Infections

Sheryl L. Henderson
Dan Danielsson
André J. Nahmias

THE TERM "HERPES" has been used in medicine for at least 25 centuries [1]. The word originates from the Greek verb ερπειν ("to creep"), which was used to describe spreading cutaneous lesions of varying causes. The "herpetic eruptions which appear about the mouth at the crisis of simple fever" (now known as cold sores or fever blisters) were first described around 100 AD, and were mentioned in Shakespeare's play *Romeo and Juliet.* In the 18th century, a French physician first described herpes of the genital tract. By the latter part of the 19th century, cytopathologic differences among various skin lesions permitted discrimination between infection of the pox- and herpes-related infections. Early in the 20th century, epidemiologic and experimental studies supported the distinction between herpes-zoster, oral herpes, and genital herpes. Infection from vesicular fluid of oral or genital herpetic lesions was found to be transmissible from human to human, from human to rabbit cornea, and later from human to other animals, *eg*, mice. Filterable infectious agents (viruses) identified in this way were then called "herpes simplex" to differentiate them from viruses causing varicella-zoster. By 1950, it was known that intraoral infections were often asymptomatic and could recur in the same individual as did fever blisters on the lips. The advent of laboratory methods to distinguish the two different types of herpes simplex viruses (HSV) in the 1960s improved understanding of the pathogenesis and clinicoepidemiologic aspects of herpetic infections [2].

Also in the 1960s, HSV1 was found to be primarily associated with nongenital infections and HSV2 with genital infections, which were also found to be commonly asymptomatic. At the same time, sexual transmission of genital herpes was confirmed, and genital herpes was found to be a common infection particularly among young adults. Maternal genital herpes was also determined to be the major source of neonatal herpes, which had been first identified clinically and virologically 30 years earlier by an Italian ophthalmologist. Cesarean section was proposed as a possible preventive method of intrapartum maternal–neonatal transmission. Further molecular and immunologic studies provided the means for characterizing different viral strains within each of the two HSV types, and to differentiate antibodies specific to each of the two HSV types. In the 1970s, new antiviral drugs became available for the treatment of the less common, clinically severe forms of the infection, and later for the milder forms. During the past 15 years, more knowledge has been obtained regarding clinicoepidemiologic, diagnostic, and therapeutic features of herpetic infections. Approximately 150 million Americans are estimated to be infected with HSV1, and 45 million with HSV2. Although the large majority of these infections are subclinical, they are still potentially transmissible to sexual partners or from mothers to neonates at delivery.

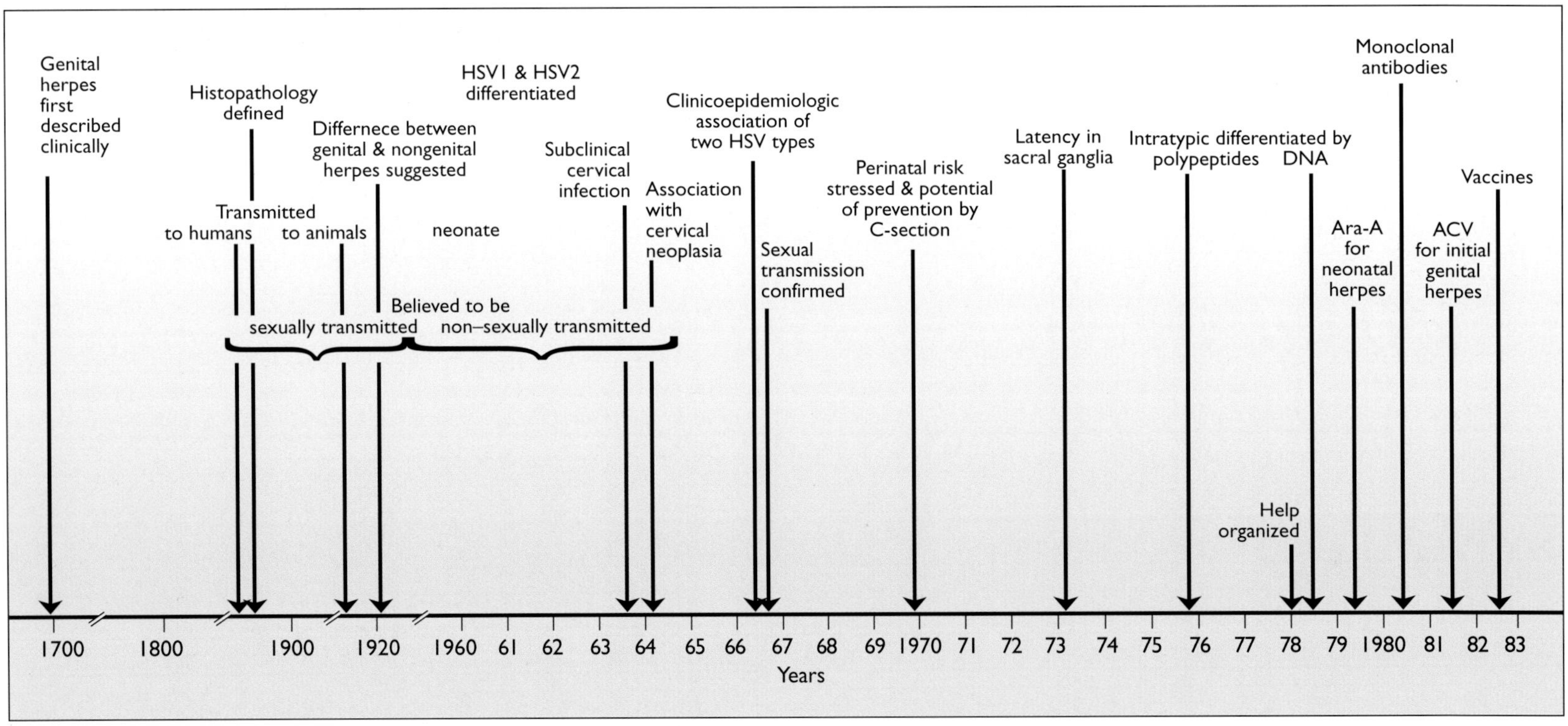

FIGURE 4-1 Historical landmarks of herpes simplex virus (HSV) infections. This figure shows important landmarks of discoveries about HSVs, with a focus on genital herpes. (*Adapted from* Becker and Nahmias [3].)

The Herpesviruses

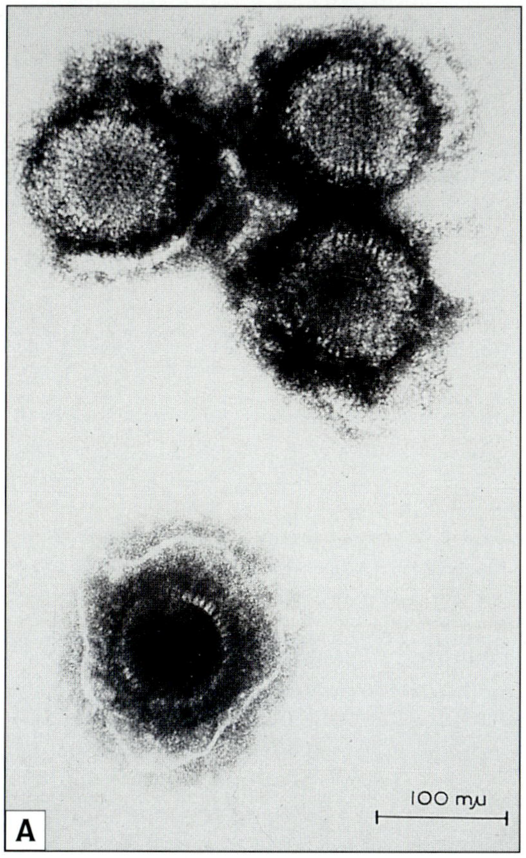

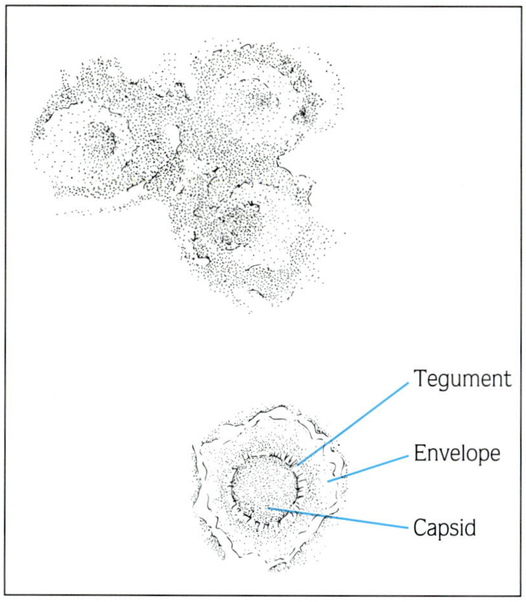

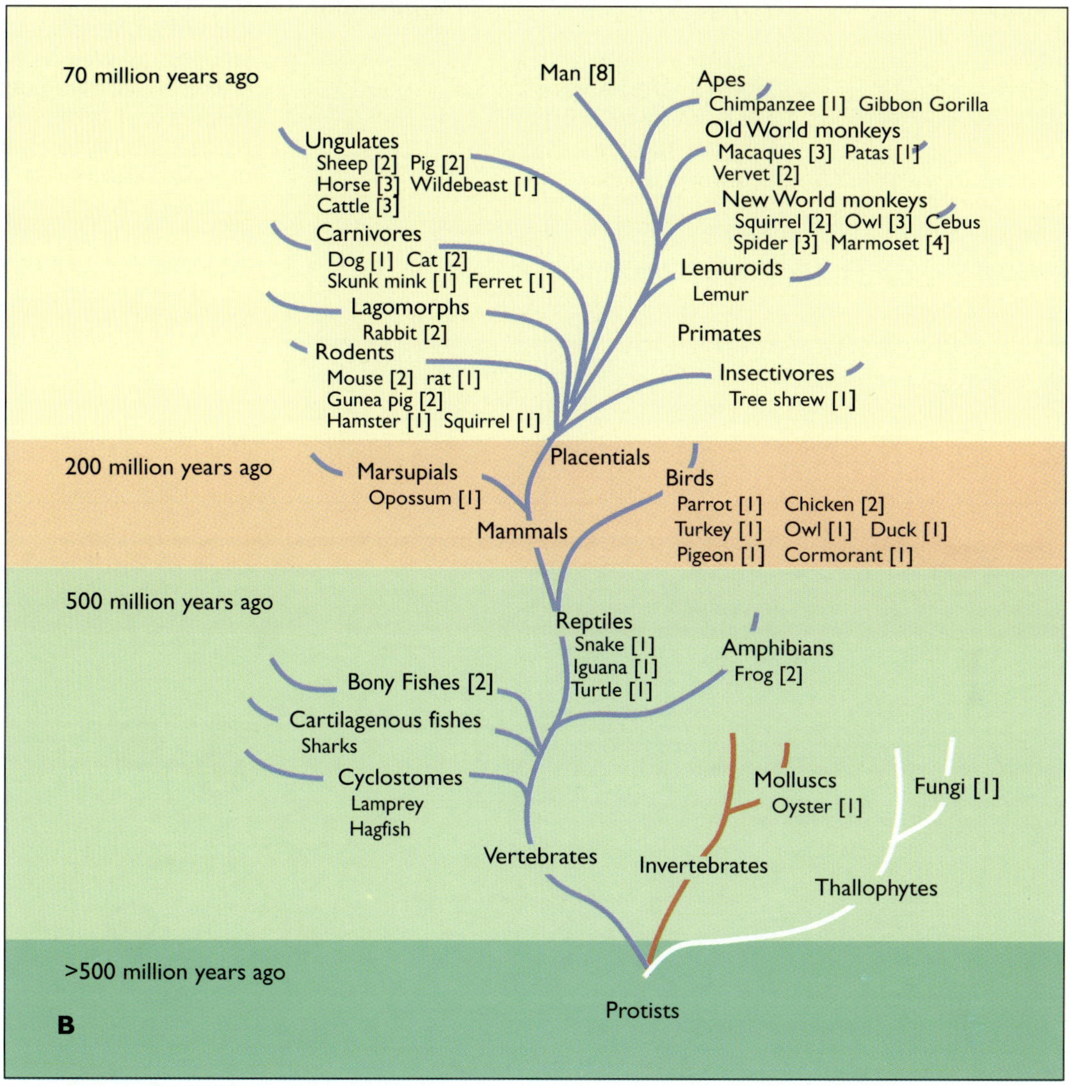

Figure 4-2 The Herpesviridae family. More than 100 double-stranded DNA viruses comprise the Herpesviridae family. The same morphology is shared among all these viruses, as demonstrated by the electron micrograph. **A,** Each virion consists of a capsid comprising 162 capsomeres arranged in an icosahedral tubular form; the capsid is surrounded in turn by the tegument [4]. The outer layer is the envelope, on which are located more than 15 glycoproteins that permit entry into the host cells and also provide mechanisms for the virus to evade host defenses. **B,** Evolution of herpesviruses. Herpesviruses have been identified in many different species and have evolved over millions of years along with the species charted. Consequently, the viruses generally cause either no or mild-to-moderate disease in their natural host; however, infection can be severe and fatal when the virus infrequently infects the natural host's brain or is transmitted to the fetus or newborn. Uncommonly, a herpesvirus of one species can cause disease that is particularly severe if it is able to infect other species. For instance, the macaque herpes B virus can cause severe encephalitis in humans.

Common names and subfamilies of human herpesviruses

Human herpesvirus number	Common name	Herpes subfamily
HHV1	Herpes simplex virus 1	α
HHV2	Herpes simplex virus 2	α
HHV3	Varicella-zoster virus	α
HHV4	Epstein–Barr virus	γ
HHV5	Cytomegalovirus	β
HHV6		β
HHV7		β
HHV8	Kaposi's sarcoma–associated herpesvirus	γ

FIGURE 4-3 Classification of the herpesviruses. The Herpesviridae family comprises three subfamilies (α, β, and γ) according to the type of cell in which latency is established and the ability of the virus to replicate in culture. Eight human herpesviruses (HHVs). The first two (HHV1 and HHV2) are more commonly known as herpes simplex viruses (HSV1 and HSV2). These two viruses, as well as HHV3 (varicella-zoster virus), belong to the α-Herpesviridae subfamily, which establishes latency in neural tissues and grows readily in culture. As will be noted later, these three human herpesviruses also share several clinicopathologic manifestations (*eg*, the ability to infect the skin and oral mucosa and, less frequently, to involve the fetus or newborn, the brain, and to cause severe disease in compromised hosts). The recent approval for use of varicella vaccines lends promise to the possible development of effective HSV vaccines.

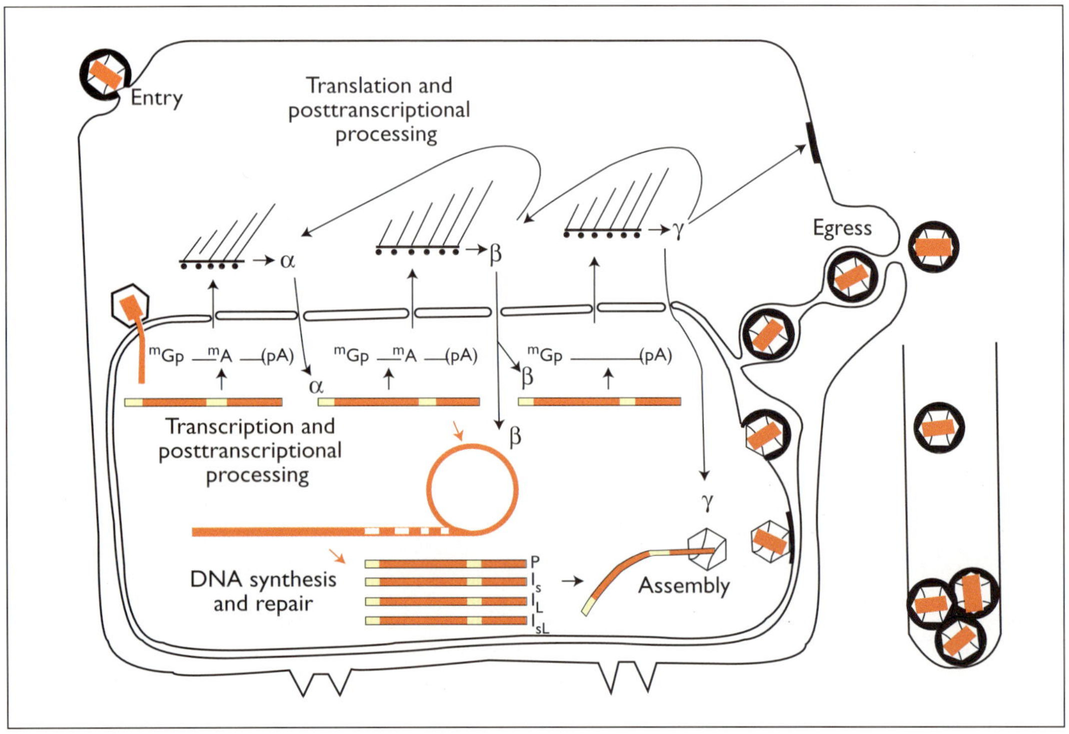

FIGURE 4-4 Replication of herpes simplex virus (HSV)1 and HSV2. Enveloped viruses of either type with their infectious DNA are able to replicate in large numbers of cells of different organs, but will primarily enter the body through skin or mucosal surfaces (mouth, genitals, anus, and conjunctiva or cornea). After absorption of the virus to the cell via viral glycoproteins, DNA is transported to the nucleus, transcribed, and translated first to α-proteins, which appear to be associated with latency [4]. The next proteins produced in the cascade (β-proteins) include thymidine kinase and DNA polymerase, which are targets for antiviral agents such as acyclovir and vidarabine (*see* Figs. 4-33 to 4-35). Thereafter, γ-proteins, the viral structural proteins, are produced. Concomitantly, new DNA is processed and then assembled with the structural proteins. These newly formed virions then exit from the cell. One cell can produce thousands of viral particles, and thus there can be millions of viral particles within a single herpetic vesicle. (Courtesy of B. Roizman, ScD).

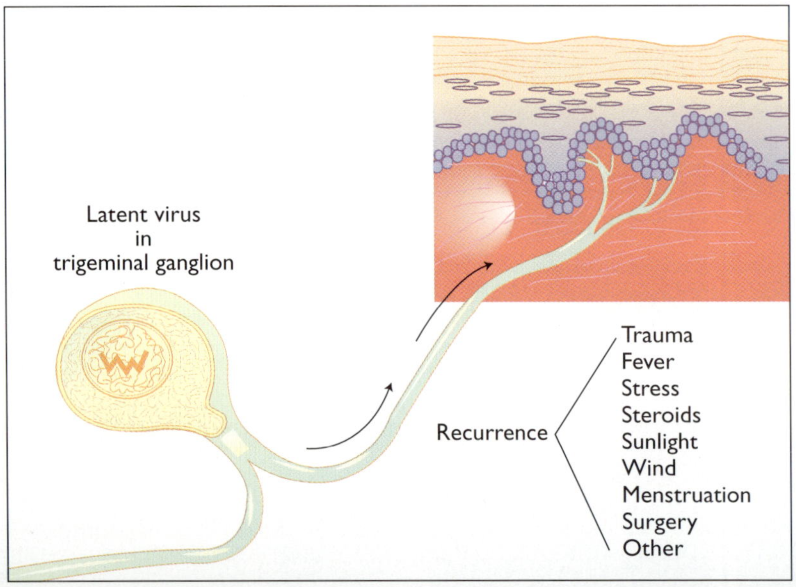

FIGURE 4-5 Latency and recurrence. The α-herpesviruses establish latency in sensory or autonomic nervous system ganglia. After a primary replicating viral infection of a mucocutaneous surface, the virus establishes a latent infection in the ganglia. A variety of stimuli can induce recurrences. Viruses are then reactivated to replicate in the ganglion and are transported to mucosal or cutaneous sites where shedding of virus occurs. Subclinical recurrences most often are only recognized by identifying virus with various laboratory methods (*see* Figs. 4-31 and 4-32). Depending on the cellular immune status of the host, recurrences may cause no signs or symptoms, or mild to severe clinical findings. Thus, transmission from a sexual partner or from a mother to her baby is most often associated with subclinical infections. Viruses causing nongenital infections most frequently establish latency in the trigeminal ganglia, and to a lesser extent in the thoracic ganglia and autonomic nervous system. Recurrences of genital infections represent most often reactivations of latent virus within the sacral ganglia.

Clinical Manifestations

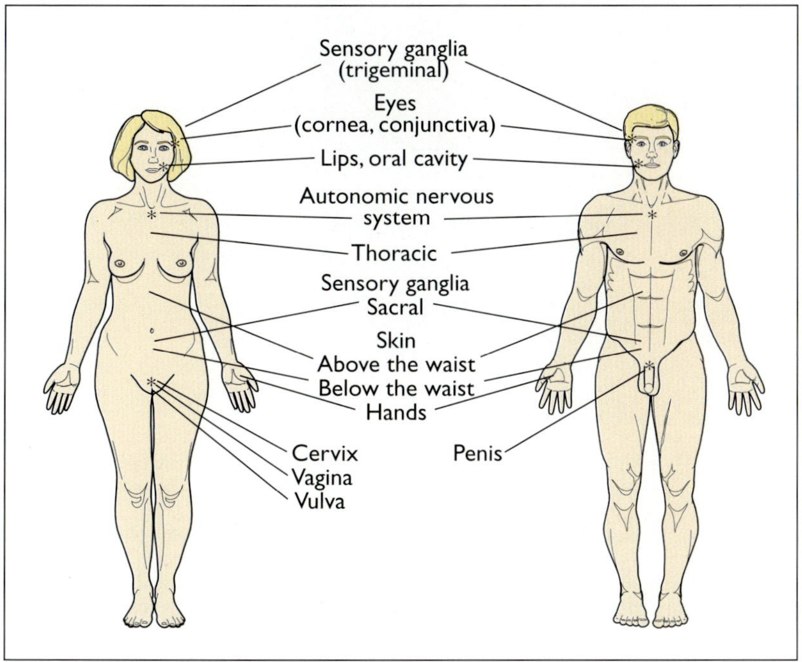

Figure 4-6 Commonly involved sites of herpes simplex virus (HSV) infection in normal children and adolescents. In children, the most commonly affected site of infection, caused almost always by HSV1, is the oral cavity followed by the skin and eyes. Genital infections in children are also caused by HSV1 (as a result of autoinoculation from oral infections) or by HSV2 (as a result of sexual abuse). HSV2 is also likely to be the most common cause of genital and anal infections in sexually active teenagers. Primary genital HSV1 infection is likely to occur predominantly in those teenagers who practice oral–genital sexual relations, often as a way to avoid other sexually transmitted diseases, including HIV.

Mild to moderately severe infections

Oral–mucosal and skin herpesvirus infections

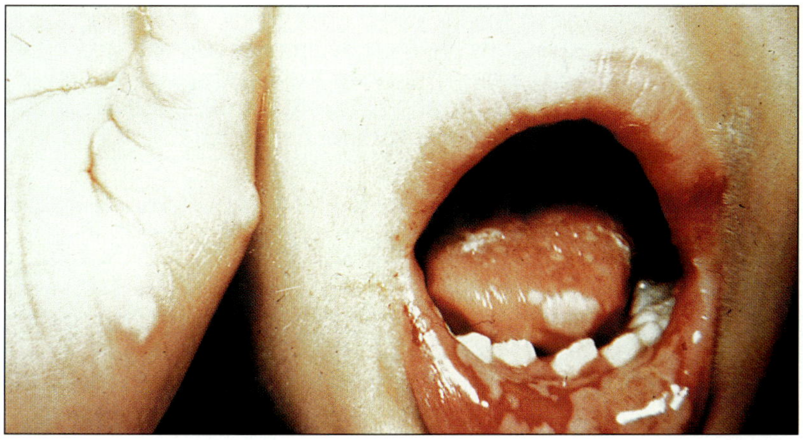

Figure 4-7 Herpesvirus oral infections. Lesions may occur in different parts of the mouth, including the inner lips, tongue, and gingiva and may also be located on the palate or posterior pharynx. Lesions in the palate and posterior pharynx. Herpetic lesions appear initially as vesicles that progress rapidly to ulcers; and may become friable and bleed. This condition can be associated with fever, irritability, regional lymphadenopathy, and significant oral pain. The child can have difficulty with eating or drinking, which may be helped by a topical anesthetic. In severe cases, intravenous fluids are required to maintain hydration. This case demonstrates the ability of a thumbsucker with gingivostomatitis to autoinoculate other areas of the body. Autoinoculation can also occur from an infected oral cavity without clinically apparent lesions, almost always as a result of a primary infection in the child.

The differential diagnosis includes aphthous ulcers, with lesions that occur and recur in various parts of the mouth. Hand, foot, and mouth (HFM) disease, usually associated with Coxsackie A16 virus, may also cause vesicles or ulcers in the anterior part of the mouth. The skin lesions of HFM as well as those of varicella-zoster virus, which can also cause oral ulcers, are most helpful in the differential diagnosis. Herpangina, which is caused by several enterovirus types, primarily affects the posterior pharynx and sometimes may be confused with HSV infection.

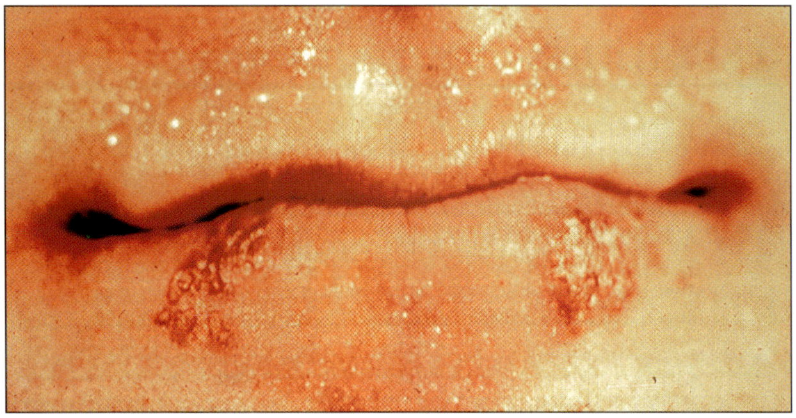

FIGURE 4-8 Recurrent orolabial herpes. Clinically manifest recurrent oral herpes simplex virus (HSV) infections are infrequently found inside the mouth of immunocompetent hosts who, however, may still shed virus in the saliva at infrequent intervals. Recurrent HSV infections may involve parts of the face other than the lips, as noted in this girl. It is particularly difficult to suspect HSV as the cause of such lesions. After a primary symptomatic or asymptomatic HSV1 oral infection, latency is usually established in the trigeminal sensory ganglia. Reactivation, which may be induced by various stimuli (*see* Fig. 4-5), most often involves the lips. Symptoms are usually mild, consisting of pain, often with a prodrome of burning or itching; the blisters may appear bilaterally as in this case. Approximately one third of school-age children (5–17 y of age) have experienced recurrent herpes labialis, which is approximately the same proportion as that found in adults.

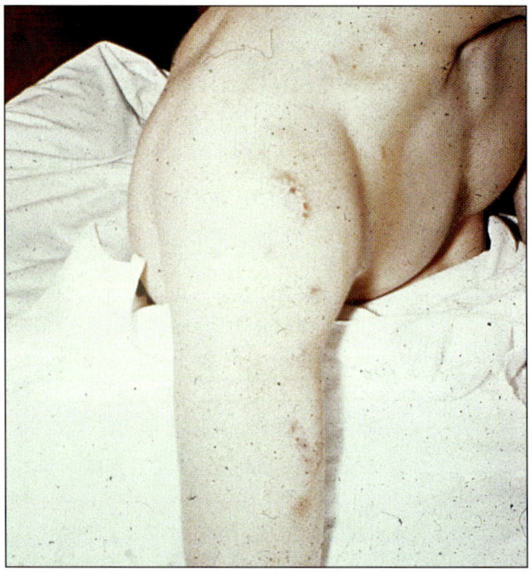

FIGURE 4-9 Herpes gladiatorum. Herpes simplex virus (HSV) can infect the cutaneous layers when there are breaks in the skin, as often occurs in wrestlers, or less frequently in others involved in contact sports. This condition has been observed in high school– and college-age wrestlers, whose broken or abraded skin comes in contact with infected saliva or skin lesions of other wrestlers. Lesions most often involve the face and arms. Wrestlers with a history of cold sores do not generally acquire such skin lesions, providing further evidence that a prior HSV1 infection usually protects one from reinfection with the same type [5].

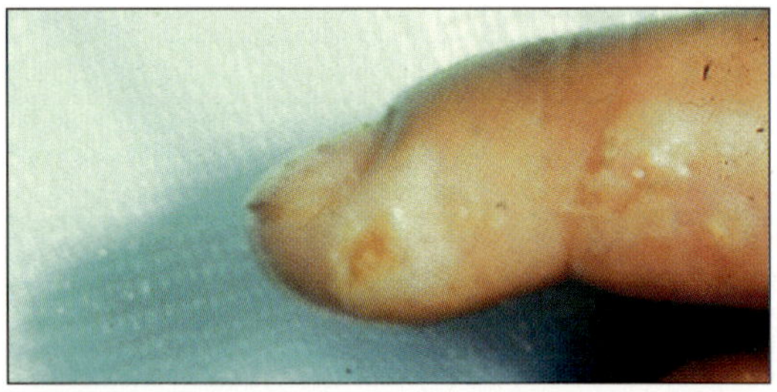

FIGURE 4-10 Herpetic whitlow. This condition is a result of a primary herpes simplex virus 1 infection caused by direct inoculation of an abrasion on the finger. A cluster of vesicles with a pustular appearance, ulceration, and erythema can be noted. Herpetic whitlows may be accompanied by fever, regional adenopathy, and occasionally by lymphangitis. They are often acquired by healthcare workers because of the increased close contact their fingers may have with infected oral secretions. These lesions are most often confused with bacterial paronychia, and treated unnecessarily with antibiotics. They may also be surgically incised, which can actually worsen the herpetic lesions. The finger lesions often recur, and in special cases (*eg*, a pianist) may require suppressive antiviral therapy (*see* Fig. 4-35).

Genital herpesvirus infections

Genital herpes in female patients

Type of infection	Duration of lesions (mean), *d*	Patients with pain, %	Duration of pain, *d*	Patients with new lesions, %	Duration of virus shedding, *d*	Patients with virus in vagina or cervix, %	Patients with type 2 infection, %
Recurrent	6.3	85	3.3	60	2.7	20	90
Initial	10.3	75	9.7	62	8.1	40	100
Primary	15.5	100	12.4	78	12.2	100	67

FIGURE 4-11 Findings associated with primary, initial, and recurrent genital herpes in female subjects. A primary genital infection is associated with longer duration of the genital lesions and viral shedding, with a greater number of new lesions, and with more pain and other clinical manifestations, including meningitis, dysuria, and adenopathy [6]. Initial infections are most commonly observed in adolescents who have experienced infection with herpes simplex virus (HSV)1 in childhood and are now having a first infection with HSV2. Because of the short duration of lesions and viral shedding during recurrences, antiviral therapy is therefore of limited value for the treatment of recurrences (*see* Fig. 4-35).

It is particularly important to distinguish among the types of external genital lesions in a pregnant woman because of differences in the concomitant viral involvement of the vagina and cervix, which correlates better with the risk of transmission to the newborn. Thus, a vaginally delivered neonate is much more likely to be infected from a maternal primary infection, when the virus is almost always present in the vagina and cervix, than when there is a recurrent vulvar ulcer.

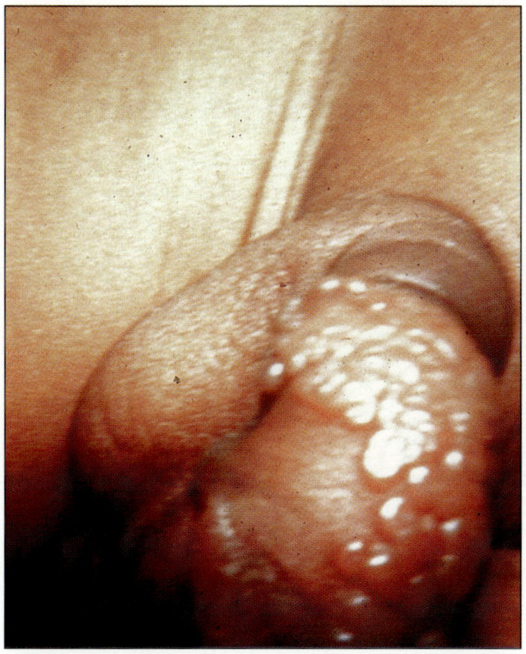

Figure 4-12 Primary herpes virus simplex (HSV)1 genital infection in a 3-year-old boy. Multiple coalescing vesicles are evident along the shaft of the penis, from which HSV1 was isolated [7]. Although sexual abuse is to be considered in a child with genital herpetic lesions, it is important to recognize the role of autoinoculation of the genitals by children with asymptomatic or symptomatic primary oral infections, who may put their hands in their mouth and transfer infected saliva to the genitals. (Such autoinoculation may also occur on the hand [*see* Fig. 4-7]). Thus, laboratory study of such children should include culture and virus typing of isolates from oral secretions and the genital lesions, as well as serologic assays.

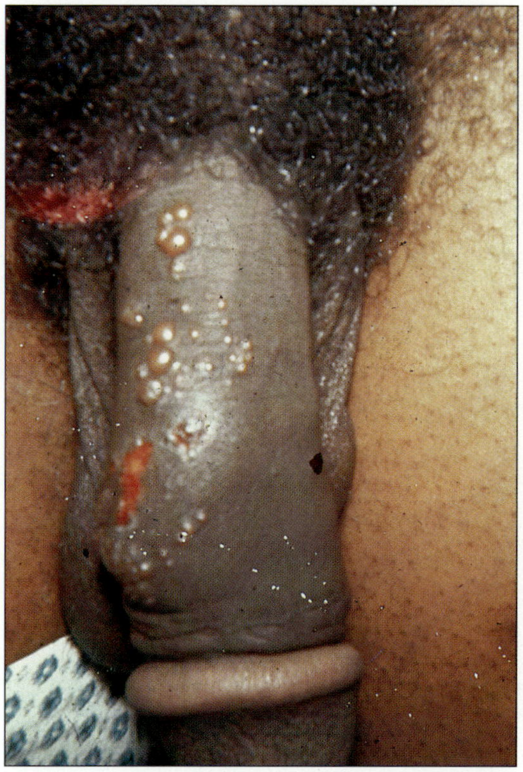

Figure 4-13 Primary genital herpes simplex virus 2 in an adolescent male patient. Multiple fluid-filled vesicles, some of which have coalesced and ulcerated, are present along the shaft of the penis. Recurrences may occur in the skin or urethra, with no visible lesions on the shaft. In patients with concomitant HIV infections, the retrovirus is often identified in the ulcerative areas, serving as a possible means of HIV transmission (*see* Fig. 4-21). Anorectal herpetic lesions are common in homosexual men.

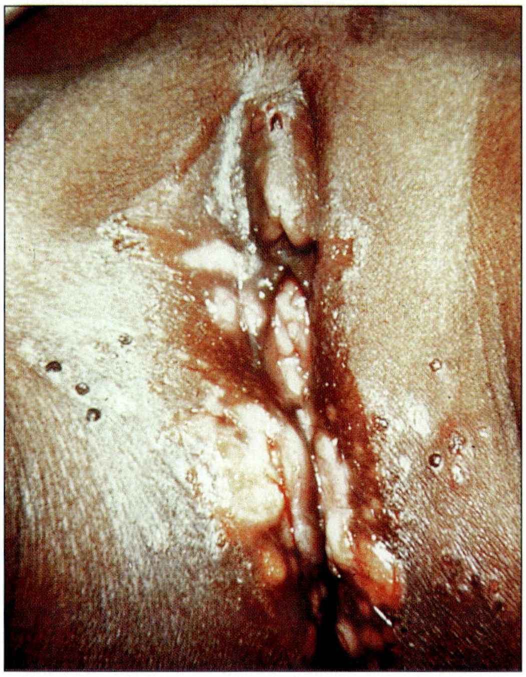

Figure 4-14 Primary genital herpes simplex virus 2 in a sexually active 12-year-old girl. In addition to clusters of crusted vesicular lesions along the labia, there are large areas of ulceration, some with yellow exudate, which may be confused with other entities. Fever, tender inguinal adenopathy, and dysuria were present. Antiviral therapy and psychosexual counseling are important in such cases.

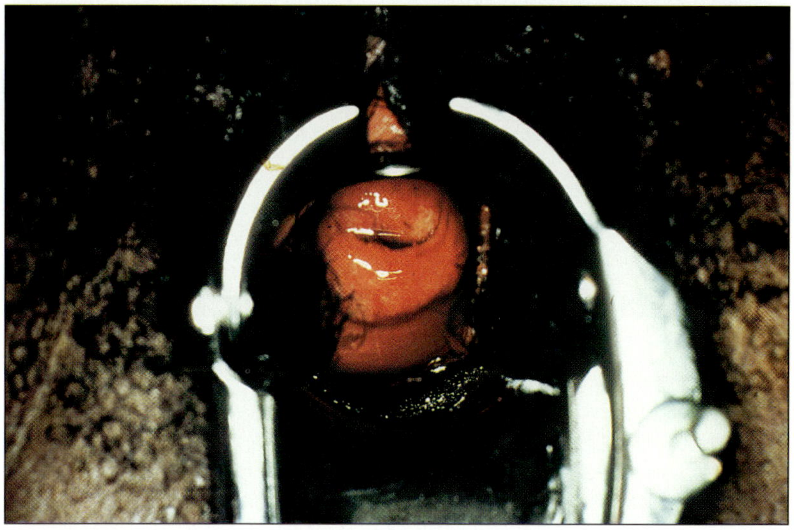

Figure 4-15 Primary herpes simplex virus 2 infection of the cervix. Infection of the cervix may occur with or without lesions, either alone or in association with clinically apparent external involvement. Cervical shedding of virus in a pregnant woman with a primary infection at the time of vaginal delivery is the setting of greatest risk of infection of the neonate (*see* Fig. 4-23). In the case of a baby suspected to have neonatal herpes, the mother's cervix should be examined in addition to serologic testing, because viral involvement may still be found as late as several weeks after delivery. A Papanicolaou smear showing the characteristic inclusions of herpes simplex virus provides a rapid method of diagnosis; confirmatory cultures of cervical secretions should also be obtained (*see* Figs. 4-31 and 4-32).

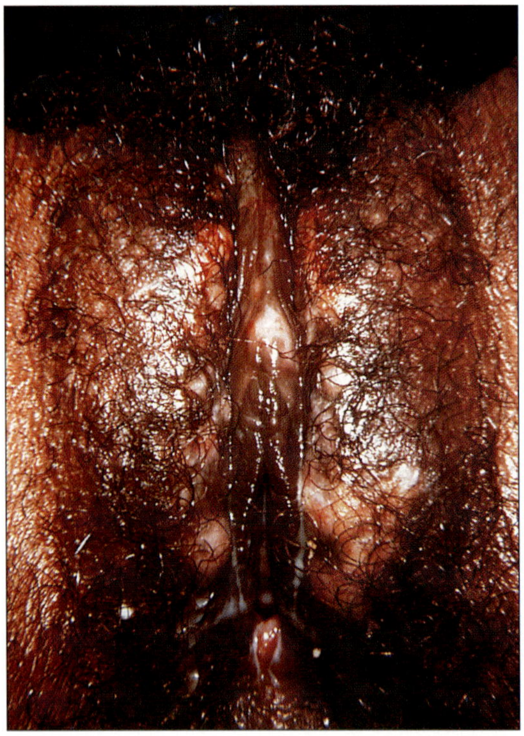

Figure 4-16 Clinical manifestations of recurrent genital herpes. When herpes simplex virus (HSV) is reactivated from the sacral ganglia, recurrent infection, which is usually asymptomatic, occurs at skin or mucosal surfaces with viral shedding. When clinically manifest, there are usually fewer and more localized signs and symptoms associated with recurrent than with primary or initial infections [6].

Recurrent genital herpes in female patients. Herpetic lesions can be found on any of the mucosal and skin areas around the genitals. These lesions are more easily diagnosed if they are multiple and a history of recurrence is obtained. The presence of one or two lesions, if any at all, requires close examination to detect them. Reactivated herpes of the cervix may be completely asymptomatic, cause few nonspecific findings, and go unnoticed by the examining physician. The viral shedding that would occur in the setting of unrecognized or nonspecific cervical lesions creates an increased risk for transmission to the newborn or to a sexual contact.

Herpesvirus ocular infection

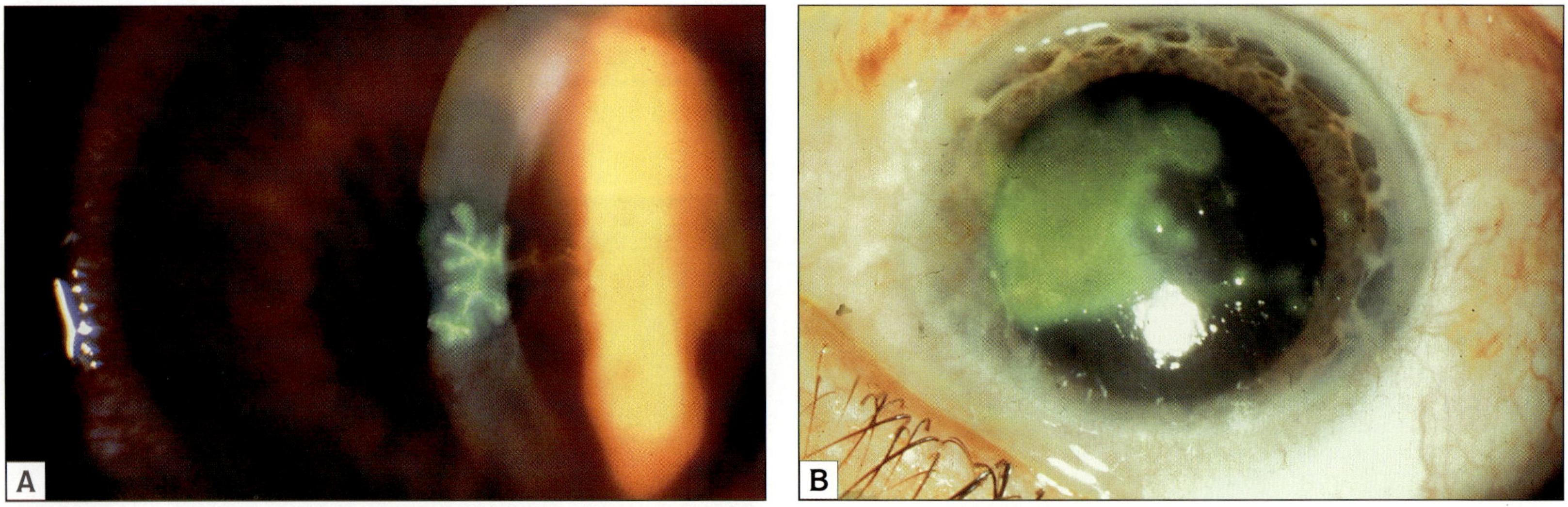

Figure 4-17 Herpes infection of the eye. Herpes simplex virus (usually type 1 after the newborn age) may cause conjunctivitis or keratitis, which can recur. Conjunctivitis is often misdiagnosed, but should be considered when recurring in the same eye. **A,** Herpes keratitis can be identified by fluorescent staining of the eye, often demonstrating the characteristic dendritic appearance. Keratitis can recur, and may eventually lead to visual impairment. **B,** A more serious complication is involvement of the corneal stroma, which requires steroid treatments in addition to antiviral therapy. It is important not to use steroids for conjunctivitis or keratitis without concomitant antiviral therapy for a disease that may be of herpetic origin, because severe ocular sequelae could ensue.

Severe herpesvirus infections and complications

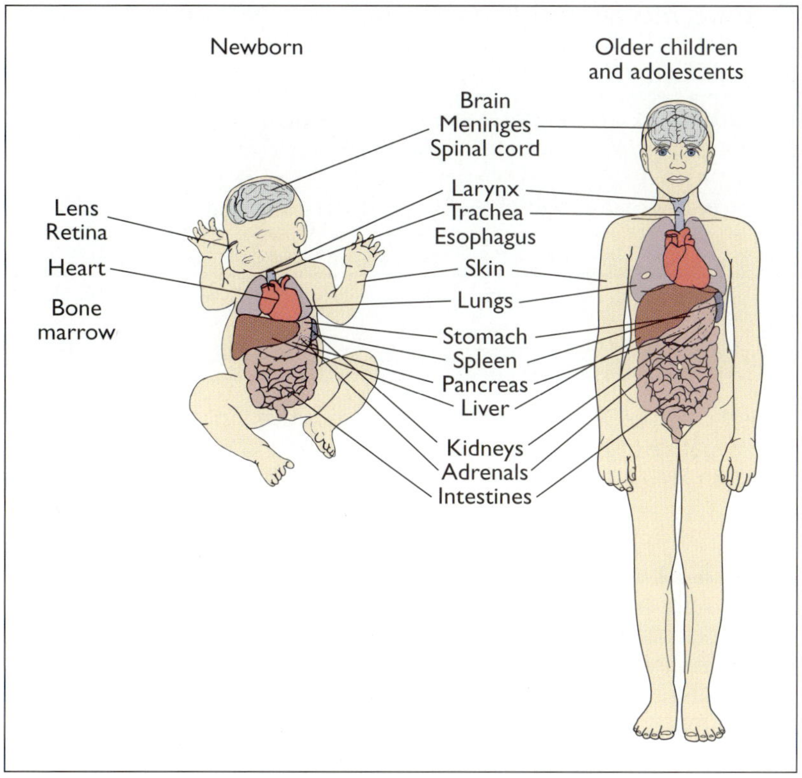

Figure 4-18 Sites of herpes simplex virus (HSV) infection in compromised hosts (children and adolescents). Although herpetic infections may infrequently cause severe complications in normal hosts, neonates and compromised hosts are more likely to experience the severe clinical manifestations. In disseminated disease, a viremia occurs and the liver and many of the visceral organs may become involved. Herpes simplex may also affect the brain—HSV2 most commonly in neonates, and HSV1 in older infants, children, and adolescents.

Herpesvirus infections in compromised pediatric hosts (excluding newborns)

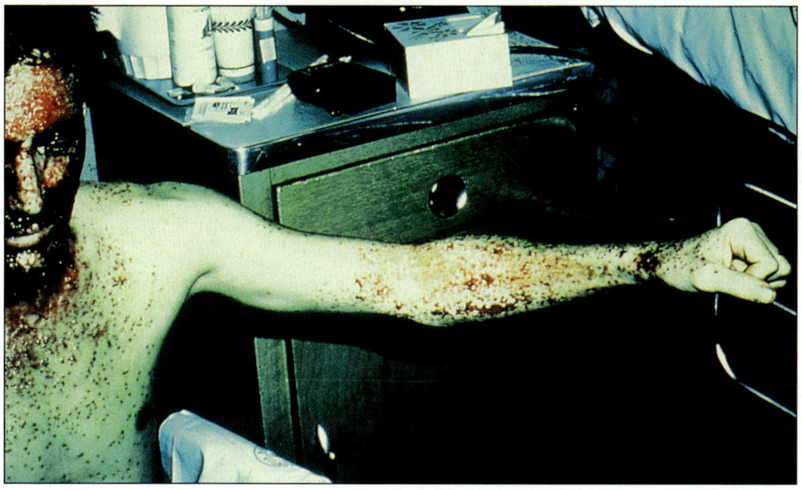

Figure 4-19 Eczema herpeticum. This form of Kaposi's varicelliform eruption occurs in patients with disruption of skin integrity, such as in those with eczema or burns. Individuals with primary herpetic infections are at risk for severe manifestations of herpes simplex virus (HSV) infections, with extensive lesions on various parts of the body. Bacterial superinfection or disseminated disease can be prevented with antibacterial and antiviral therapy. HSV recurrences tend to cause less severe clinical manifestations of eczema herpeticum. Kaposi's varicelliform eruption was also caused in earlier years by smallpox vaccination (eczema vaccinatum). However, we observed a case of eczema coxsackium in an eczematous child with hand and mouth disease attributed to Coxsackie A16 [8].

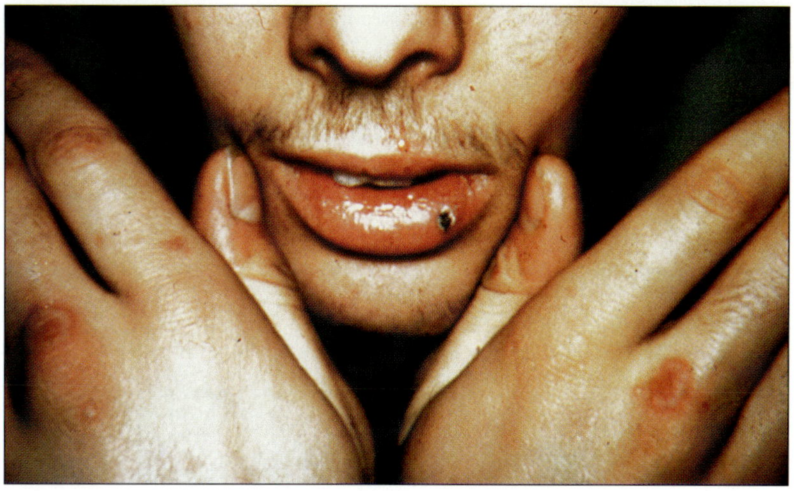

Figure 4-20 Erythema multiforme (EM). The target lesions of EM are seen on the hands of this teenager with recurrent herpes labialis. It is now believed that symptomatic or asymptomatic herpes simplex virus (HSV)1 or HSV2 infections represent a major cause of EM. Recurrent EM associated with HSV may be suppressed with antiviral agents.

Genital herpes as a facilitator of HIV1 sexual transmission

Favoring increased risk of viral acquisition by an HIV-negative individual with genital herpes from an HIV-positive sexual partner*	Favoring increased risk of transmitting to HIV-negative sexual partner by an HIV-positive individual with genital herpes†
HSV2 is a very common (perhaps the most common) cause of genital ulcers and of recurrent ulcers throughout the world	HSV amplifies HIV1 replication in cell culture
Seven case-control studies and two of three prospective studies concur that HSV2 likely has a role in facilitating the acquisition of HSV1	HIV1 can be identified in 90% of genital herpetic ulcers of HIV-positive subjects
	Recurrences of genital herpes increase HIV viral load in plasma

* Mostly based on clinical and serologic epidemiologic studies.

† Mostly based on virologic studies

Figure 4-21 Genital herpes simplex virus and its relationship to transmission of HIV. Several clinical, seroepidemiologic, and virologic studies indicate that genital herpes may facilitate sexual transmission of HIV-1 from 1) an HIV-positive individual to an HIV-negative individual with genital herpes, or 2) an individual who has both HIV-1 and genital herpes to his or her sexual contacts [9].

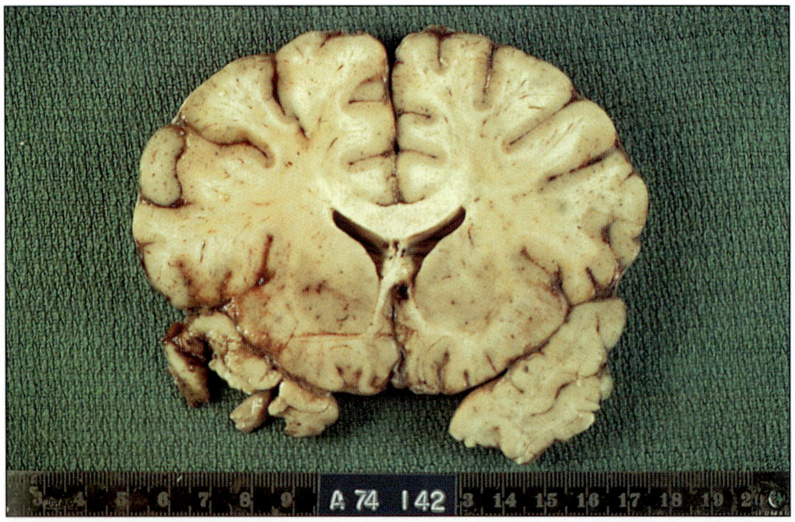

Figure 4-22 Herpes involvement of the central nervous system (CNS). Approximately 20% of cases of encephalitis with known cause, outside the newborn age, are caused by a herpes simplex virus (usually type 1) primary or reactivated infection. The temporoparietal sites of the brain are most often affected, as noted in this figure. A patient may present with fever, mental status or behavioral changes, headache, generalized or focal seizures, and various signs of neurologic impairment. In children with CNS involvement, association with gingivostomatitis is more suggestive of a herpetic cause than is the presence of fever blisters, because a nonspecific reactivation of herpes labialis may accompany any febrile illness. Examination of the CSF often shows a pleocytosis, normal to decreased glucose concentration, and elevated protein levels that continue to rise, in contrast to many other entities. Cultures of the CSF are of poor sensitivity (<5%). Diagnosis by polymerase chain reaction to detect the HSV DNA is now available to most clinicians, although sensitivity and specificity are not 100% [10]. Early treatment with antiviral agents is indicated to prevent severe sequelae or death, because a bad prognosis can occur even in treated patients, particularly those who present with advanced neurologic manifestations (*eg*, coma). It should be noted that HSV2 is the usual cause of benign meningitis, which may recur with genital herpetic recrudescences. Also, HSV encephalitis in immunocompromised hosts (*eg*, those with Hodgkin's disease or AIDS) has a more chronic course, probably because of the decreased immunopathologic effects on the brain by inflammatory cells and their products.

Congenital and neonatal herpesvirus infections

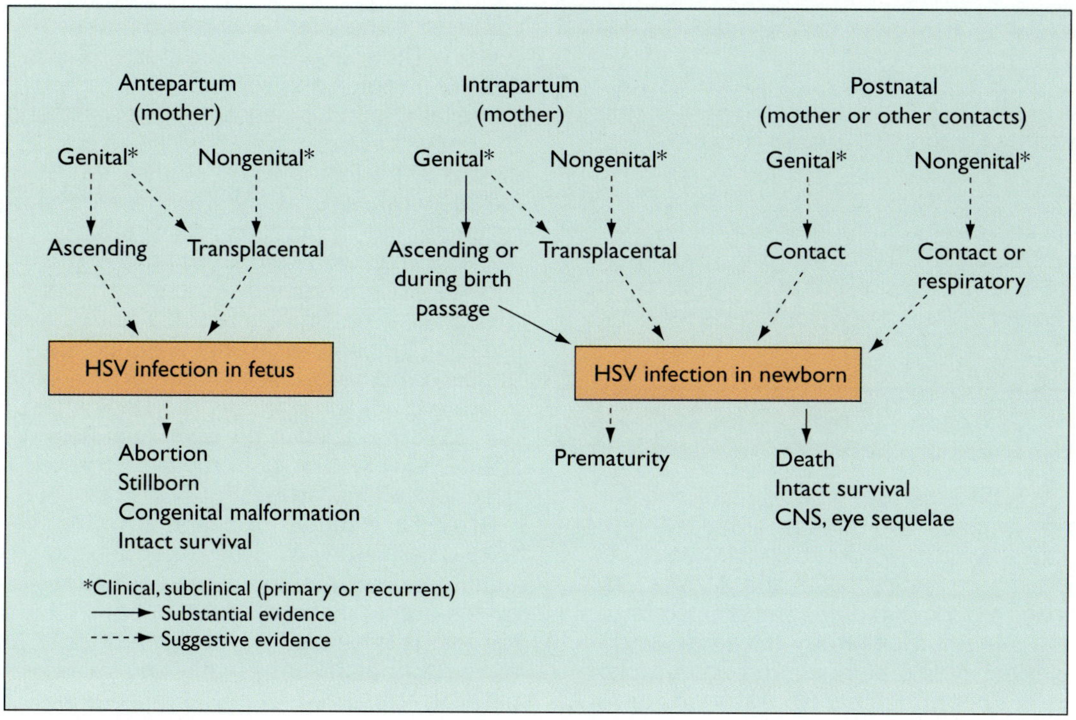

FIGURE 4-23 Possible sources and modes of transmission of neonatal herpes simplex virus (HSV) infection. There are three time periods during which a fetus or newborn may become infected by a mother shedding virus in her cervix or elsewhere: antepartum, intrapartum, and postpartum.

Primary maternal infections that occur antepartum may cause abortion or premature delivery. Transplacentally transmitted infection is very uncommon, with only a few live births reported with congenital anomalies of the central nervous system or the eyes. An ascending maternal genital infection late in gestation is more common, resulting from recognized or unrecognized breaks in the amniotic membranes or associated chorioamnionitis (5% to 10% of all neonatal HSV cases are noted in the first day of life and are from this source). Most frequently, the herpetic infection is acquired around the time of delivery from a pregnant woman with virus in her cervical secretions, with the baby becoming infected by an ascending infection, or on passage through an infected birth canal. Sometimes the virus is introduced through a break in the skin at the site of a fetal scalp electrode. Infection may also occur postnatally from a mother with lesions on her breasts or hands, or viral shedding from other sites. Neonates, primarily premature infants in intensive care units, can also acquire a nosocomial infection, necessitating isolation of all suspect cases of neonatal herpes. To our knowledge, there is only one case of neonatal infection caused by a healthcare worker with fever blisters who was sucking amniotic fluid by mouth with a De Lee device (no longer used due to the HIV threat). The outcome of infection of neonates with HSV, unlike other TORCH (toxoplasmosis, other, rubella, cytomegalovirus, and herpes simplex) agents, is almost always clinically manifest.

In a pregnant woman with an active HSV infection at the time of delivery, it is important to determine the risk of transmission to the neonate. Infants born vaginally to mothers with primary genital infection have approximately a 50% risk of infection. These neonates are more likely to be exposed to a large viral inoculum, and do not have the maternal transplacental antibodies, which are more likely to protect from acquisition of the infection and from disseminated neonatal disease. If the lesion represents a recurrence, the likelihood of neonatal infection drops to 5% or less, and disseminated disease of the neonate is much less likely. The risk is higher when membranes have been ruptured for prolonged periods, and if the baby is born prematurely.

It is now a standard of obstetrical care to perform a cesarean section, if possible, on a mother with an active HSV lesion at the time of delivery, to reduce the risk of exposing the infant to concomitantly infected cervical secretions. Fetal scalp monitoring introduces a possible portal of entry for the virus, and might be avoided in a woman with a history of recurrent disease. Because the major maternal site of neonatal infection is the cervix, we recommend that the vagina and cervix, as well as any suspect lesions, be cultured at the time of delivery. HSV genital infection occurs at a rate of approximately 1% at any time during gestation but is approximately 50 times less often identified at the time of delivery. It should be recognized that approximately two thirds of neonates with herpes simplex disease are born to a mother without clinical evidence of infection and who has no past history of genital herpes in herself or in a sexual partner [11]. (*From* Nahmias and Visintine [12]; with permission.)

Classification of herpes simplex virus disease in neonates

Clinical group	Definition
Disseminated	Newborns with evidence of visceral disease (*eg*, hepatitis, pneumonitis) with or without CNS involvement
Localized (no evidence of visceral dissemination)	
CNS	CNS disease is evidenced by compatible neurologic signs and cerebrospinal fluid findings; may also have involvement of the skin, eye, or mouth
Skin, eye, or mouth	Localize involvement of one or more of three sites without evidence of CNS findings

Figure 4-24 Classification of herpes simplex virus (HSV) disease in neonates. Neonatal herpes has been classified into three nonexclusive forms of HSV disease with varying prognosis, whether untreated or treated. Clinical findings, which can occur up to 6 weeks of age, will also differ according to the form of disease (*see* Figures 4-25 and 4-27) [13].

Because many cases of neonatal herpes may have a poor outcome, it is important to identify possible cases as early as possible, and to use empiric therapy for a few days until other diagnoses are ruled in or out. Every effort should be made to obtain cogent information to increase suspicion of neonatal herpes because initial laboratory diagnostic tests may be negative. These efforts include 1) checking repeatedly for skin, ocular, and oral lesions and obtaining an ophthalmologic evaluation; 2) obtaining repeated cultures of the infant's eyes and mouth (even without lesions) and cultures of the mother's vagina and cervix (even if speculum examination is negative postnatally and the baby presents several weeks after birth); 3) performing CSF studies, which include viral cultures and polymerase chain reaction; and 4) obtaining serial brain scans or magnetic resonance images to ascertain diagnosis and subsequently prognosis. Serologic studies for HSV antibodies are of diagnostic value only when no antibodies are detected in the mother's serum, indicating a likely primary infection. A test for IgM antibodies in the baby may help after 2 to 4 weeks, but only if performed in research laboratories.

Great care should be taken in trying to elicit a history of genital herpes and talking to parents about the possibility or the actual diagnosis of neonatal herpes. It is particularly important not to cause guilt feelings in already stressed parents. (*Adapted from* Nahmias *et al.* [13]; with permission.)

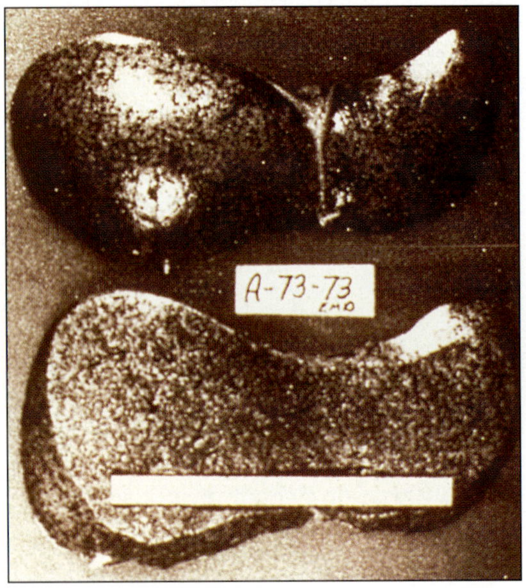

Figure 4-25 Neonates with disseminated herpes simplex virus (HSV) disease. The infant with disseminated disease presents early (within 1–2 wk), often with fever and irritability, followed by severe systemic signs such as disseminated intravascular coagulation and shock. The primary organ involved is the liver (*see* figure), and transaminase levels are usually extremely elevated and are most helpful to suspect this diagnosis of any neonate presenting with signs of sepsis. These infants are usually born to mothers with primary genital infection with cervical involvement, and thus, they do not receive protective transplacental antibody. Examination of the mother around the time of delivery may elicit findings of primary infection and postnatal speculum examination of the cervix may be useful in noting lesions and for attempting to culture HIV.

Untreated, the mortality in infants with disseminated disease is 80% to 90%; thus, cases are often only diagnosed postmortem. The gross pathology of the liver of this infant who died of disseminated HSV disease shows focal areas of necrosis. Some infants with severe hepatic involvement may require antiviral therapy for several months.

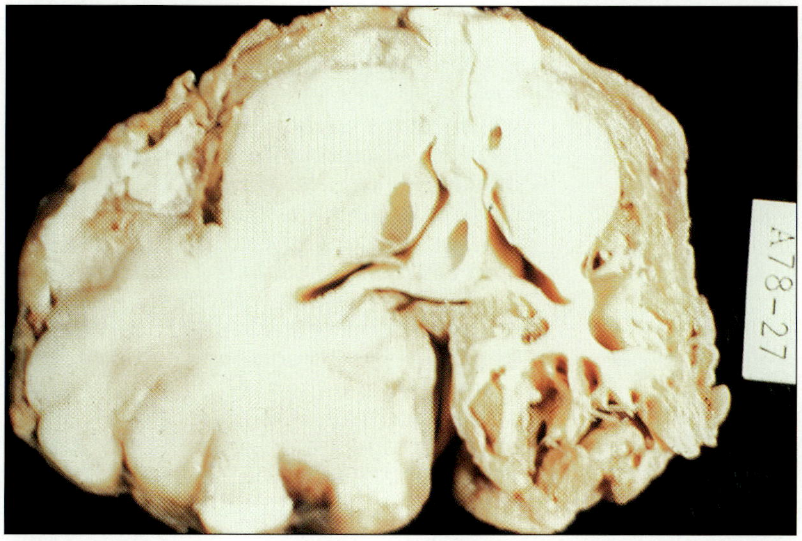

Figure 4-26 Herpes encephalitis in a newborn. Herpes simples virus (HSV) can be one of the most destructive infections of the neonatal brain, even if treated. Encephalitis most commonly occurs by neurogenic spread of HSV, unlike infection in older individuals in which disease usually remains localized to one area of the brain. In the neonate, infection initially may be located in the temporoparietal area, but there is then rapid progression to involve other parts of the brain. In contrast, central nervous system (CNS) disease associated with disseminated infection is likely to be due to the embolization of virus to different parts of the brain. It usually occurs late in the course of the disease, and neurologic sequelae are likely to be less severe than local CNS encephalitis.

Neurogenic encephalitis occurs most commonly with maternal recurrent infection and usuall presents after the 10th to 14th day of life. These infants may present with fever, intractable seizures, irritability, a bulgin fontanel, or poor feeding. However, they may have no neurologic signs, even if the brain scans show marked cortical involvement. The changes seen with brain imaging may not be present early enough to use as a diagnostic tool with which to make decisions about therapy. The presence of skin, eye, or mouth lesions help to confirm the diagnosis. When such lesions are absent, the diagnosis should be suspected when the cerebrospinal fluid shows significant cell numbers, a normal or low glucose concentration, a rising protein level on repeat lumbar puncture, and negative bacterial cultures (even with prior antibacterial therapy). The fatality rate of untreated neonates with CNS disease is approximately 50%. Although mortality may be reduced by the use of antiviral therapy, sequelae still occur in a significant proportion of the infected babies (*see* Figure 4-33).

Neonatal HSV should be suspected throughout the year, but it becomes even more likely as the cause of nonbacterial neonatal meningoencephalitis and, together with arboviruses, accounts for the majority of CNS involvement during the warmer months. The differential diagnosis also includes brain abscesses as well as partly treated bacterial meningitis. Noninfectious conditions to consider include congenital defects and CNS bleeding, particularly in the choroid plexus.

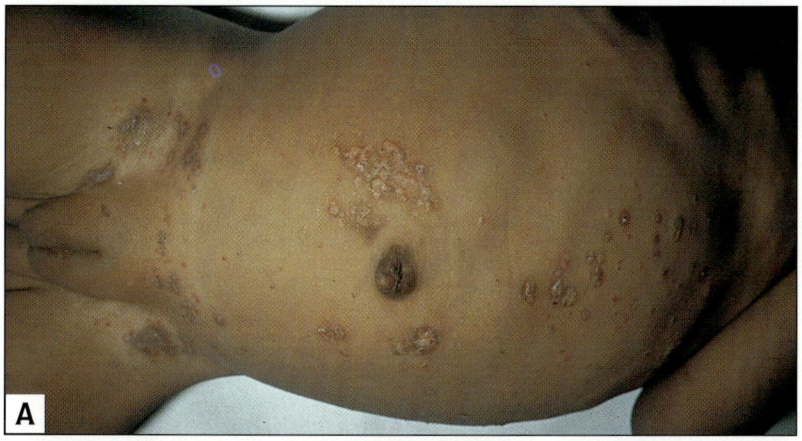

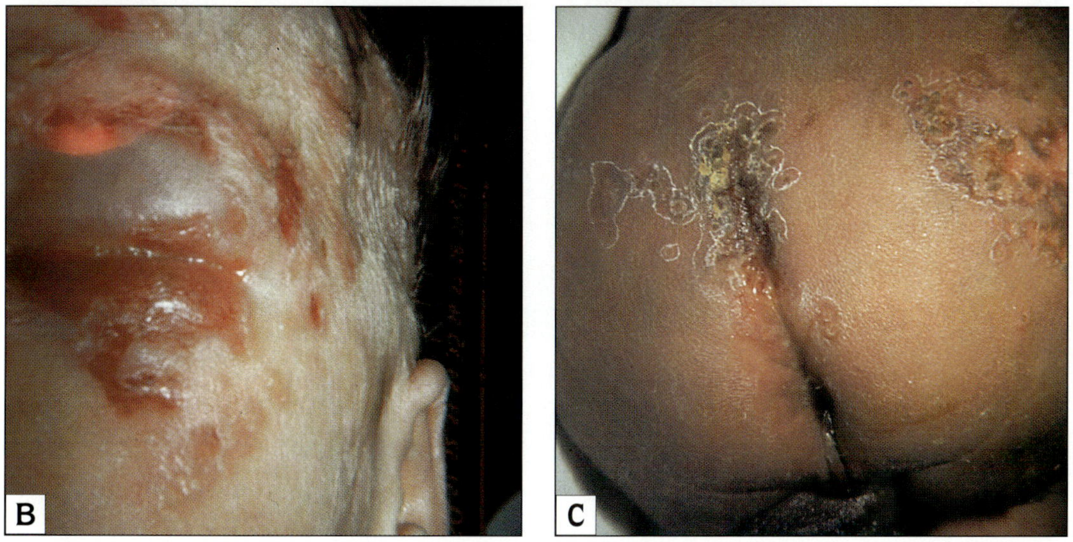

Figure 4-27 Skin manifestations of neonatal herpes simplex virus (HSV). The cutaneous lesions in HSV infection are characteristically vesicular and sometimes appear in clusters. **A**, The lesions may be limited to one site or extend to cover many skin surfaces. The location of lesions depends on the presentation at delivery or the use of fetal scalp monitors, which introduce breaks in the skin. **B** and **C**, The presenting part is most often involved; therefore, lesions may be found in the scalp, face (*panel B*), buttocks (*panel C*), scrotum, or feet. The vesicular lesions of cutaneous herpes simplex virus infection may coalesce to form bullae, and erosions may develop. Denuded areas (*panel B*) may then appear. Cultures and smears taken directly from the lesions, in addition to the eyes and mouth, can confirm the diagnosis. When present alone, skin, eye, or mouth disease is rarely fatal; however, if untreated, it may progress to disseminated or central nervous system infection. In one study, 20% of infants with skin, eye, or mouth disease (who had three or more recurrences withing the first 6 months of life) were shown to have a greater risk of developmental problems than those with less than three recurrences [14]. Differential diagnoses of skin lesions to consider in neonates include benign conditions (*eg*, erythema toxicum, miliaria, transient neonatal pustular melanosis, bullous impetigo, and candidal infection) as well as the more severe ones (*eg*, epidermolysis bullosa, incontinentia pigmenti, and scalded skin syndrome).

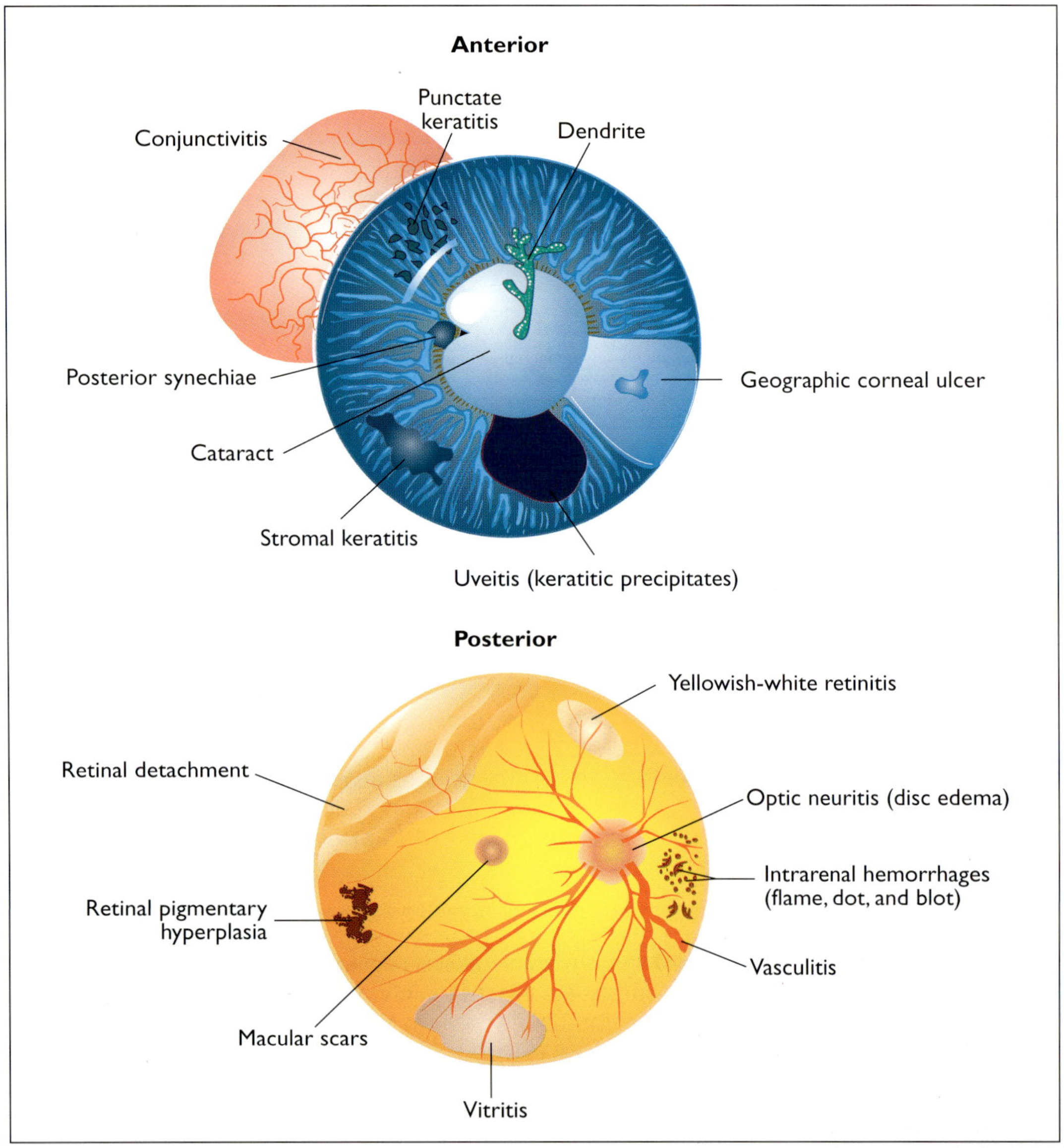

FIGURE 4-28 Ocular findings in herpes infections of the newborn. Herpes simplex virus infection of the eyes in neonates may involve a wide spectrum of ocular structures. Disease may range from mild conjunctivitis to chorioretinitis and optic neuritis, which is unlike the usual infection in older individuals, in whom the cornea or conjunctivae are usually involved. In newborns, ocular disease is often associated with central nervous system or disseminated disease; therefore it is helpful to use a topical ocular antiviral medication as prophylaxis in addition to systemic therapy. Viral cultures of the eyes in babies may be positive in the absence of evident clinical lesions. (*Adapted from* Gammon and Nahmias [15]; with permission.)

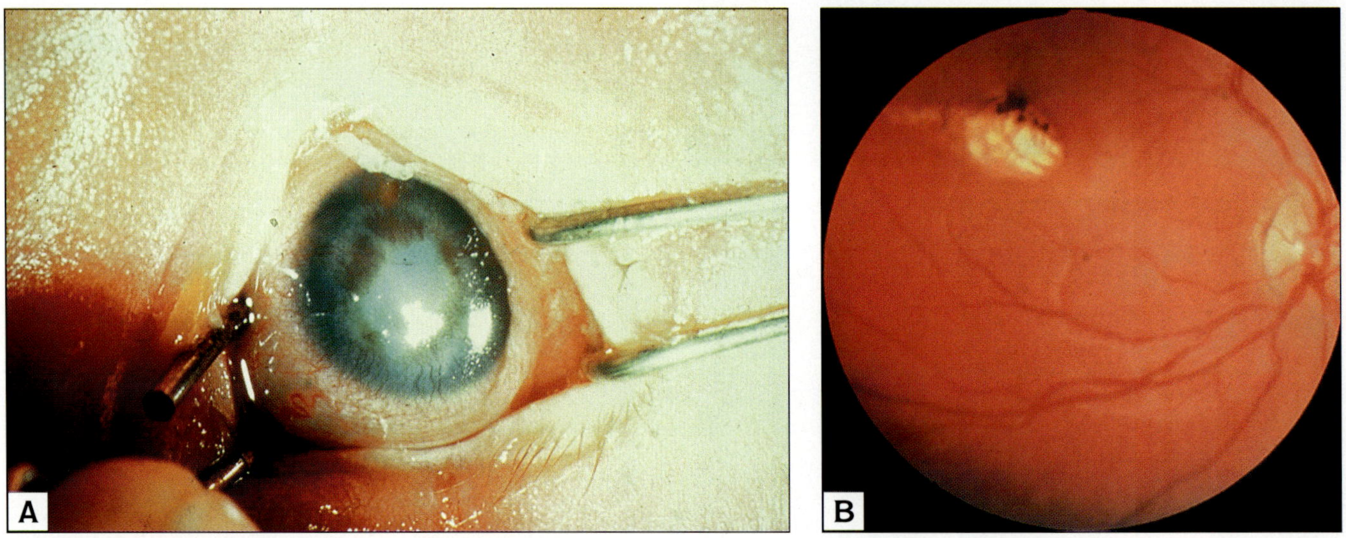

FIGURE 4-29 Herpes simplex virus infection of the eye in neonates. **A,** Opacification of the cornea. This condition can be extensive soon after birth, and responds well to topical antiviral therapy. **B,** Chorioretinitis. This condition may not be observed until several weeks after birth. It is important that ophthalmologists be involved early and provide follow-up examinations in neonates with suspected herpes, particularly because these specialists can assist in the diagnosis and prognosis of cases of neonatal herpes. Systemic antiviral therapy is now also recommended in any neonate with ocular herpes.

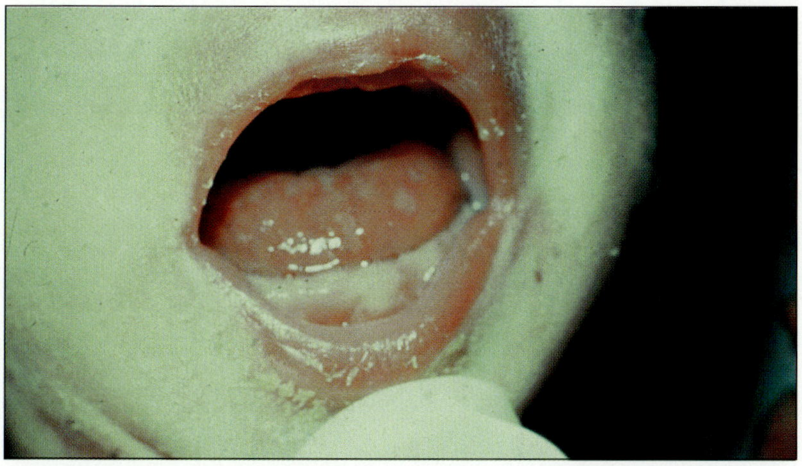

Figure 4-30 Herpes simplex virus infection of the mouth of a neonate. In evaluating an exposed infant, it is important to examine repeatedly all skin sites and possible portals of entry, including all mucosal sites. The mouth may be the only site of infection in localized skin, eyes, or mouth disease; lesions may be single or multiple. Cultures of the saliva should always be obtained, because they can often determine a positive result even in the absence of visible lesions.

Laboratory Diagnosis

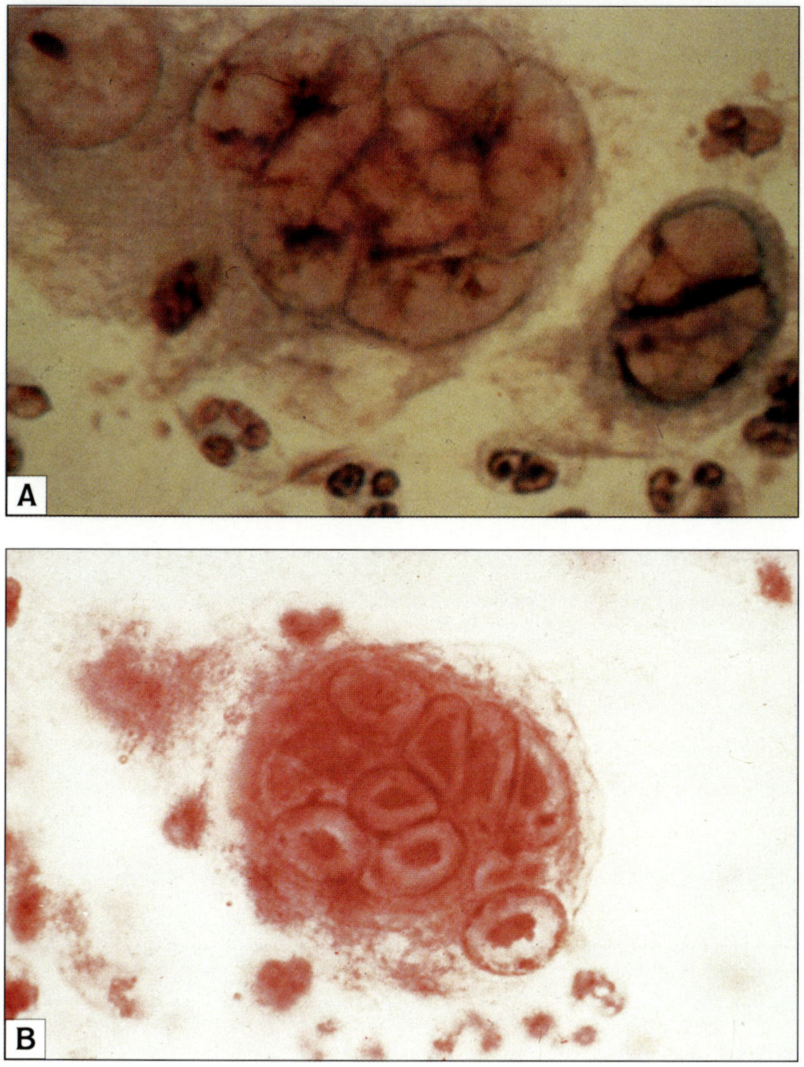

Figure 4-31 Cytologic diagnosis. A Giemsa-stained slide of a scraping of an herpetic lesion can reveal the multinucleated giant cells (*panel A* [Tzanck preparation]). In obtaining a smear, the vesicle is unroofed and cultured, and a scraping performed at the base of the lesion near the edges to obtain the infected epithelial cells. Erroneous readings of multinucleated cells can be made when cells are on top of each other. Most experts prefer to use the Papanicolaou (*panel B*) or hematoxylin and eosin preparations, which also reveal the characteristic intranuclear inclusions with multinucleation [16]. Other causes of intranuclear inclusions are varicella-zoster virus (VZV), which is unlikely to present in the neonatal period without other findings of congenital VZV infection, as well as cytomegalovirus, which usually does not cause multinucleation and may also have cytoplasmic inclusions.

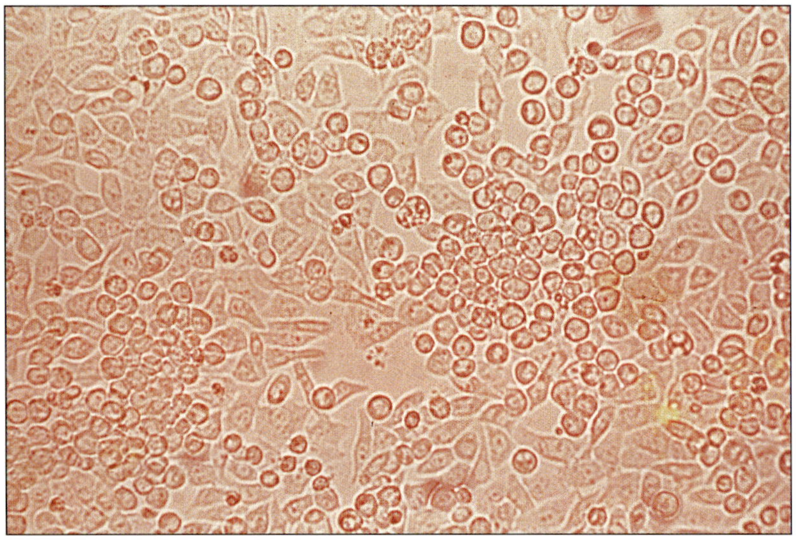

FIGURE 4-32 Viral identification methods. The gold standard for the diagnosis of herpes simplex virus infection is still a positive culture, which is made easier by the ability of the virus to affect a wide variety of cultured cells. Observation of such cultures reveals a distinct cytopathic effect on the cell monolayer. A positive viral culture, particularly in susceptible cells such as rabbit kidney cultures, are often evident within 1 to 2 days, and are infrequently positive after 4 days.

Fluorescent microscopy can help to characterize and type the herpes simplex virus, which is isolated in culture. However, it is unreliable for direct examinations of clinical materials by inexperienced individuals. A false-positive direct fluorescent microscopy test in a baby, with no other confirmation, may result in a large amount of unnecessary hospitalization, treatment, and undue concern for the family.

Molecular methods have added information to the diagnostic examinations. The polymerase chain reaction (PCR) method is currently being used in the diagnosis of herpes encephalitis in a newborn or older individuals. When compared with brain biopsy culture, the sensitivity of PCR is 98% and specificity is 94% [10]. However, because these tests are not 100% sensitive or specific, caution is needed. The decision to use or continue antiviral therapy should not be based solely on this criterion. Another useful molecular method is restriction enzyme analysis, which distinguishes viral strains within the same herpes simplex virus type [17].

ANTIVIRAL THERAPY

Assessment of morbidity after 12 months in infants with neonatal herpes simplex virus infection treated with vidarabine or acyclovir

	Infant morbidity after 12 mo							
Extent of disease	Normal	Mild	Moderate	Severe	Subtotal	Infants alive after 12 mo (morbidity unknown), *n*	Dead within 12 mo, *n*	Total, *n*
Skin, eye, or mouth infection								
Vidarabine	22	1	1	1	25	6	0	31
Acyclovir	45	0	1	0	46	8	0	54
Central nervous system infection								
Vidarabine	13	1	5	11	30	1	5	36
Acyclovir	8	5	6	9	28	2	5	35
Disseminated disease								
Vidarabine	7	1	0	4	12	2	14	28
Acyclovir	3	1	0	1	5	2	11	18
Total	98	9	13	26	146	21	35	202

FIGURE 4-33 Effect of treatment of neonatal herpes with vidarabine or acyclovir. Results of the first studies conducted by the National Institutes of Health Herpes Antiviral Collaborative Group demonstrated the efficacy of an antiviral agent, vidarabine, in a placebo-controlled study of herpes simplex disease in newborns [18]. Later comparisons of vidarabine and acyclovir showed no significant difference between the two drugs in the extent of morbidity and mortality. *Adapted from* Whitley *et al.* [14]; with permission.)

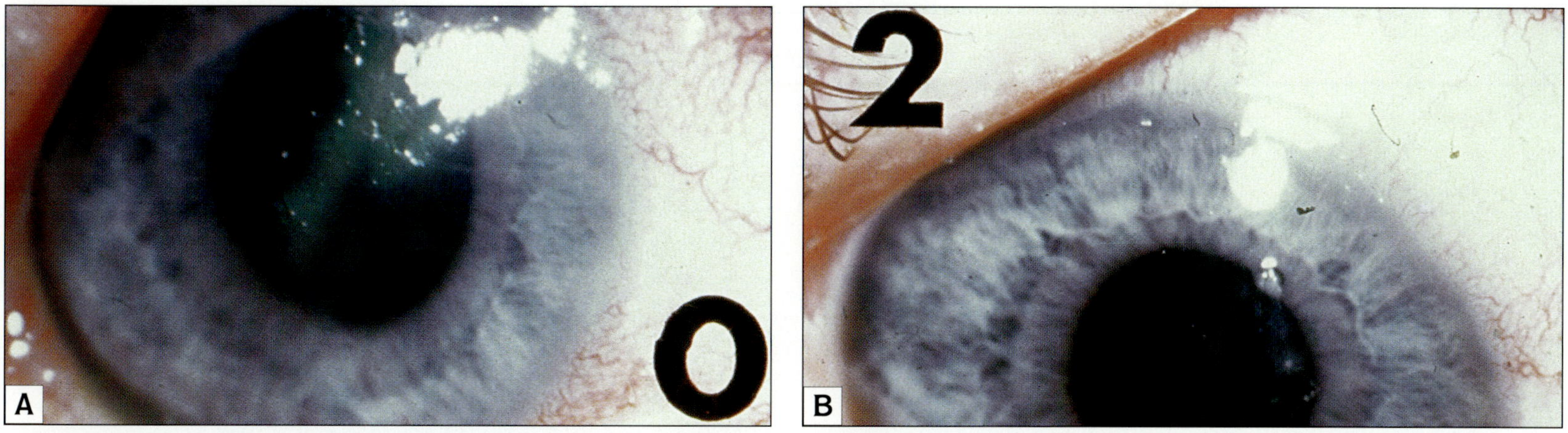

Figure 4-34 Response of the eye to topical antiviral treatment with trifluorothymidine in a child. **A,** This patient with herpetic keratitis received topical trifluorothymidine therapy every 2 to 3 hours. **B,** The response was very noticeable at 48 hours. It should be noted that in neonates, concomitant systemic therapy is most often needed.

Indications for use of acyclovir in pediatric herpes simplex virus infections
Intravenous acyclovir*
Neonatal herpes
Older pediatric, immunocompromised, or normal patients with the following indications:
Herpes encephalitis or other severe CNS disease
Disseminated herpes
Severe mucocutaneous infection (*eg*, herpes esophagitis, eczema herpeticum, herpetic whitlow)
Oral acyclovir†‡
Moderately severe initial episodes of the following conditions:
Genital or anorectal herpes
Primary HSV stomatitis, herpetic whitlow, herpes gladiatorum
Recurrent erythema multiforme or eczema herpeticum
Daily suppressive oral therapy†
Infrequent pediatric indications for psychosocial reasons or in patients with 6 to 8 clinical recurrences of genital herpes per year
Prophylacitc therapy†
Primarily used for transplant patients with positive HSV serology

* Confirm diagnosis as rapidly as possible to determine duration of therapy.
† Outside newborn age.
‡ Infrequently indicated for cases of recurrent oral, skin, or anogenital herpes in normal host.

Figure 4-35 Indications for acyclovir therapy in pediatric herpes simplex virus (HSV) infection. As noted earlier, the use of intravenous acyclovir is indicated in any clinically suspect case of neonatal herpes. Most authorities will use parenteral acyclovir in neonates born to women with a first episode of genital herpes around the time of delivery, because the risk of neonatal infection is approximately 50%. Babies born to mothers with recurrent genital herpes, or who are at risk from other postnatal maternal or nosocomial sources, should be watched clinically carefully for approximately a month for any possible herpetic manifestations and have weekly eye and mouth cultures. Older children or adolescents with suspect HSV encephalitis or other severe central nervous system manifestations, and those with disseminated herpes and severe mucocutaneous infections, would benefit from early intravenous acyclovir therapy. The decision between the use of intravenous or oral acyclovir will depend on the severity of mucocutaneous manifestations in immunocompetent or immunocompromised hosts, *eg*, severe stomatitis with poor fluid intake, first episode genital lesions with severe dysuria, or herpetic skin lesions in an AIDS patient. Once the diagnosis is confirmed in such cases, acyclovir is to be continued according to the severity of the disease and its likely prognosis. Thus, intravenous therapy may be needed for 21 days or longer in cases of neonatal herpes encephalitis or of disseminated herpes with severe hepatic involvement.

Treatment with oral acyclovir, usually for approximately a week, may be used in first episodes of moderately severe genital herpes, and for moderately severe stomatitis. The large majority of recurrent mucocutaneous infections in normal hosts do not require therapy. However, in pediatric patients with recurrent laboratory-confirmed genital herpes with 6 to 8 episodes per year, or with herpetic infections with psychosocial impact, continuous oral suppressive therapy for several months, if not longer, might be considered (although experience in pediatric patients is very limited) [19]. Intermittent therapy given early, if possible in the prodromal stage, might be useful for cases of erythema multiforme triggered by HSV recurrences. It may also be given in some cases of recurrent mucocutaneous infections with psychosocial implications. It is important to recognize that such therapy is only slightly better than placebo for most recurrent episodes.

Topical acyclovir therapy (as an ointment) is no longer indicated for mucocutaneous herpetic lesions, because it is generally less effective than oral therapy. The exception is topical use of trifluorothymidine or topical acyclovir for ocular involvement (conjunctivitis or uncomplicated keratitis).

Prophylactic intravenous or oral therapy has proven useful in pediatric patients who are seropositive for HSV (no matter the virus type), and who are undergoing bone marrow or various types of organ transplantation [20]. Current information does not suggest the need for prophylactic treatment of pregnant women with a history of genital herpes to avoid transmission to her baby. However, in case of serious illness caused by HSV in a pregnant woman, *eg*, herpes encephalitis, intravenous acyclovir becomes necessary for her benefit.

Antiviral agents other than acyclovir that have effectiveness against HSV1 and HSV2 have become available during the past two decades. However, compared with acyclovir, these drugs have received relatively little clinical experience or controlled studies in pediatric patients (*eg*, famciclovir and valacyclovir), are more difficult to administer, and have worse side effects or greater toxicity in neonates (*eg*, vidarabine, ganciclovir, or foscarnet). For oral or systemic treatment, acyclovir currently remains the drug of choice. However, when there is evidence of acyclovir resistance in clinical isolates, which primarily occurs in immunocompromised hosts, other agents may be needed. In such situations, intravenous foscarnet appears to be more effective than vidarabine.

Conclusions

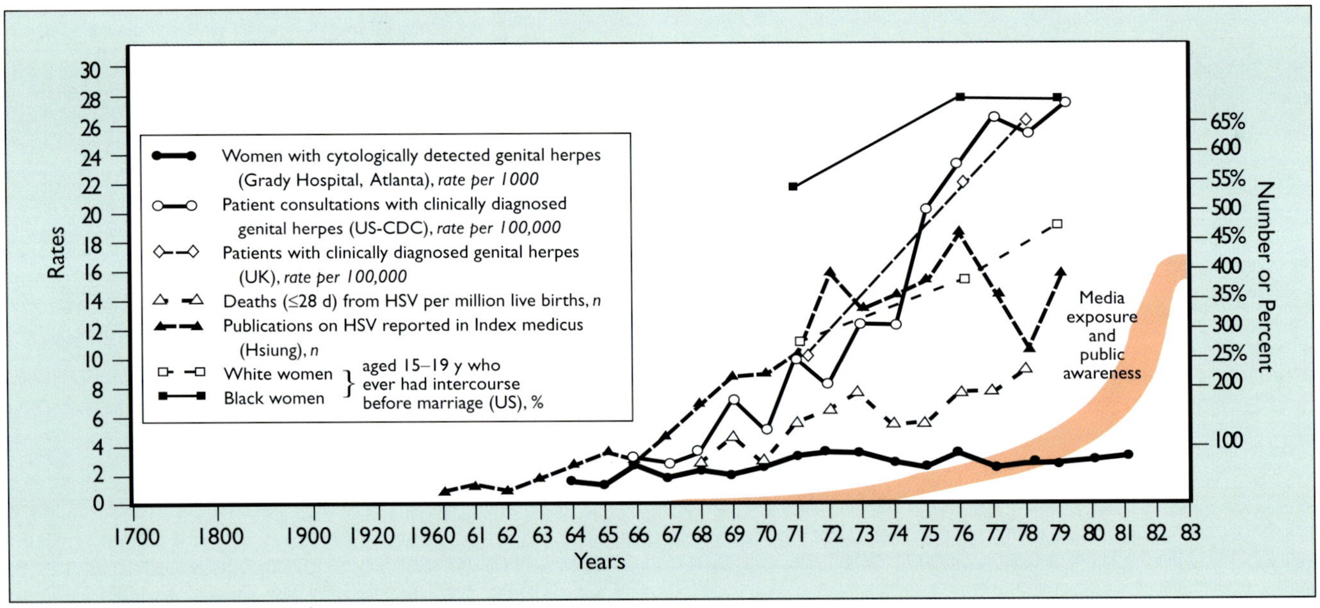

Figure 4-36 Past epidemiologic trends and expectations for pediatric herpes simplex virus (HSV) in the next decade. The epidemiologic information noted presents patterns of HSV infection between 1960 and 1980 that were not readily understandable. The presentations made so far serve as a base for discussing these patterns, and for indicating remaining challenges for the future.

Public concern and education related to HSV infections. As noted by the *thick increasing line* in this figure (and in Fig. 4-1), there was great public concern about genital herpes in the 1970s. The recognition of a persistent and recurring sexually transmitted disease with severe impact on babies primarily affected middle-class white Americans, whose sexual liberation by the contraceptive pill and antibacterial agents was now challenged. The newest survey (the US National Health and Nutrition Examination Survey [NHANES] III) suggests no similar concern among young white Americans regarding the much more clinically devastating HIV. This finding is probably based on the belief that this group is not at high risk for HIV infection. In addition to this erroneous belief, because heterosexual and homosexual activities are well-recognized risk factors for teenagers, there is the likelihood (*see* Fig. 4-21) that HSV can facilitate HIV transmission. Another erroneous belief is that HSV2 is the herpetic infection of greatest medical concern. As also noted earlier, outside the neonatal age, HSV1 infection actually represents a greater problem overall, and particularly in relation to the brain, skin, and eyes, and the more severe herpetic infection in compromised hosts. Public concern with genital herpes led to the formation of community herpes awareness (HELP) groups for afflicted individuals in the 1970s, which are still active in many communities. Such groups and others are helping to educate about all sexually transmitted diseases, including HIV and HSV. Pediatricians and other healthcare workers dealing with children and adolescents have a special role in this educational effort. Information on herpes can be received through national hotlines at the Centers for Disease Control and Prevention (1-800-227-8922) and the American Social Health Associaton (1-919-361-8488).

Along with the mounting medical and scientific awareness of HSV infections occurring since the mid 1960s (then the subject of only a handful of investigators in this area), publications have also greatly increased. As noted by the *yellow line*), their number rose greatly between 1960 and 1980 and, together with rising numbers of media reports and public awareness, are likely to be partly responsible for the physician reports of the 1970s of marked increases in clinically manifest genital herpes. It was also believed that black Americans had less genital herpes than white Americans, because they had fewer clinically manifest infections. It has since been found that only 3% to 5% of black Americans with HSV2 antibodies give a history of genital herpes, compared with 10% to 20% of white Americans. Further, by adolescence there is a twofold higher prevalence of HSV1 antibodies in black Americans than in white Americans. Because HSV1 has been noted to diminish many of the clinical manifestations of genital HSV2 infection, whites therefore tend to have more primary infections, with more frequent clinical manifestations. This characteristic is likely to have contributed also in bringing more patients to the attention of American and British physicians in the 1970s and beyond. This figure also shows that the proportion of adolescent girls, aged 15 to 19 years, who had sexual intercourse before marriage increased twofold for whites during the 1970s, and stabilized for black Americans. The recent NHANES III results concur with other surveys in the 1990s, indicating increasing sexual encounters among young white Americans.

A rising awareness of neonatal herpes was also partly responsible for the increased reported US cases of neonatal deaths (*purple line*). However, in a municipal hospital in Atlanta with approximately 8000 deliveries a year, no such increase was observed in either cytologically detected genital herpes in women, or in cases of neonatal herpes, since the early 1960s. Neonatal herpes in our Atlanta hospital was both less frequent and included fewer disseminated cases than other institutions, *eg*, in Seattle. This is because the prevalence of HSV2 antibodies in pregnant women in the Atlanta hospital is twice that of hospitals evaluated.

The likely somewhat dismal future of herpetic infections in our pediatric population emphasizes the need to suspect, diagnose accurately, and treat optimally the various clinical forms of HSV1 and HSV2 infections in neonates, children, and adolescents. For more information on the future of herpetic infections, please refer to Becker and Nahmias [3]. (*Adapted from* Becker and Nahmias [3].)

Acknowledgments

The studies that provided the information presented here were supported by various grants since 1962 from the National Institutes of Health, the Centers for Disease Control and Prevention, and the National Foundation–March of Dimes.

References

1. Stanberry LR, Jorgenson DM, Nahmias AJ:Herpes simplex viruses 1 and 2. In *Viral Infections of Humans:Epidemiology and Control*, edn 4. Edited by Evans AS, Kaslow RA. New York:Plenum Medical Book Company; 1997:419–454.
2. Nahmias A, Dowdle W:Antigenic and biologic differences in herpesvirus hominis. *Prog Med Virol* 1968, 10:110–159.
3. Becker T, Nahmias A:Genital herpes:yesterday, today, and tomorrow. *Ann Rev Med* 1985, 36:185–193.
4. Whitley RJ, Kimberlin DW, Roizman B:Herpes simplex viruses. *Clin Infect Dis* 1998, 26:541–555.
5. Becker TM, Kodsi R, Bailey P, *et al.*:Grappling with herpes:herpes gladiatorum. *Am J Sports Med* 1988, 16:665–669.
6. Corey L, Adams HG, Brown ZA, Holmes KK:Genital herpes simplex virus infections:clinical manifestations, course, and complications. *Ann Intern Med* 1983, 98:958–972.
7. Nahmias A, Dowdle W, Naib Z, *et al.*:Genital infections with herpesvirus hominis types 1 and 2 in children. *Pediatrics* 1968, 42:659–666.
8. Nahmias A, Froeschle J, Feorino P, McCord G:Generalized eruption in a child with eczema due to coxsackie virus A16. *Arch Dermatol* 1968, 97:147–148.
9. Nahmias AJ, Lee FK, Keyserling, HK:The epidemiology of genital herpes. In *Genital and Neonatal Herpes*. Edited by Stanberry LR. Chichester, England:John Wiley and Sons; 1996:93–138.
10. Lakeman FD, Whitley RJ:Diagnosis of herpes simplex encephalitis:application of polymerase chain reaction to cerebrospinal fluid from brain-biopsied patients and correlation with disease. *J Infect Dis* 1995, 171:857–863.
11. Whitley RJ, Arvin AM:Herpes simplex virus infections. In *Infectious Diseases of the Fetus and Newborn Infant*. Edited by Remington JS, Klein JO:Philadelphia:WB Saunders Company; 1995:354–376.
12. Nahmias A, Visintine A:Herpes simplex. In *Infectious Diseases of the Fetus and Newborn Infant*. Edited by Remington J, Klein J:Philadelphia:WB Saunders Co; 1976:156–190.
13. Nahmias A, Alford C, Korones S:Infection of the newborn with herpesvirus hominis. In *Advances in Pediatrics*. Edited by Schulman I. Chicago:YearBook Medical Publishers; 1970:185–226.
14. Whitley R, Arvin A, Prober C, and the National Institute of Allergy and Infectious Diseases Collaborative Antiviral Study Group:Predictors of morbidity and mortality in neonates with herpes simplex virus infections. *N Engl J Med* 1991, 324:450–454.
15. Gammon JA, Nahmias AJ:Herpes simplex ocular infections in the newborn. In *Viral Diseases of the Eye*. Edited by Darrel RW. Philadelphia:Lea and Febiger; 1985:46–58.
16. Naib ZM, Nahmias AJ, Josey WE:Cytology and histopathology of cervical herpes simplex. *Cancer* 1966, 19:1026–1030.
17. Buchman TG, Simpson T, Nosal C, *et al.*:The structure of herpes simplex virus DNA and its application to molecular epidemiology. *Ann N Y Acad Sci* 1980, 354:279–290.
18. Whitley RJ, Nahmias AJ, Soong S-J, *et al.*:Vidarabine therapy of neonatal herpes simplex virus infection. *Pediatrics* 1980, 66:495–501.
19. Whitley RJ, Kimberlin DW:Prophylaxis and Treatment of herpesvirus infections in children. *Semin Pediatr Inf Dis* 1997, 8:196–204.
20. Frenck RW, Kohl S.:Herpes simplex virus in the immunocompromised child. In *Infection in Immunocompromised Infants and Children*. Edited by Patrick CC. New York:Churchill-Livingstone; 1992:604–624

Selected Bibliography

Stanberry LR, Jorgenson DM, Nahmias AJ:Herpes simplex viruses 1 and 2. In *Viral Infections of Humans-Epidemiology and Control*, edn 3. Edited by Evans AS. New York:Plenum Publishing Corporation; 1989:393–417.

Stanberry L (ed.):*Genital and Neonatal Herpes*. Chichester, England:John Wiley and Sons; 1996:93–138.

Starr SE (guest ed.):Herpes virus infections. *Semin Pediatr Inf Dis* 1997, 8:125–204.

Whitley RJ, Arvin AM:Herpes simplex virus infections. In *Infectious Diseases of the Fetus and Newborn Infant*. Edited by Remington JS, Klein JO. Philadelphia:WB Saunders Company; 1995:354–376.

CHAPTER 5

Varicella and Herpes Zoster

Ann M. Arvin

VARICELLA-ZOSTER VIRUS (VZV) is a human alpha herpesvirus that causes varicella and herpes zoster. Varicella (or chickenpox), which results from primary VZV infection, is a common childhood illness associated with fever and a generalized, pruritic vesicular rash. After primary infection, VZV establishes latency in cells of the dorsal root ganglia. Reactivation from latency results in herpes zoster, commonly referred to as "shingles." Herpes zoster is a localized, painful, vesicular rash involving one or adjacent dermatomes. The incidence of herpes zoster increases with age or immunosuppression. Advances have been made in understanding VZV that have led to new ways to treat and prevent VZV infections. Antiviral agents that modify the severity of varicella and herpes zoster have been developed, and a live attenuated varicella vaccine that protects against primary VZV infection is now licensed for clinical use.

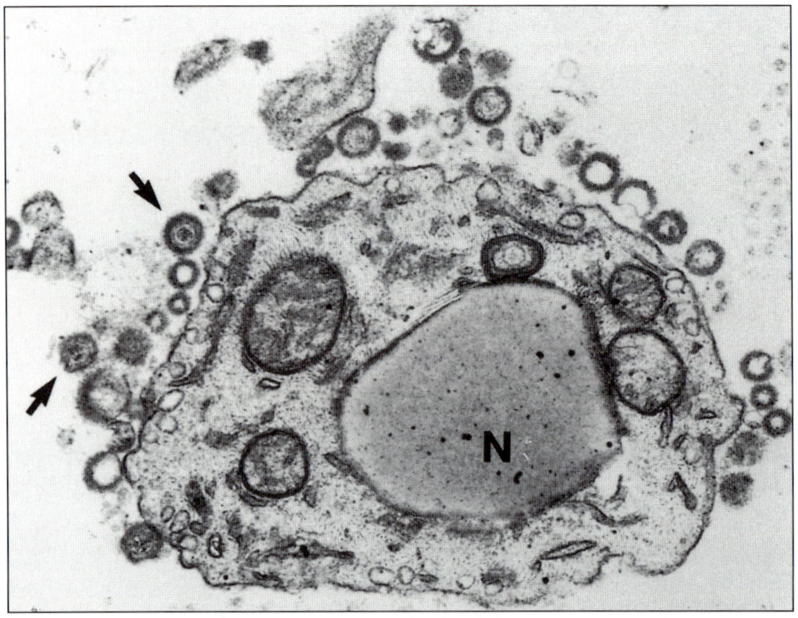

FIGURE 5-1 Varicella-zoster virus (VZV) replication in human skin cells. The VZV virion consists of an icosahedral nucleocapsid that surrounds a core that contains the linear, double-stranded DNA genome; a protein tegument separates the capsid from the lipid envelope that incorporates the major viral glycoproteins . The IE62 protein is the major transactivator for VZV replication and is a major component of the tegument . Other VZV proteins with gene regulation activities include the products of open reading frames 4, 10, 61, 62, and 63. Electron microscopy studies show that most VZV virions are enclosed in cytoplasmic vacuoles within infected cells. VZV is highly temperature sensitive, with inactivation occurring at 56° to 60°C; it is not infectious if the virion envelope is disrupted by detergents or freeze-thawing [1].

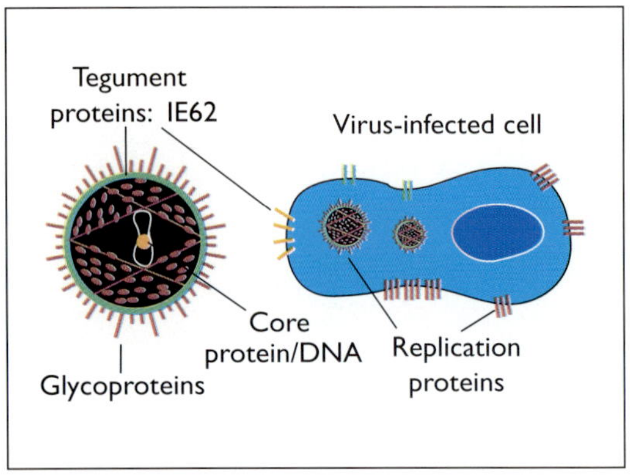

FIGURE 5-2 Host recognition of host varicella-zoster virus (VZV). VZV is the smallest of the human herpesviruses. VZV DNA consists of approximately 125,000 base pairs with genes coding for at least 69 proteins. VZV produces regulatory and structural proteins and glycoproteins that are also expressed on cell membranes during viral replication. The viral thymidine kinase of VZV is inhibited by acyclovir and related antiviral drugs.

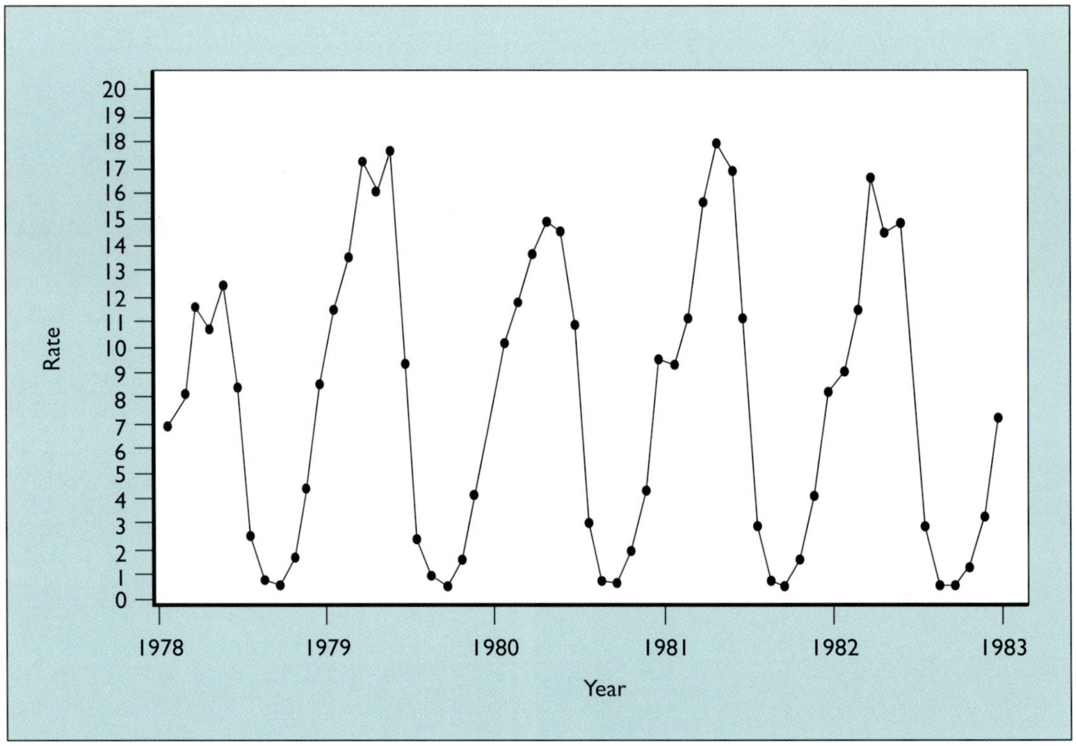

FIGURE 5-3 Epidemiology of varicella zoster virus (VZV). VZV is found in a world-wide geographic distribution, but annual epidemics are more prevalent in temperate climates (most often during late winter and spring). Varicella attack rates among susceptible household contacts are approximately 90%. Epidemiologically distinct VZV strains exhibit little antigenic variation. Restriction endonuclease analyses of viral DNA are identical for VZV isolates from a common source. True reinfection, causing second episodes of varicella, is very rare. VZV is highly species-specific for humans in its infectivity.

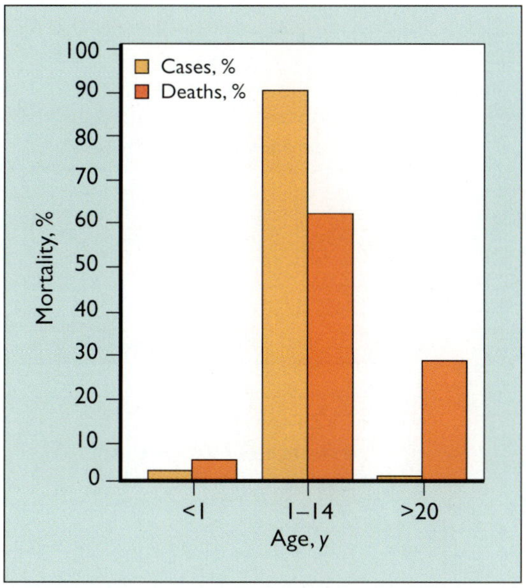

FIGURE 5-4 Age-related increase in the mortality of varicella in children and adults. Although the incidence of varicella is low in adults, adults have excessive rates of mortality associated with primary varicella zoster virus infection compared with children. (*Adapted from* Preblud [2]; with permission).

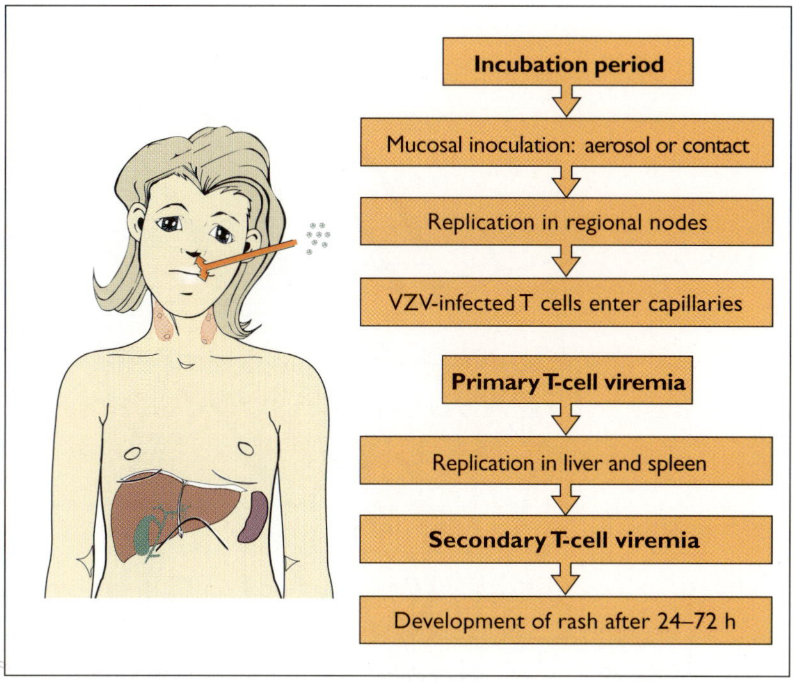

FIGURE 5-5 Pathogenic events during the incubation period of varicella. In the first phase of varicella, infectious virus present in respiratory droplets or vesicular fluid from an infected contact is inoculated at mucous membrane sites. Primary varicella-zoster virus (VZV) infection is characterized by a relatively prolonged incubation period, ranging from 10 to 21 days, with a usual duration of 14 to 16 days. The virus is thought to spread to regional lymph nodes, resulting in a primary viremic phase that permits the transport of the virus to the liver or other cells of the reticuloendothelial system. The virus is transmissible for 24 to 48 hours before the onset of the rash. (*Adapted from* Arvin [3]; with permission.)

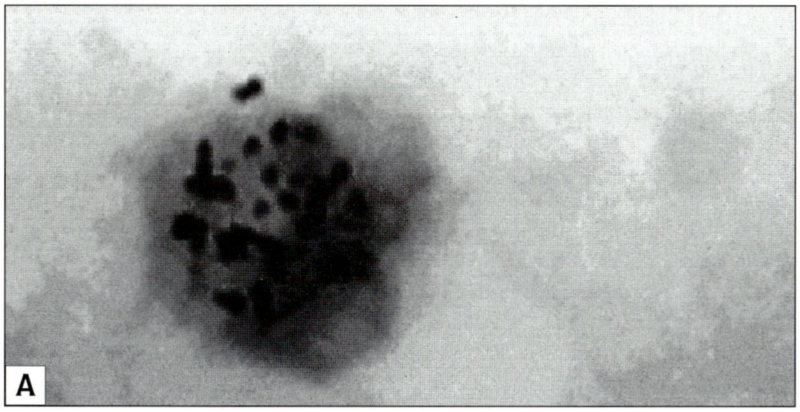

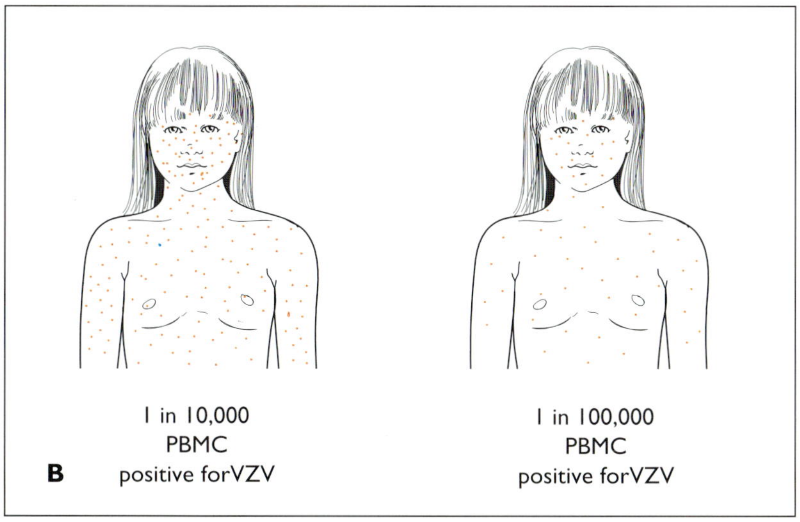

FIGURE 5-6 Lymphotropism in the pathogenesis of varicella. Varicella-zoster virus (VZV) is a lymphotropic herpesvirus with the capacity to infect $CD4^+$ and $CD8^+$ T cells [4]. Cell-associated VZV viremia can be detected during in the last 4 or 5 days before the onset of symptoms and for a few days after the appearance of the varicella rash. Approximately 1:10,000 to 1:100,000 peripheral blood mononuclear cells (PBMC) contain VZV DNA.

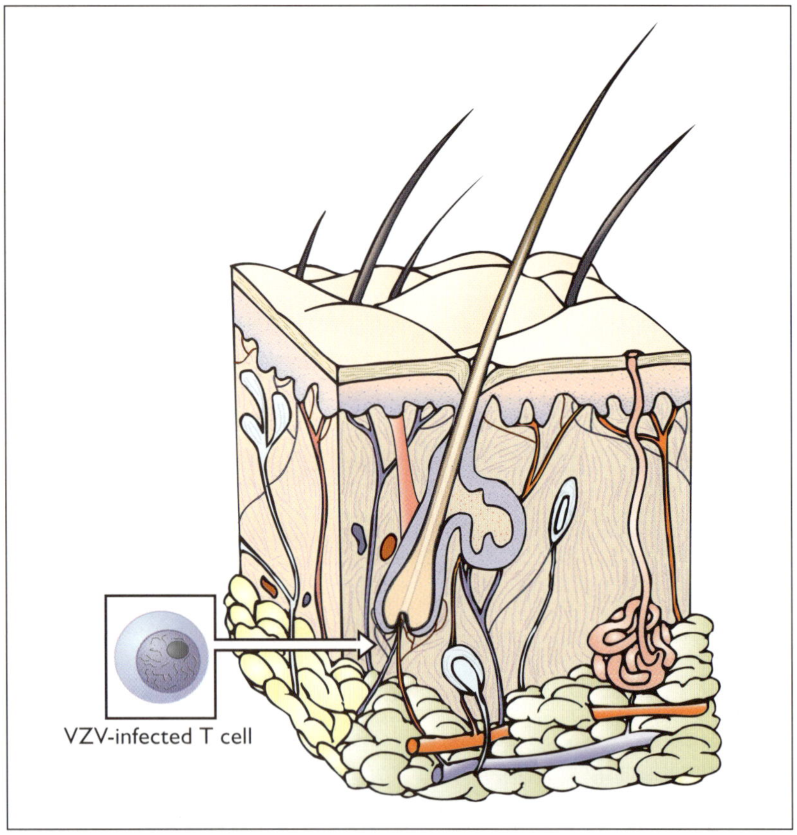

Figure 5-7 The pathogenesis of cutaneous infection in varicella. Cell-associated viremia provides the virus with access to epidermal cells, and replication in these cells causes the typical varicella rash. Infected T cells can migrate out of the capillaries into cutaneous tissue and release infectious virions that enter skin cells. Varicella-zoster virus may also infect cells forming the capillary walls before spread to adjacent skin cells.

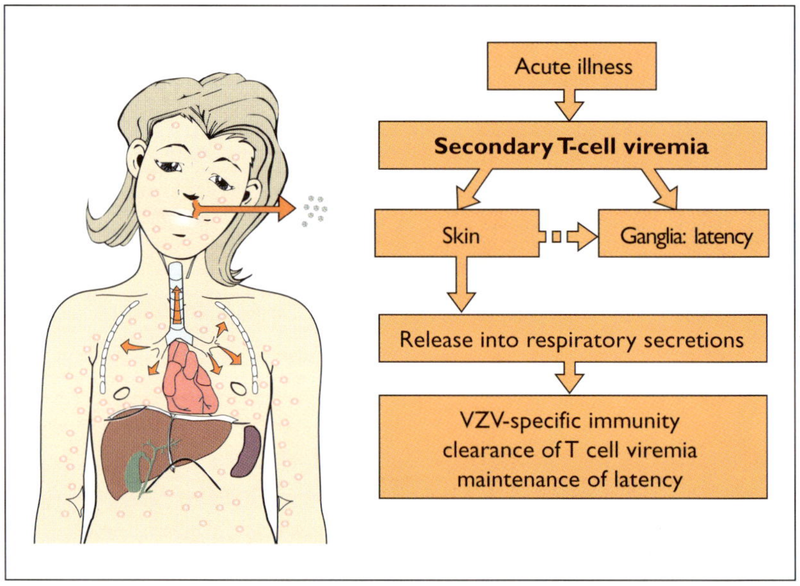

Figure 5-8 The clinical course of acute varicella. Varicella often begins with a prodrome of fever and malaise about 24 to 48 hours before the appearance of the first skin lesions. Fever, fatigue, and anorexia occur in the early, viremic phase of the illness. Varicella is usually associated with mild lymphopenia and granulocytopenia and often slight abnormalities of liver function tests. The initial lesions typically involve the scalp, face, or trunk and are pruritic, erythematous macules; the maculopapular phase evolves to a vesicular phase. The lesions are described as resembling a "dew drop on a rose petal." Ulcerative lesions appear on mucous membranes. New lesions develop for 3 to 5 days (range, 1 to 7 days). Lesions begin to crust by 24 to 48 hours, noted first as clouding of vesicular fluid; some lesions become umbilicated. Several "crops" appear with later lesions on the arms and legs. The number of lesions varies from as few as 10 to more than 1500, with a usual range of 100 to 300. The rash is more extensive in older children, secondary household cases, and patients with skin trauma, such as sunburn or eczema. Lesions heal as new epithelial cells form at the base of the lesion; hypopigmentation is common during healing. Scarring is rare except for the initial lesions.

During acute varicella, varicella-zoster virus (VZV) reaches cells of the dorsal root ganglia and establishes latency. Infectious virus is released in respiratory secretions and can be transmitted to susceptible contacts by airborne spread. Acute varicella resolves when VZV-specific immunity is elicited. The host response clears T-cell viremia and controls viral infection within dorsal root ganglia. (*Adapted from* Moffat *et al.* [4]; with permission.)

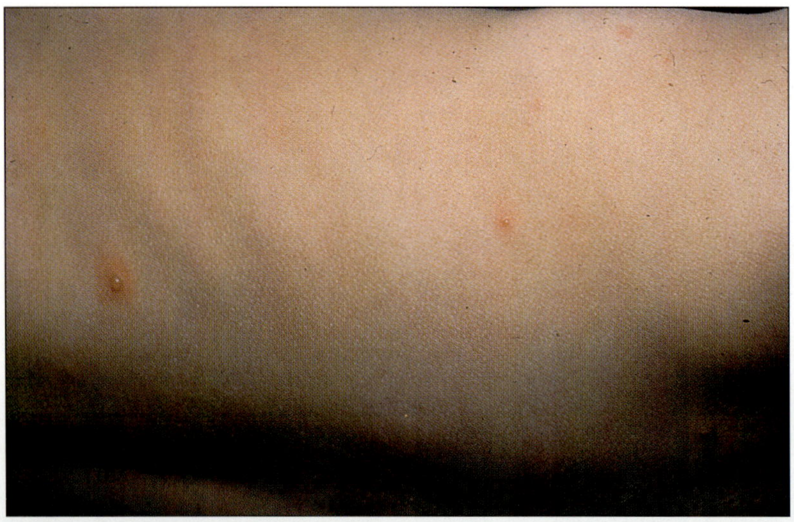

Figure 5-9 Varicella skin lesions. Cutaneous varicella lesions evolve through maculopapular, vesicular, and crusting phases. The histologic changes associated with the maculopapular stage include vasculitis involving small blood vessels and the appearance of multinucleated epithelial cells with intranuclear inclusions. The evolution to vesicles is associated with progressive "ballooning" degeneration of epithelial cells, coalescence of fluid-filled vacuoles between cells, and increased numbers of infected cells at the base of the lesion. Deep, ulcerated lesions are characterized by necrosis through the whole dermal layer. Keratinocyte infection is associated with release of cell-free virus into vesicular fluid. Direct contact with infectious virus in cutaneous lesions allows varicella-zoster virus transmission.

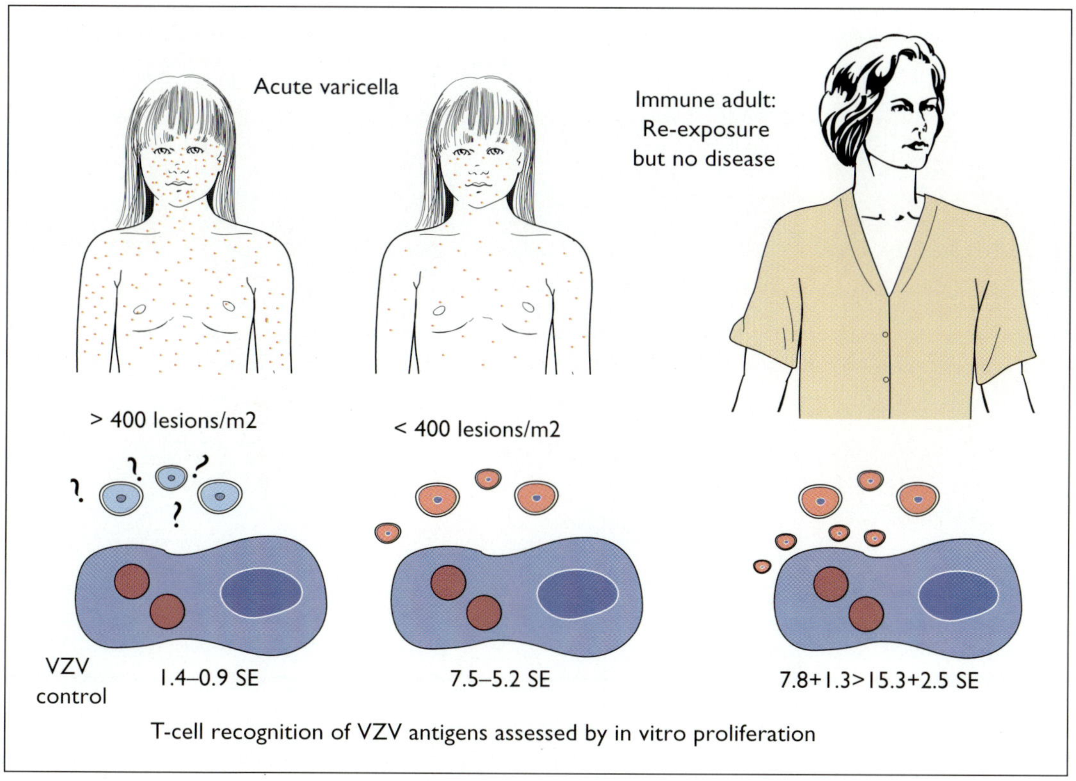

FIGURE 5-10 The immune response to varicella-zoster virus (VZV). Primary VZV infection elicits IgG, IgM, and IgA antibodies. VZV antibodies have neutralizing activity against the virus and lyse infected cells via antibody-mediated cellular cytotoxicity. VZV antibodies are usually detectable within 3 days after the onset of acute varicella. IgM antibodies decline within a few months but IgG antibodies persist for years after primary VZV infection. Cell-mediated responses to VZV eliminate virus-infected T cells and restrict virus replication in skin lesions. Varicella is mild when VZV-specific T cells (*red*) are detected within 72 hours. VZV-specific T cells produce cytokines of the T helper-1 type, including interleukin-2 and interferon gamma. Cytotoxic $CD4^+$ and $CD8^+$ T-cells that recognize VZV-infected cells are elicited during primary VZV infection. Reexposure to varicella boosts T-cell responses (*red*) in individuals with preexisting immunity.

Complications of varicella-zoster virus
Complications
Bacterial infection
Cellulitis
Sepsis
Pneumonia
Adenitis
Arthritis
Encephalitis (1.7 per 100,000 cases)
Reye's syndrome (3.2 per 100,000 cases)
Hospitalizations per year (~10,000 per 4 million cases)
Deaths per year (~100 per 4 million cases)

FIGURE 5-11 Complications of varicella-zoster virus (VZV). The most common complication of varicella is secondary bacterial infection. VZV can disseminate to lungs, liver, central nervous system, and other organs if the host response is inadequate to terminate cell-associated viremia . Extensive viral replication in the liver with widespread hepatocellular destruction is a complication of progressive varicella and causes fulminant hepatic failure. Meningoencephalitis and cerebellar ataxia are the major clinical manifestations of central nervous system involvement. Neurologic complications usually occur from 2 to 6 days after the onset of the rash. Permanent sequelae are rare. Children with varicella who are given salicylates are at risk for Reye's syndrome. Unusual complications of varicella include thrombocytopenia, adrenal damage, glomerulonephritis, viral arthritis, uveitis, retinal necrosis, myocarditis, pancreatitis and orchitis.

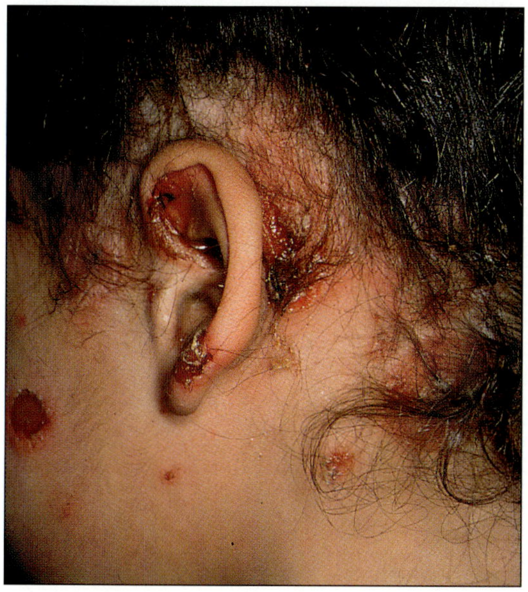

FIGURE 5-12 Secondary staphylococcal infection. Secondary bacterial infections, usually caused by *Staphylococcus aureus* or *Streptococcus pyogenes* (group A β-hemolytic streptococcus) are the most frequent complications of varicella. Secondary bacterial infection is recognized as bullous progression or cellulitis surrounding one or more lesions. Regional lymphadenitis and subcutaneous abscesses may occur. Deep tissue sites of bacterial infection, usually caused by *S. aureus* or *S. pyogenes*, may follow subclinical bacteremia in children with varicella. The common manifestations include staphylococcal or streptococcal pneumonia, arthritis, or osteomyelitis. This child has *S. aureus* superinfection of varicella lesions.

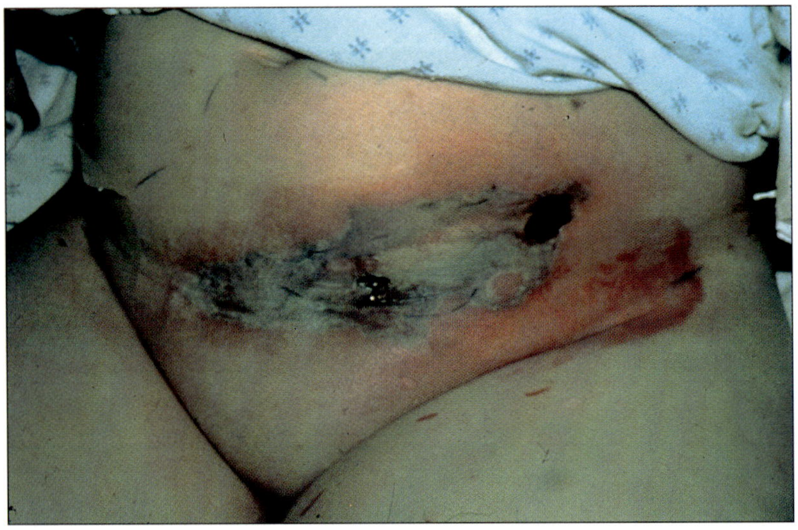

Figure 5-13 Secondary streptococcal infection. Varicella gangrenosa, which is usually caused by *Streptococcus pyogenes*, is diagnosed when an area of rapidly extending erythema, pain, and induration appear around a single lesion, often on the trunk or an extremity. This child has *S. pyogenes* superinfection of varicella lesions. (*From* Smith *et al.* [5]; with permission.)

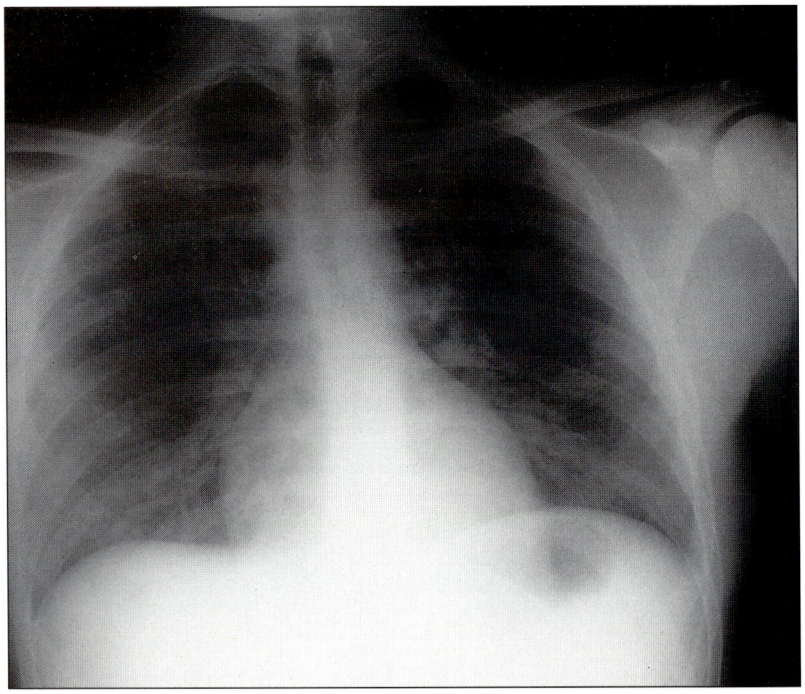

Figure 5-14 Varicella pneumonia. Varicella pneumonia is caused by varicella-zoster virus infection of epithelial cells of the pulmonary alveoli, with mononuclear cell infiltration and edema of the alveolar septae. The interstitial inflammatory process impairs oxygen transfer. Cough and dyspnea develop within 1 to 6 days after the rash appears. Varicella pneumonia can be mild and transient, or progress to severe hypoxemia and respiratory failure. Physical abnormalities may be limited to fever and tachypnea, with few rales. As illustrated in this adult who had pneumonia 72 hours after the onset of varicella, chest radiography usually shows interstitial pneumonitis with diffuse bilateral infiltrates and perihilar, nodular densities.

Consequences of varicella exposure in pregnancy

Immune	Susceptible
No consequences for fetus or newborn	Maternal Varicella pneumonia Premature labor Fetus Congenital varicella syndrome (rare, < 2%) Newborn Perinatal varicella

Figure 5-15 Varicella in pregnancy. Varicella can cause morbidity and mortality in the pregnant woman, the fetus, or newborn infant, but it is a rare complication of pregnancy in the United States because most adults are immune. The incidence was 0.7 per 1000 women in a study of 30,000 pregnancies. The risk of varicella pneumonia appears to be increased during pregnancy. Varicella embryopathy is most often associated with maternal varicella during the first 20 weeks of gestation, but the risk is low, with an incidence of only about 2% based on combined data from available studies. Varicella-zoster virus is transmitted to the fetus in later gestation as shown by immunologic evaluation of infants and the occurrence of herpes zoster during the first few years of life.

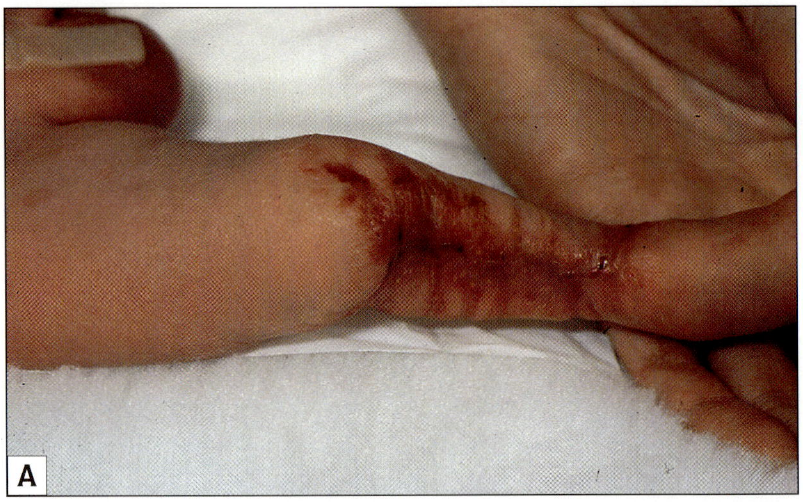

Figure 5-16 Congenital varicella. The congenital varicella syndrome, or varicella embryopathy, is characterized by microcephaly with cortical atrophy and calcifications caused by intrauterine encephalitis, limb hypoplasia, unusual cicatricial skin scars, cutaneous defects and hypopigmentation, chorioretinitis, microophthalmia, cataracts, and damage to the autonomic nervous system. Limb anomalies and other sequelae of intrauterine varicella may be apparent by sonographic evaluation of the fetus. Damage to the autonomic nervous system results in neurogenic bladder, hydroureter, hydronephrosis, and severe gastroesophageal reflux with recurrent aspiration pneumonia. **A,** Unusual skin lesions and limb anomalies that characterize this syndrome.

(continued on next page)

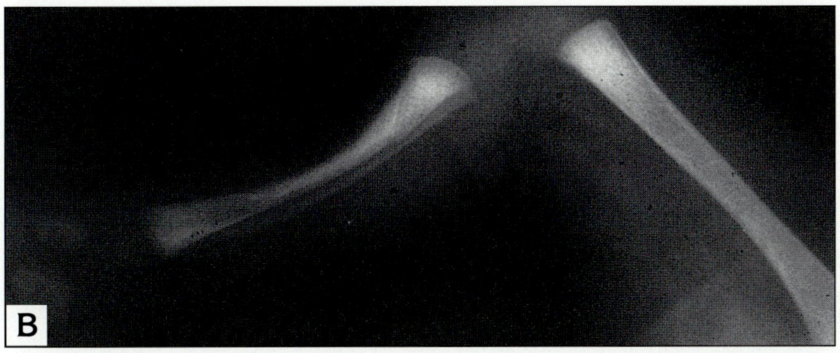

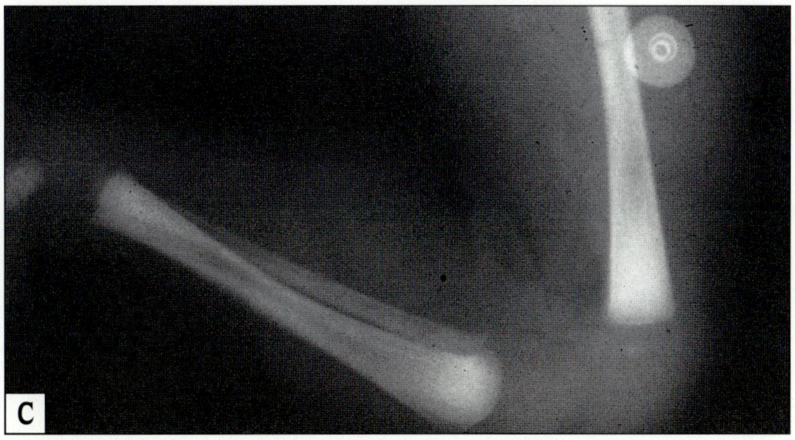

Figure 5-16 *(continued)* **B** and **C**, Radiograph of abnormalities of the long bones and foot in an infant who was exposed to maternal varicella at 13 weeks gestation.

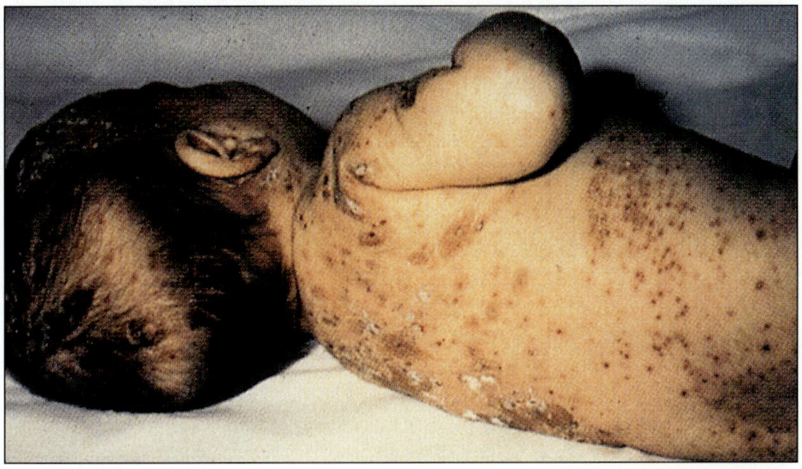

Figure 5-17 Perinatal varicella. Transplacentally acquired IgG antibodies to varicella-zoster virus usually prevent or modify the severity of varicella during the first 6 months of life. Infants whose mothers develop varicella in late gestation are at risk for neonatal varicella. Without passive antibody prophylaxis, the attack rate is about 20% and the mortality rate is about 30% when the mother develops varicella from 4 days before to 2 days after delivery . Infants of mothers with varicella more than 5 days before delivery may have cutaneous varicella lesions at birth or develop lesions within the first 5 days, but they are usually protected by maternal IgG antibodies. Infants exposed to varicella by nonmaternal contact rarely have neonatal disease because most are born to seropositive mothers. This infant had neonatal varicella after maternal infection beginning 24 hours before delivery. (*From* the International Herpes Management Forum [6]; with permission.)

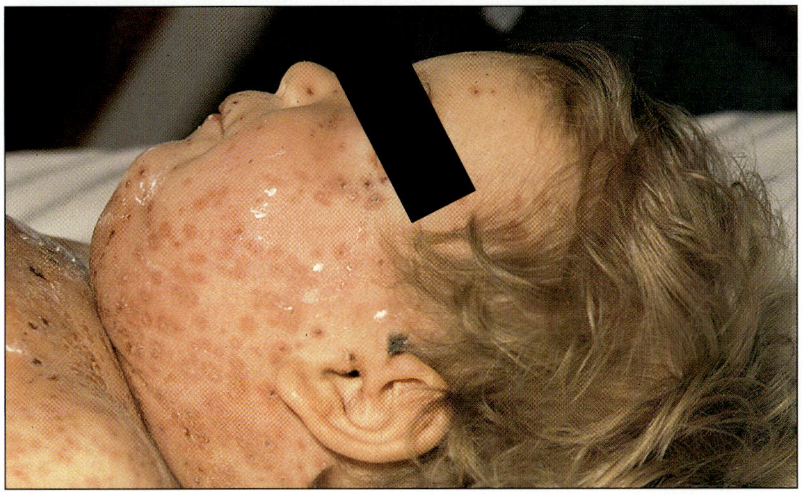

Figure 5-18 Varicella in the immunocompromised child. Before antiviral drugs were available, 30% to 50% of children with lymphoproliferative malignancies or solid tumors developed disseminated varicella, 20% had varicella pneumonia and 7% to 17% had fatal infection. Immunocompromised children who have absolute lymphopenia (<500 mm^3) and delayed cellular immunity are at high risk for progression. Immunocompromised children have prolonged new lesion formation, increased numbers of lesions, and may develop pneumonia, hepatitis, encephalitis, and disseminated intravascular coagulopathy. Children with congenital T-cell immunodeficiencies are at risk for fatal varicella. This child developed varicella while receiving immunosuppression for nephrotic syndrome.

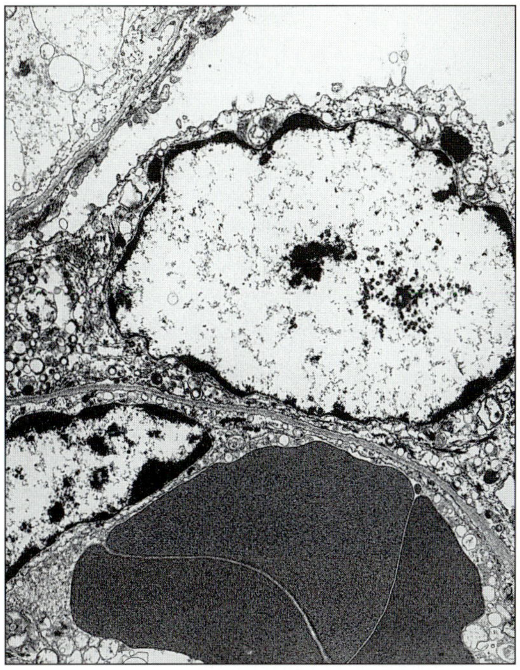

Figure 5-19 Varicella pneumonia in an immunocompromised child. Fatal varicella in immunocompromised children is usually related to pneumonia and respiratory failure. This electron microscopy photograph illustrates the presence of many varicella-zoster virus virions within an alveolar cell of the lung at autopsy from a child with leukemia who died from varicella.

A. Outline of treatment using acyclovir for varicella in healthy children

Rationale: varicella morbidity is unpredictable
Enrollment: 2–12 y, lesions < 24 h
Dosage: 20 mg/kg four times daily

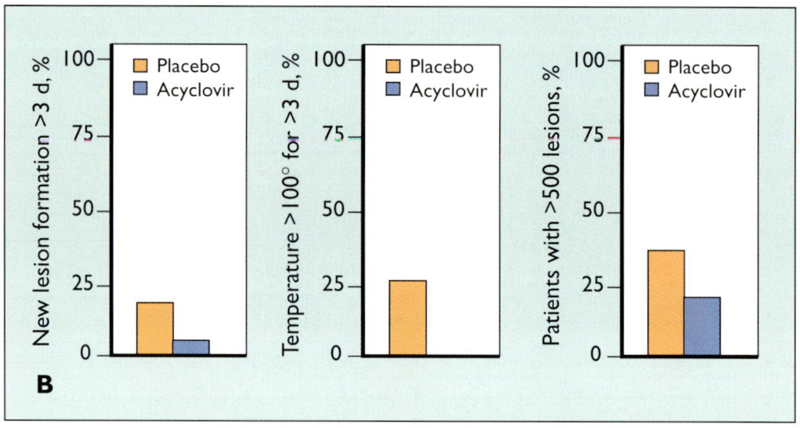

FIGURE 5-20 Treatment of varicella in healthy children. Oral acyclovir is licensed for the treatment of varicella in healthy children and adults. **A,** Treatment rationale, enrollment, and dosage of acyclovir therapy. **B,** Efficacy of acyclovir. Acyclovir decreases the severity of primary varicella-zoster virus infection in otherwise healthy children, adolescents, and adults as long as treatment is started within 24 hours after the appearance of the first cutaneous lesions . Oral acyclovir given at 20 mg/kg four times a day for 5 days reduced the occurrence and number of days of fever, the number of days of new lesion formation, and the total number of cutaneous lesions and pruritis in healthy children (2 to 12 years of age) with varicella. Oral acyclovir treatment also modifies the clinical course of varicella in adolescents and adults. (*Adapted from* Dunkle *et al.* [7]; with permission.)

Treatment of varicella in immunocompromised children

Acyclovir indicated
- Patients
  - Malignancy, bone marrow or organ transplantation, high-dose steroid therapy
  - Congenital T-cell immunodeficiencies
  - Human immunodeficiency virus detection
  - Neonatal varicella after maternal varicella beginning within 5 d before or 2 d after delivery
  - Associated pneumonia or encephalitis
- Administration
  - Initiate as soon as possible after initial lesions appear
  - Intravenous route
  - Dose
    - < 1 y of age: 30 mg/kg/d divided into 8-h doses given as 1-h infusion
    - > 1 y of age: 1.5 g/m^2/d divided into 8-h doses given as 1-h infusion
  - Duration: 7 d or until no new lesions have appeared for 48 h

FIGURE 5-21 Treatment of varicella in immunocompromised children. Acyclovir therapy compensates for the diminished host response in immunocompromised children with varicella, terminating cell-associated viremia and limiting visceral dissemination. The mortality rate of primary varicella-zoster virus infection is decreased by treatment primarily because spread of the virus to lungs is reduced. Acyclovir should be initiated within 24 to 72 hours after the onset of the rash when possible. Because of limited oral absorption, the drug is given intravenously at a dose of 500 mg/m^2 per dose every 8 hours and continued for 7 days or until no new lesions have appeared for at least 48 hours. Intravenous acyclovir is indicated for healthy as well as high-risk patients who have pneumonia, hepatitis, thrombocytopenia or encephalitis. Supportive therapy improves survival significantly because tissue damage to lungs, liver, and other organs caused by varicella-zoster virus is reversible in many cases. (*Adapted from* the American Academy of Pediatrics [8]; with permission.)

Use of varicella-zoster immunoglobulin for prophylaxis in high-risk populations

Patients at risk
- Immunocompromised children with no history of varicella
- Pregnant women with no history of varicella and no antibodies to VZV*
- Infants born to mothers whose varicella begins within 5 d before or 2 d after delivery
- Premature infants < 28 wk of gestation or < 1000 g and hospitalized premature infants with no maternal history of varicella, antibodies to VZV, or both

Criteria for exposure
- Varicella
  - Household contact
  - Close indoor contact defined as face-to-face exposure to playmate, schoolmate, or other infected individual
  - Hospital contact with an index case in the same room, open ward, or nursery
  - Hospital contact by face-to-face exposure to an infected patient, staff member, visitor, or other individual
  - Newborn exposure to maternal varicella
- Herpes zoster
  - Intimate, direct contact with infected individual
- Administration of VZIG
  - VZIG must be given within 96 h and, when possible, within 48 h after the exposure
  - Dose: 1 vial (125 U)/10 kg body weight (maximum 5 vials) by intramuscular injection†

* Serologic testing is recommended when results can be obtained immediately because most adult women with no history of varicella are immune.

† VZIG must not be given intravenously.

Figure 5-22 Varicella-zoster immunoglobulin (VZIG). Passive antibodies present during the early incubation period can modify the acquisition or severity of varicella. VZIG is made from immunoglobulin with high titers of IgG antibodies against varicella-zoster virus (VZV). VZIG prophylaxis is indicated for susceptible high-risk individuals, including immunocompromised children and pregnant women, who have had a close exposure to an individual with varicella or herpes zoster and who can be given VZIG within 96 hours after the exposure; newborns exposed to maternal varicella should also receive VZIG. Some high-risk patients develop varicella despite VZIG prophylaxis and may require acyclovir therapy. (*Adapted from* the American Academy of Pediatrics [8]; with permission.)

Recommendations concerning varicella immunization

Indications
- Age 12 mo–13 y: susceptible by history; one dose
- Age 13 y–young adult: consider serologic testing; two doses with 4–8-wk interval

Precautions
- With susceptible immunocompromised patients
- With pregnant women
- With newborns

Contraindications
- Exposure: varicella or herpes zoster within previous 21 d
- Acute febrile illness
- Underlying diseases
  - Congenital and acquired immunodeficiencies, blood dyscrasias
  - Leukemia, lymphoma, other malignancies*
  - Symptomatic HIV infection
- Immunosuppression
  - Radiation or chemotherapy
  - Steroid therapy: prednisone ≥ 2 mg/kg/d for ≥ 1 mo or equivalent
- Allergy: neomycin, gelatin, or other vaccine components
- Treatment
  - Immunoglobulin or other blood products within 5 mo
  - Salicylates within previous 6 wk†
- Pregnancy

* Available for children with acute leukemia in remission at least 1 y on clinical study protocol coordinated by Merck and Co., Inc., West Point, PA.

† Unless the risk of natural varicella outweighs the theoretical concern of possible Reye's syndrome.

Figure 5-23 Recommendations regarding live attenuated varicella vaccination. The live attenuated varicella vaccine preparations contain the Oka strain of varicella-zoster virus, a clinical isolate that was passaged in guinea pig embryo fibroblasts and expanded for vaccine production in human diploid cells. The vaccine induced protection against household exposure with an efficacy rate of more than 95% in an initial placebo-controlled study and vaccine efficacy has been documented in open trials based on the predicted annual attack rates. Herpes zoster is less frequent among vaccines than expected with natural infection, but long-term surveillance is required to confirm this observation. (*Adapted from* Arvin [9]; with permission.)

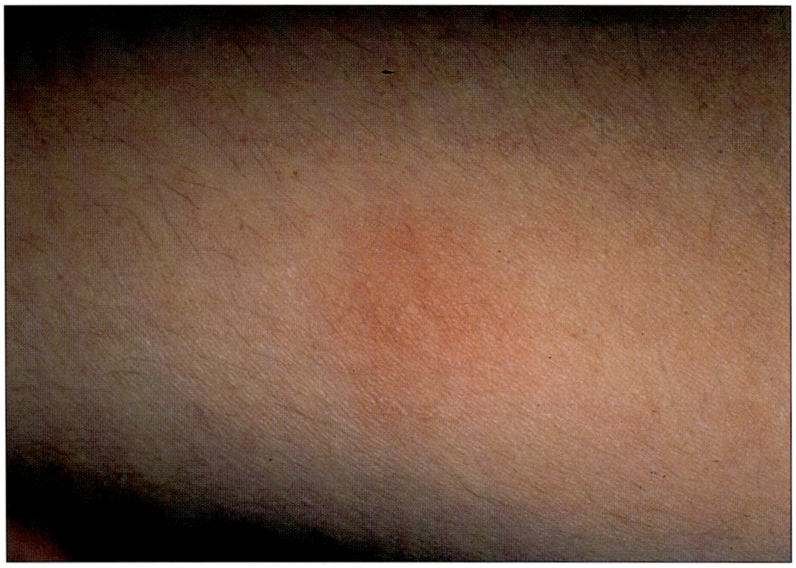

FIGURE 5-24 Vaccine rash. Varicella vaccine is tolerated well by healthy children. Some recipients have a vaccine-associated rash, with an average of six lesions (range, one to 47). This vesicular rash occurred at the injection site in an adult vaccinee from whom the vaccine virus was isolated. (*Adapted from* Arvin [9]; with permission.)

Protective efficacy of varicella immunization in healthy children by active surveillance

		Incidence of breakthrough varicella/y, %				
Vaccine lot	**PFU/dose**	**1**	**2**	**3**	**4**	**5**
1987	1000–1625	3.0 (*n*=2994)	3.3 (*n*=2415)	4.4 (*n*=911)	4.3 (*n*=538)	4.5 (*n*=376)
1991	2900–9000	0.6 (*n*=955)	0.8 (*n*=717)			

FIGURE 5-25 Protective efficacy of varicella vaccine. Immunization with Oka strain vaccines effectively prevents primary varicella-zoster virus infection in most healthy children. Vaccine-induced immunity is less likely than natural immunity to be completely protective against symptoms after close exposure, but the clinical course of varicella is altered significantly in most cases. This table provides a comprehensive analysis of the protective efficacy of the Oka/Merck vaccine as submitted to the U.S. Food and Drug Administration in support of licensure. PFU—plaque-forming unit. (*Adapted from* Krause and Klinman [10]; with permission.)

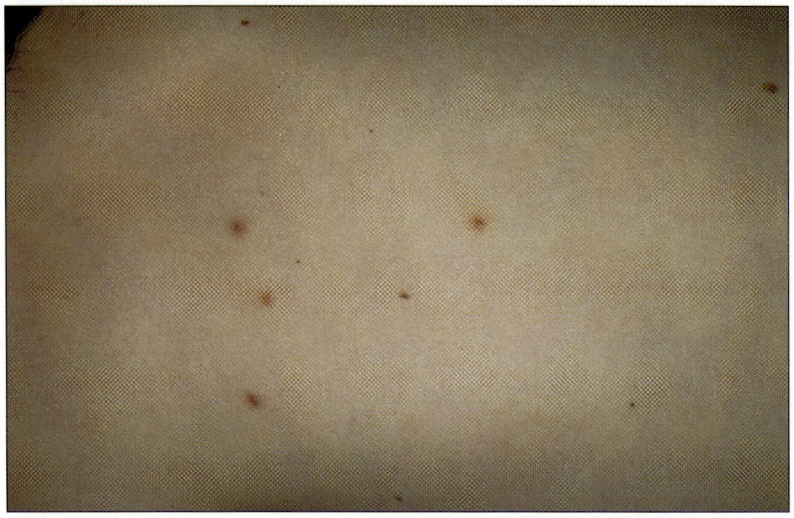

FIGURE 5-26 Modified varicella in vaccine recipients. Some children and adults with vaccine-induced immunity develop mild breakthrough infections after exposure to natural virus, but the illness is characterized by fewer than 50 cutaneous lesions with no fever in most cases. Symptoms of varicella are modified substantially by vaccine-induced immunity. This photograph illustrates the scattered lesions of modified breakthrough varicella.

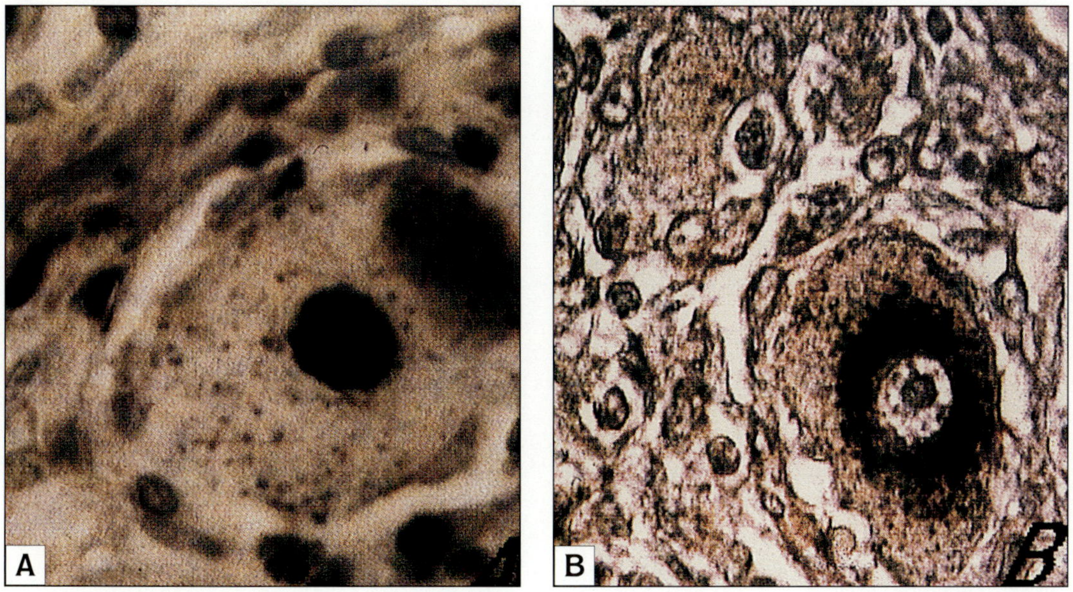

FIGURE 5-27 Varicella-zoster virus (VZV) latency. Persistent infection of cells in the dorsal root ganglia is probably a consequence of all primary VZV infections . VZV may reach dorsal root ganglia from mucocutaneous lesions by an ascending route along neuronal cell axons or the virus may be carried to these sites by infected T cells before cutaneous lesions appear. Current studies indicate that VZV persists in satellite cells that surround neurons in ganglia as well as some neurons. Low-level transcription of some viral genes appears to persist during latent VZV infection. During latency, memory T cells that recognize VZV proteins are maintained at frequencies of approximately 1:40,000 peripheral blood mononuclear cells in immune adults. These responses may persist because of periodic reexposures of immune individuals to VZV or by subclinical reactivations of latent virus. **A,** *In situ* hybridization of right T11 illustrates AP signal in the nucleus and cytoplasm of neurons and in the nucleus of satellite cells. **B,** *In situ* hybridization of left L4 illustrating AP signal in the nucleus of neurons and satellite cells but not in the cytoplasm of neurons. (*From* Lungu *et al.* [11]; with permission.)

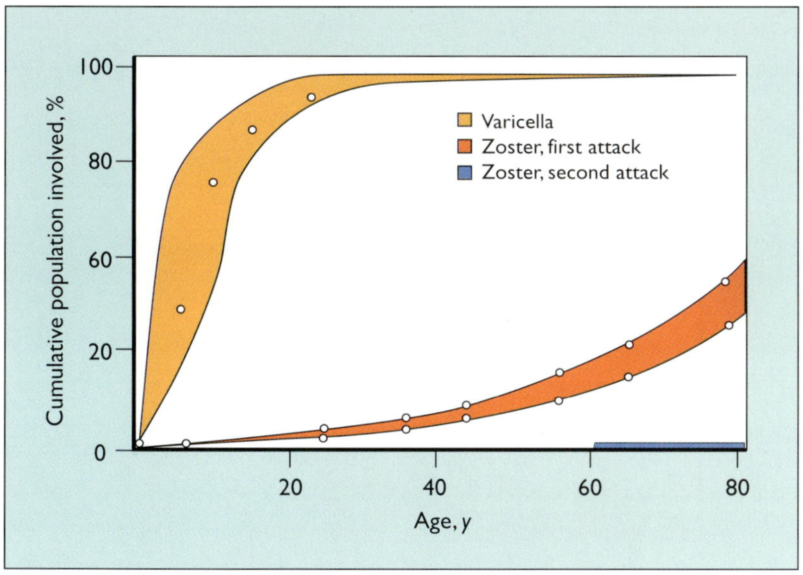

FIGURE 5-28 The epidemiology of herpes zoster. Herpes zoster occurs only in individuals who have had primary varicella-zoster virus infection and results from the reactivation of endogenous, latent virus. Early studies defined the incidence of herpes zoster as 3.4 cases per 1000 persons per year in the United Kingdom. The incidence increases with age, to more than 10 cases per 1000 persons by 75 years. Herpes zoster is very unusual in children. (*Adapted from* Hope-Simpson [12]; with permission.)

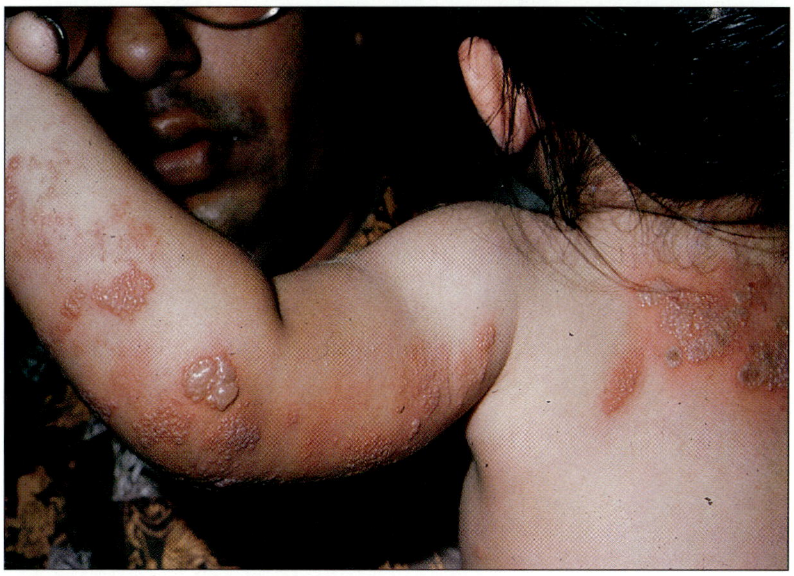

FIGURE 5-29 Herpes zoster rash. Varicella-zoster virus reactivation from latency causes a localized, unilateral, pruritic vesicular rash involving the dermatomal distribution of one or more adjacent sensory nerves. The rash is often preceded by several days of pain, and acute pain and hypersensitivity accompany the rash. The vesicles coalesce into larger, fluid-filled lesions as the infection progresses. Scattered cutaneous lesions outside the primary dermatome are observed occasionally.

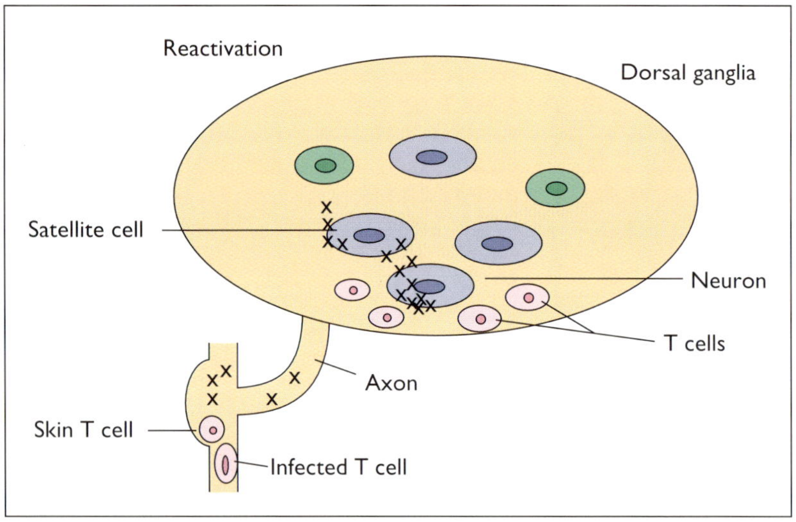

Figure 5-30 Host–virus interactions in herpes zoster. Host as well as viral factors determine whether symptomatic varicella-zoster virus (VZV) reactivation occurs. Diminished T-cell responses to VZV in the elderly and immunocompromised patients result in an increased risk of herpes zoster. Histopathologic studies of ganglia during VZV reactivation show extensive inflammation and necrosis. The virus probably reaches the skin after cell-to-cell spread in ganglia transfers it into sensory neural axons for transport to cutaneous cells. Infectious virus may be transported along multiple axons because clusters of lesions appear in scattered areas of the involved dermatome. Inflammation and necrosis from VZV reactivation sometimes extend into the anterior horn cells, producing myelitis and deficits of motor function. The histopathologic changes in the skin resemble varicella lesions .

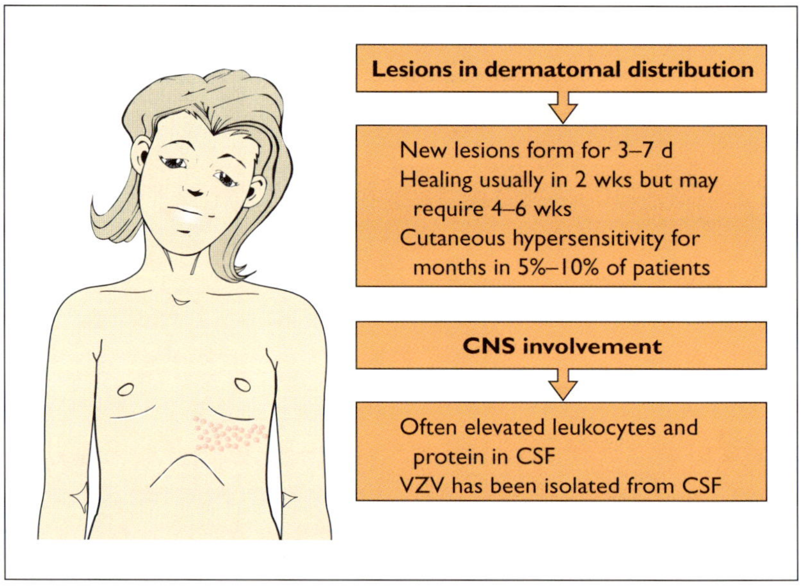

Figure 5-31 Clinical course of herpes zoster. New lesion formation usually stops within 3 to 7 days; cutaneous healing usually occurs within 2 weeks but may require 4 to 6 weeks. Patients often have elevated leukocyte counts and protein level in cerebrospinal fluid (CSF), and varicella-zoster virus (VZV) has been isolated from the CSF. Cutaneous hypersensitivity persists for several months among 5% to 10% of patients.

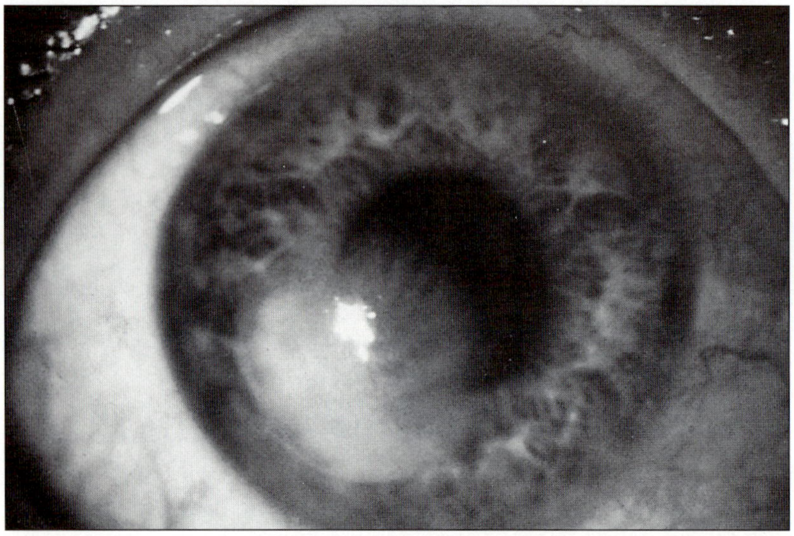

Figure 5-32 Ocular manifestations of herpes zoster. Although varicella-zoster virus reactivation involving the ophthalmic branch of the trigeminal nerve may be associated with conjunctivitis, dendritic keratitis, anterior uveitis, iridocyclitis, and panophthalmitis, blindness following herpes zoster ophthalmicus is rare. Vision loss following herpes zoster is usually caused by retrobulbar neuritis and optic atrophy. Varicella-zoster virus retinitis occurs in severely immunocompromised patients. (*From* Liesegang [13]; with permission.)

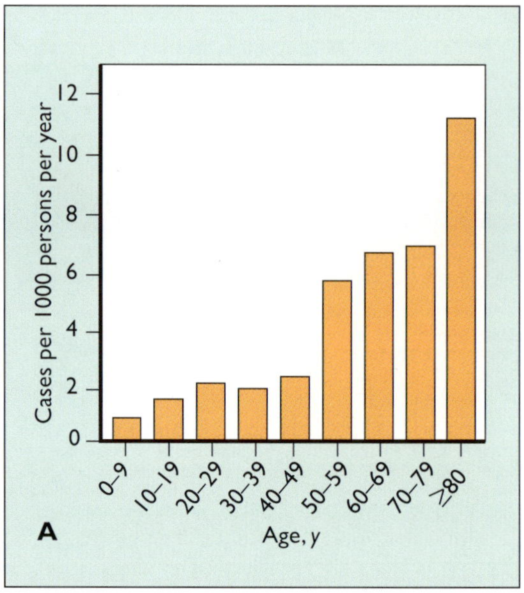

Figure 5-33 Postherpetic neuralgia. Postherpetic neuralgia is the most common and debilitating complication of herpes zoster. The risk of postherpetic neuralgia increases with increasing age. Postherpetic neuralgia persists after resolution of the cutaneous rash. **A,** Annual incidence of herpes zoster per 1000 persons in a general medical practice.

(continued on next page)

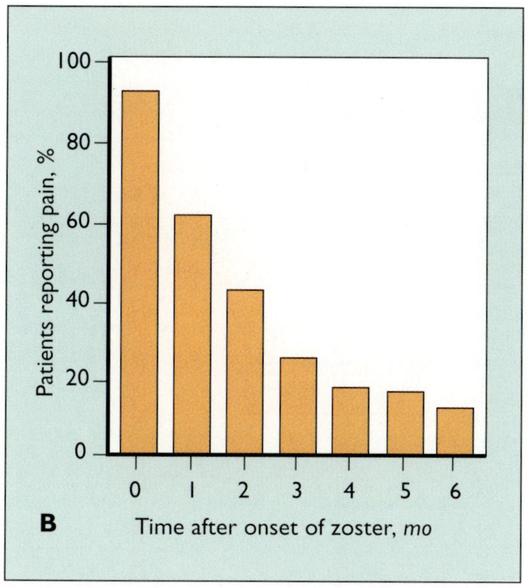

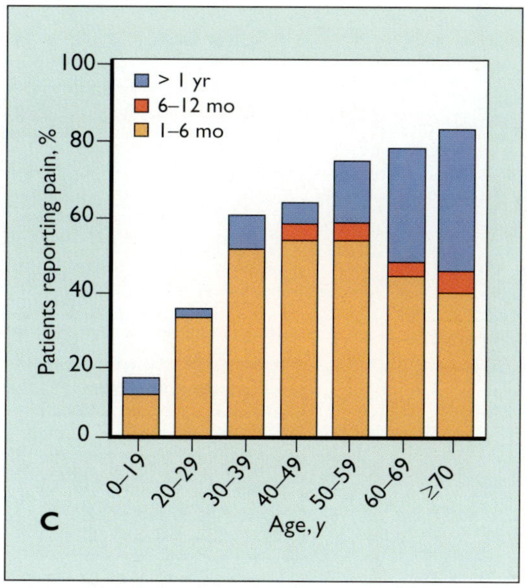

FIGURE 5-33 *(continued)* **B**, Percentage of patients with pain persisting after the onset of the zoster-associated rash (data are from the placebo group in one large, double-blind treatment study). **C**, Proportion of patients with postherpetic neuralgia according to age. (*Adapted from* Kost and Straus [14]; with permission.)

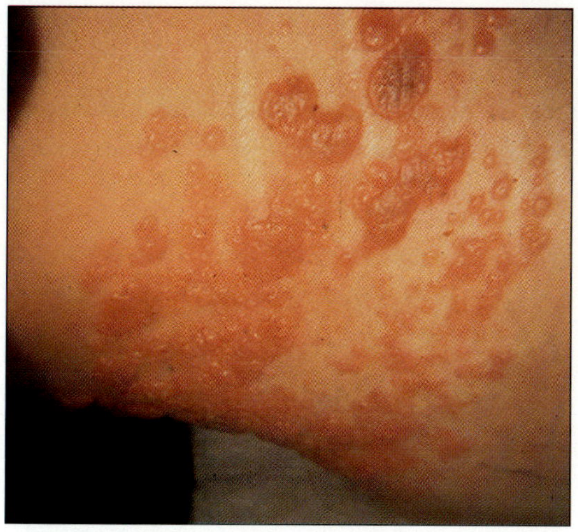

FIGURE 5-34 Herpes zoster in an immunocompromised patient. Herpes zoster is common among patients who are treated with immunosuppressive drugs for cancer, to prevent rejection of bone marrow or organ transplants, for chronic inflammatory diseases, and among individuals with HIV infection. This photograph shows the local rash in a patient with cancer.

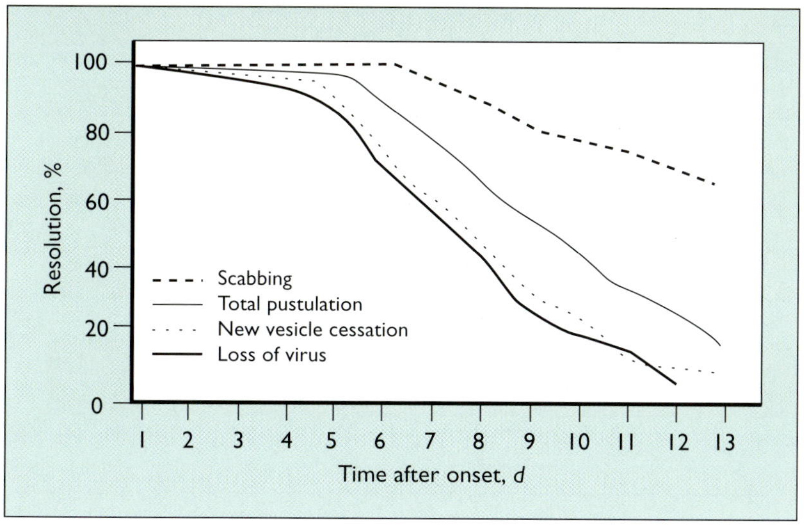

FIGURE 5-35 Clinical course of herpes zoster in immunocompromised patients. Herpes zoster in immunocompromised patients is often associated with a more extensive and prolonged local rash. Immunosuppression increases the morbidity and mortality associated with herpes zoster, primarily caused by the occurrence of pneumonia, but the overall risk of fatal recurrent varicella-zoster virus is less than 1%. Some immunocompromised patients develop relapsing or chronic varicella-zoster virus reactivation. (*Adapted from* Whitley [15]; with permission.)

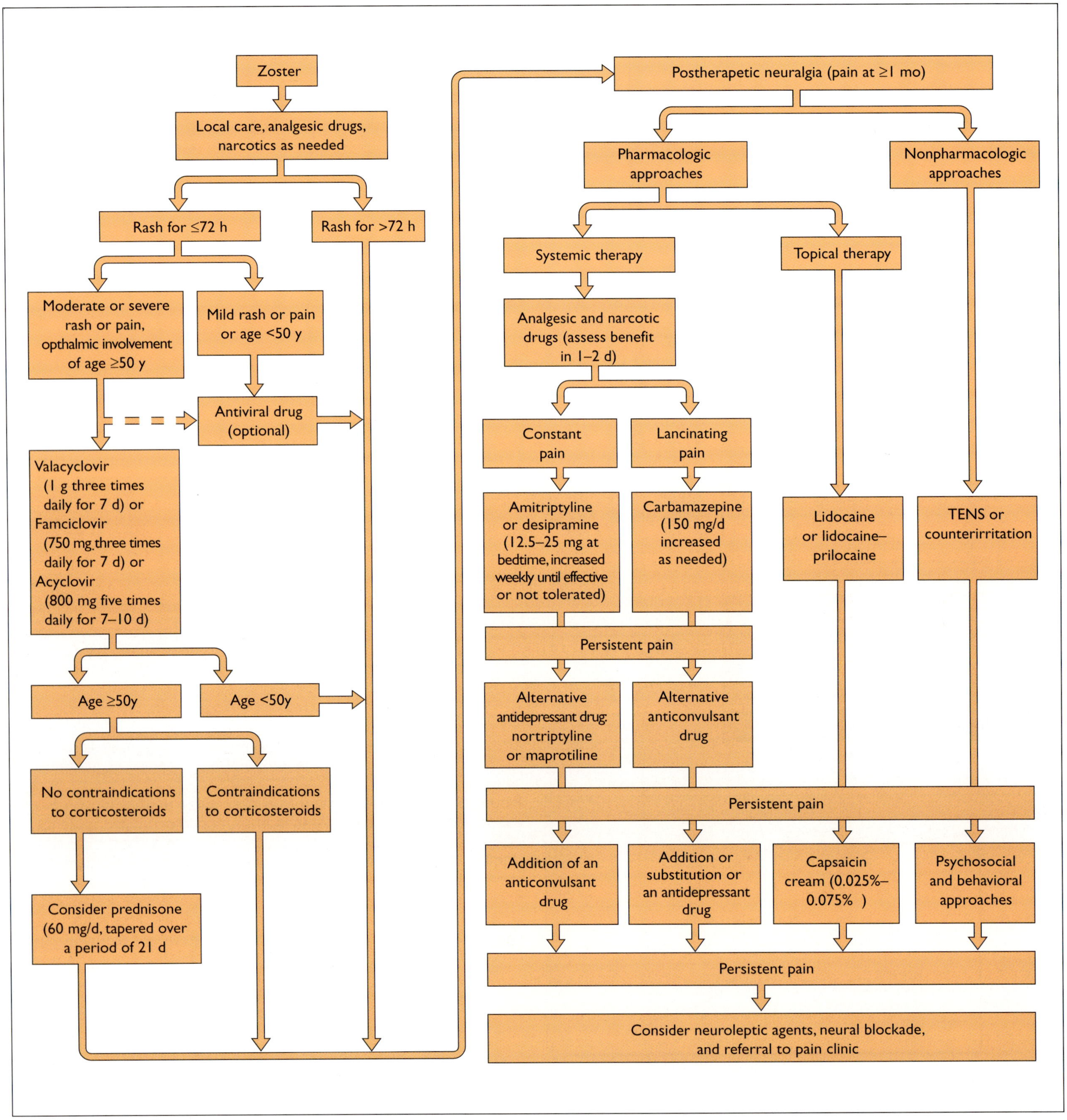

FIGURE 5-36 Treatment of herpes zoster. Herpes zoster in healthy and immunocompromised patients can be treated effectively with acyclovir, valacyclovir, or famciclovir. Herpes zoster in healthy individuals does not always require antiviral treatment. Elderly individuals who are 60 years of age or older are most likely to benefit; ophthalmic zoster should be treated because of the risk of acute uveitis and chronic keratitis. The number of days of new lesion formation, extent of dermatomal involvement, and the time to crusting and healing are shortened with antiviral therapy. Acute pain is also less severe. Recurrent episodes of herpes zoster occur in some immunocompromised patients within a few days or weeks after acyclovir therapy is stopped, but most patients respond to treatment with a second course of acyclovir. As is true in other herpesvirus infections, antiviral therapy does not eliminate varicella-zoster virus (VZV) from the host. Prolonged acyclovir therapy can select for thymidine kinase–negative VZV mutants. Newer agents, such as famciclovir and valacyclovir, inhibit VZV by the same mechanisms as acyclovir and are therefore not effective against thymidine kinase–negative VZV strains. Foscarnet and interferon alfa are unrelated agents that have some clinical efficacy in high-risk patients and are current alternative agents for treatment of acyclovir-resistant VZV infections. TENS—transcutaneous electrical nerve stimulation. (*Adapted from* Kost and Straus [14]; with permission.)

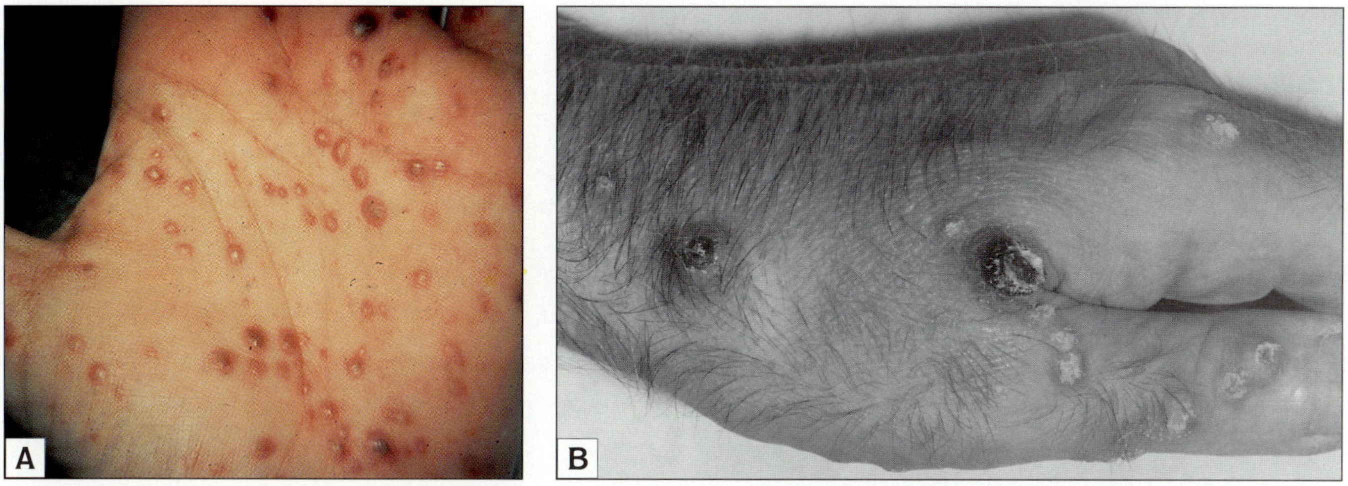

FIGURE 5-37 Herpes zoster in patients with HIV infection. **A**, Rash in disseminated herpes zoster. Immunocompromised patients with VZV reactivation may develop VZV viremia with dissemination to lung, liver, central nervous system and other organs. Visceral dissemination may occur in immunocompromised patients without cutaneous herpes zoster. This photograph illustrates the cutaneous rash of disseminated herpes zoster in a bone marrow transplant recipient. The rash cannot be differentiated from varicella lesions by clinical appearance unless it is accompanied by lesions in the typical localized, dermatomal distribution. **B**, Epidermal hyperplasia in a patient with AIDS. Herpes zoster is an early clinical sign of HIV infection in high-risk populations. These patients are at risk for progressive, disseminated, or chronic varicella-zoster virus (VZV) reactivation. Some episodes of retinitis and progressive central nervous system infection in patients with AIDS are caused by VZV. The unusual complications of VZV in these patients may occur in the absence of or after the resolution of cutaneous lesions. As shown in this photograph, recurrent VZV lesions in patients with AIDS are characterized by epidermal hyperplasia. VZV reactivation is also a cause of retinitis in HIV-infected patients. (*Panel B from* Arvin [3]; with permission.)

Prevention of herpes zoster

Reconstitution by inactivated varicella vaccine after bone marrow transplantation

	Vaccine	No vaccine
Total lesions	13 (3–24)	400 (100– > 500)
New lesions	6 d (2–21)	5 d (3–9)
Crusting	8 d (1–28)	11 d (7–20)
Acute pain	4 d (0–7)	18 d (7–21)
Acyclovir	1/5*	3/5*
PHN	0/5*	4/5*
Severity score	6.4±1.0	11.8±1.1 (*P*=0.007)

*Number of patients affected/total.

FIGURE 5-38 Prevention of herpes zoster. The efficacy of acyclovir prophylaxis for varicella-zoster virus (VZV) suppression has been evaluated in bone marrow transplant recipients who are at high risk for recurrent VZV infections. An inhibitory effect can be shown during acyclovir administration, but VZV reactivation occurs when acyclovir is discontinued. Because the increased occurrence of herpes zoster with age is caused by waning immunity to VZV, therapeutic vaccination with varicella vaccine may provide a strategy to prevent herpes zoster in otherwise healthy elderly patients. Immunization with inactivated varicella vaccine reduced the severity of herpes zoster in immunocompromised patients. PHN—postherpetic neuralgia. (*Adapted from* Redman *et al.* [16]; with permission.)

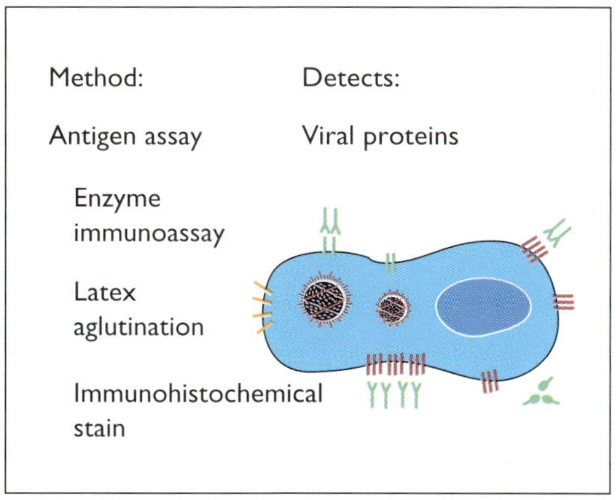

FIGURE 5-39 Diagnosis of varicella-zoster virus (VZV) by virus detection. Virologic methods for the laboratory diagnosis of VZV detect the presence of infectious virus, viral DNA, or viral protein in clinical specimens. Immunofluorescence or immunoperoxidase stains allow rapid identification of VZV in specimens of epithelial cells from suspected VZV lesions. Optimal sensitivity of these methods requires obtaining cells from the base of the lesion after unroofing a fresh vesicle or vesicles. Viral culture is less useful because of the relatively prolonged time required to detect cytopathic changes. Hybridization and polymerase chain reaction methods are sensitive and specific for the detection of VZV in clinical specimens.

REFERENCES

1. Arvin AM: Varicella-zoster virus. In *Virology*, edn 3. Edited by Fields BN, Knipe DM, Howley PH: Philadelphia/New York: Lippincott-Raven; 1995:2547–2586.
2. Preblud SR: Varicella: complications and costs. *Pediatrics* 1986, 78:728–735.
3. Arvin AM: Varicella-zoster virus. In *Principles and Practices of Pediatric Infectious Diseases.* Edited by Long S, Prober C, Pickering L. Philadelphia/New York: Lippincott-Raven; 1997:1144–1153.
4. Moffat J, Zerboni L, Stein M, *et al.*: The attenuation of the vaccine Oka strain of varicella-zoster virus and the role of glycoprotein C in alphaherpesvirus virulence demonstrated in the SCID-hu mouse. *J Virol* 1998, 72:965–974.
5. Smith EW, Garson A, Bolyston JA, *et al.*: Varicella gangrenosa due to beta-hemolytic group A steptococci. *Pediatrics* 1976, 57:306–310.
6. International Herpes Management Forum: *Diagnosis of Herpesvirus Infections.* West Sussex, UK: PPS Europe; 1994.
7. Dunkle LM, Arvin AM, Whitley RJ, *et al.*: A controlled trial of acyclovir for chickenpox in normal children. *N Engl J Med* 1991, 325:1539–1544.
8. American Academy of Pediatrics: Varicella-zoster infections. In *Report of the Committee on Infectious Diseases*, edn 24. American Academy of Pediatrics; 1997:573–585.
9. Arvin AM: The varicella vaccine. In *Current Clinical Topics in Infectious Diseases.* Edited by Remington J, Swartz M, Malden MA: Blackwell Science; 1997:100–137.
10. Krause P, Klinman DM: Efficacy, immunogenicity, safety, and use of live attenuated chickenpox vaccine. *J Pediatr* 1995, 127:518–525.
11. Lungu O, Annunziato PW, Gershon A, *et al.*: Reactivated and latent varicella-zoster virus in human dorsal root ganglia. *Proc Natl Acad Sci U S A* 1995, 92:10980–10984.
12. Hope-Simpson RE: The nature of herpes zoster: a long-term study and a new hypothesis. *Proc R Soc Med* 1965, 58:9–20.
13. Liesegang TJ: Ocular viral infections: varicella-zoster virus. In *Antiviral Agents and Viral Diseases of Man.* Edited by Galasso G, Whitley R, Merigan T. New York: Lippincott-Raven; 1997:229–255.
14. Kost RG, Straus SE: Postherpetic neuralgia: pathogenesis, treatment and prevention. *N Engl J Med* 1996, 335:32–42.
15. Whitley RJ: Varicella zoster virus infections. In *Antiviral Agents and Viral Diseases of Man.* Edited by Galasso G, Whitley R, Merigan T. New York: Lippincott-Raven; 1997:279–304.
16. Redman RL, Nader S, Zerboni L, *et al.*: Early reconstitution of immunity and decreased severity of herpes zoster in bone marrow transplant recipients immunized with inactivated varicella vaccine. *J Infect Dis* 1997, 176:578–585.

CHAPTER 6

Enteroviruses

Mark J. Abzug
Eric A.F. Simoes

ENTEROVIRUSES ARE positive-stranded RNA viruses that are ubiquitous and cause more morbidity than mortality. There are approximately 70 enteroviruses, which are so named because the primary site of viral replication is the gastrointestinal tract. However, they cause a variety of infections in distant sites due to their spread (viremia) to other organs. These infections may be nonspecific (febrile illnesses) or affect multiple organ systems (liver, central nervous system, heart) or localize to a single organ system (poliomyelitis). The best-studied enteroviruses are the polioviruses (three types). Enteroviruses are notorious for the significant morbidity that they cause in the newborn, and they are frequent causes of viral illnesses with rash or ulcers, myocarditis, aseptic meningitis, hemorrhagic conjunctivitis, and encephalomyelitis. Because of the large number of enterovirus serotypes that cause disease and the poor understanding of the pathogenesis of some of the immune-mediated manifestations of enterovirus infections, vaccines have not been developed for nonpolio enteroviruses. However, the understanding of the virus at the molecular and ultrastructural level has resulted in the development of a class of antiviral compounds (the "WIN" compounds) that show promise in the treatment of some of these severe infections. The significant disease caused by polioviruses in adolescents in developing countries in the 1950s led to development of two types of vaccines: a live attenuated oral poliovirus vaccine (Sabin) and a killed injectable vaccine (Salk). Because there are only three serotypes and immunity is long-lasting, vaccines have been successful in eradicating the disease from the Western hemisphere; it is hoped that the strategy of "National Immunization Days" will eradicate this once-dreaded disease from the world within the next 5 to 10 years.

VIROLOGY

Classification of human enteroviruses

Family: Picornaviridae
Genus: Enterovirus
Subgroups:
- Polioviruses (serotypes 1–3)
- Coxsackieviruses A (serotypes A1–A22, A24*)
- Coxsackieviruses B (serotypes B1–B6)
- Echoviruses (serotypes 1–9, 11–27, 29–33†)
- Numbered enteroviruses (serotypes 68–71‡)

* Coxsackievirus A23 was previously identified as echovirus 9

† Echoviruses 10 and 28 have been reclassified as nonenteroviruses; echovirus 34 was previously identified as coxsackievirus A24.

‡ Enterovirus 72 (hepatitis A virus) has been reclassified.

FIGURE 6-1 Classification of human enteroviruses. The human enteroviruses are within the family Picornaviridae, so named because they are small (pico), RNA-containing viruses. The Picornaviridae family also includes the genus *Rhinovirus* (which includes the human rhinoviruses), the genus *Hepatovirus* (which includes hepatitis A virus), and other genera containing related animal viruses. The genus *Enterovirus* is divided into subgroups based on replication patterns in tissue culture and animals. Newer enteroviruses are now simply numbered. Species (serotypes) are distinguished by antigenic differences.

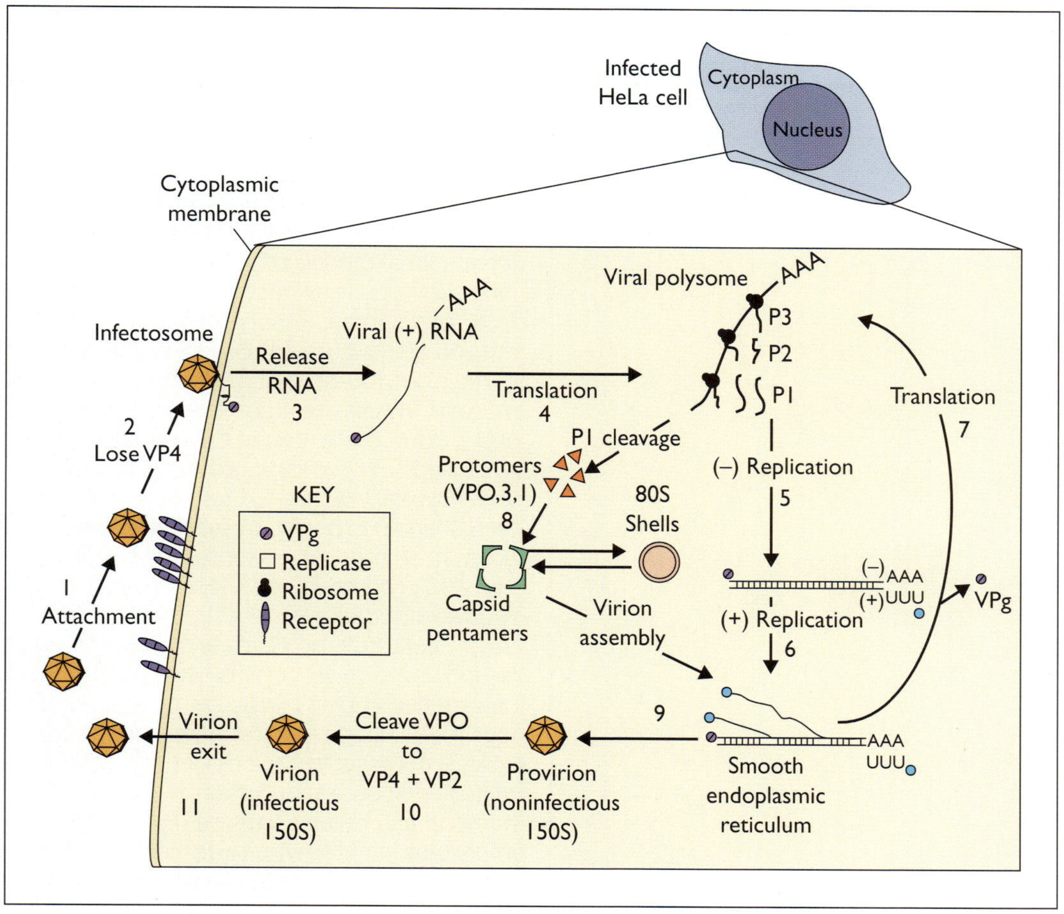

FIGURE 6-2 The cycle of infection of enteroviruses. After attachment of the enterovirus (1) to the surface receptor, a conformational change occurs in the surface capsid proteins (2), resulting in release of viral RNA into the cytoplasm of the cell (3) where all further multiplication occurs. Because all enteroviruses are positive-stranded RNA viruses, translation of viral RNA occurs immediately (4). This viral strand directs the synthesis of a polyprotein that undergoes self-cleavage by proteinases encoded in the polyprotein. The first fragment released is the precursor protein (P1), followed by the midpiece precursor protein (P2) and, eventually, the terminal segment (P3). These segments undergo self-cleavage into 10 to 11 proteins that are involved in replication, including synthesis of complementary negative-stranded RNA (5), which then serves as a template for synthesis of further positive strands (6). These strands are then cycled into the pool of translating positive-stranded RNA species (7). Cleavage of P1 (8) triggers assembly of the products (protomers) into capsid pentamers (8) that package the positive-stranded RNA into noninfectious provirion particles (9). Cleavage of one of the capsid protomers (VPO) at this stage into VP4 and VP2 result in the production of infectious virions (10), which are released from the cell by cytolysis (11). (*Adapted from* Rueckert [1]; with permission.)

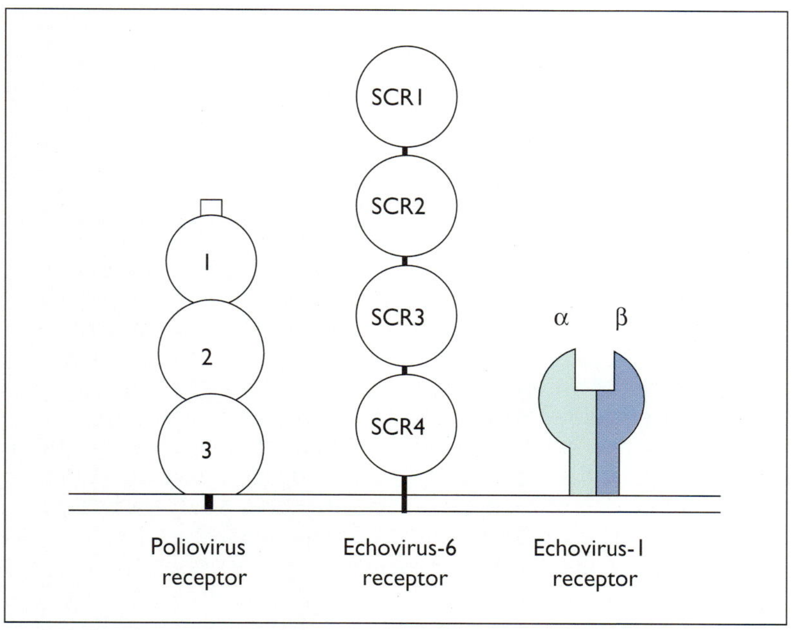

FIGURE 6-3 Three classes of enterovirus receptors. The poliovirus receptor (PVR) is a member of the immunoglobulin super-family with three structural domains (1 to 3) in a single chain. Domain 1 of the PVR binds poliovirus and is responsible for infection. Domain 2 is *N*-glycosylated, and is also responsible for attachment, but glycosylation may modify poliovirus–PVR affinity. Echoviruses (6,7,13,21,29,33) use the decay-accelerating factor (DAF/CD55) complement regulatory protein as a receptor. DAF has four short consensus repeat sequences (SCRs) approximately 60 amino acids long that show significant homology to each other. Internalization of the virus receptor complex may occur after interaction with a secondary (as yet unidentified) factor. Certain echoviruses (1,8) use the integrin VLA-2 as a receptor. VLA-2 consists of two polypeptide chains, the α chain and the β chain, which are anchored in the membrane by their α chain. The identity of receptors for other echoviruses that use neither DAF or VLA-2 is unknown. Intercellular adhesion molecule-1 may be the receptor for coxsackie A viruses.

Pathogenesis

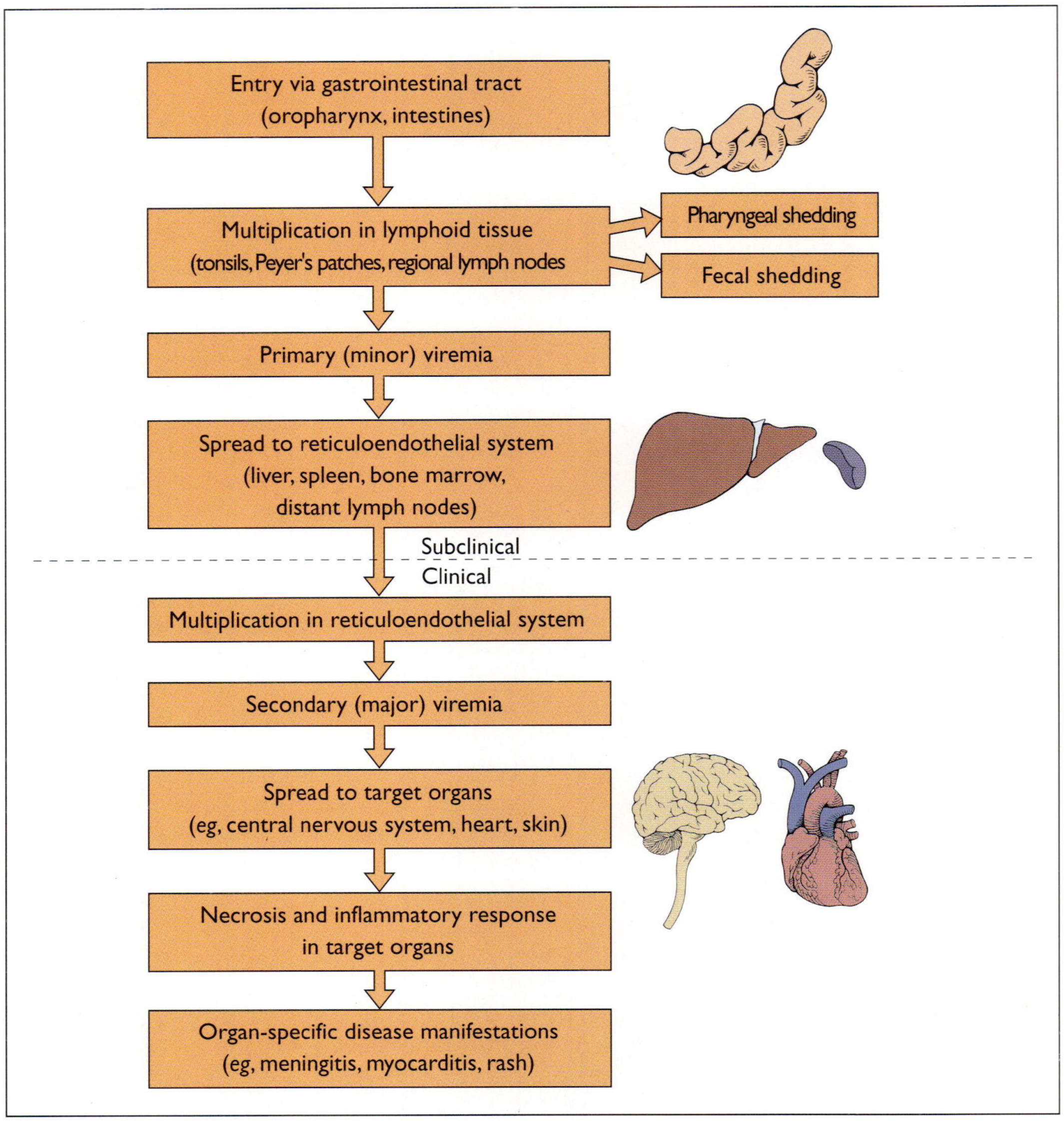

Figure 6-4 Pathogenesis of enterovirus infections. This outline of the presumed pathogenesis of enterovirus infections is largely based on experimental data derived from animal models of infection. Enterovirus infections are transmitted primarily by fecal–oral spread, although respiratory transmission also occurs. Initial replication occurs in the pharynx and gastrointestinal tract; mucosal M cells are a possible site of viral entry. Local replication in the gastrointestinal tract leads to oropharyngeal shedding of virus (typically lasting <4 wk) and prolonged fecal shedding (6 wk). In subclinical infections, host immune responses limit replication and progression of infection beyond the reticuloendothelial system. In clinical infections, replication proceeds and virus spreads to additional target organs, with tropism determined in part by the serotype of infecting virus. Disease manifestations are a result of local necrosis and the responding inflammatory response to infection. Although both humoral and cellular defenses appear to be important in enterovirus infections, humoral immunity appears to be the predominant arm in the control and recovery from enterovirus infections.

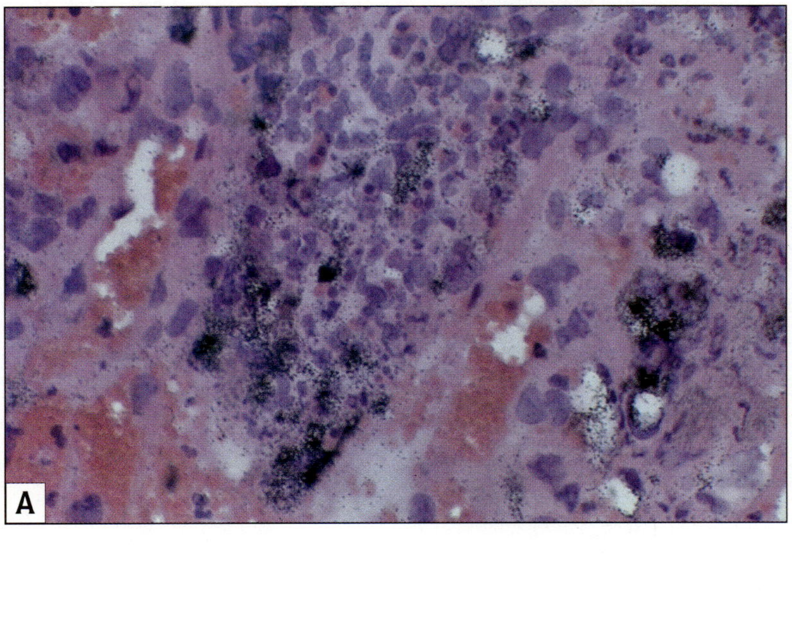

Figure 6-5 Animal models of enterovirus infection. Numerous models of poliovirus and nonpoliovirus enterovirus infections have been established in animals ranging from mice to primates to study mechanisms of viral spread, tissue damage, host response, and treatment of enterovirus diseases such as paralytic disease, meningoencephalitis, myocarditis, and intrauterine infection. Newer virologic methods, including immunofluorescence, in situ hybridization, and the polymerase chain reaction have aided in these studies. One murine model established to study vertical transmission uses Theiler's murine encephalomyelitis virus (TMEV), a picornavirus that biologically behaves similarly to enteroviruses and is a natural pathogen of mice. Infection of pregnant mice in early gestation produces both extensive viral infection and damage in the vascular labyrinth layer of the murine placenta. **A,** Areas of hyalinization and hemorrhage in an infected placenta (× 40). *Black grains* indicate the presence of TMEV RNA detected by in situ hybridization. Transplacental infection occurs following maternal inoculation in early pregnancy, producing infection of various fetal organs (heart, great vessels, lung, liver, and brain) and an increase in fetal abnormalities.

(continued on next page)

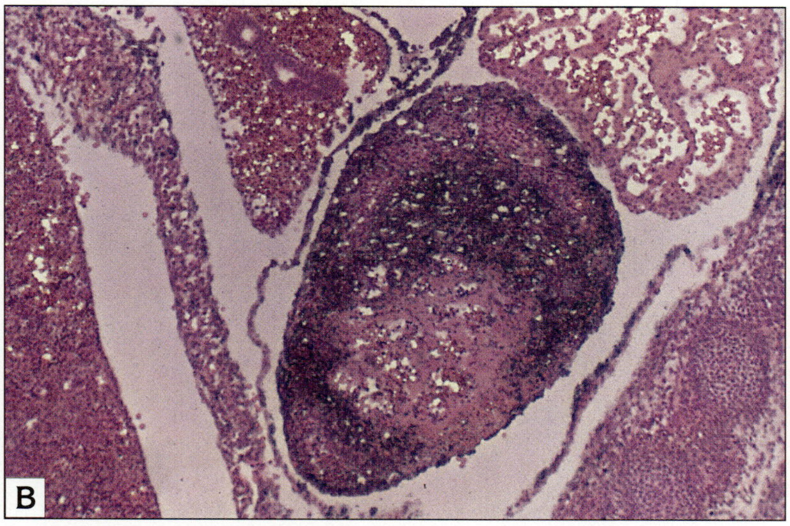

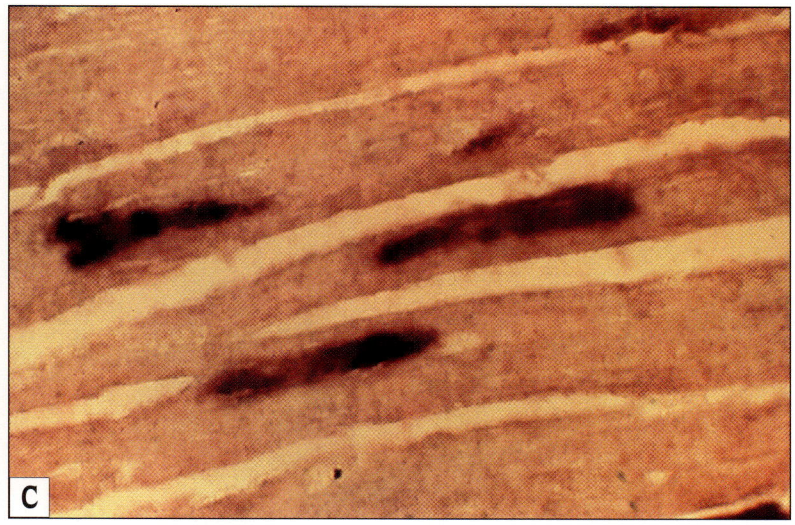

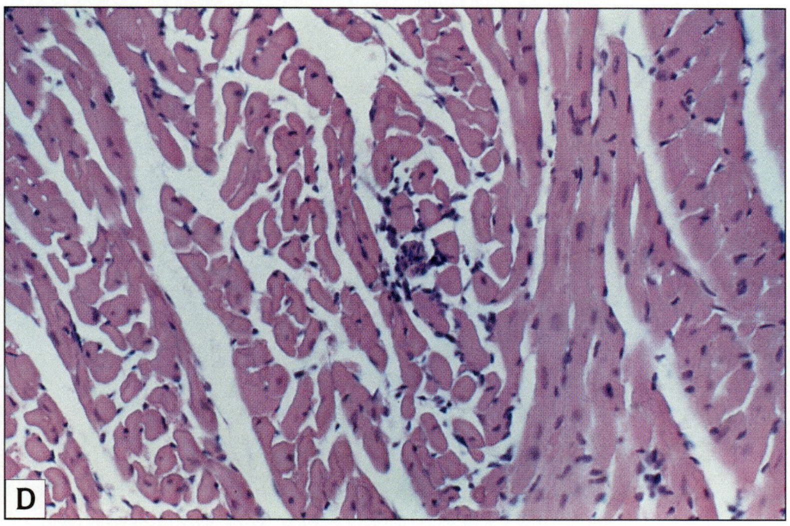

Figure 6-5 *(continued)* **B,** In situ hybridization of fetal heart (× 10). *Black signal* demonstrates TMEV infection. Maternal cardiac infection has been studied in this model to investigate the role of viral myocarditis in peripartum cardiomyopathy. **C,** In situ hybridization of maternal heart (× 40). *Purple staining* indicates viral infection of cardiac myocytes. **D,** Hematoxylin and eosin stain (× 20) demonstrating inflammation in the infected heart of a gravid female. (*Panels A and B from* Abzug *et al.* [2]; *panels C and D courtesy of* A. Palmer, MD)

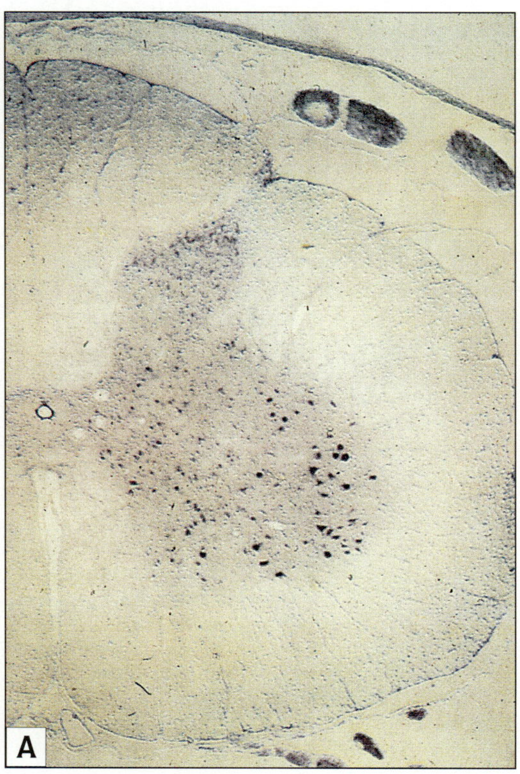

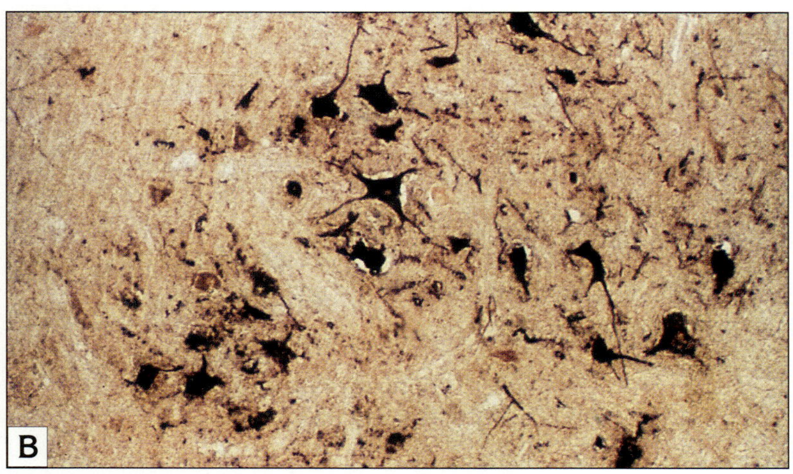

Figure 6-6 Normal anatomy of the human midlumbar spinal cord. **A,** A cresyl fast violet stain of a transverse section of the left half of the human spinal cord demonstrates the posterior (*top*) and anterior (*bottom*) gray matter, with the commissural gray matter surrounding the central canal (× 10). The motor neurons are large and grouped in the anterior gray horns. **B,** Demonstration of poliovirus RNA by in situ hybridization in anterior horn cells (× 10). This low-power view of the anterior horn demonstrates virally infected (*deep purple stain*) motor neurons in the anterior horn of the lumbar region. Sections were obtained from spinal cord sections of Bonnet monkeys (*Macaca radiata*) injected intraneurally with Mahoney type 1 poliovirus, necropsied 6 days post-infection. Poliovirus initially infects the M cells of the Peyer's patches in the intestine, and then causes a viremia. During this viremia, other reticuloendothelial cells are infected from which, in a few cases, poliovirus reaches the central nervous system, probably via the muscles and then the axons of the motor neurons. Further spread in the central nervous system appears to be intraneural. (*Panel A from* Williams *et al.* [3]; with permission; *panel B courtesy of* E. Ponnuraj, PhD.)

EPIDEMIOLOGY

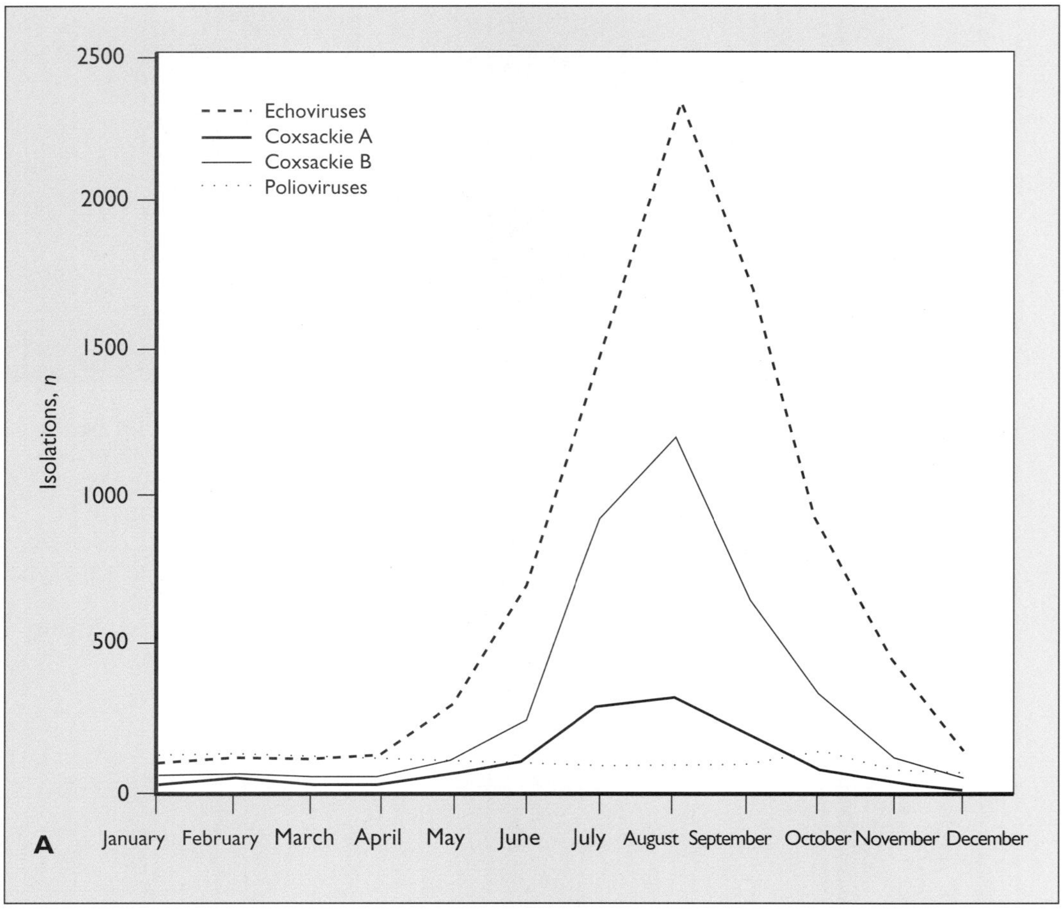

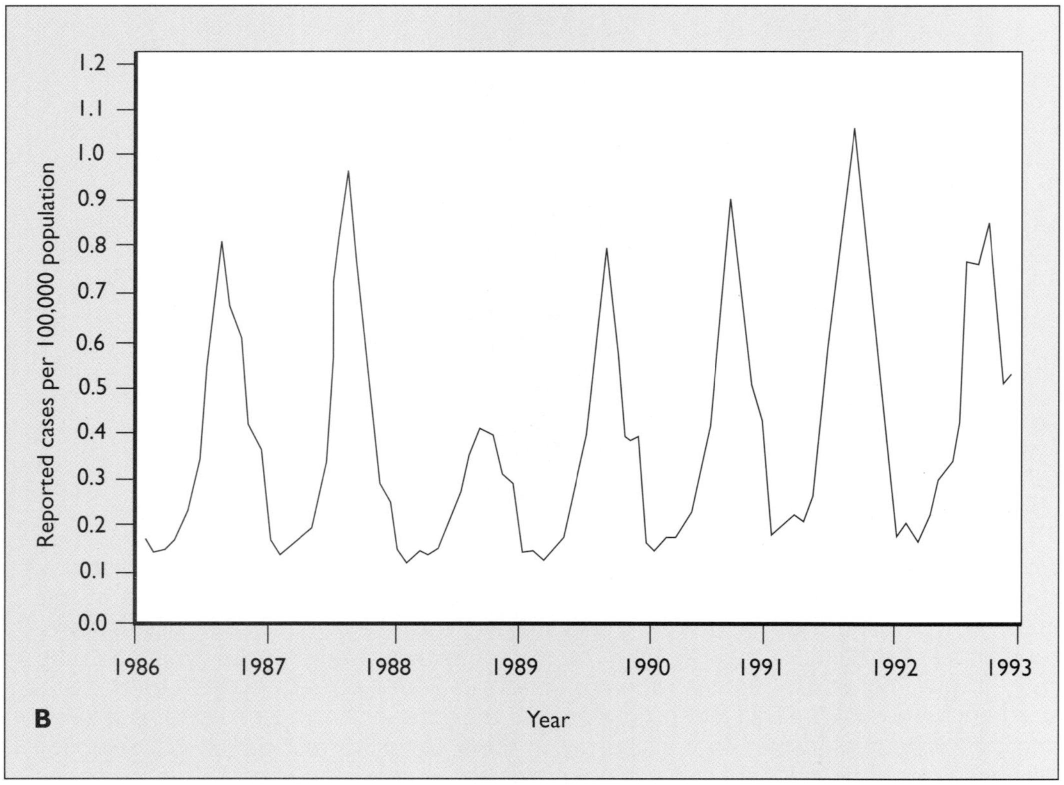

FIGURE 6-7 Seasonality of enterovirus infections. One feature of the epidemiology of enterovirus infections is their striking seasonality. Annual peaks occur during the summer and fall in temperate climates; infections occur throughout the rest of the year at a much lower incidence rate. This seasonal pattern is not apparent in tropical regions. **A,** Reported enterovirus infections in the United States between 1970 and 1979 plotted by month of occurrence, demonstrating large peaks in the summer and fall months with a low baseline incidence for the remainder of the calendar year. **B,** Reported aseptic meningitis cases between 1986 and 1992 in the United States by month of occurrence. Because enteroviruses account for the majority of these cases, the seasonality of aseptic meningitis in the United States mirrors the seasonality of enterovirus infections. A total of 35,251 cases of polio were reported in 1988. No cases were reported from Australia, United States, Canada, Japan, or parts of Europe and South America. Fewer than 10 cases each were reported from France, Spain, Mongolia, some Middle Eastern countries, and some North African and South American countries. However, more than 10 cases each were reported from most of Asia and Africa and some of South America. By 1996, only 3995 cases of polio were reported in the world. The Americas were certified polio-free in 1994; since this time there have been no indigenous cases of poliomyelitis acquired in the Americas and no transmission or detection of wild-type poliovirus in sewage. Most of Europe, China, Australia and New Zealand, and parts of Africa had no reports of poliomyelitis in 1996. It is possible that by the year 2005 the world will be free of non–vaccine-associated paralytic poliomyelitis. (*Data from* J. Hombach, Global Programme on Vaccines, World Health Organization, Geneva, Switzerland. (*Panel A adapted from* Melnick [4]; *panel B adapted from* Rotbart [5]; with permission.)

Clinical Manifestations

Clinical manifestations of enterovirus infections

	Coxsackieviruses group A*	Coxsackieviruses group B*	Echoviruses*
Illness associated with many enteroviruses	Asymptomatic infection	Asymptomatic infection	Asymptomatic infection
	Febrile illness with or without respiratory symptoms	Febrile illness with or without respiratory symptoms	Febrile illness with or without respiratory symptoms
	Aseptic meningitis (1–11, 14, 16–18, 22, 24)	Aseptic meningitis (1–6)	Aseptic meningitis (all except 24, 26, 29, 32)
	Encephalitis (2,5–7, 9)	Encephalitis (1–3, 5, 6)	Encephalitis (2–4, 6, 7, 9, 11, 14, 17–19, 25)
	Paralysis (4, 6, 7, 9, 11, 14, 21)	Paralysis (1–6)	Paralysis (1–4, 6, 7, 9, 11, 14, 16, 18, 19, 30)
Illness more characteristic of particular groups or serotypes	Herpangina (2–6, 8, 10, 22)	Exanthem (1, 3, 4, 5)	Exanthem (especially 9 and 16 but also 1–8, 11, 14, 18, 19, 25, 30, 32, 33)
	Hand-foot-and-mouth syndrome (5, 7, 9, 10, 16)	Pleurodynia (1–5)	Generalized disease of newborn (4, 6, 7, 9, 11, 12, 14, 19, 21, 51)
	Lymphonodular pharyngitis (10)	Pericarditis (1–5)	Neonatal diarrhea (11, 14, 18)
	Exanthem (2, 4, 5, 9, 16)	Myocarditis (1–5)	Chronic meningoencephalitis in agammaglobulinemic patients (2, 3, 5, 9, 11, 19, 24, 25, 30, 33)
	Epidemic conjunctivitis (24)	Generalized disease of newborn (1–5)	
Etiologic role undefined or uncertain	Diarrhea	Diarrhea	Diarrhea
	Hemolytic uremic syndrome	Myositis (2, 6)	Hemolytic uremic syndrome (22)
	Guillain–Barré (2, 5, 9)	Diabetes mellitus	Reye's syndrome
	Reye's syndrome	Hemolytic uremic syndrome (2, 4)	Myositis (9, 11)
	Mononucleosis-like syndrome (5, 6)	Mononucleosis-like syndrome (5)	Guillain–Barré (6, 22)
	Infectious lymphocytosis	Reye's syndrome	Infectious lymphocytosis (25)

*Numbers in parentheses indicate serotypes implicated.

Figure 6-8 Clinical manifestations of enterovirus infections. The clinical manifestations of enterovirus infections are protean, ranging from mild flu-like or respiratory illnesses to more serious manifestations including meningoencephalitis, myopericarditis, and disseminated neonatal disease. As indicated in this table, certain diseases are preferentially associated with particular subgroups of enteroviruses or even specific serotypes; however, there is great overlap and most clinical manifestations can be caused by a variety of serotypes. (*Adapted from* Modlin [6]; with permission.)

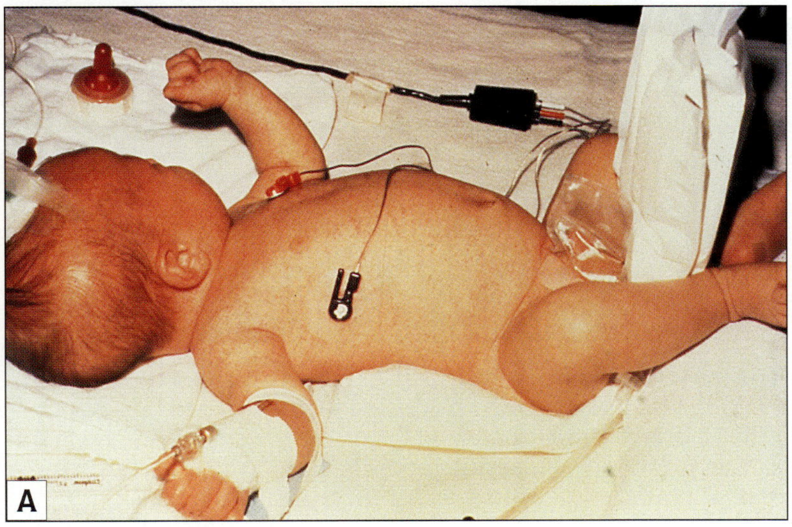

A

Figure 6-9 Mucocutaneous manifestations of enterovirus infections. Exanthems and enanthems are frequent findings in children with enterovirus infections. A variety of rashes are common, including macular, maculopapular, vesicular, petechial, and urticarial exanthems. **A,** An enterovirus-infected newborn with a generalized, fine maculopapular eruption..

(continued on next page)

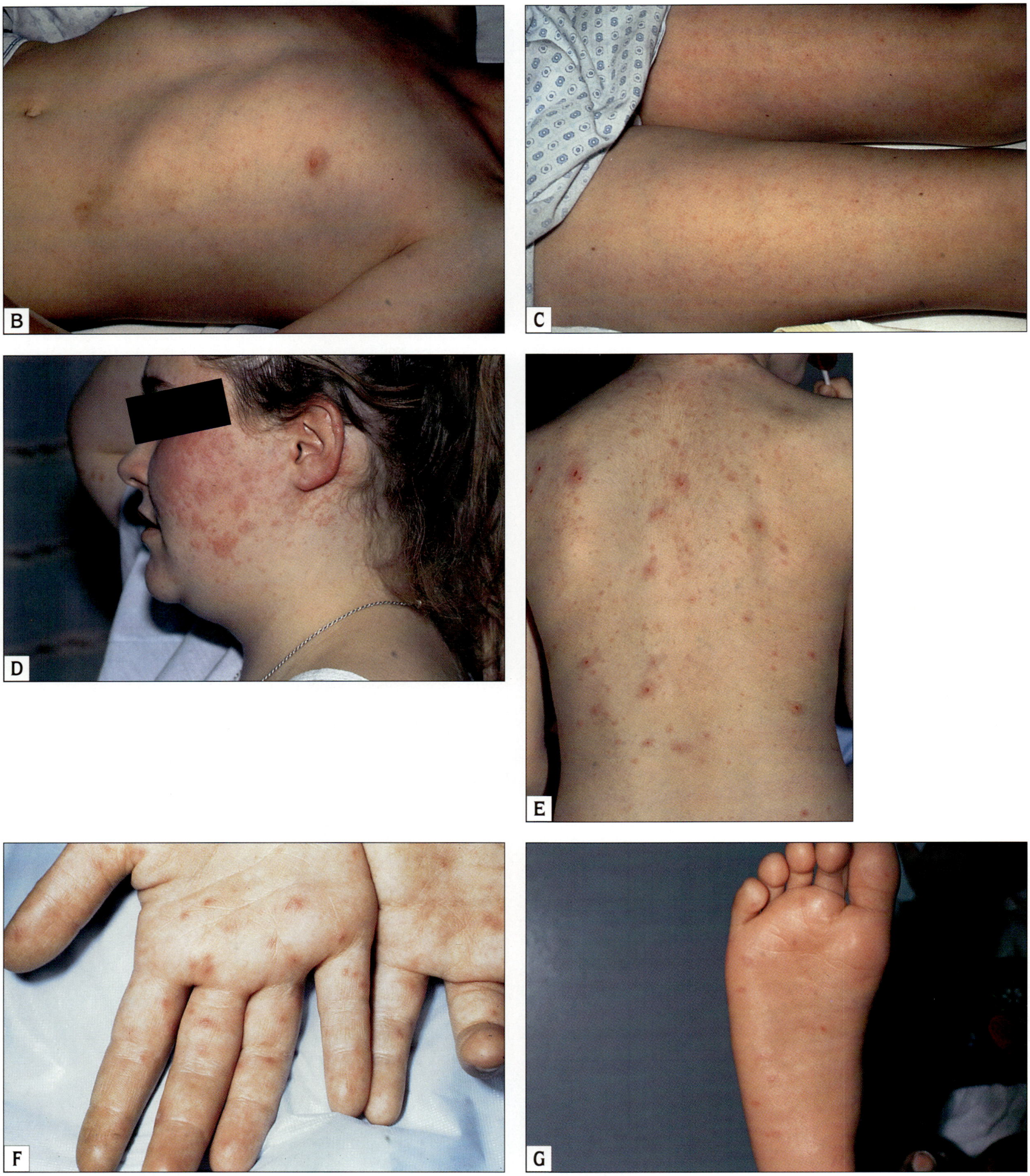

Figure 6-9 *(continued)* **B** and **C,** Similar, fine maculopapular rashes on the trunk and lower extremities, respectively, on older children with enterovirus infections. **D,** A more confluent, blotchy rash located on the face. **E,** A varicella-like exanthem consisting of vesicles with surrounding erythema on the back. Echovirus 9, an enterovirus serotype known to frequently cause exanthems, caused the rashes in **D** and **E.** Hand-foot-and-mouth disease is characterized by vesiculopustular lesions on the hands and fingers, feet, or buttocks and in the oropharynx; it is commonly caused by infection with coxsackie A16 virus. **F,** characteristic lesions on hands. **G,** Lesions on foot.

(continued on next page)

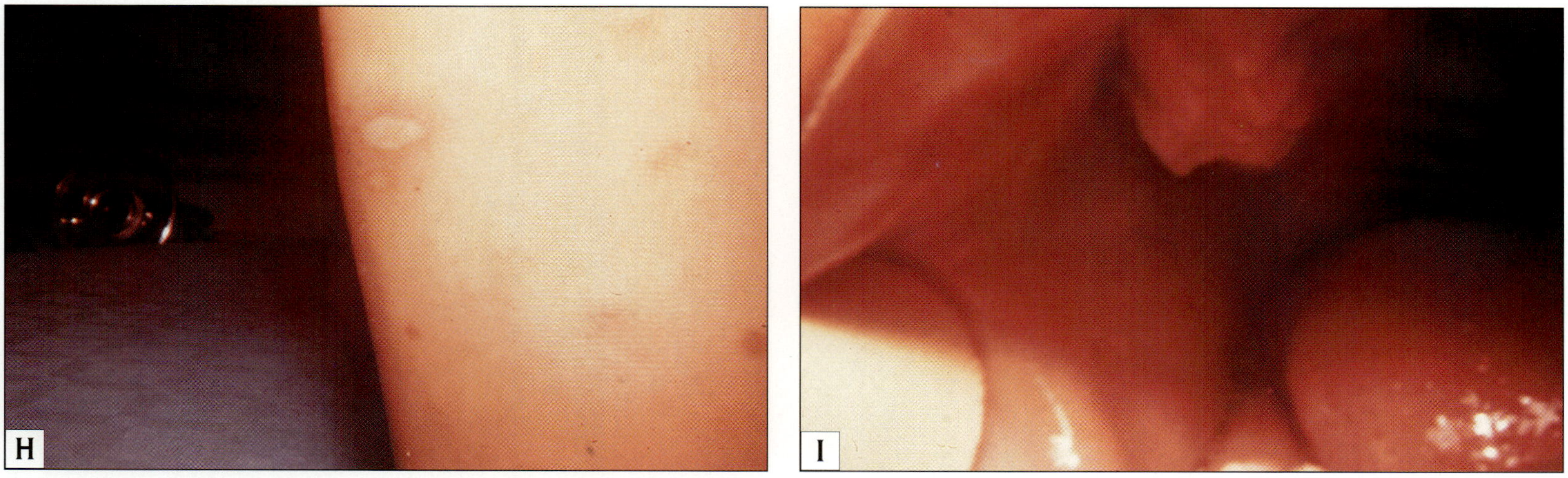

Figure 6-9 *(continued)* **H,** Lesions on foot. **I,** Lesions on buccal mucosa. In contrast to hand-foot-and-mouth disease, the vesiculoulcerative lesions of herpangina are typically located in the posterior oropharynx and are caused by many different enterovirus serotypes. (*Panel A from* Abzug [7] and *courtesy of* HA Rotbart, MD; *panels B, C, and F–I courtesy of* JV Lustig, MD; *panels D and E courtesy of* JE Shira, MD).

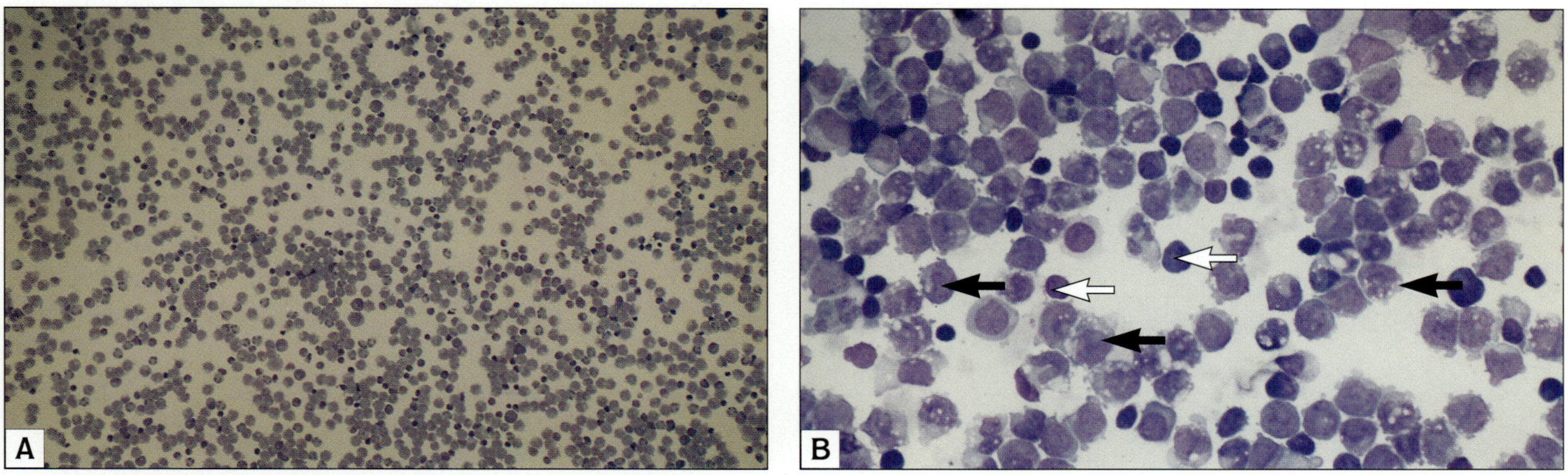

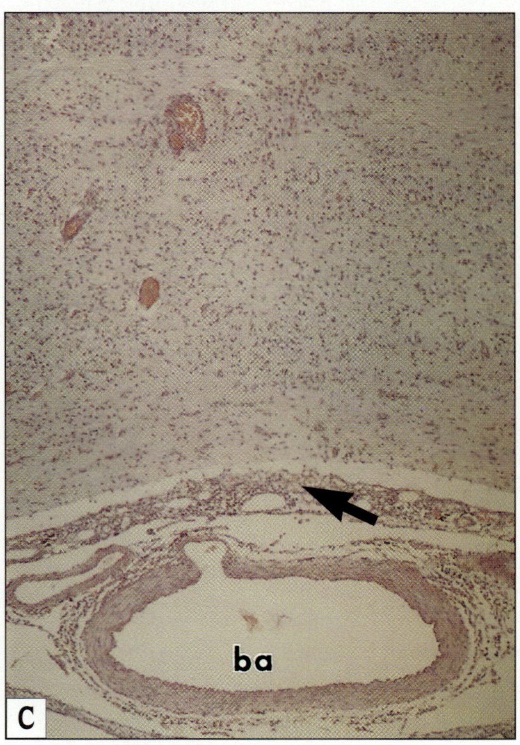

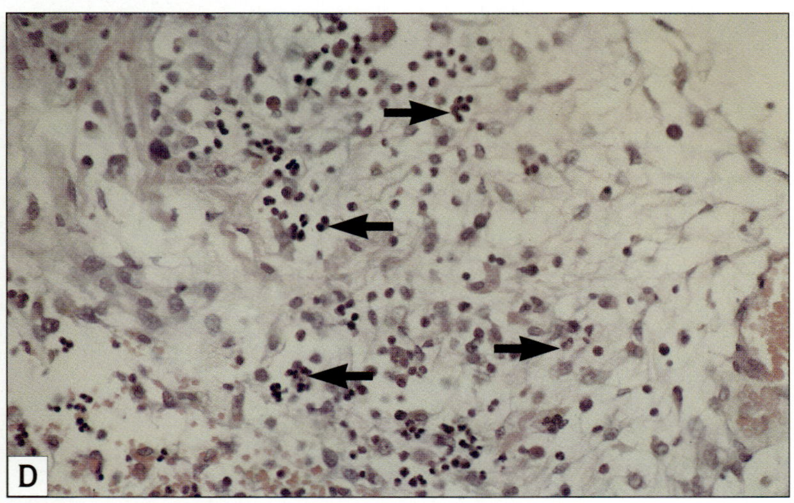

Figure 6-10 Central nervous system pathology of enterovirus infections. Enteroviruses are frequent causes of central nervous system infections, including meningitis, encephalitis, and myelitis. **A,** Typical cytospin preparation of cerebrospinal fluid from a child with enterovirus meningitis (Wright's stain, × 100). There is a marked increase in cellularity, with many vacuolated macrophages. **B,** Vacuolated macrophages seen at high power (*closed arrows*), along with numerous lymphocytes (*open arrows*) (Wright's stain, × 400). **C,** Meningeal inflammation (*arrow*) at the base of the pons, near the basilar artery (ba) (hematoxylin and eosin, × 100). **D,** Higher power reveals a cellular infiltrate containing neutrophils, lymphocytes, and plasma cells within the meninges (*arrows*) (hematoxylin and eosin, × 200). Brain parenchyma may be affected at multiple sites, including cerebral white and gray matter, cerebellum, basal ganglia, and brain stem.

(continued on next page)

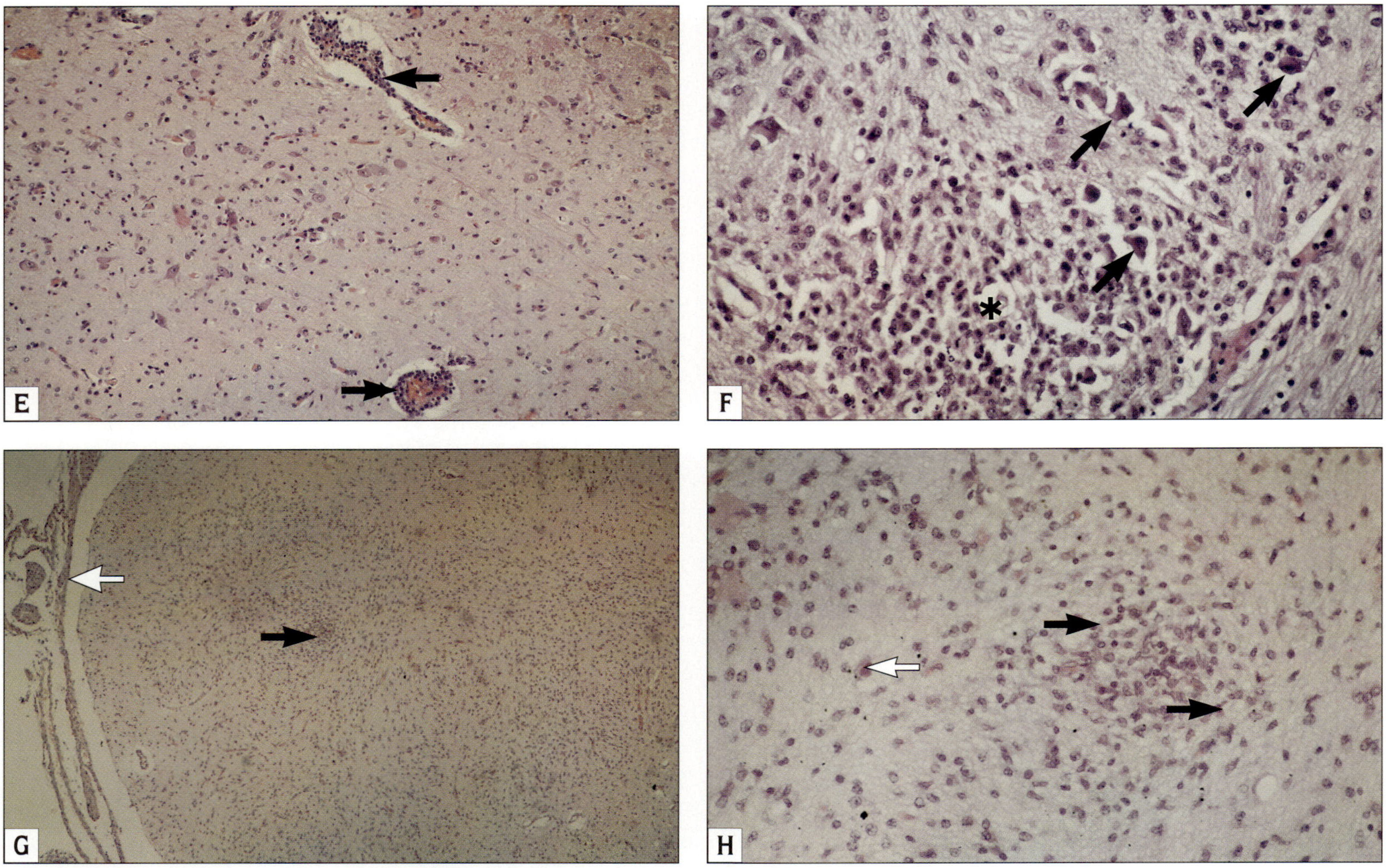

Figure 6-10 *(continued)* **E,** Characteristic perivascular lymphocytic infiltrates (*arrow*) and mild increases in lymphocytic cellularity and gliosis within the parenchyma of cerebral deep gray matter (hematoxylin and eosin, × 100). **F,** A large focus of inflammation (*asterisk*) and nearby degenerating neurons (*arrows*) are seen in the brain stem (hematoxylin and eosin, × 200). **G,** Infection in the spinal cord and its meninges; increased cellularity is present in both white matter (*arrow*) and meninges (*open arrow*) (hematoxylin and eosin, × 40). **H,** At higher power, an increase in the number of glial cells and lymphocytes (*arrows*) and a degenerating neuron (*open arrow*) are found within white matter tracts (hematoxylin and eosin, × 200). (*Courtesy of* RW Tyson, MD.)

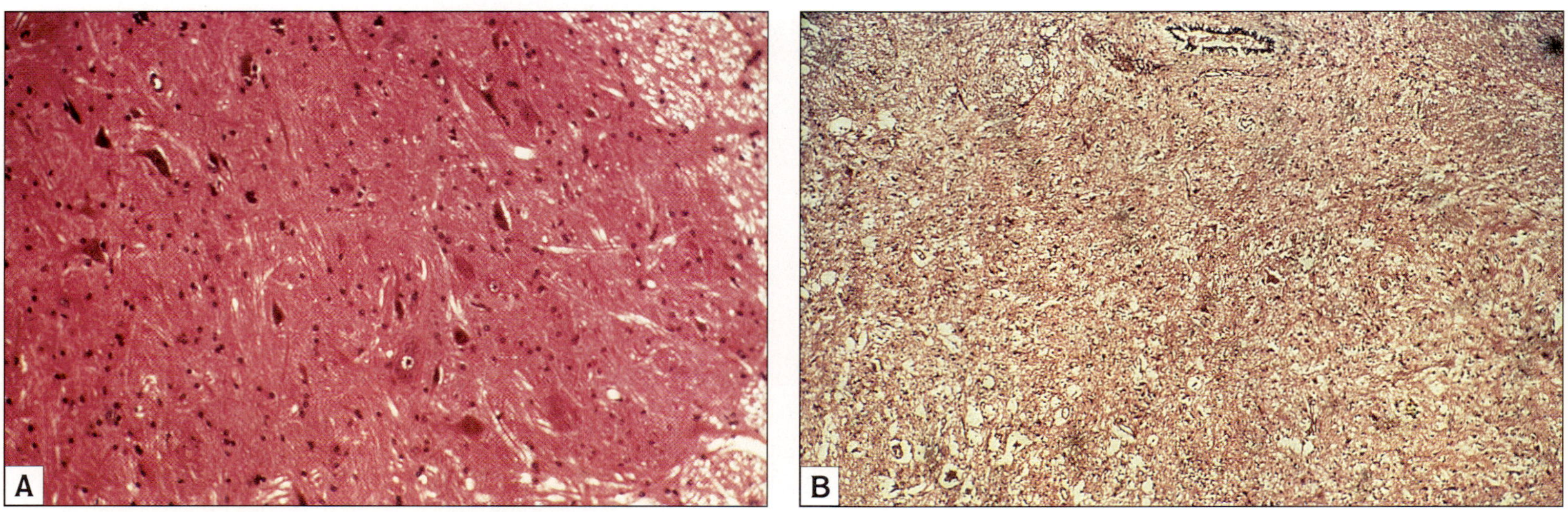

Figure 6-11 Central nervous system pathology of experimental polio virus infection: transverse sections of the spinal cord of normal and Mahoney strain poliovirus–infected *Macaca radiata*. **A,** Anterior horn region of a normal uninfected monkey showing the anterior horn with normal neurons (hematoxylin and eosin, × 10). **B,** Anterior horn of the lumbar spinal cord of a Mahoney infected monkey, demonstrating loss of anterior horn morphology and infiltration with inflammatory cells and loss of motor neurons (hematoxylin and eosin, × 10).

(continued on next page)

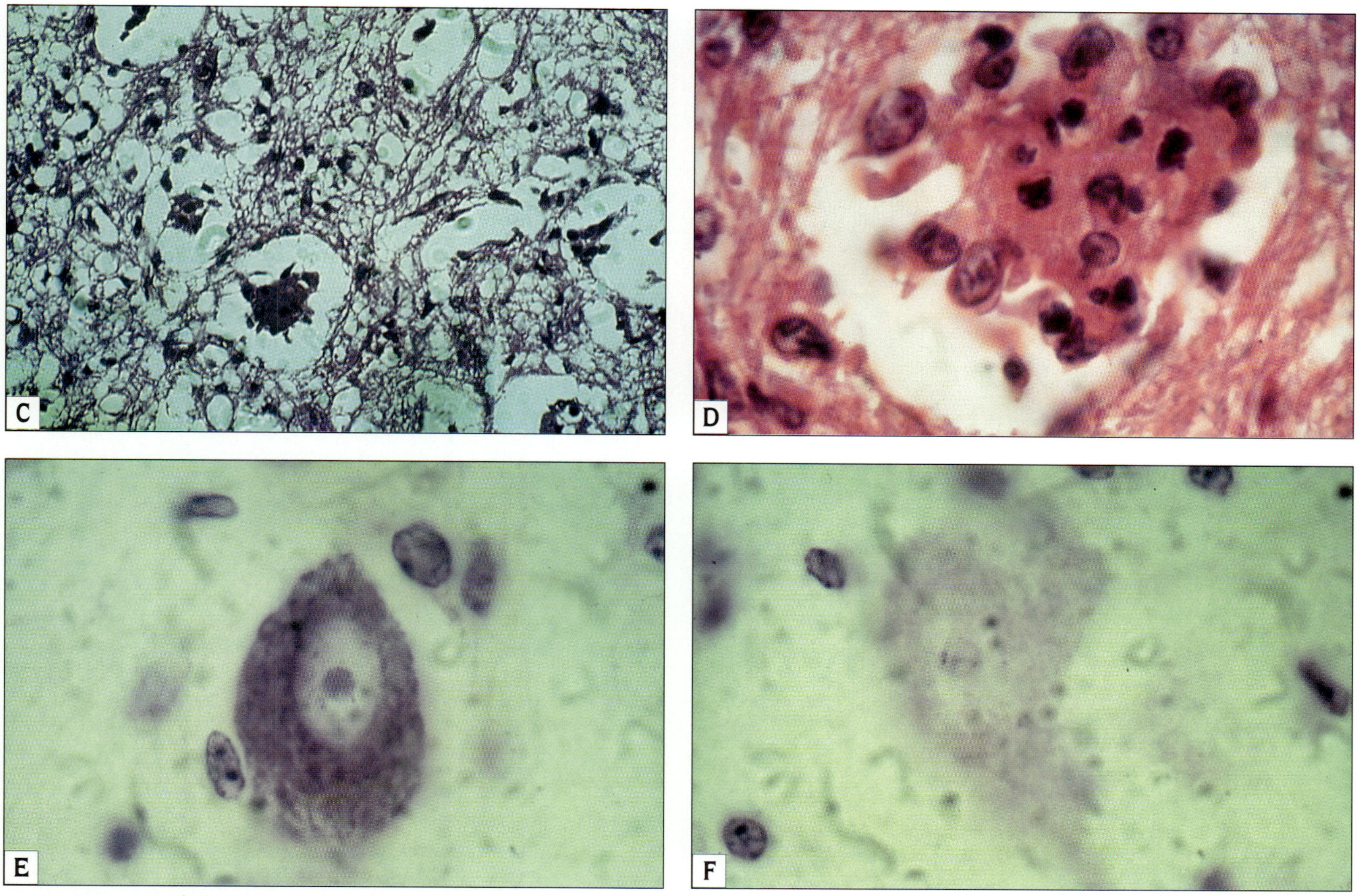

Figure 6-11 *(continued)* **C,** Lumbar region of the spinal cord from a Mahoney-infected monkey demonstrating degenerating anterior horn neurons and neuronal drop out (hematoxylin and eosin, × 25). **D,** Anterior horn from a Mahoney-infected monkey showing neuronophagia (hematoxylin and eosin, × 100). **E,** Normal neurons from noninfected monkey showing Nissl substance throughout the cytoplasm (*purple dots*) (cresyl violet, × 100). **F,** Anterior horn neuron from the cervical region of a Mahoney-infected *Macaca radiata* demonstrating loss of Nissl substance (cresyl violet, × 100) [8]. (*Courtesy of* E. Ponnuraj, PhD.)

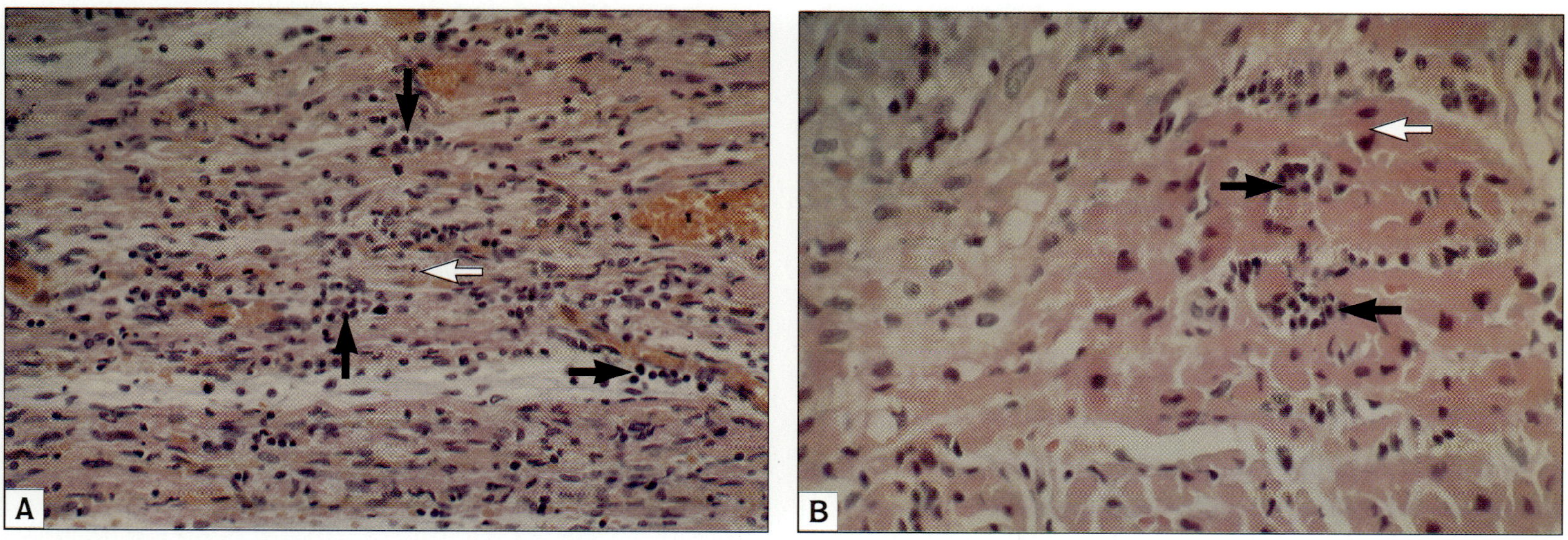

Figure 6-12 Cardiac pathology of enterovirus infections. Another relatively frequent target of enteroviruses is the heart. Cardiac infection can be a part of a severe, disseminated infection (*eg*, in neonatal infection), or it can occur as an isolated finding, resulting in acute myocarditis or pericarditis. Chronic myocarditis and dilated cardiomyopathy may follow acute myocarditis. **A,** Cardiac tissue has prominent interstitial and perivascular neutrophilic and monocytic inflammatory infiltrates (*arrows*) and apparent myocyte damage (*open arrow*) (hematoxylin and eosin, × 200). **B,** At higher power, myocyte damage (*open arrow*) and interstitial inflammation (*arrows*) are readily apparent (hematoxylin and eosin, × 400). (*Courtesy of* RW Tyson, MD.)

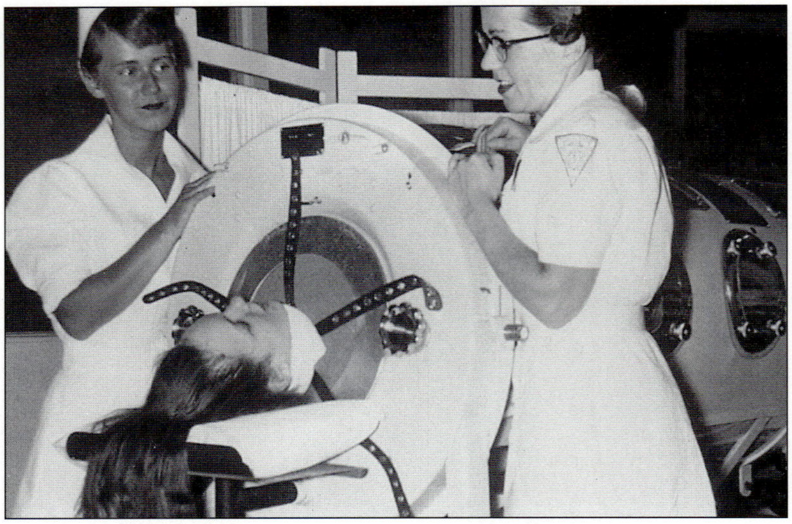

Figure 6-13 Adolescent with paralytic poliomyelitis in a respirator. The poliomyelitis epidemic rose to such heights in 1949 that patients with the disease took the majority of beds at The Children's Hospital in Denver. Lou Shannon, a physical therapist, recalled her first day at The Children's Hospital: "The hospital was taken over by polio-afflicted patients. Occupied beds lined several of the corridors. It is important to recognize the dedication of the staff. At times, they spent many 12 hour days caring for their patients, knowing that the next morning it would start all over again." Respirators, like the one pictured here, did all the breathing for those patients whose chest and abdominal muscles were affected by polio. These children slept, ate, bathed, and lived in these breathing machines.

Chronic conditions caused by enteroviruses
Proven
Progressive postpoliomyelitis muscle atrophy
Chronic dilated cardiomyopathy
Recurrent pericarditis, chronic constrictive pericarditis
Chronic meningoencephalitis (humoral immune deficiency)
Chronic myositis (humoral immune deficiency)
Chronic hepatitis (humoral immune deficiency)
Possible?
Congenital anomalies (*eg*, central nervous system, cardiac, urogenital, gastrointestinal)
Postviral fatigue syndrome
Dermatomyositis/polymyositis
Diabetes mellitus
Amyotrophic lateral sclerosis

Figure 6-14 Long-term complications of enterovirus infections. Enteroviruses have been shown to be definitely responsible for a number of chronic conditions, including progressive post-poliomyelitis muscle atrophy following poliovirus infection and residual cardiac disease following enteroviral myopericarditis. For other conditions, including congenital anomalies, chronic fatigue syndrome, dermatomyositis and polymyositis, diabetes mellitus, and amyotrophic lateral sclerosis, a role for enteroviruses has been proposed, but experimental data are not conclusive. Likewise, viral persistence in some of these syndromes has been suggested but not definitively proven. Chronic enterovirus infections of the central nervous system, and occasionally also of muscle and liver, are well-described in patients with antibody deficiencies.

Laboratory Diagnosis

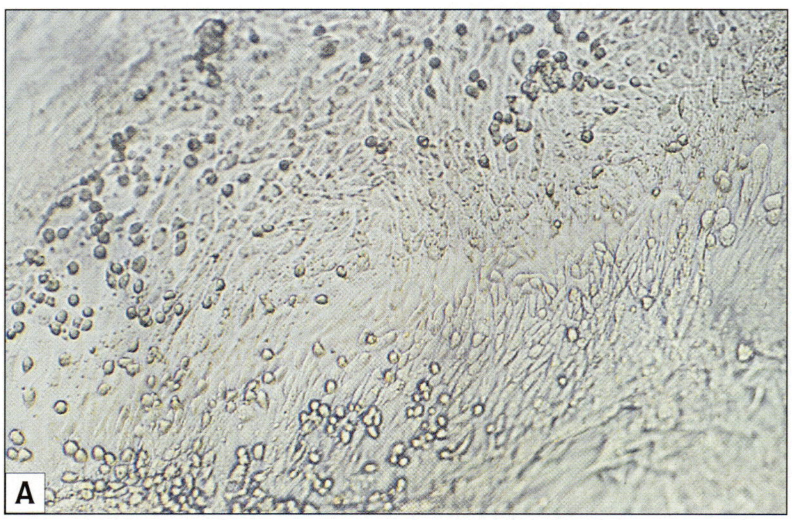

Figure 6-15 Laboratory diagnosis of enterovirus infections. The discovery of tissue culture for viral cultivation in the 1950s supplanted animal inoculation as the mainstay of laboratory diagnosis of enterovirus infections. Enteroviruses produce characteristic cytopathic effect (CPE) in tissue culture cell lines, including monkey kidney lines and human cell lines (*eg*, fibroblast and rhabdomyosarcoma cell lines). **A,** Photomicrograph (× 100) of CPE of enterovirus in a primary rhesus monkey kidney cell line; refractile cells are infected with coxsackievirus A9. Notice normal cells in the upper left and lower right hand corners, whereas cells showing CPE are refractile and rounded up. More recently, indirect viral detection methods have been developed to detect enteroviral antigens (immunoassays) or nucleic acid (solid and liquid phase hybridization, in situ hybridization, and polymerase chain reaction). The polymerase chain reaction (PCR) amplifies target nucleic acid, thereby increasing sensitivity as compared with direct nucleic acid hybridization.

(continued on next page)

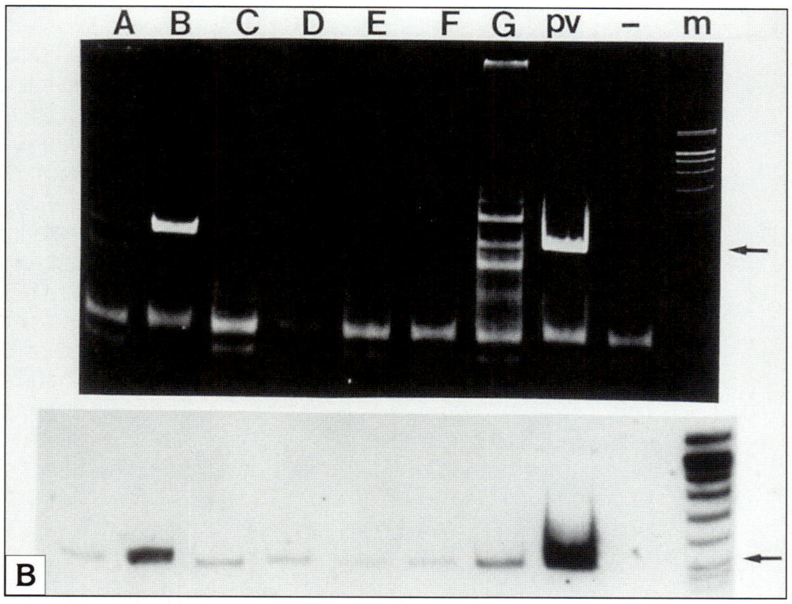

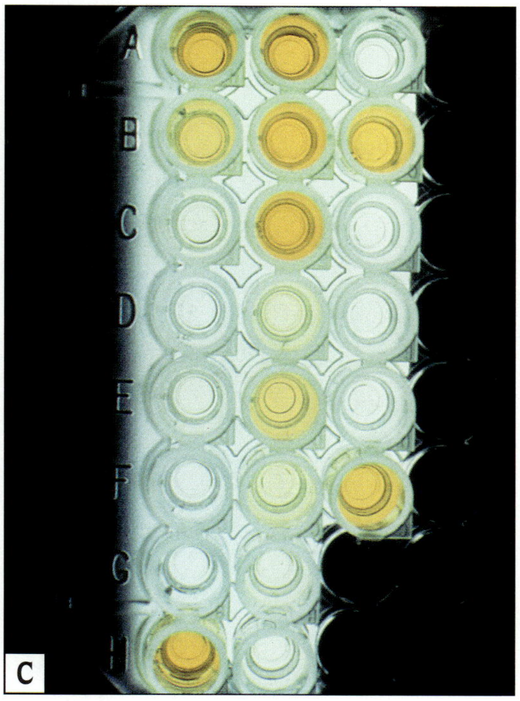

FIGURE 6-15 *(continued)* **B,** *Top half* demonstrates an agarose gel electrophoresis of enterovirus PCR-amplified cerebrospinal fluid specimens from patients with agammaglobulinemia and chronic enterovirus meningoencephalitis; *bottom half* shows a Southern blot hybridization of the same agarose gel. *Arrows* indicate bands of 154 nucleotides in length, the size of the enterovirus PCR product. Lanes A to G contain patient specimens, lane PV contains poliovirus RNA, lane "–" contains cerebrospinal fluid from an uninfected patient, and lane m contains marker nucleic acid of varying sizes. **C,** Detection of enterovirus PCR-amplified nucleic acid via a microtiter plate colorimetric assay. Microtiter wells contain reaction products of PCR assays performed on neonatal serum and urine specimens. *Colored wells* are positive samples; the color reaction is produced following hybridization of bound probe with biotin-labeled amplified enterovirus nucleic acid. This colorimetric PCR assay takes approximately 5 hours to complete. (*Panel A courtesy of* C. Robinson, PhD; *panels B and C courtesy of* HA Rotbart, MD.)

THERAPY

A. Neutralization titers in study intravenous immune globulin lots for viral isolates from 15 enterovirus-infected neonates

	Reciprocal neutralization titer	
Isolate	**IVIG lot 1**	**IVIG lot 2**
Echovirus 6	400	200
Echovirus 6	3200	3200
Echovirus 9	800	400
Echovirus 9	100	100
Echovirus 11	400	800
Echovirus 11	1600	1600
Echovirus 11	800	800
Coxsackievirus B2	1600	1600
Coxsackievirus B2	1600	1600
Coxsackievirus B4	100	100
Coxsackievirus B4	100	100
Coxsackievirus B4	<100	<100
Coxsackievirus B4	3200	3200
Coxsackievirus B4	100	100
Untyped	200	400
Geometric mean titer	439 (107–1793)*	439 (107–1793)*

* Numbers in parentheses are the range of ± 1 SD around the geometric mean derived from logarithmic scale.

FIGURE 6-16 Immune globulin therapy of enterovirus infections. Antibodies appear to be the most important host defense against enteroviruses, and antibody-deficient patients may suffer severe or prolonged enterovirus infections. Immune globulin has been used therapeutically for antibody-deficient patients with chronic meningoencephalitis with some success. Maintenance prophylactic intravenous immune globulin (IVIG) for antibody-deficient patients has reduced the incidence of chronic meningoencephalitis in this population. IVIG contains neutralizing antibody to many common enterovirus serotypes, and it has been used in a modest number of cases of neonatal enterovirus infection. **A,** Neutralization titers (NTs) in two lots of IVIG for enterovirus isolates from 15 infected neonates.

(continued on next page)

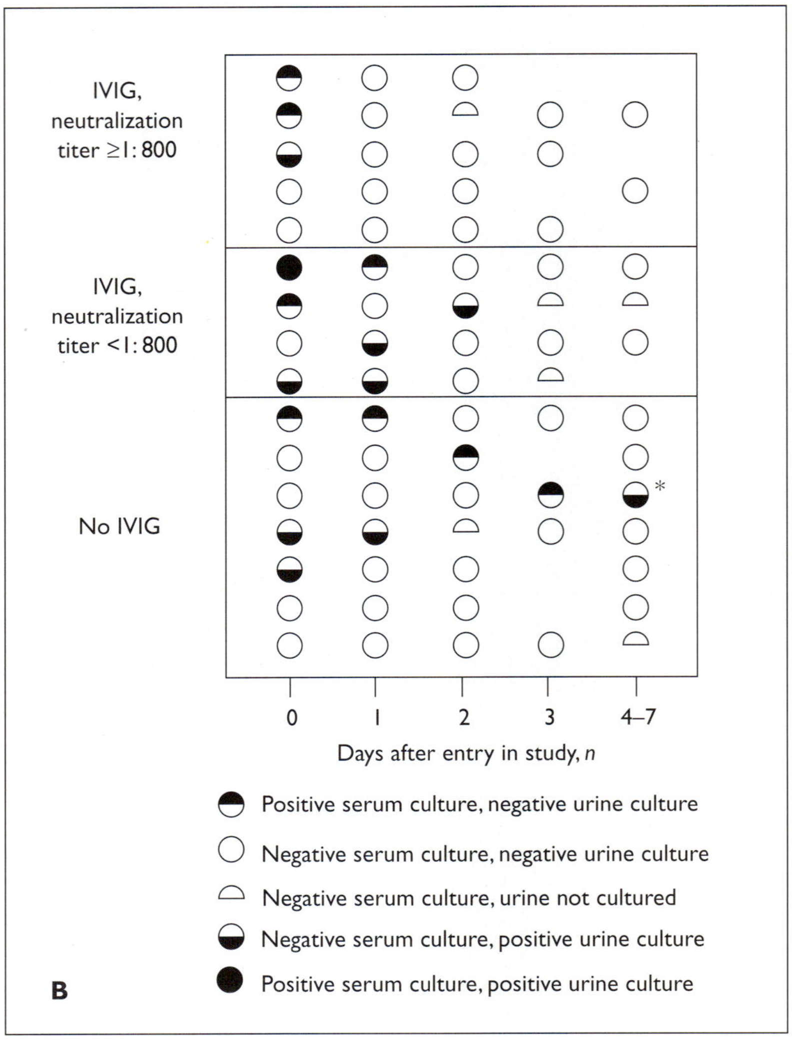

Figure 6-16 *(continued)* The only randomized trial to study therapy with IVIG in neonatal enterovirus disease was too small to demonstrate clinical efficacy, but it did show a trend toward faster resolution of viremia and viruria in newborns who received immune globulin containing high neutralization titers to their own infecting viral serotypes. **B,** Serial viral cultures of serum and urine from 16 enterovirus-infected neonates. Patients are divided into three groups: those who received IVIG containing an NT of 1:800 or more to their own viral isolates, those who received IVIG containing an NT of less than 1:800 to their own isolates, and those who did not receive IVIG (control subjects). Results of daily serum and urine viral cultures for each enterovirus-infected patient are depicted horizontally. Entry into the study is indicated as day 0. Data for days 4 to 7 after entry into the study have been combined; in some cases, multiple samplings during this period are represented by one circle. The *top half* of each circle refers to serum culture, and the bottom half of each circle refers to urine culture. The *shaded areas* indicate culture positivity and *open areas* indicate culture negativity. *No circle* indicates that cultures were not obtained on that study day. *Asterisk* indicates positive urine culture 5 days after entry in study. (*Panels A and B from* Abzug *et al.* [9]; with permission.)

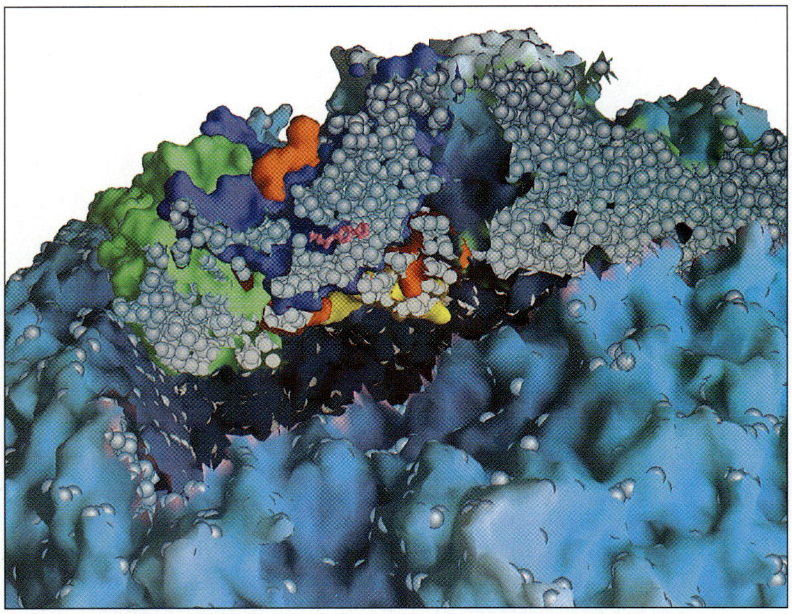

Figure 6-17 Pharmaceutical therapies for enterovirus infections. Several compounds have been developed to combat infection caused by enteroviruses and the closely related rhinoviruses. These include agents that interfere with attachment of the virus to cell receptors or uncoating of the viral RNA, inhibit RNA replication, or inhibit protein synthesis. The greatest clinical experience exists with agents in the former category, particularly the series of "WIN" compounds, which bind to hydrophobic pockets located beneath canyons formed at the junctions of the VP1 and VP3 proteins on the enterovirus capsid. The crystallographic structure of a portion of the rhinovirus 14 capsid containing the drug WIN 52035 (*pink*) within a hydrophobic pocket is shown in the figure. *Dark blue* indicates VP1; *green* indicates VP2; *orange* indicates VP3; *yellow* indicates VP4. Pleconaril (VP 63843, ViroPharma, Inc., Exton, PA) is a WIN compound that is now in clinical development. It has broad activity against enteroviruses and rhinoviruses and has been shown in human trials to be efficacious for coxsackievirus A21 upper respiratory infections and for enteroviral meningitis. Clinical trials for other enteroviral diseases are currently in progress. (*Courtesy of* J. Sgro.)

Prevention

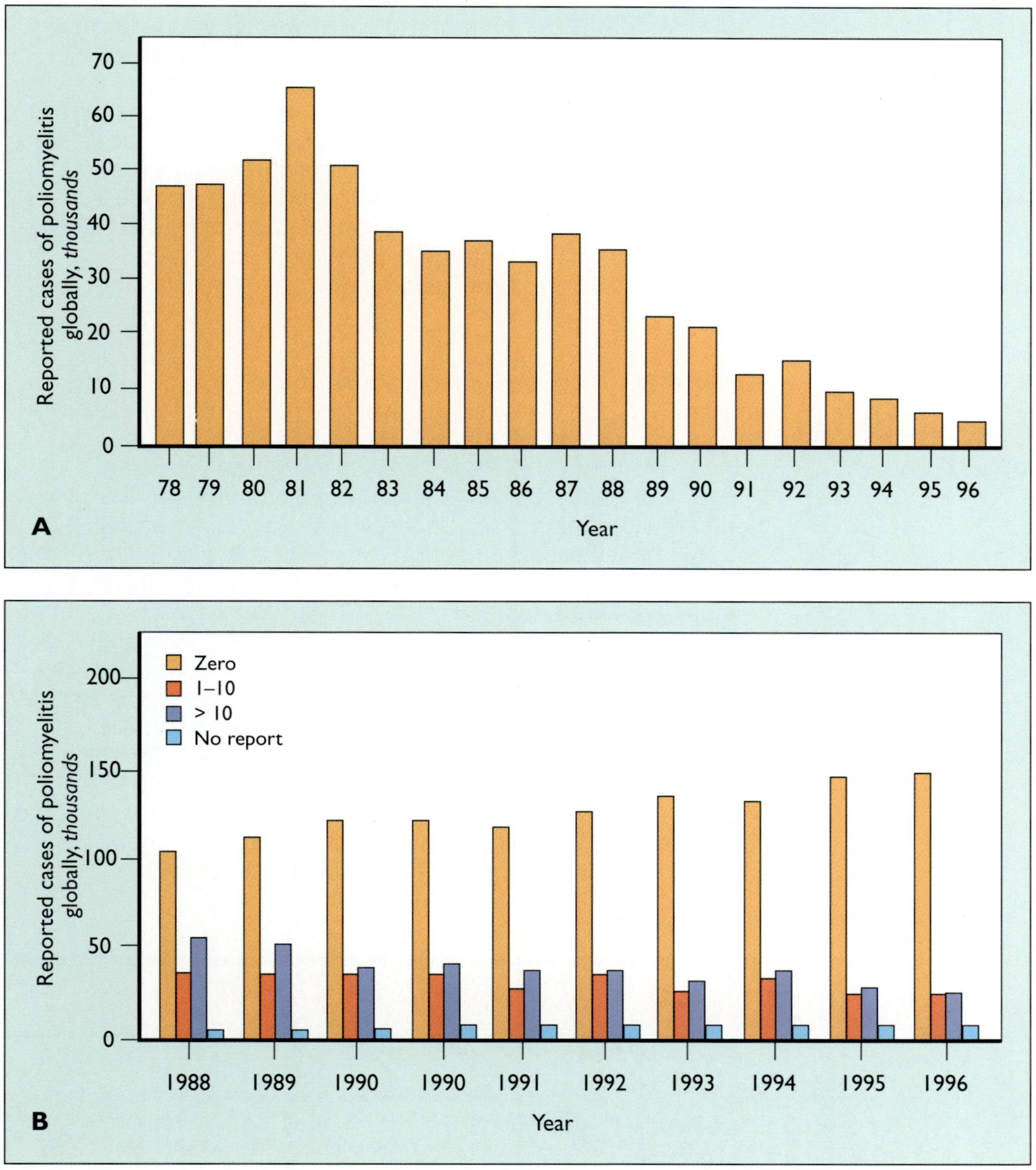

Figure 6-18 Global eradication of poliomyelitis. The strategy used by the World Health Organization has been the use of National Immunization Days (NIDs). This strategy encompasses routine immunization with the addition of two NIDs in the year when all children under 5 years of age are actively sought out and administered a dose of oral poliovirus vaccine regardless of prior immunization status. By the end of 1997, with the success of NIDs in eradicating poliomyelitis in the Americas, 117 countries are now using NIDs in an effort to eradicate poliomyelitis globally. **A**, A dramatic decline in reported cases of poliomyelitis globally. In some countries where poliomyelitis was eradicated prior to the start of NIDs, routine immunizations have been used to eradicate poliomyelitis (*eg*, Australia, Europe, United States, and Canada). **B**, Dramatic increase in the number of countries reporting zero or less than 10 poliomyelitis cases per year between 1988 and 1996, with a decrease in number of countries reporting greater than 10 poliomyelitis cases per year. It has been estimated that by 2005, poliomyelitis will be eradicated globally.

A. Characteristics of the total reported cases of vaccine-associated paralytic poliomyelitis between 1980 and 1994
Otherwise healthy (49/125)
Healthy close contacts (40/125)
Community acquired (6/125)
Immune compromise (30/125)

Figure 6-19 Studies on vaccine-associated paralytic poliomyelitis (VAPP). In the United States, where oral poliovirus vaccine has been routinely used since the mid-1960s, an average of eight to 10 children with VAPP occur per year. The vaccine strains of poliovirus revert to a neurovirulent phenotype on passage through the gastrointestinal tract. These passaged strains can infect either the vaccinee or a contact. **A**, The characteristics of the total reported cases of VAPP between 1980 and 1994. Ninety-five of the 125 cases occurred in otherwise healthy recipients or contacts and 30 occurred in immune-compromised patients.

(continued on next page)

B. Incidence of vaccine-associated paralytic poliomyelitis among three case categories

Case category	First dose	Subsequent dose	Ratio
Recipient	1:1.4	1:27.2	21-fold
Contact	1:2.2	1:17.5	7-fold
Immunocompromise	1:5.8	1:12.9	2-fold

Figure 6-19 *(continued)* **B.** The number of cases of VAPP per million doses of oral poliovirus vaccine distributed, comparing the rate with first doses versus subsequent doses. Most cases occurred with the first dose of vaccine. In recipients, there is a 21-fold higher incidence of VAPP in recipients of first doses; likewise, there is a sevenfold higher incidence in contacts and a twofold higher incidence in immune-compromised patients following administration of the first dose. This finding suggested a strategy of sequential injectable killed poliovirus vaccine followed by oral poliovirus vaccine.

Acceptable combinations of injectable killed polio vaccine* and oral poliovirus vaccine†

	2 mo	4 mo	12–18 mo	4–6 y
IPV-OPV	IPV	IPV	OPV	OPV
OPV	OPV	OPV	OPV	OPV
IPV	IPV	IPV	IPV	IPV

* 40-8-32 D-antigen units of types 1, 2, and 3, respectively.

† Trivalent.

Figure 6-20 Acceptable combinations of injectable poliovirus vaccine (IPV) and oral poliovirus vaccine (OPV) for routine vaccination in infants and children in the United States. In order to avoid approximately 50% of cases of VAPP, the American Academy of Pediatrics and the Advisory Committee on Immunization Practices, Centers for Disease Control and Prevention have both recommended as an option the use of a sequential IPV–OPV schedule. The IPV produces good humoral immunity and less gut immunity, whereas live attenuated OPV produces more gut immunity and equivalent humoral immunity. However, the danger (albeit small) of VAPP is a disadvantage of OPV. Two doses of enhanced IPV would induce enough humoral immunity to protect nonimmunocompromised recipients from developing VAPP on subsequent receipt of OPV. The use of two doses of IPV in children with immune compromise would allow the detection of immune deficiency prior to the age of 12 to 18 months when the first dose of OPV would be given to these recipients. Four doses of either OPV or IPV are also acceptable combinations.

References

1. Rueckert RR: Picornaviridae: the viruses and their replication. In *Fields Virology*, ed 3. Edited by Fields BN, Knipe DM, Howley PM, *et al.* Philadelphia: Lippincott-Raven Publishers; 1996:609–654.
2. Abzug MJ, Rotbart HA, Magliato SA, Levin MJ: Evolution of the placental barrier to fetal infection by murine enteroviruses. *J Infect Dis* 1991, 163:1336–1341.
3. *Gray's Anatomy*, ed 37. Edited by Williams PL, Warwick R, Dyson M, Bannister LH. New York: Churchill-Livingstone; 1989.
4. Melnick JL: Enteroviruses: polioviruses, coxsackieviruses, echoviruses, and newer enteroviruses. In *Fields Virology*, ed 3. Edited by Fields BN, Knipe DM, Howley PM, *et al.* Philadelphia: Lippincott-Raven Publishers; 1996:655–712.
5. Rotbart HA: Meningitis and encephalitis. In *Human Enterovirus Infections*. Edited by Rotbart HA. Washington, DC: ASM Press; 1995:271–289.
6. Modlin JF: Coxsackieviruses, echoviruses, and newer enteroviruses. In *Principles and Practice of Infectious Diseases*, ed 4. Edited by Mandell GL, Bennett JE, Dolin R. New York: Churchill-Livingstone; 1995:1620–1636.
7. Abzug MJ: Perinatal enterovirus infections. In *Human Enterovirus Infections*. Edited by Rotbart HA. Washington, DC: ASM Press; 1995:221–238.
8. Ponnuraj EM, Levin MJ, John TJ, Simoes EAF: Cell-to-cell spread of poliovirus in the spinal cord of Bonnet monkeys (*Macaca radiata*). *J Gen Virol*, 1998: in press.
9. Abzug MJ, Keyserling HL, Lee ML, *et al.*: Neonatal enterovirus infection: virology, serology, and effects of intravenous immune globulin. *Clin Infect Dis* 1995, 20:1201–1206.

CHAPTER 7

Streptococcal Infections

Adnan S. Dajani
Patricia Ferrieri

Pathogenesis

Group A streptococcal suppurative/invasive diseases	
Tonsillopharyngitis	Bone/joint infections
Soft-tissue infections	Osteomyelitis
Impetigo	Pyogenic arthritis
Necrotizing fasciitis	Sinusitis
Cellulitis	Mastoiditis
Lymphangitis	Pulmonary infections
Lymphadenitis	Pneumonitis
Thrombophlebitis	Empyema
Abscess formation	Postpartum infections
Septicemia	Puerperal sepsis
Toxic shock–like syndrome	Myometritis
Meningitis	Breast abscesses

Figure 7-1 Group A streptococcal suppurative/invasive diseases.

Group A streptococcal nonsuppurative diseases
Rheumatic fever
Glomerulonephritis
Others
Toxic shock–like syndrome
Scarlet fever
Kawasaki syndrome (?)

Figure 7-2 Group A streptococcal nonsuppurative diseases.

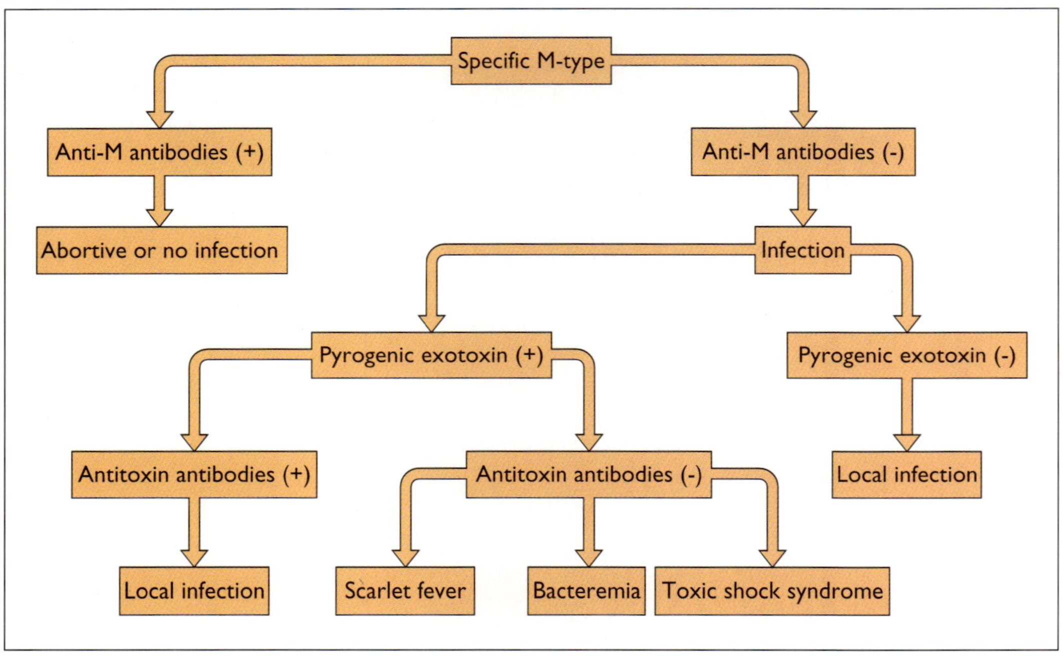

Figure 7-3 Model for group A streptococcal infections. Group A streptococci contain or produce a number of products that may contribute to disease production. If a human host is exposed to a particular M type of group A streptococci, infection may or may not ensue, depending on the absence or presence of antibodies to the specific M protein. Infection may be localized or may spread; the exact mechanism for invasiveness is not well defined, but invasiveness is associated with certain M types (*eg*, M1, M3). If the infecting strain is capable of producing pyrogenic exotoxins (especially exotoxin A), then scarlet fever, bacteremia, or toxic shock syndrome may occur, particularly if the host lacks antistreptococcal pyrogenic exotoxin antibodies.

Group A streptococcal constituents or extracellular products that may contribute to pathophysiology of sepsis and shock

Constituent/product	Pathogenic property
M protein	Antiphagocytic (anti-M antibody promotes bacterial opsonization, uptake, and PMN killing)
Pyrogenic exotoxins A, B, C	Pyrogenicity
	Suppresses Ig production
	Induces monokines (*eg*, interleukin-1β, TNF-α)
	T-cell mitogen
	Alters reticuloendothelial cell function
	Inhibits neutrophil chemotaxis through TNF-α
	Enhances delayed hypersensitivity, leading possibly to skin findings
Hyaluronidase	Cleaves hyaluronic acid in tissue matrix
Protease	Proteolytic, damaging to proteins
Streptolysin O	May act synergistically with exotoxin to influence monocyte and macrophage monokine production

PMN—polymorphonuclear cells; TNF—tumor necrosis factor.

FIGURE 7-4 Group A streptococcal constituents or extracellular products that contribute to pathophysiology of sepsis and shock. Group A streptococci produce large numbers of extracellular products. Some of these have been shown to play a role in the pathophysiology of disease production.

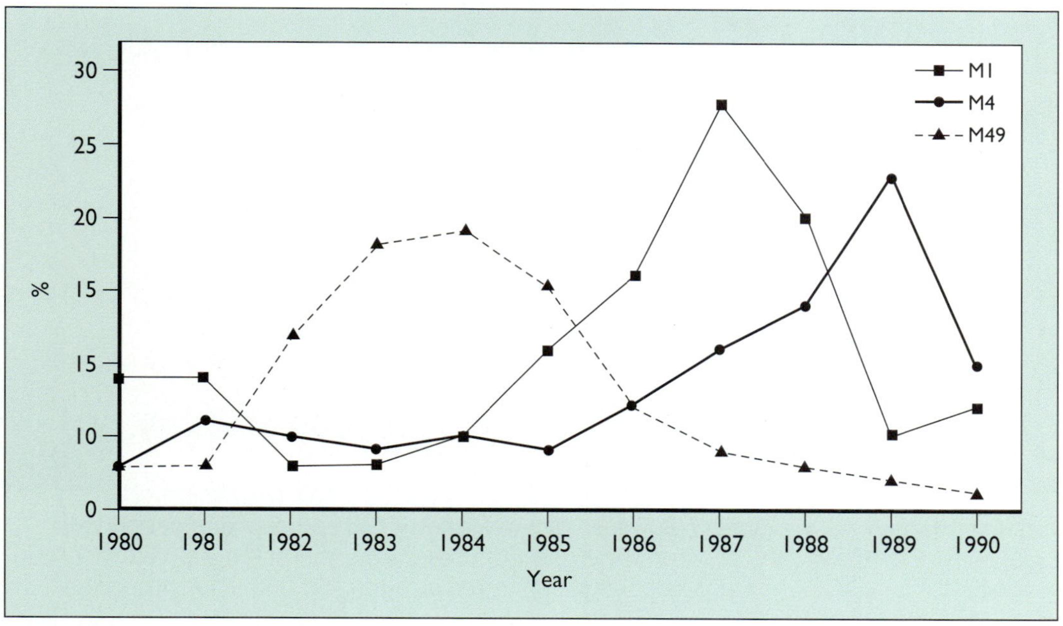

FIGURE 7-5 Changes in group A streptococcal serotypes in Britain between 1980 and 1990. Extensive epidemiologic investigations of group A streptococcal serotypes in Britain between 1980 and 1990 indicated that some serotypes (such as M3 and M12) showed no great variations from year to year; some other strains caused nationwide epidemics. The figure represents the frequency of three distinct serotypes (M1, M4, and M49) during the observation period. Types M1 and M3 were associated with invasive disease and fatal infections. Type M4 accounted for 50% of erythromycin-resistant strains [1].

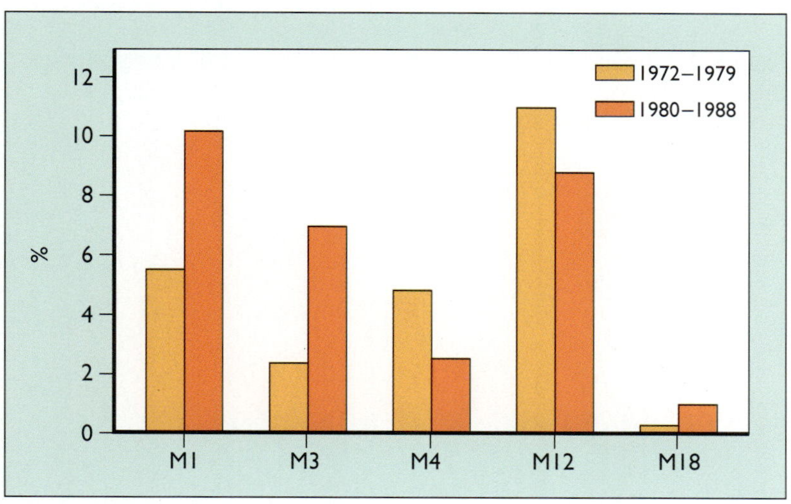

FIGURE 7-6 Changes in proportion of M types in the United States between 1972 and 1988. The proportions of M types in various parts of the United States vary at different times. The figure compares the frequency of five distinct M types over two periods: 1972 to 1979 and 1980 to 1988. Between 1980 and 1988, a relative increase was noted in types M1, M3, and M18, whereas a relative decrease was observed for types M4 and M12. Types M1 and M3 are known to be associated with invasive (bacteremic) infections. Indeed, an increase in invasive group A streptococcal infections has been observed since the early 1980s in the United States. Type M1, M3, and M18 are all implicated as "rheumatogenic" streptococci [2].

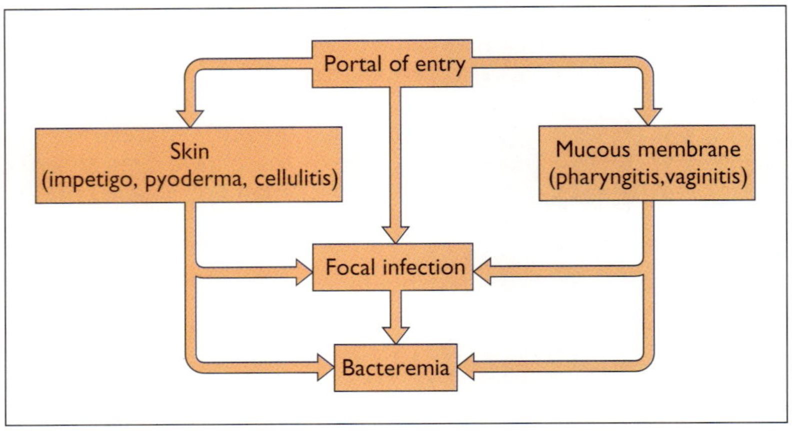

FIGURE 7-7 Pathogenesis of invasive group A streptococcal infections. Organisms enter via the skin or mucous membranes and may lead to local infection. This may progress to focal infection, or it may spread to systematic bacteremia.

CLINICAL CONDITIONS

Impetigo

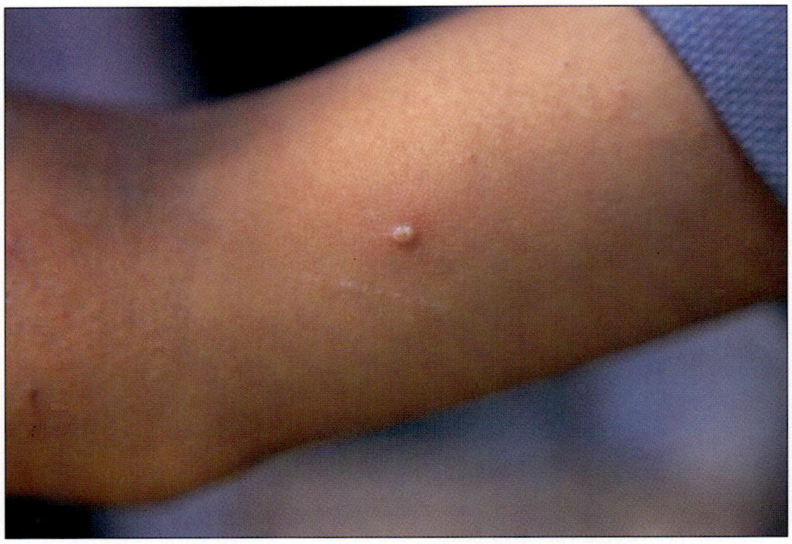

FIGURE 7-8 Pustular lesion on the skin characteristic of early stages of streptococcal impetigo. During this stage, culture of the lesion usually yields pure growth of group A streptococci. Usually, minimal or no erythema surrounds the lesion. The vesicular stage usually lasts 1 to 2 days.

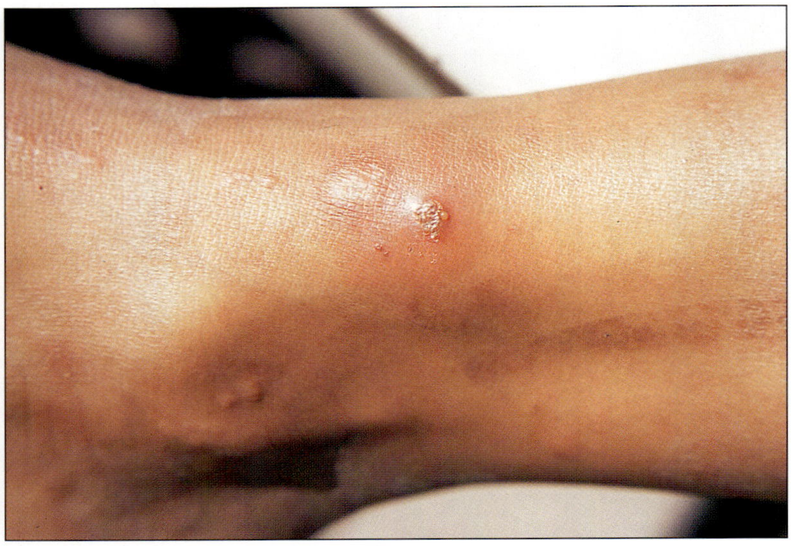

FIGURE 7-9 Three-day-old lesion of streptococcal impetigo with amber, crumbly crust. Cultures during this stage yield either group A streptococci alone or mixed streptococci and staphylococci.

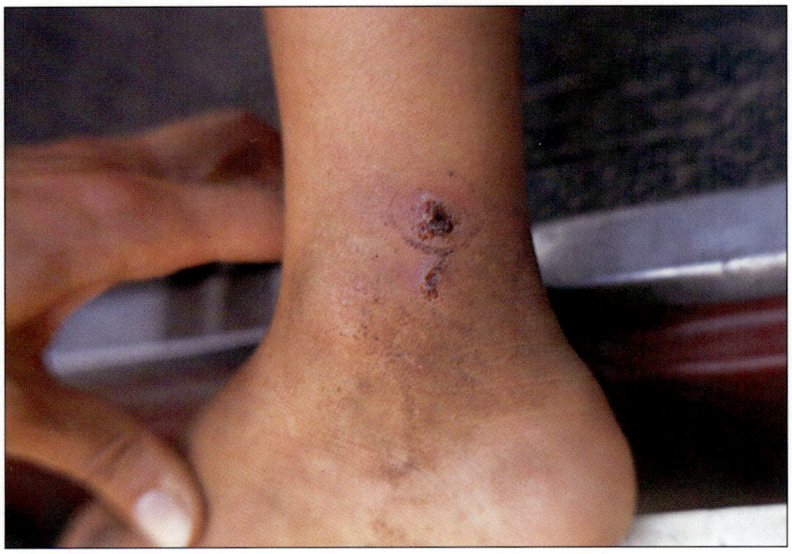

FIGURE 7-10 One-week-old lesion of streptococcal impetigo with thick, reddish-brown crust. Cultures at this stage usually yield mixtures of group A streptococci and staphylococci.

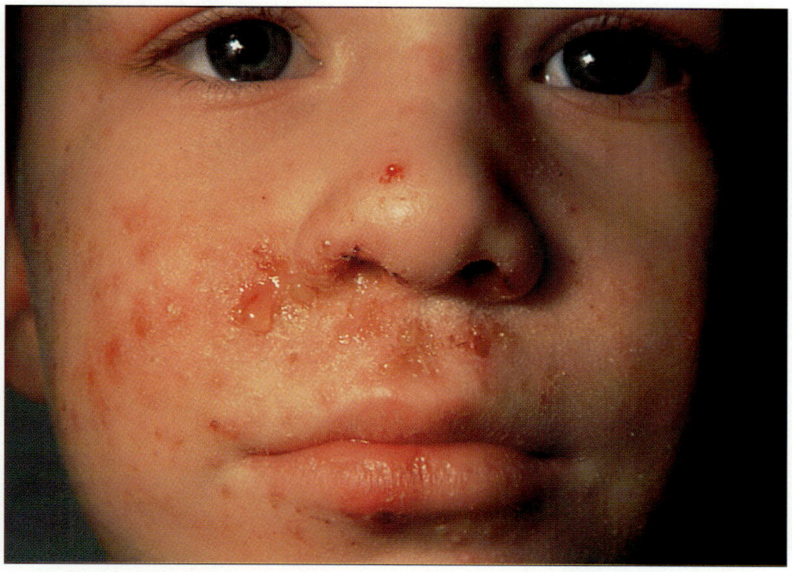

Figure 7-11 Facial impetigo 3 days after onset. Serous, oozing, honey-yellow crusts with a "stuck-on" appearance below the nares and pustules below the lips are apparent in this child aged 5 years with classic impetigo. Culture yielded group A streptococci. (*Courtesy of* A.M. Margileth, MD).

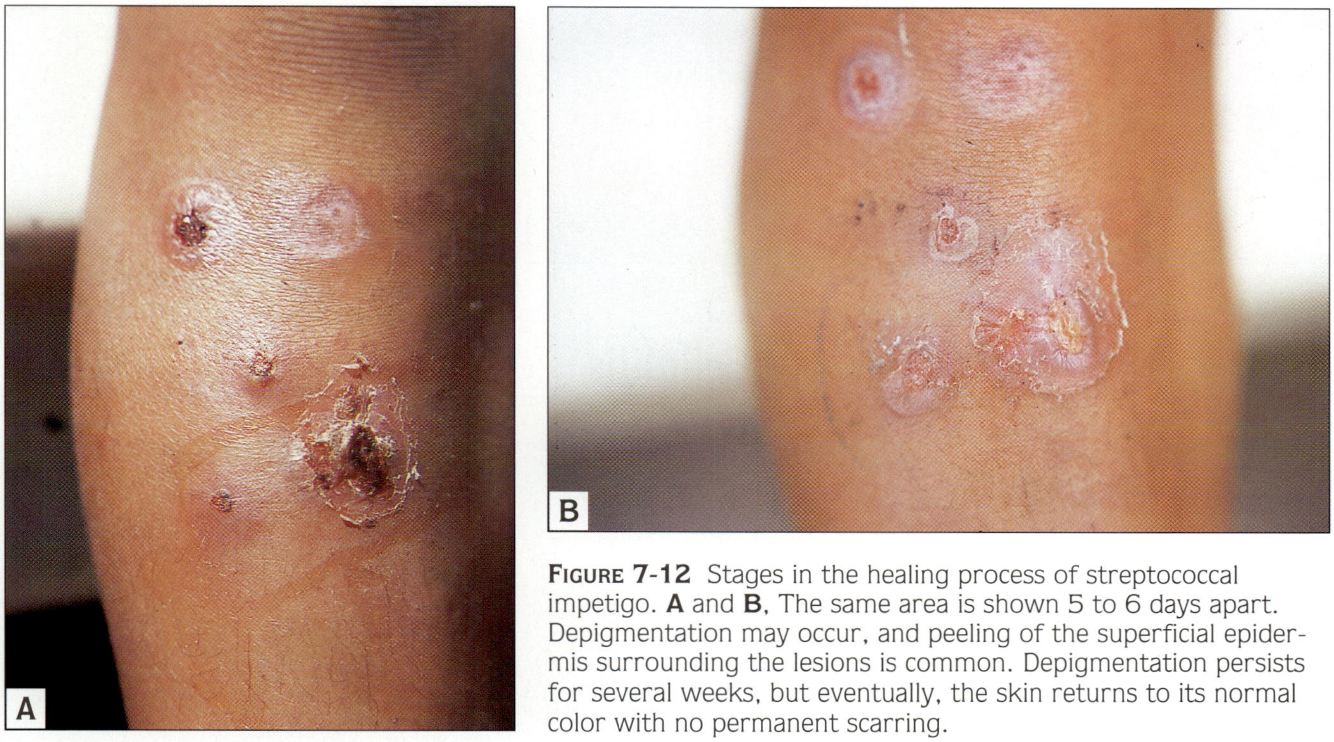

Figure 7-12 Stages in the healing process of streptococcal impetigo. **A** and **B**, The same area is shown 5 to 6 days apart. Depigmentation may occur, and peeling of the superficial epidermis surrounding the lesions is common. Depigmentation persists for several weeks, but eventually, the skin returns to its normal color with no permanent scarring.

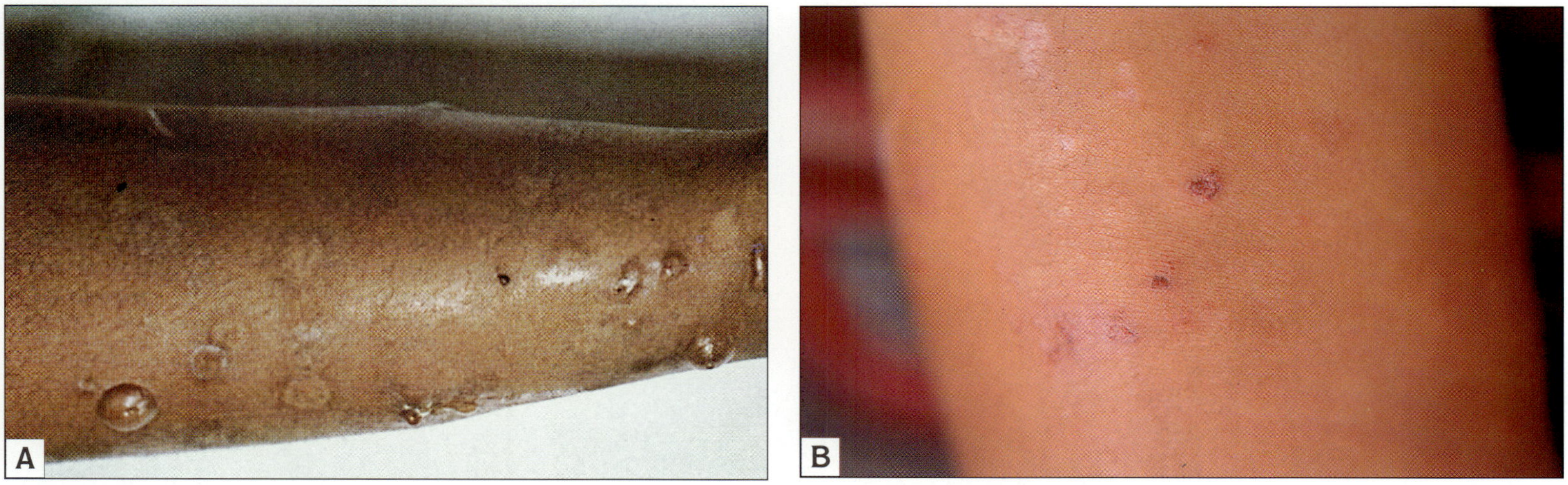

Figure 7-13 Staphylococcal impetigo. *Staphylococcus aureus* also may cause impetigo, and recent studies suggest that staphylococcal impetigo may be more common than the streptococcal variety. Clinically, staphylococcal impetigo presents in two forms: **A**, Bullous impetigo appears as thin-walled, fluid-filled lesions that vary in size from a few millimeters to several centimeters. Bacteria can be recovered from the fluid. **B**, In the second form, lesions have thin, varnishlike, light-brown crusts.

Ecthyma

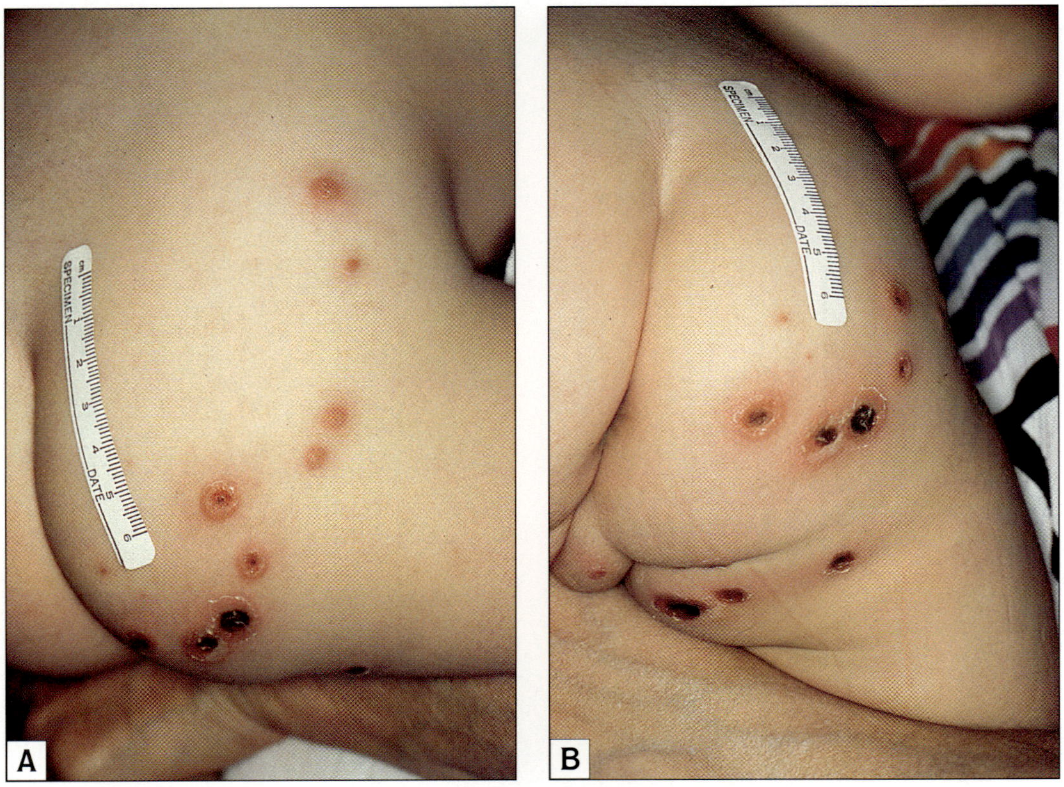

FIGURE 7-14 Streptococcal ecthyma. **A** and **B**, Ecthyma is a deeper lesion than impetigo. The lesion starts as a pustular eruption, usually seated on a hardened base, and surrounded by an inflammatory area. Pigmented scarring often occurs after healing.

Cellulitis

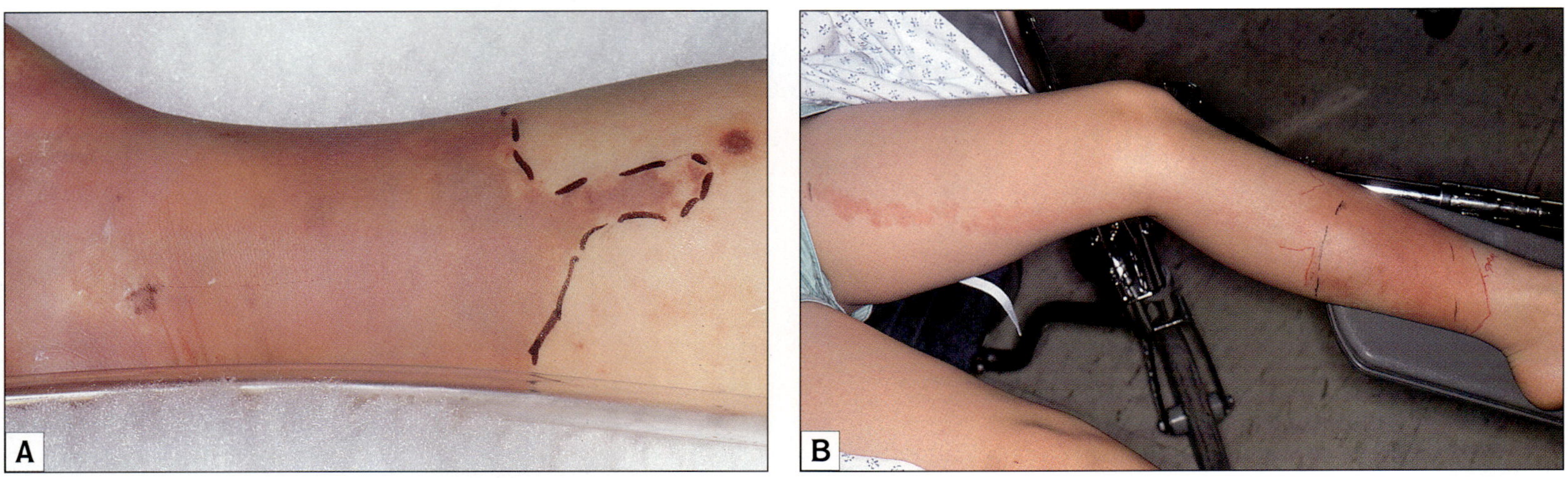

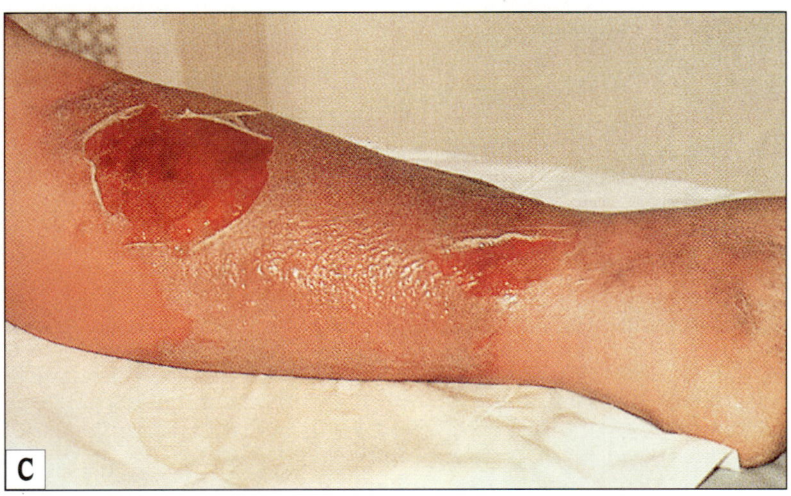

FIGURE 7-15 Streptococcal cellulitis. Group A streptococci are a common cause of cellulitis. Infection is often secondary to blunt or penetrating injury, usually on exposed skin. **A**, Infection may spread to involve a large area. **B**, Phlebitis or lymphangitis also may be noted. **C**, Infection may be very extensive and results in tissue necrosis and gangrene.

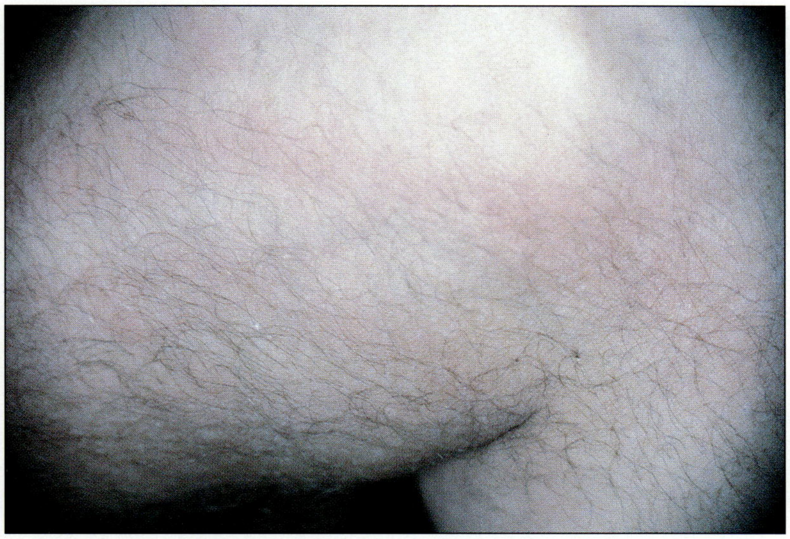

FIGURE 7-16 Lymphangitis. Reddened streaks extending proximally from an infected wound or cellulitis are invariably caused by group A streptococci. Prompt antibiotic treatment is mandatory because bacteremia and systemic toxicity develop rapidly. (*Courtesy of* D.L. Stevens, MD, PhD.)

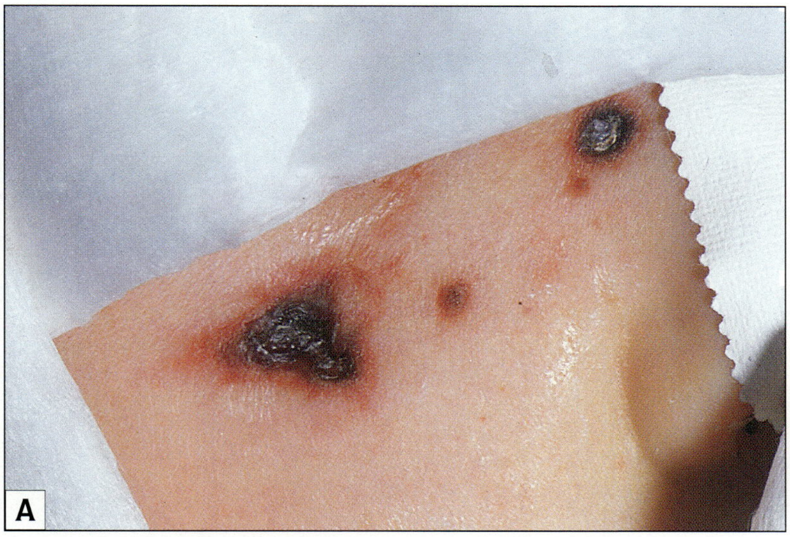

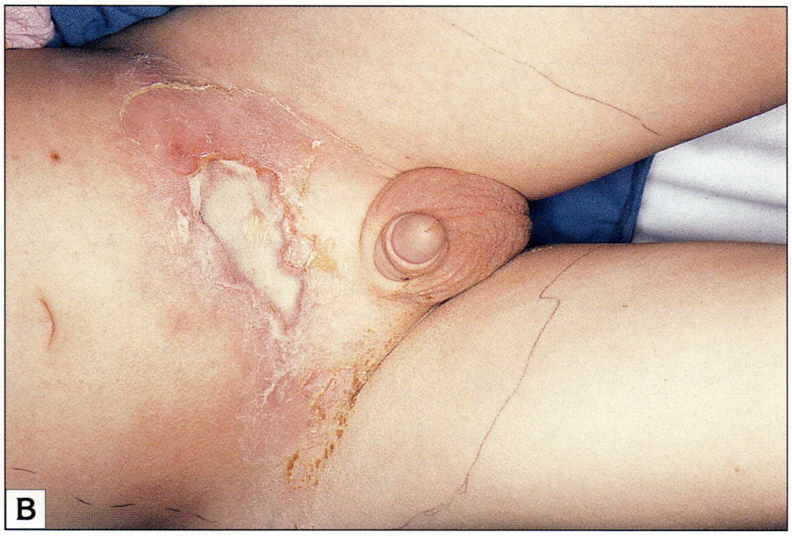

FIGURE 7-17 Varicella secondarily infected by streptococci. **A** and **B**, Varicella (chickenpox) lesions may sometimes become secondarily infected, and group A streptococci are a very common cause of secondary infection. Such infection may be severe and associated with bacteremia.

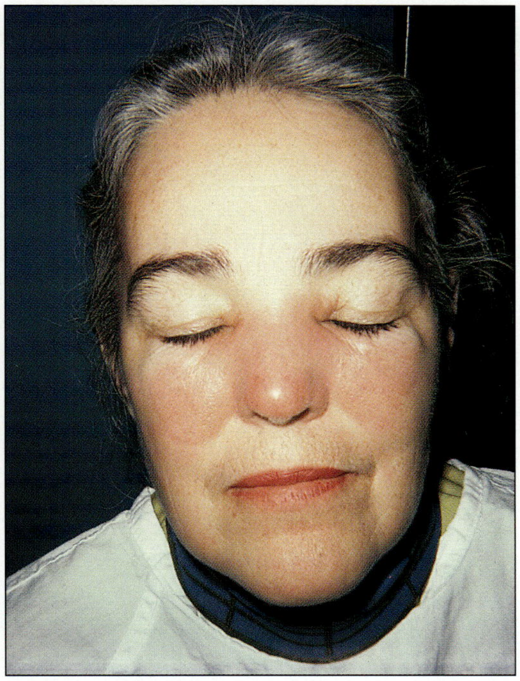

FIGURE 7-18 Erysipelas. Erysipelas is a form of streptococcal cellulitis that usually occurs on the face. There is commonly a leading edge of the infection as it spreads from the involved area. Constitutional symptoms (fever, malaise, chills) are not uncommon.

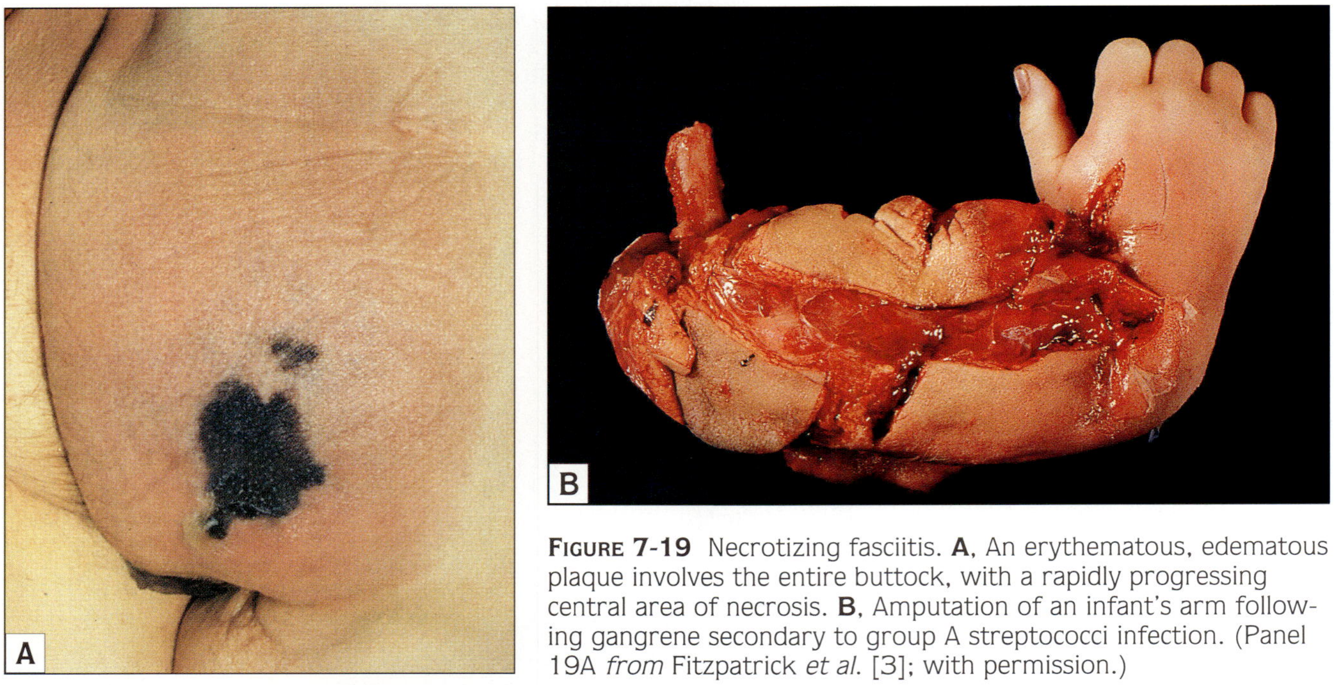

Figure 7-19 Necrotizing fasciitis. **A**, An erythematous, edematous plaque involves the entire buttock, with a rapidly progressing central area of necrosis. **B**, Amputation of an infant's arm following gangrene secondary to group A streptococci infection. (Panel 19A *from* Fitzpatrick *et al.* [3]; with permission.)

Pharyngitis

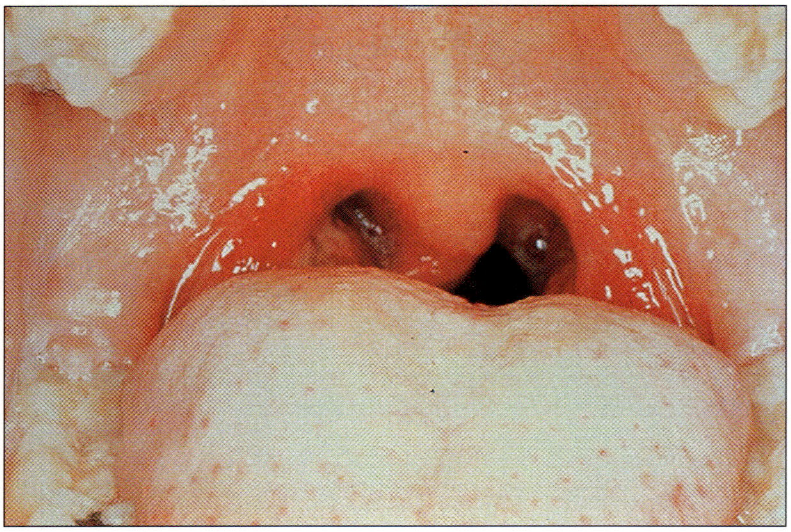

Figure 7-20 Streptococcal pharyngitis. Group A streptococci are the most common cause of bacterial pharyngitis. There is usually tonsillopharyngeal erythema, swelling, and exudate. Soft palate petechiae also may be noted. Anterior cervical adenitis and scarlatiniform rash are other findings. Sore throat usually is sudden and associated with fever, pain on swallowing, and other constitutional symptoms. These findings, however, are not diagnostic. Definitive diagnosis is made by means of a positive rapid streptococcal antigen test or a throat culture.

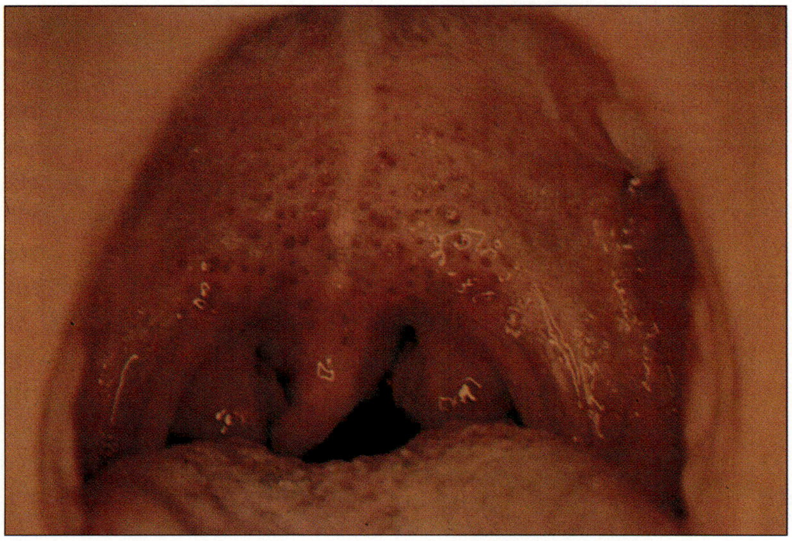

Figure 7-21 Marked petechial stippling of the soft palate in streptococcal pharyngitis. The typical appearance of the pharynx—severe erythema with exudate and palatal petechiae also is seen in scarlet fever. (*From* Stillerman and Bernstein [4]; with permission.)

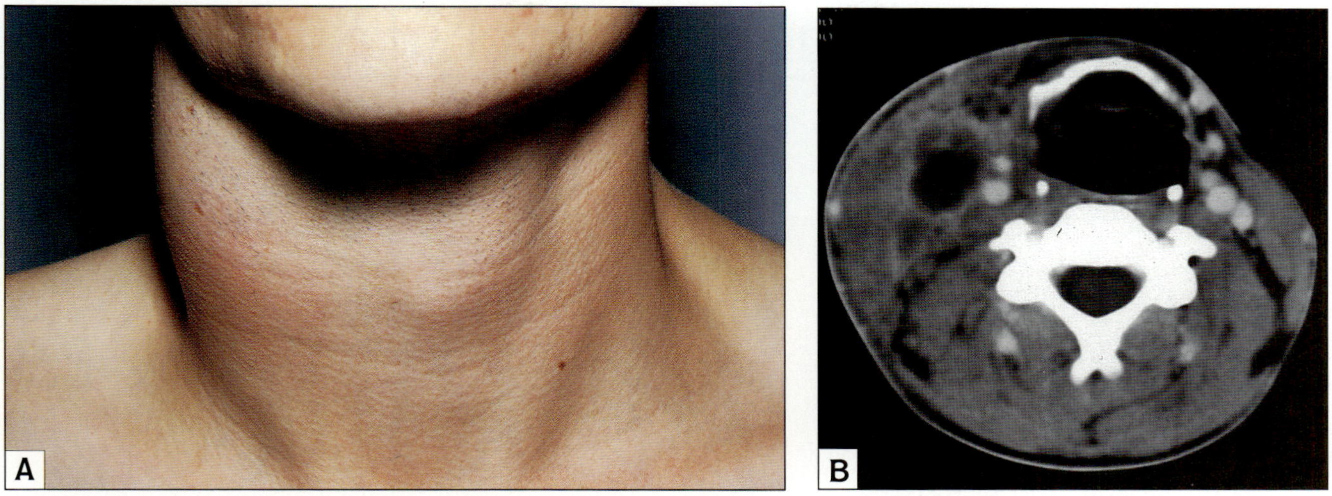

Figure 7-22 Peritonsillar abscess with extension to deep tissues of the neck, complicating streptococcal pharyngitis. **A**, Swelling of the neck with loss of definition of the sternocleidomastoid muscle is shown. **B**, A computed tomography scan of the neck shows a deep collection of inflammatory material. (*Courtesy of* D.L. Stevens, MD, PhD.)

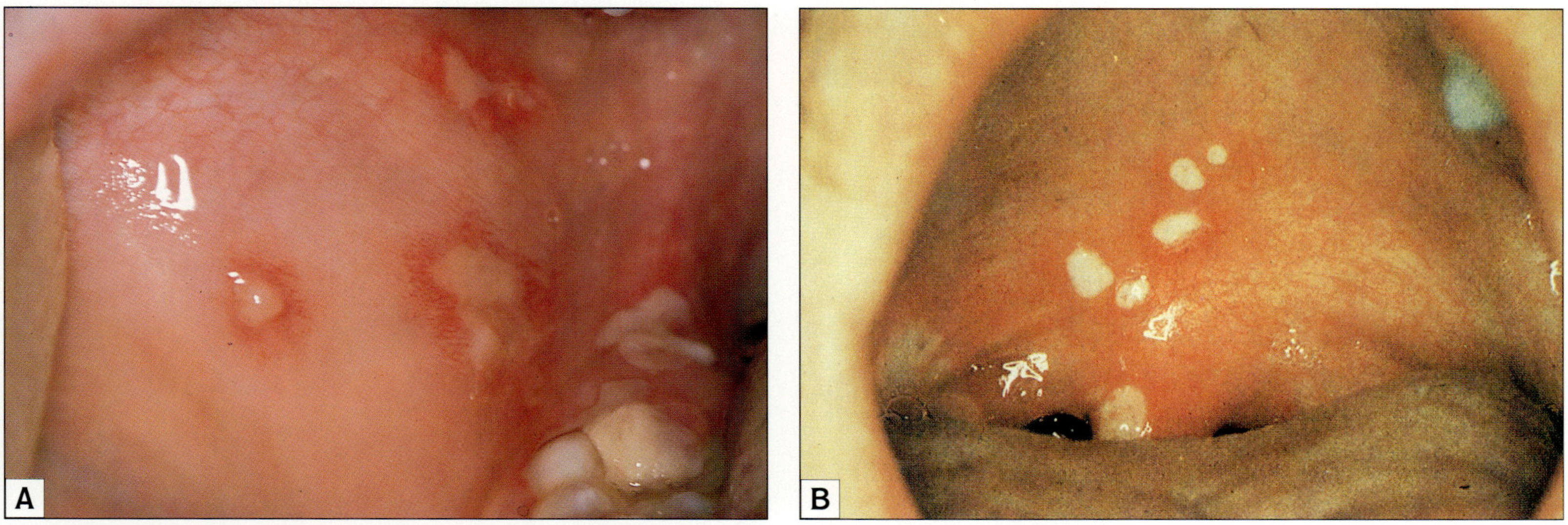

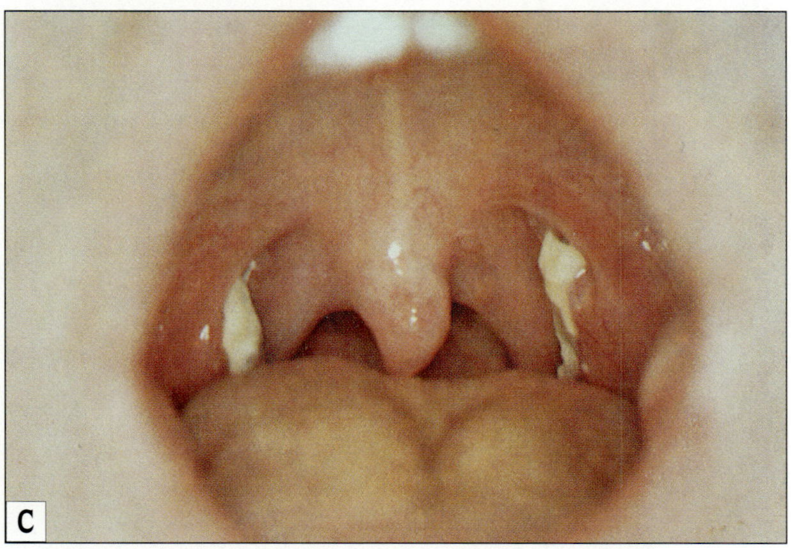

Figure 7-23 Viral causes in the differential diagnosis of streptococcal pharyngitis. Other common causes of pharyngitis include a number of viruses. **A**, Herpes simplex usually causes ulcerative lesions that may involve the tonsils and pharynx, but more commonly these lesions are anterior in the oral cavity. **B**, Herpangina (caused by many different enteroviruses) appears as ulcerative lesions on the anterior tonsillar pillars, soft palate, tonsils, pharynx, and posterior buccal mucosa. **C**, Infectious mononucleosis is caused by Epstein-Barr virus. In addition to the pharynx, multiple other organs also are involved.

Nonsuppurative Complications

Scarlet Fever

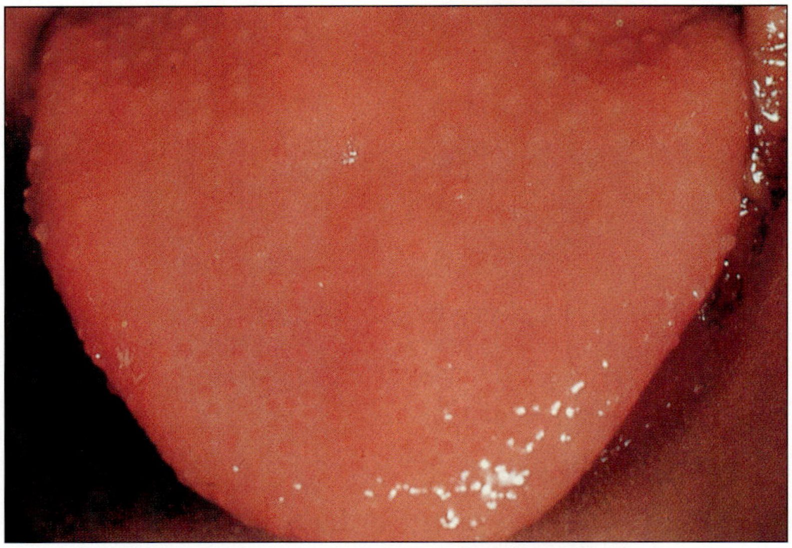

Figure 7-24 Strawberry tongue. Strawberry tongue is sometimes seen in cases of scarlet fever. During the first few days of illness, the tongue is covered with a thick white material through which the enlarged red papillae protrude. The white material peels in a few days, resulting in the red strawberry stage shown here. Strawberry tongue also is seen in patients with Kawasaki disease.

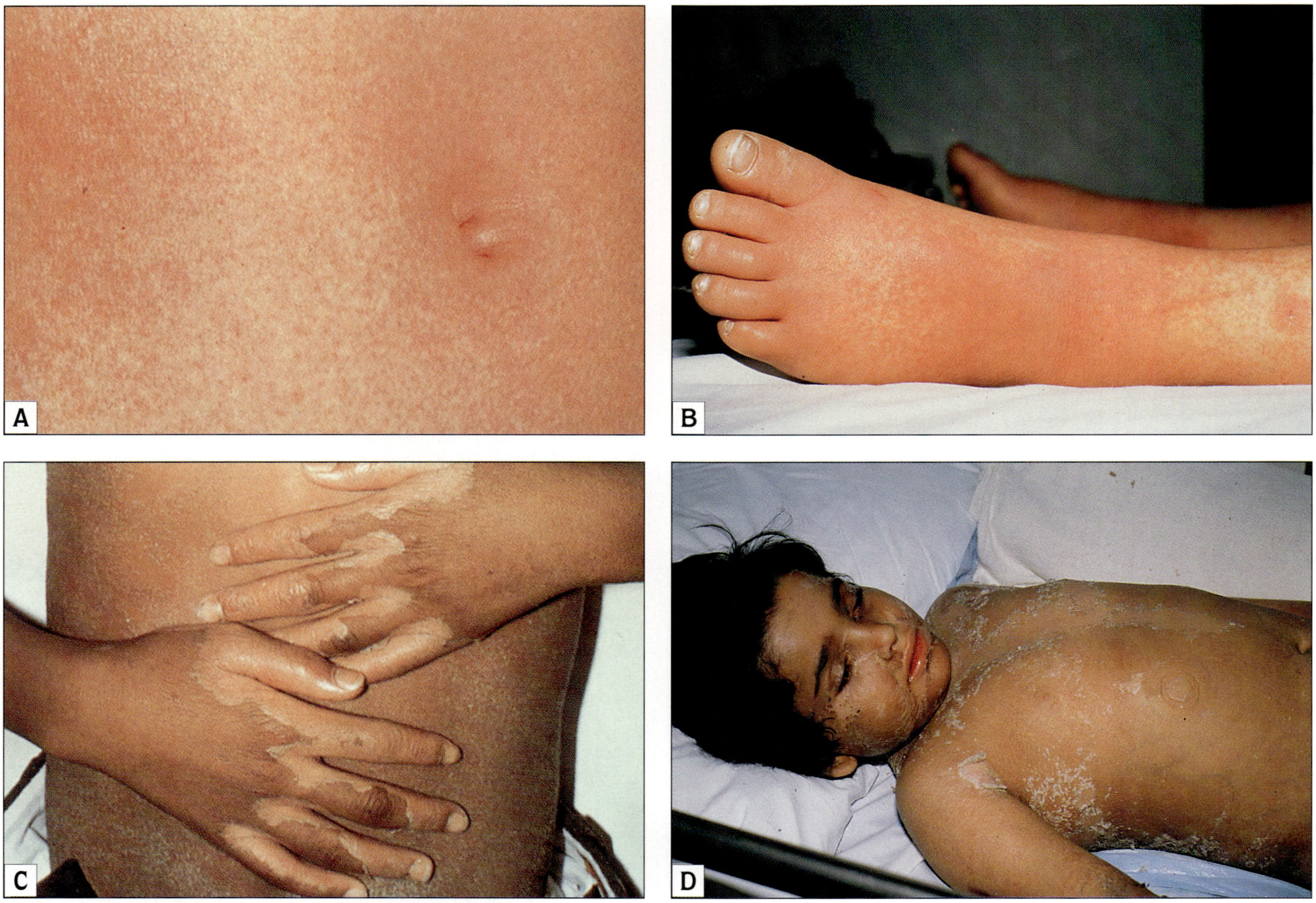

Figure 7-25 Rash of scarlet fever. **A** and **B**, The rash of scarlet fever is typically discrete, pinhead-sized, and erythematous, and it may have the feel of sandpaper. The rash blanches on applying pressure to the skin. **C** and **D**, Later in the course of scarlet fever, desquamation occurs.

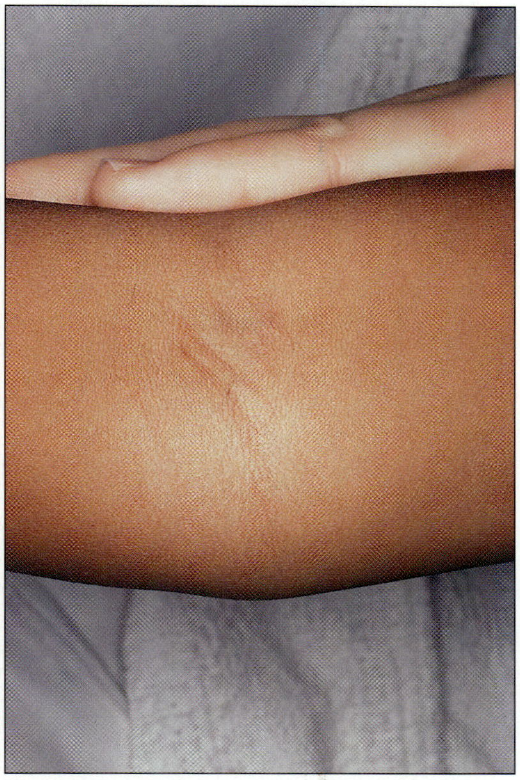

FIGURE 7-26 Pastia's lines in scarlet fever. The rash of scarlet fever is accentuated in the skin folds, especially the antecubital fossa (as seen here), but also in the neck, axillae, and groin. These lines persist for a day or two after desquamation of the rash.

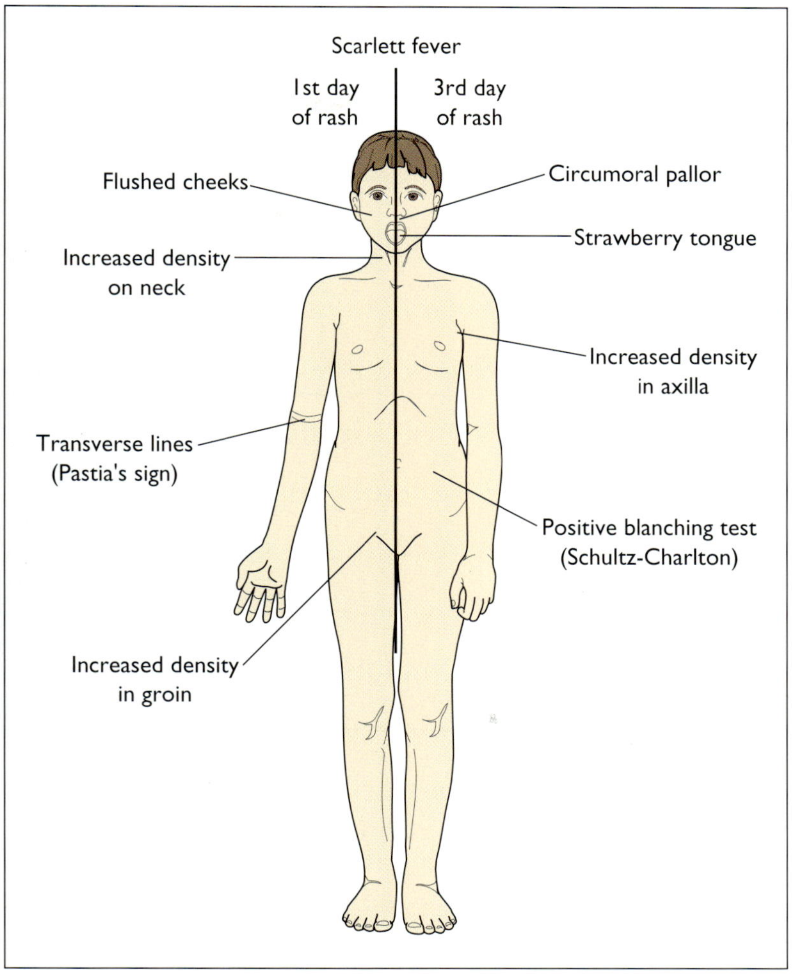

FIGURE 7-27 Development and distribution of scarlet fever rash. The exanthem of scarlet fever becomes generalized very quickly, usually within 24 hours. The punctate rash commonly does not involve the face, although the forehead and cheeks are red, smooth, and flush. There is an area of paleness around the mouth (circumoral pallor). The tongue changes as the disease progresses, resulting in the distinctive strawberry tongue by the fourth or fifth day. (*Adapted from* Krugman and Ward [5].)

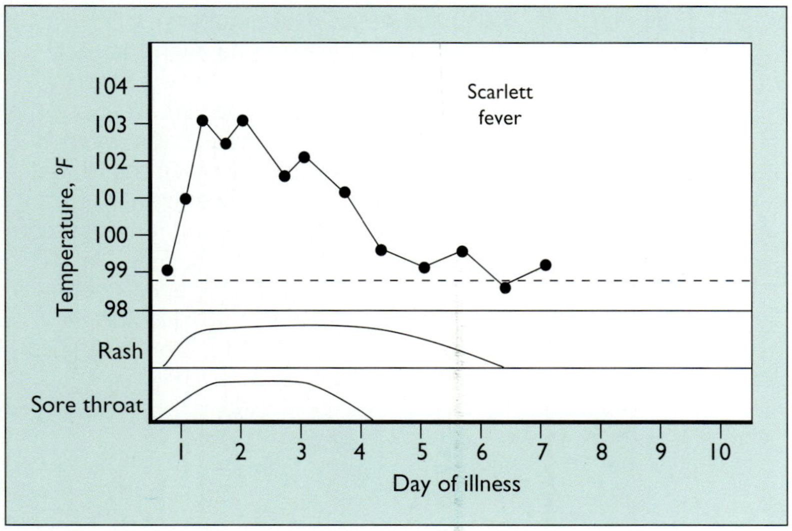

FIGURE 7-28 Typical course of untreated, uncomplicated scarlet fever. The rash usually appears within 24 hours of onset of fever and sore throat. In the typical case, the fever rises rapidly to 103° F and reaches its peak on the second day. It resolves gradually over 4 to 5 days. (*Adapted from* Krugman and Ward [5].)

Rheumatic Fever

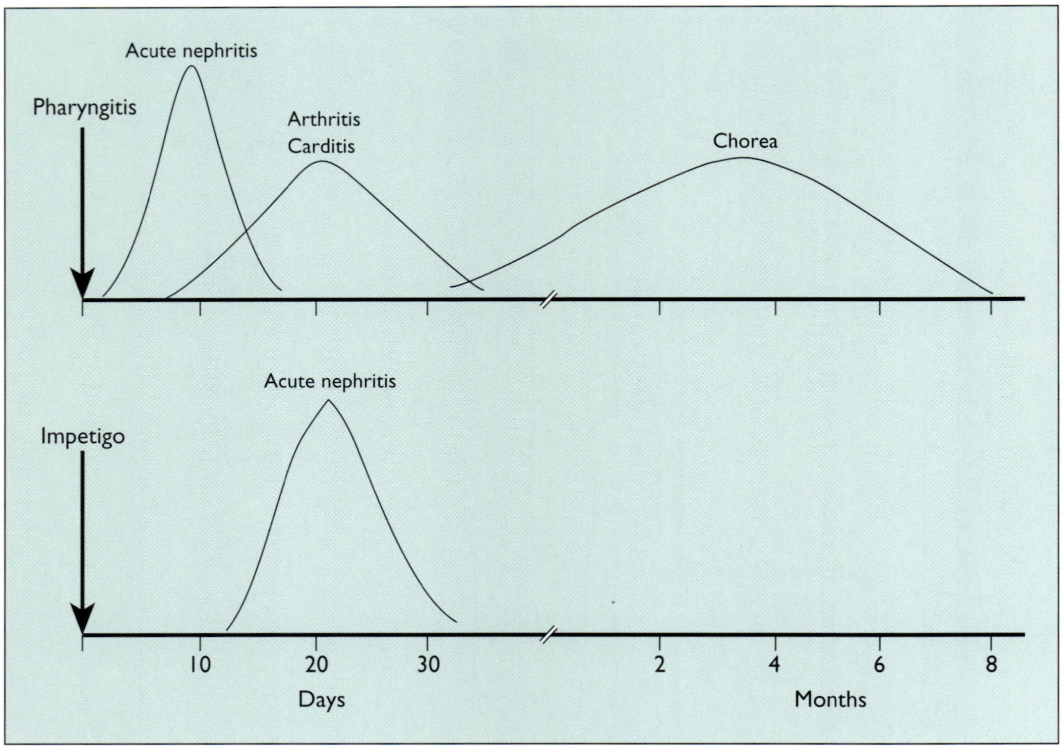

FIGURE 7-29 Occurrence of complications following group A streptococcal (GAS) infections. The major nonsuppurative complications of GAS infections are rheumatic fever and glomerulonephritis. Acute poststreptococcal nephritis may follow streptococcal pharyngitis or streptococcal impetigo. The latent period for nephritis following pharyngitis is shorter. Rheumatic fever does not occur after impetigo. It may occur in up to 3% of individuals with untreated GAS pharyngitis. Onset of acute rheumatic fever is usually at least 7 to 10 days after the onset of pharyngitis. The latent periods for arthritis and carditis are much shorter than the latent period for chorea.

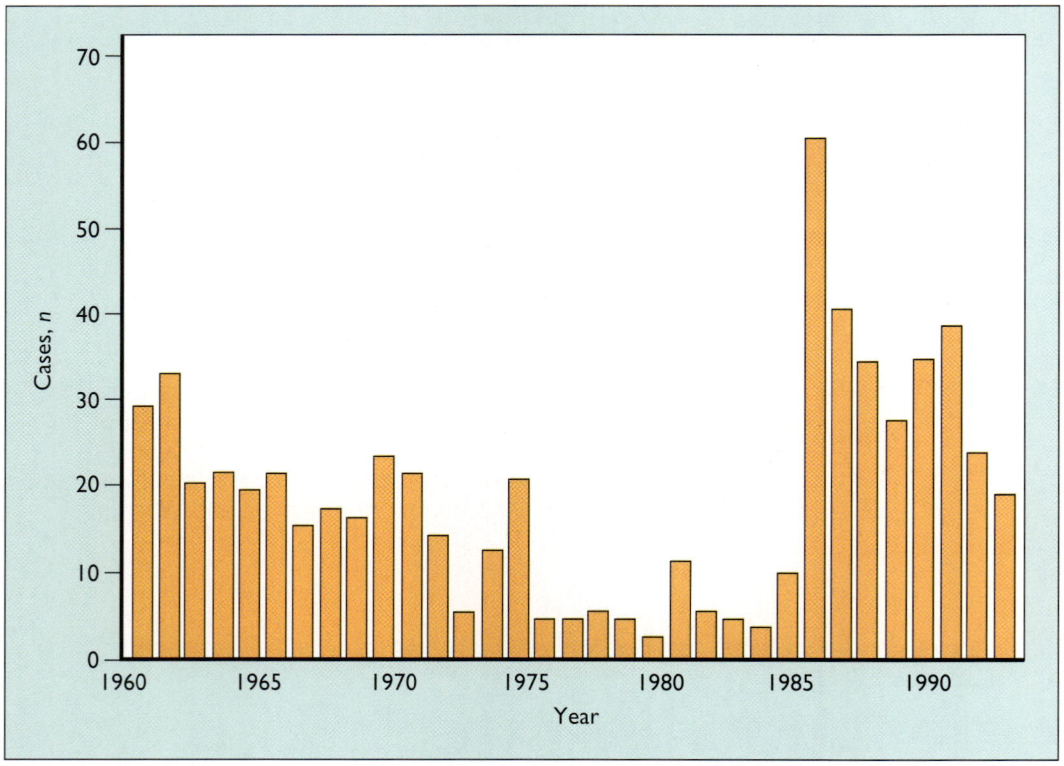

FIGURE 7-30 Frequency of acute rheumatic fever in Salt Lake City between 1960 and 1992. The incidence of rheumatic fever and prevalence of rheumatic heart disease vary in different countries. At the turn of the century, the incidence of rheumatic fever in the United States was over 100 per 100,000 population, but it declined to 40 to 65 per 100,000 between 1935 and 1960 and is currently estimated at < 2 per 100,000. Data shown in the figure reflect the fluctuations in cases of acute rheumatic fever observed in Salt Lake City between 1960 and 1992. The numbers of cases were declining through the early 1980s, but beginning in 1985, a sharp increase in cases was observed. At about the same time, a similar increase was noted in some other geographic areas in the United States. The increase has been related to the reappearance of specific group A streptococcal serotypes (notably M1, 3, 5, 6, 14, 18, 19, 27, and 29). Rheumatic fever continues to be the major cause of acquired heart disease in many parts of the world, particularly in developing countries [6].

Guidelines for the diagnosis of initial attack of rheumatic fever (Jones Criteria, updated 1992)
Major manifestations
Carditis
Polyarthritis
Chorea
Erythema marginatum
Subcutaneous nodules
Minor manifestations
Clinical findings
Arthralgia
Fever
Laboratory findings
Elevated acute phase reactants
Erythrocyte sedimentation rate
C-reactive protein
Prolonged PR interval
Supporting evidence of antecedent group A streptococcal infection
Positive throat culture or rapid streptococcal antigen test
Elevated or rising streptococcal antibody titer

FIGURE 7-31 Modified Jones criteria for rheumatic fever. Because there is no single pathognomonic feature for the diagnosis of rheumatic fever, a set of diagnostic guidelines were developed by Jones in 1944, and these have been updated regularly by the American Heart Association, most recently in 1992. The diagnosis of an initial attack of acute rheumatic fever is strongly suggested in patients with two major or one major and two minor criteria and documentation of recent streptococcal infection (positive throat culture or elevated serum streptococcal antibodies) [7].

Streptococcal Toxic Shock Syndrome

Features of streptococcal toxic shock syndrome
Hypotension/shock
Fever
Rash—diffuse erythroderma (may be absent)
Desquamation, 1–2 wks after onset of illness
Involvement of ≥ 3 organ systems:
Gastrointestinal (vomiting and/or diarrhea)
Mucous membrane (erythema)
Renal
Hepatic
Hematopoietic (coagulopathy)
Musculocutaneous (soft-tissue necrosis)
Central nervous system
Pulmonary (acute respiratory distress syndrome)
Isolation of group A streptococci from a normally sterile site (definite) or nonsterile site (probable)

FIGURE 7-32 Features of streptococcal toxic shock syndrome.

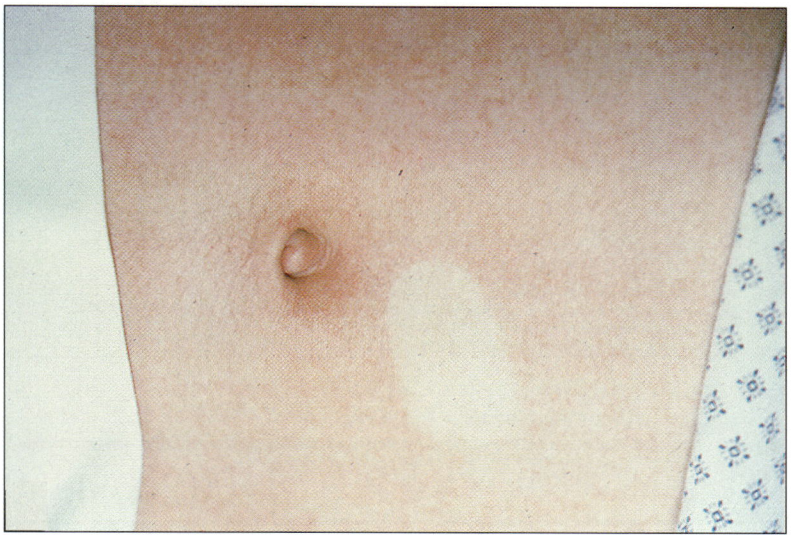

FIGURE 7-33 Blanching of petechial rash in streptococcal toxic shock syndrome. Sudden onset of high fever (to 40° C, 104° F), erythroderma, petechial rash, conjunctival hemorrhages, pharyngitis, and abdominal pain is typical of toxic shock syndrome, as seen in this girl aged 13 years 6 hours after onset. Shock may develop along with hypotension, very poor capillary filling, marked malaise, lethargy, and jaundice. In this patient, a throat culture was positive for group A streptococci and her antistreptolysin titer was elevated to 1:1360 (although most cases of toxic shock syndrome are due to *Staphylococcus aureus*). Desquamation of her fingers and toes developed after 3 to 7 days on antibiotic therapy, with recover following. (*Courtesy of* A.M. Margileth, MD.)

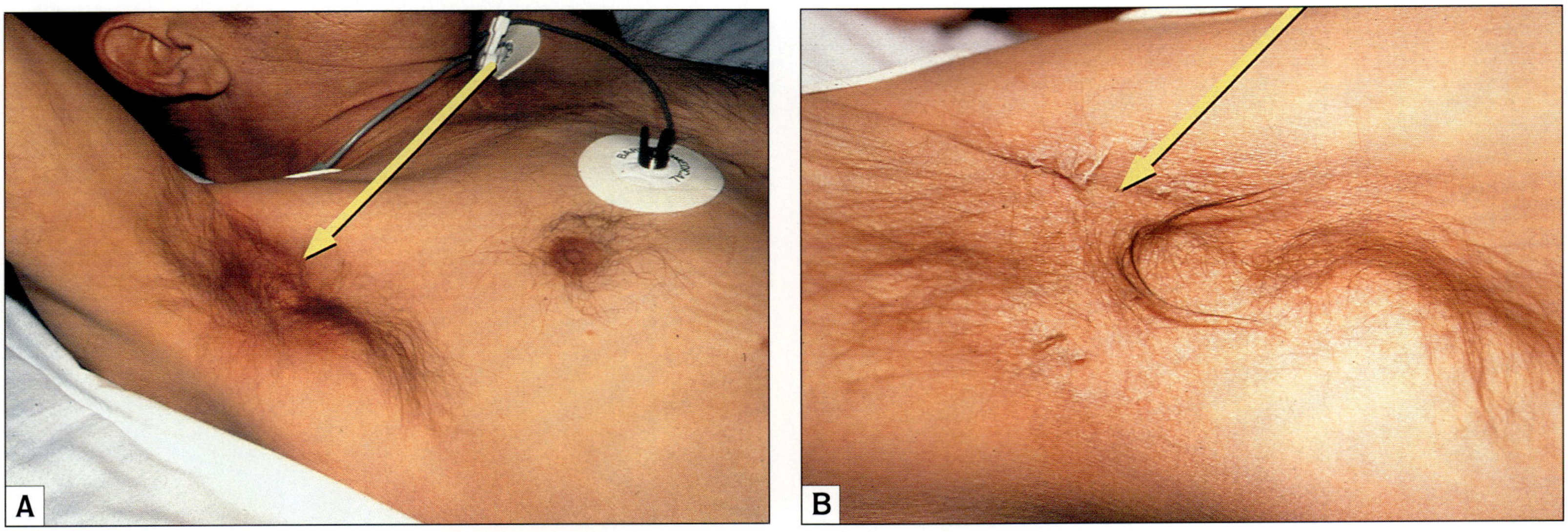

Figure 7-34 Erythematous rash in streptococcal toxic shock syndrome. The rash (*arrows*) may occur anywhere and is transient. **A**, Erythema of the axillae in a patient. **B**, Desquamation of the erythematous skin 10 to 14 days after the rash appeared. (*Courtesy of* D.L. Stevens, MD, PhD.)

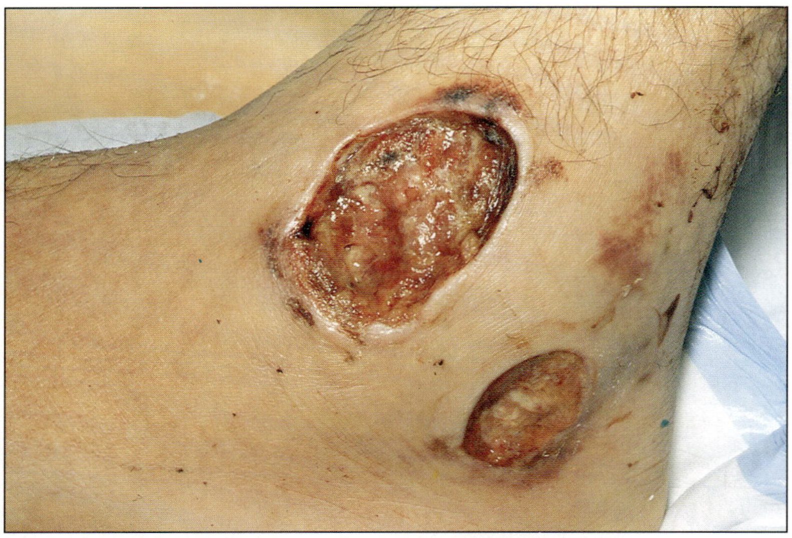

Figure 7-35 Localized cutaneous gangrene in a patient with group A streptococcal bacteremia. The well-circumscribed necrotic areas are likely due to vascular occlusion and tissue infarction. (*Courtesy of* D.L. Stevens, MD, PhD.)

Diagnosis and Treatment

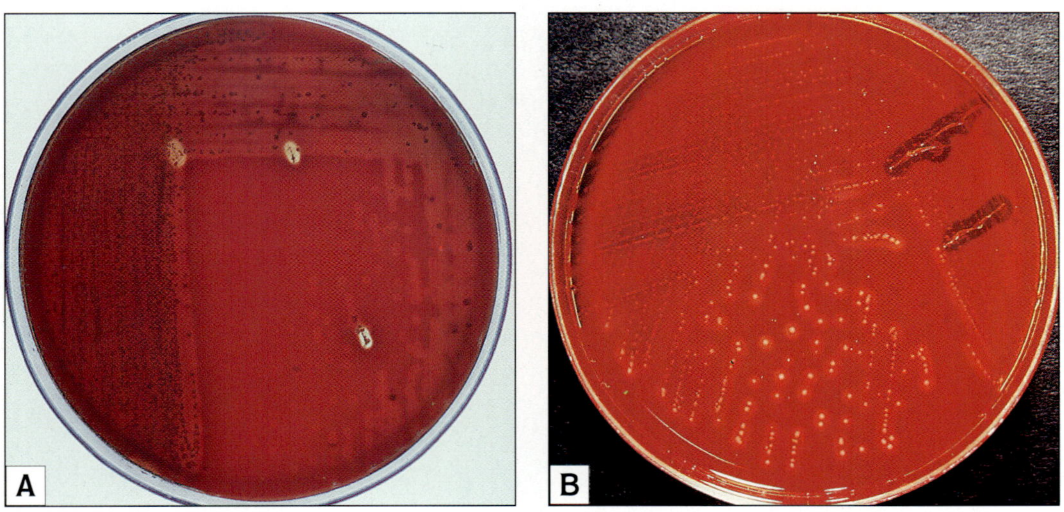

Figure 7-36 Throat cultures for group A streptococci (GAS). The "gold standard" for diagnosing GAS pharyngitis is to obtain an appropriate throat culture. A swab of both tonsils and the posterior pharynx should be plated on a blood agar plate (5% sheep blood in trypticase soy agar), the plate streaked and "stabbed," and incubated at 35° to 37° C for 18 to 24 hours. **A**, GAS colonies are usually small and slightly whitish and are surrounded by a clear zone of hemolysis (β-hemolysis). Sometimes, the hemolysis is accentuated or occurs only in subsurface growth (where the agar had been stabbed). **B**, Single β-hemolytic colonies are then picked and streaked onto a fresh blood agar plate to obtain a pure culture.

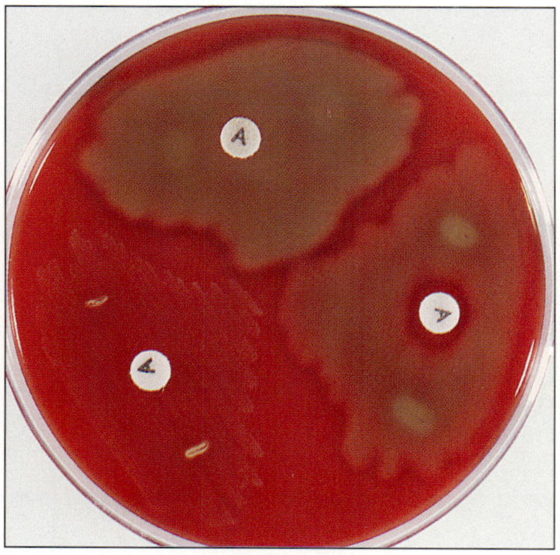

FIGURE 7-37 Bacitracin inhibition test for group A streptococci (GAS). GAS can be differentiated from other β-hemolytic colonies by determining if they are inhibited by an "A" disc (disc containing 0.02 units of bacitracin) after an additional overnight incubation. Strains inhibited by the bacitracin disc are presumptively identified as group A; strains not inhibited by bacitracin are presumed to be nongroup A. Alternatively, serologic tests may be performed to identify GAS.

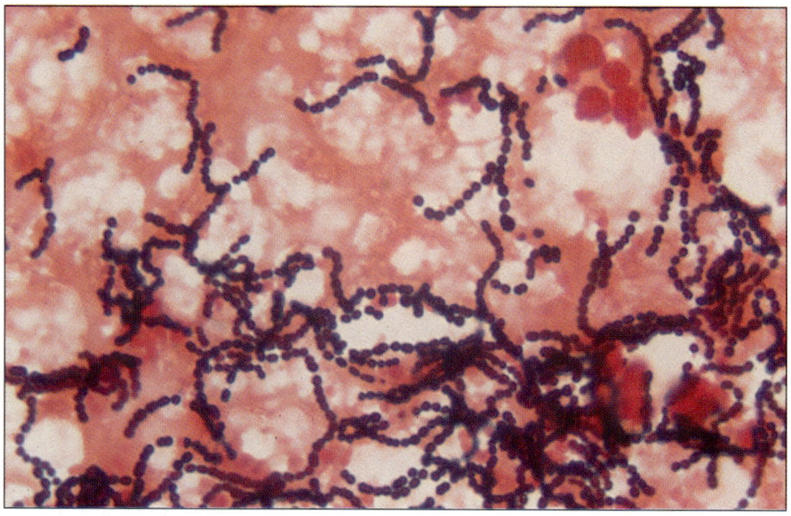

FIGURE 7-38 Gram stain of group A streptococci (GAS). GAS can be suspected when a Gram stain of material obtained from normally sterile body site or of pus shows gram-positive cocci in chains. The identity of the organisms should be confirmed by appropriate cultures. Gram stains of material obtained from the respiratory (throat, pharynx), gastrointestinal, or genitourinary tracts or from the skin are less helpful because other organisms (α-hemolytic streptococci, enterococci, pneumococci) may resemble GAS on Gram smears.

Choice of antibiotics in the treatment of group A streptococcal infections
First choice
Penicillin
Other acceptable choices
Other penicillins (ampicillin, amoxicillin, oxacillin, etc.)
Cephalosporins
Macrolides (erythromycin, azithromycin, clarithromycin)
Clindamycin
Unacceptable
Tetracyclines
Chloramphenicol
Sulfonamides, including trimethoprim-sulfamethoxazole

FIGURE 7-39 Choice of antibiotics in the treatment of group A streptococcal infections. Macrolides and clindamycin are recommended for individuals allergic to penicillin. Cephalosporins should not be used in individuals with immediate (anaphylactic-type) hypersensitivity to penicillin.

Usual doses for penicillin for the treatment of group A streptococcal infections
Streptococcal pharyngitis
Penicillin V, 250–500 mg 2–3 times daily orally × 10 days, *or*
Benzathine penicillin, 600,000 U im once for children < 60 lbs *or* 1.2 MU for patients > 60 lbs
Other infections
Penicillin G, 50,000–100,000 U/kg/day (im or iv)
Duration of treatment depends on illness and clinical response
im—intramuscularly; iv—intravenously.

FIGURE 7-40 Usual dosages for penicillin for group A streptococcal infections. Duration of treatment depends on an individual's severity of illness and clinical response.

References

1. Colman G, Tanna A, Efstratiou A, Gaworzewska E: The serotypes of *Streptococcus pyogenes* present in Britain during 1980–1990 and their association with disease. *J Med Microbiol* 1993, 39:165–178.
2. Schwartz B, Facklam RR, Breiman RF: Changing epidemiology of group A streptococcal infection in the USA. *Lancet* 1990, 336:1167–1171.
3. Fitzpatrick TB, Johnson RA, Polano MK, *et al.*: *Color Atlas and Synopsis of Clinical Dermatology: Common and Serious Diseases*, 2nd ed. New York: McGraw-Hill; 1992.
4. Stillerman M, Bernstein SH: Streptococcal pharyngitis: Evaluation of clinical syndromes in diagnosis. *Am J Dis Child* 1961, 101:476–489.
5. Krugman S, Ward R: *Infectious Diseases of Children and Adults*, 5th ed. St. Louis: Mosby; 1973.
6. Veasey LG, Tani LY, Hill HR: Persistence of acute rheumatic fever in the intermountain area of the United States. *J Pediatr* 1994, 124:9–16.
7. Dajani AS, Ayoub E, Bierman FZ, *et al.*: Guidelines for the diagnosis of rheumatic fever: Jones criteria, 1992 update. *JAMA* 1992, 268:2069–2073.

Selected Bibliography

Cleary PP, Kaplan EL, Handley JP, *et al.*: Clonal basis for resurgence of serious *Streptococcus pyogenes* disease in the 1980s. *Lancet* 1992, 339:518–521.

Dajani AS, Ayoub E, Bierman FZ, *et al.*: Guidelines for the diagnosis of rheumatic fever: Jones criteria, 1992 update. *JAMA* 1992, 268:2069–2073.

Dajani AS, Taubert K, Ferrieri P, *et al.*: Treatment of acute streptococcal pharyngitis and prevention of rheumatic fever: A statement for health professionals. *Pediatrics* 1995, 96:758–764.

Schwartz B, Facklam RR, Breiman RF: Changing epidemiology of group A streptococcal infection in the USA. *Lancet* 1990, 336:1167–1171.

Stevens DL: Invasive group A streptococcus infections. *Clin Infect Dis* 1992, 14:2–13.

CHAPTER 8

Staphylococcal Infections

James K. Todd

THE STAPHYLOCOCCI are gram-positive, aerobic organisms commonly found in the nose and on the skin of most individuals. There are two major organism groups—*Staphylococcus aureus* (which is often pathogenic and causes localized abscesses and toxin-mediated diseases) and coagulase-negative staphylococci (which usually cause infection only associated with foreign bodies, *eg*, vascular catheters).

Within the *S. aureus* species there are many different strains distinguished by their ability to cause local infection and produce a variety of toxins, which mediate the clinical manifestations associated with scalded-skin syndrome, toxic shock syndrome, or food poisoning. Disease manifestations in patients will depend on the infecting strain of *S. aureus* and the patient's immunity, especially to toxins. Treatment often requires drainage of focal infections (*eg*, abscesses) and antibiotics. Most strains are resistant to penicillin G and ampicillin but are susceptible to the beta-lactamase-resistant penicillins (*eg*, oxacillin). There are an increasing number of strains that are resistant to the methicillin group of antibiotics (including oxacillin and the cephalosporins) that are referred to as methicillin-resistant *S. aureus*. These are usually susceptible to vancomycin, but recently, resistance has been reported.

Coagulase-negative staphylococci are usually found on the skin, and except for their ability to attach to indwelling foreign bodies (*eg*, vascular catheters, prosthetic valves), they are much less pathogenic. They are the most common cause of vascular catheter–associated sepsis and central nervous system shunt infections; they also may be difficult to treat without removing the foreign body. Coagulase-negative staphylococci are usually resistant to the penicillins and cephalosporins and are usually susceptible to vancomycin and rifampin (which should never be used as a single drug).

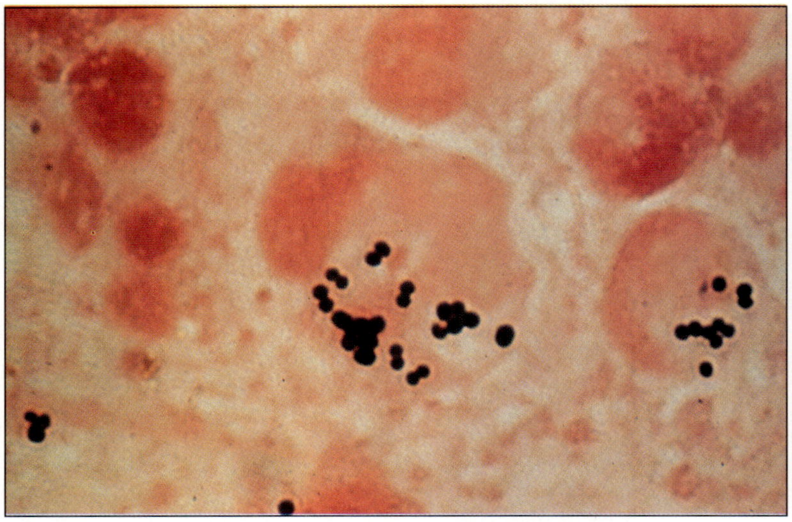

FIGURE 8-1 Gram stain of *Staphylococcus* organisms. Staphylococci are gram-positive cocci that are configured in pairs and clusters ("staphylo" means "grape-like"). These organisms are common causes of wound and skin infections and abscesses.

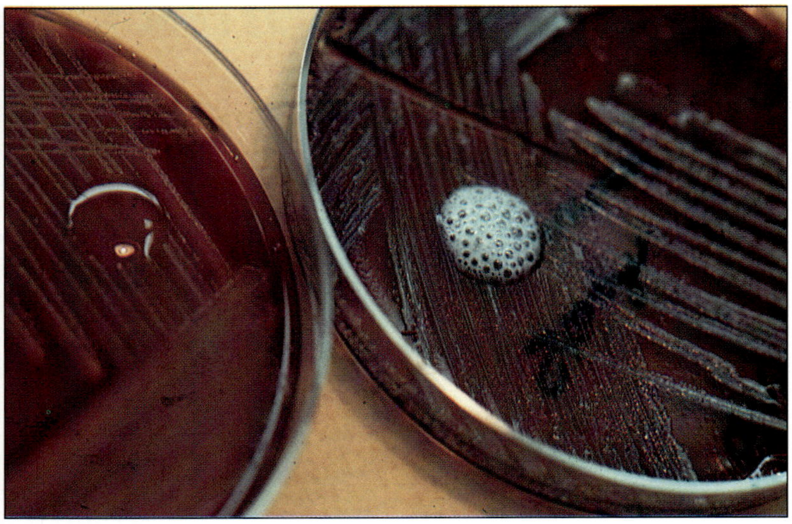

FIGURE 8-2 Staphylococci (*right*) and streptococci (*left*) on a blood agar plate. These organisms may each produce beta-hemolysis on blood agar plates. They are distinguished by the catalase reaction, which produces vigorous bubbles when a drop of peroxide comes in contact with the colony. Staphylococci are catalase-positive.

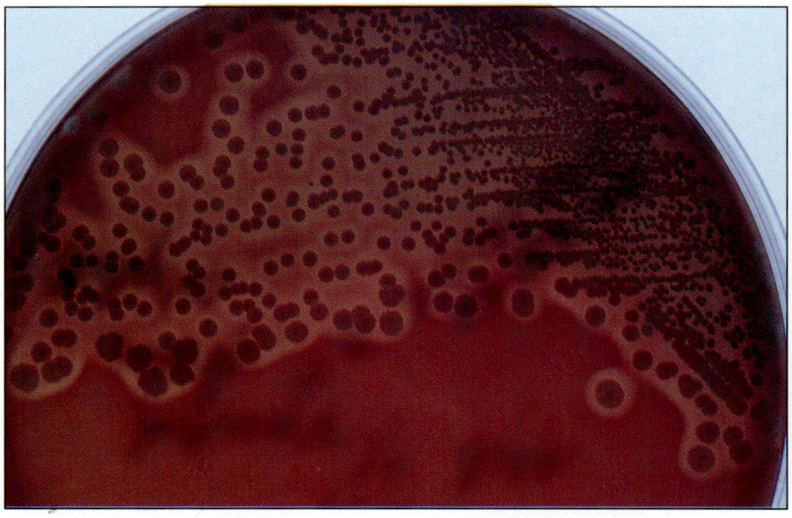

FIGURE 8-3 Growth of staphylococci. Staphylococci grow well on blood agar but not MacConkey agar. *Staphylococcus aureus* colonies are often (but not always) b-hemolytic and golden in color. Coagulase-negative staphylococci are often (but not always) nonhemolytic and white in color.

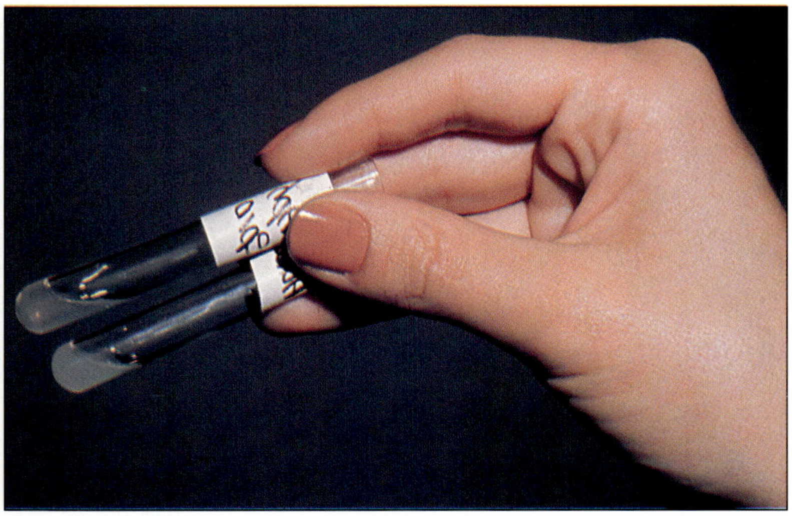

FIGURE 8-4 Coagulase test and *Staphylococcus aureus*. *S. aureus* is coagulase-positive: it causes clotting of plasma in vitro (*lower tube*). The coagulase enzyme produced by *S. aureus* may play a role in localizing infections by creating a wall of fibrin that results in abscess formation.

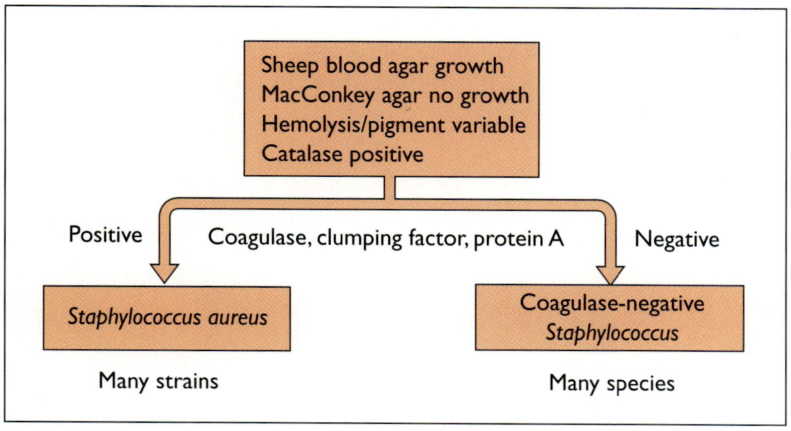

FIGURE 8-5 Microbiologic identification of staphylococcal species. Organisms that cause coagulation or clumping in plasma or produce protein A are considered to be *Staphylococcus aureus*; all others are called coagulase-negative staphylococci (many species).

Prevalence of staphylococci in humans

	Nose	Skin	Other
Staphylococcus aureus	+++	+	Throat, vagina
Coagulase-negative *Staphylococcus*	+	+++	Throat

FIGURE 8-6 Prevalence of staphylococci in humans. Staphylococci are common elements of the normal flora in most humans. *Staphylococcus aureus* is most commonly found in the anterior nares, whereas various strains of coagulase-negative staphylococci can be cultured from the skin.

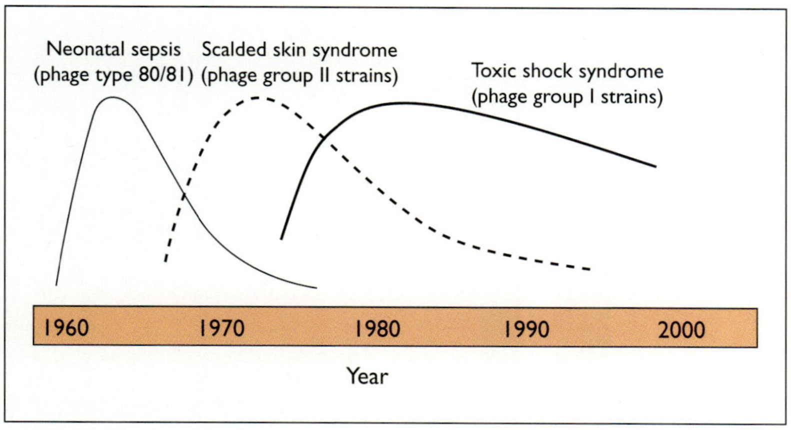

FIGURE 8-7 Epidemiology of *Staphylococcus aureus* diseases. There are many strains of *S. aureus* with differing virulence factors. The strain predominance varies over time such that some disease may be more prevalent.

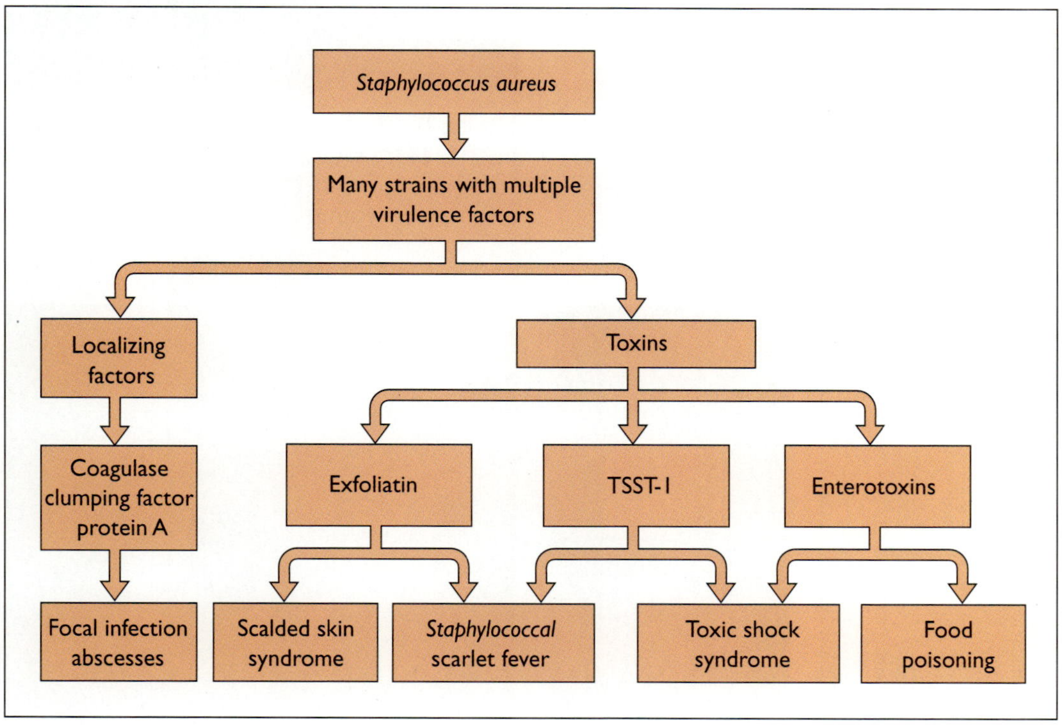

FIGURE 8-8 Relationship of staphylococcal virulence factors and resultant diseases. There are many different strains of *Staphylococcus aureus* that produce various virulence factors. These toxins and enzymes determine the disease symptoms. TSST-1—toxic shock syndrome toxin-1.

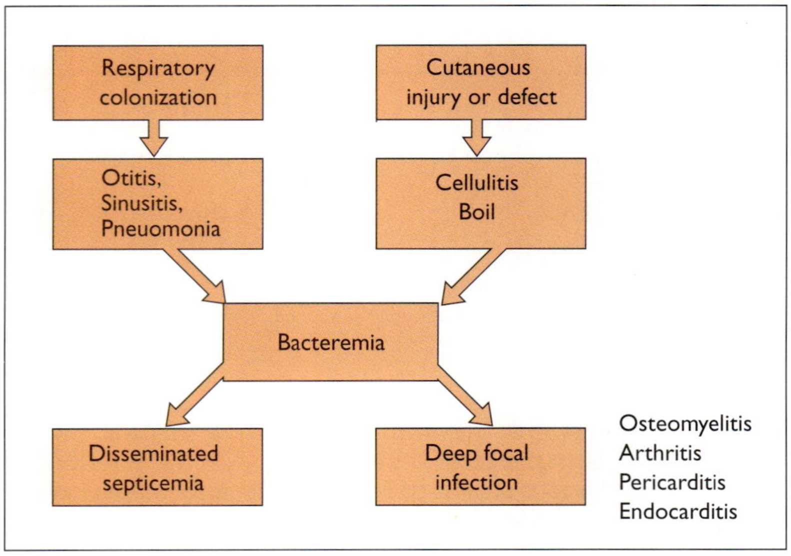

Figure 8-9 Pathogenesis of focal and invasive staphylococcal infections. Although *Staphylococcus aureus* infections often remain localized, the organism may cause bacteremia and deep infection (*eg*, osteomyelitis).

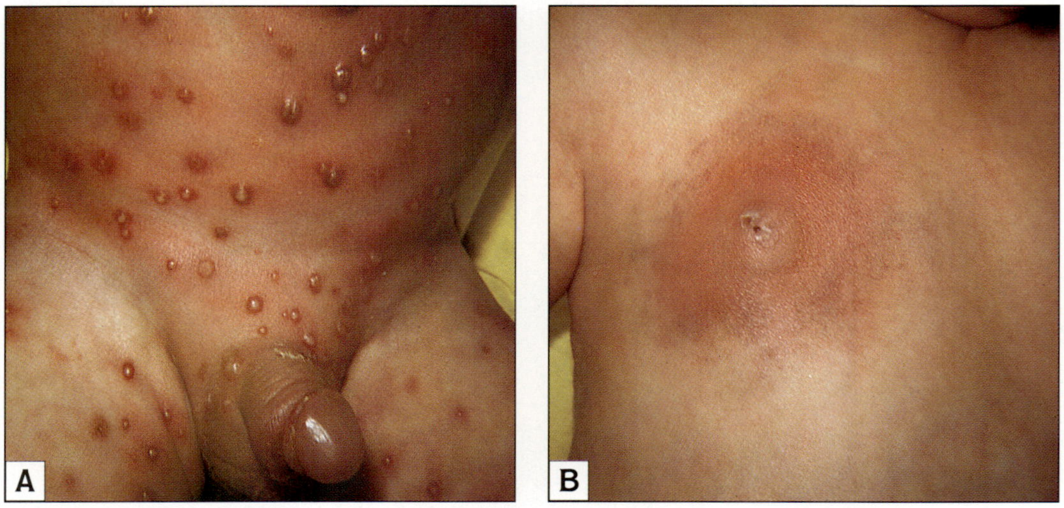

Figure 8-10 Examples of localized sites of *Staphylococcus aureus* infection in an infant who also had bacteremia. **A,** Multiple furuncles (boils). **B,** Breast abscess.

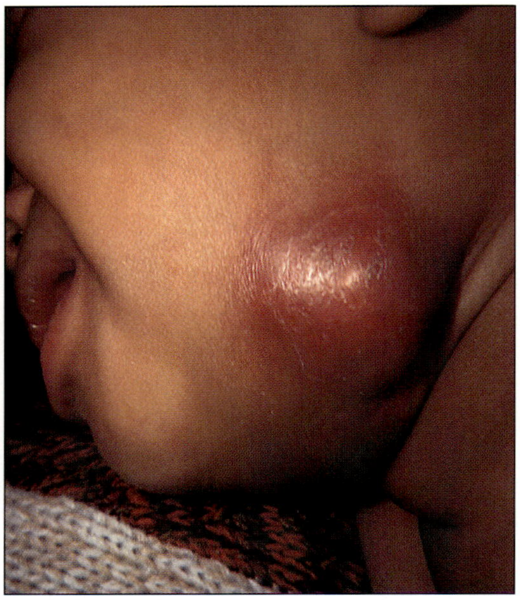

Figure 8-11 Cervical lymphadenitis in an infant. *Staphylococcus aureus* is the most common cause of bacterial adenitis in infants and young children.

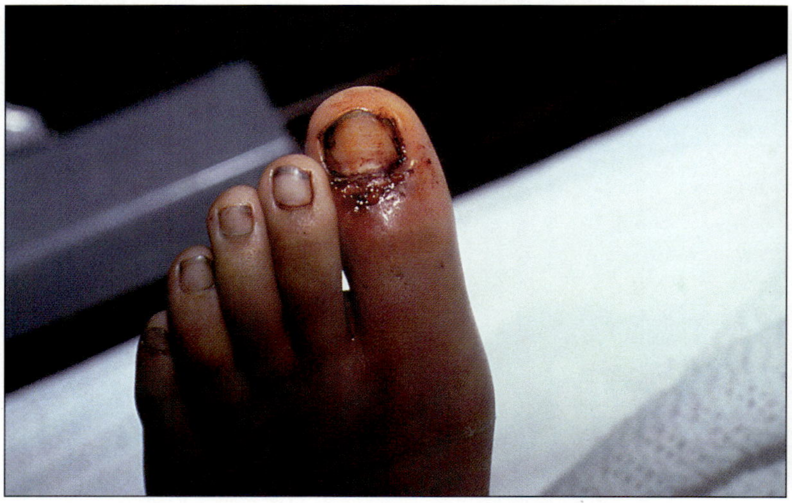

Figure 8-12 Paronychia of toe secondary to *Staphylococcus aureus* infection.

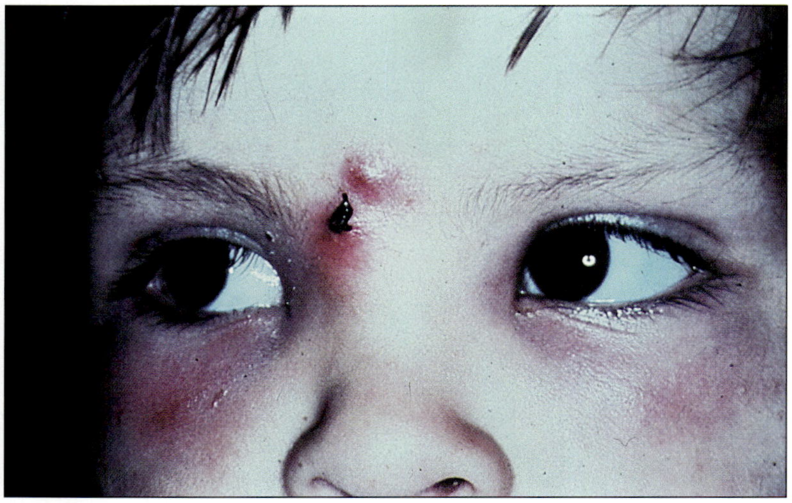

Figure 8-13 Wound infection with adjacent furuncle and periorbital cellulitis. Sometimes *Staphylococcus aureus* infection is not contained well by the abscess and can spread to adjacent tissues.

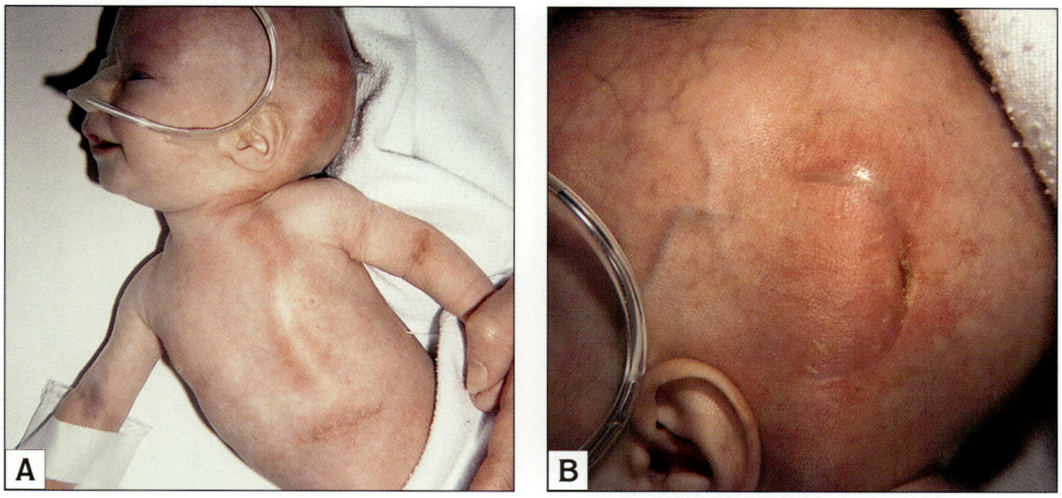

Figure 8-14 *Staphylococcus aureus* infection of ventriculoperitoneal shunt. **A,** Inflammation along entire shunt catheter. **B,** Wound dehiscence at shunt insertion site. Most shunt infections are caused by coagulase-negative staphylococci. *Staphylococcus aureus* is more aggressive when it infects foreign bodies and causes more tissue damage.

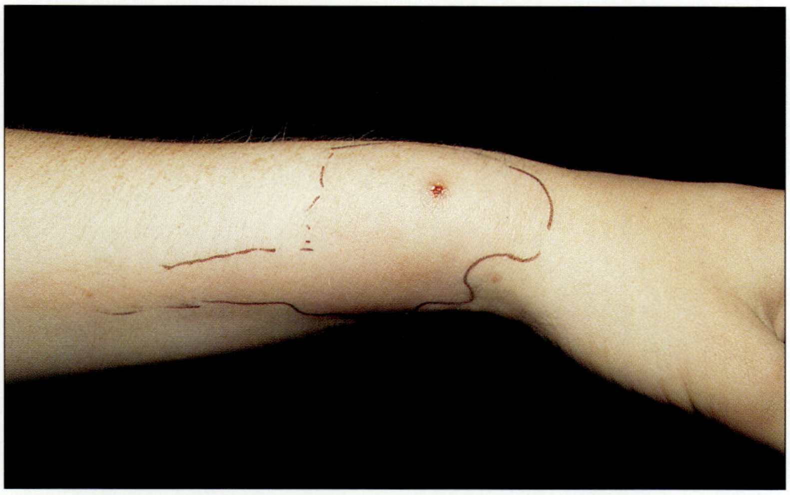

Figure 8-15 Septic thrombophlebitis at site of intravenous infusion with secondary bacteremia. Phlebitis is commonly caused by *Staphylococcus aureus* and may lead to septicemia.

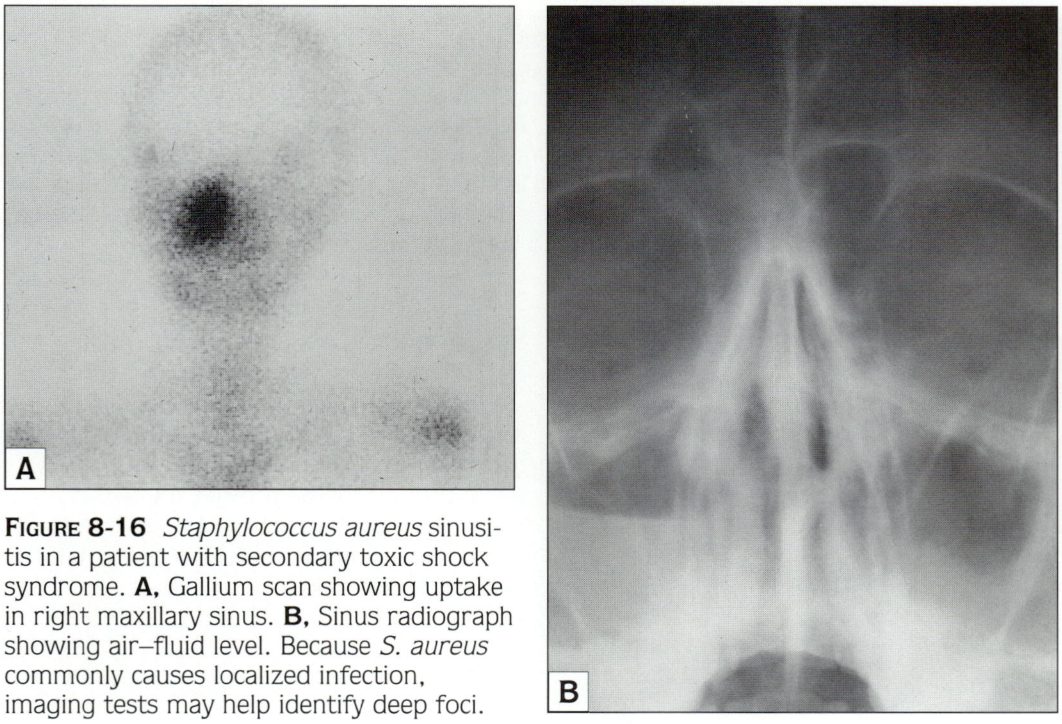

Figure 8-16 *Staphylococcus aureus* sinusitis in a patient with secondary toxic shock syndrome. **A,** Gallium scan showing uptake in right maxillary sinus. **B,** Sinus radiograph showing air–fluid level. Because *S. aureus* commonly causes localized infection, imaging tests may help identify deep foci.

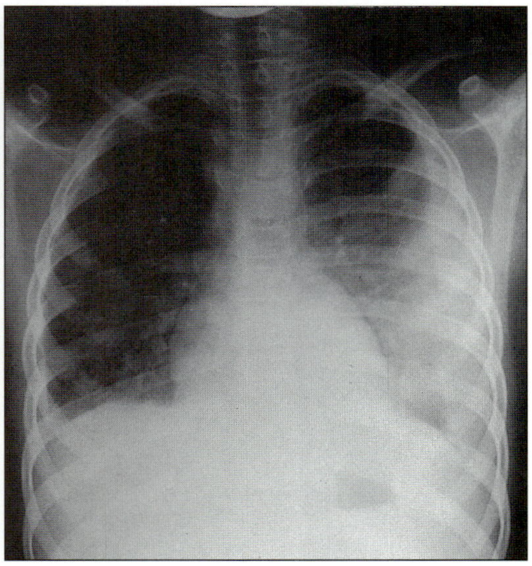

Figure 8-17 Staphylococcal pneumonia and empyema in a 12-year-old boy. *Staphylococcus aureus* pneumonia may be rapidly progressive, with pneumatoceles and tension pyopneumothorax.

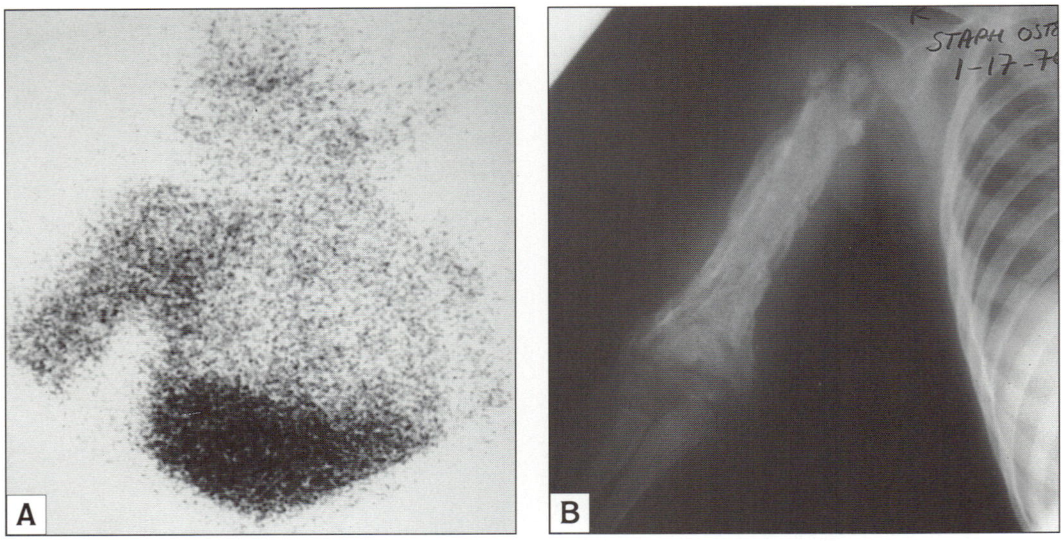

FIGURE 8-18 Severe untreated osteomyelitis secondary to *Staphylococcus aureus* infection in the right humerus. **A,** Bone scan showing increased uptake. **B,** Radiograph showing severe bone destruction (sequestra) and periosteal new bone formation. *S. aureus* is the most common cause of spontaneous osteomyelitis. It can usually be treated with long-term antibodies and drainage.

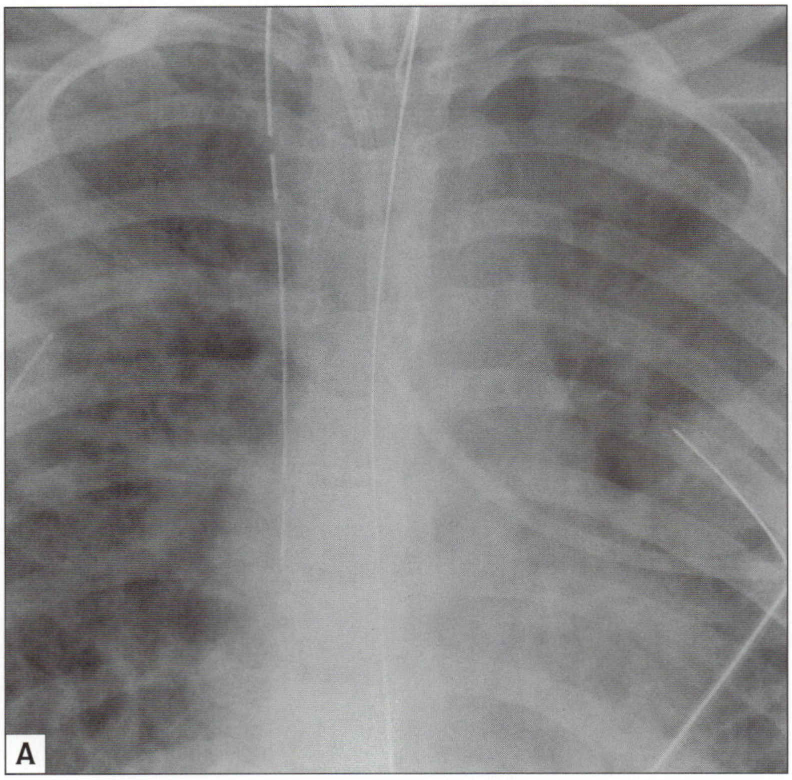

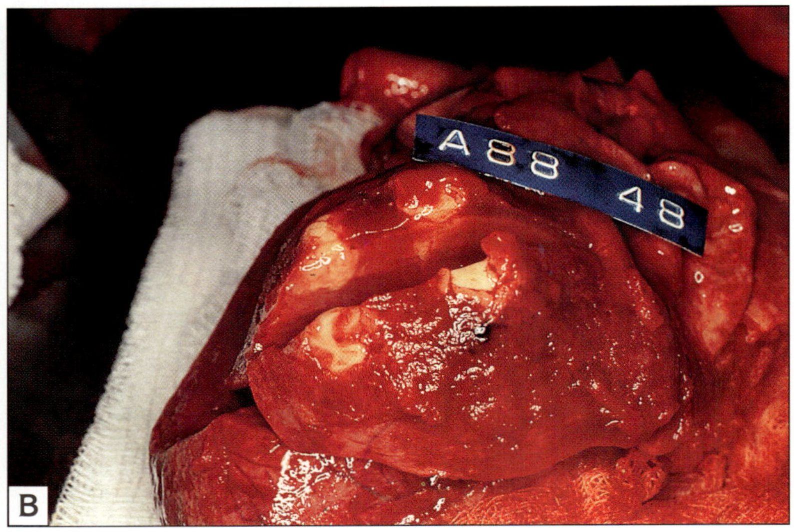

FIGURE 8-19 Fatal disseminated staphylococcal septicemia in a 13-year-old girl with bacteremia and multiple foci of infection (pyoderma, arthritis, pneumonia, endocarditis, myocardial abscesses, and hepatic abscesses). **A,** Chest radiograph showing multifocal pneumonia. **B,** Heart with multiple myocardial abscesses. Disseminated *Staphylococcus aureus* disease is uncommon but can be devastating. Adolescents seems to be the highest risk group, but multifocal disease can occur in infants and immunocompromised children as well.

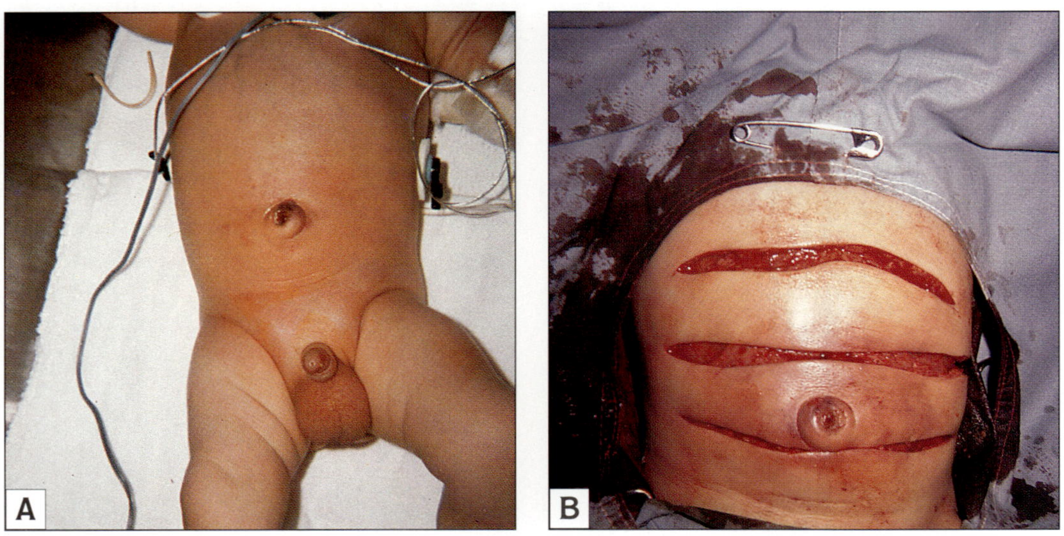

FIGURE 8-20 Newborn with necrotizing fasciitis secondary to *Staphylococcus aureus* infection of umbilicus. **A,** Fasciitis prior to surgery. **B,** After fasciotomy. Necrotizing fasciitis is uncommon. In the newborn, *S. aureus* is often the cause, whereas *Streptococcus pyogenes* is more common thereafter. Fasciotomy is a critical part of treatment.

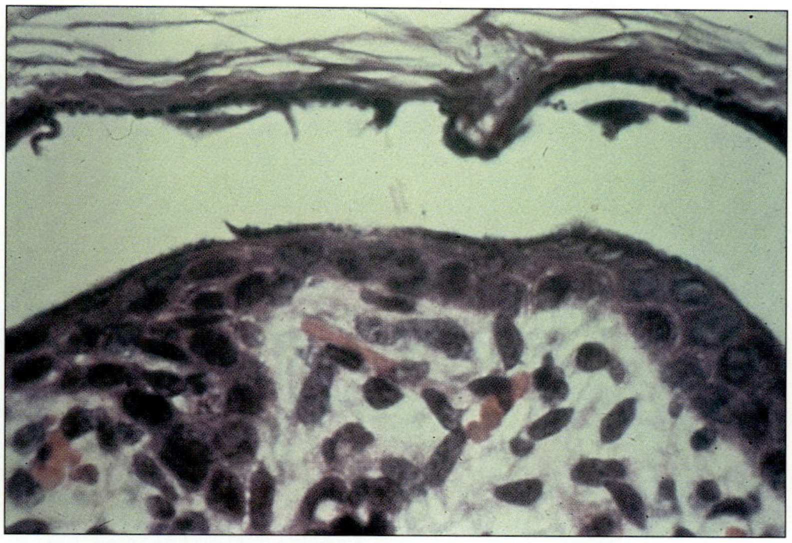

FIGURE 8-21 Exfoliatin toxin produced by phage group II *Staphylococcus aureus* causing separation of granular cell layer in mouse. This is the toxin that causes scalded skin syndrome. It causes skin cleavage at the granular cell layer.

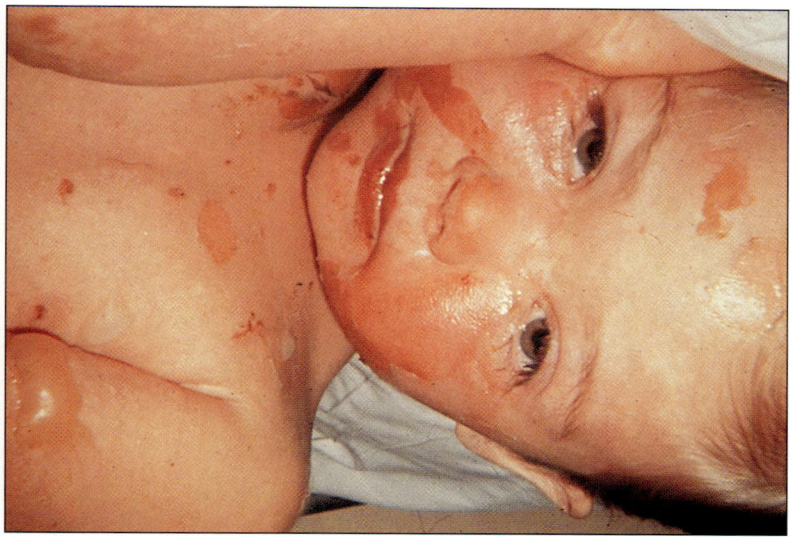

FIGURE 8-22 Classic scalded skin syndrome secondary to systemic toxemia from a *Staphylococcus aureus* nasopharyngitis. Accompanying symptoms include fever, painful erythroderma, sterile bullous lesions, and positive Nikolsky's sign (sloughing of skin secondary to tangential pressure).

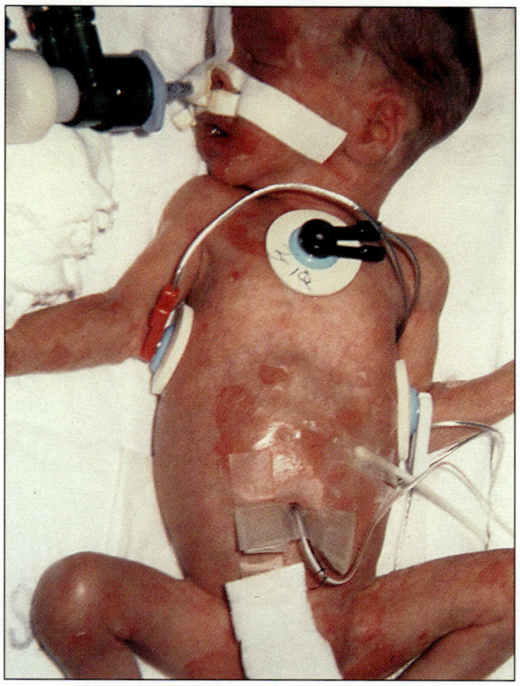

FIGURE 8-23 Ritter's disease (scalded skin syndrome in a newborn) secondary to *Staphylococcus aureus* bacteremia. This variant of scalded skin syndrome in a newborn is often more severe because of the young age.

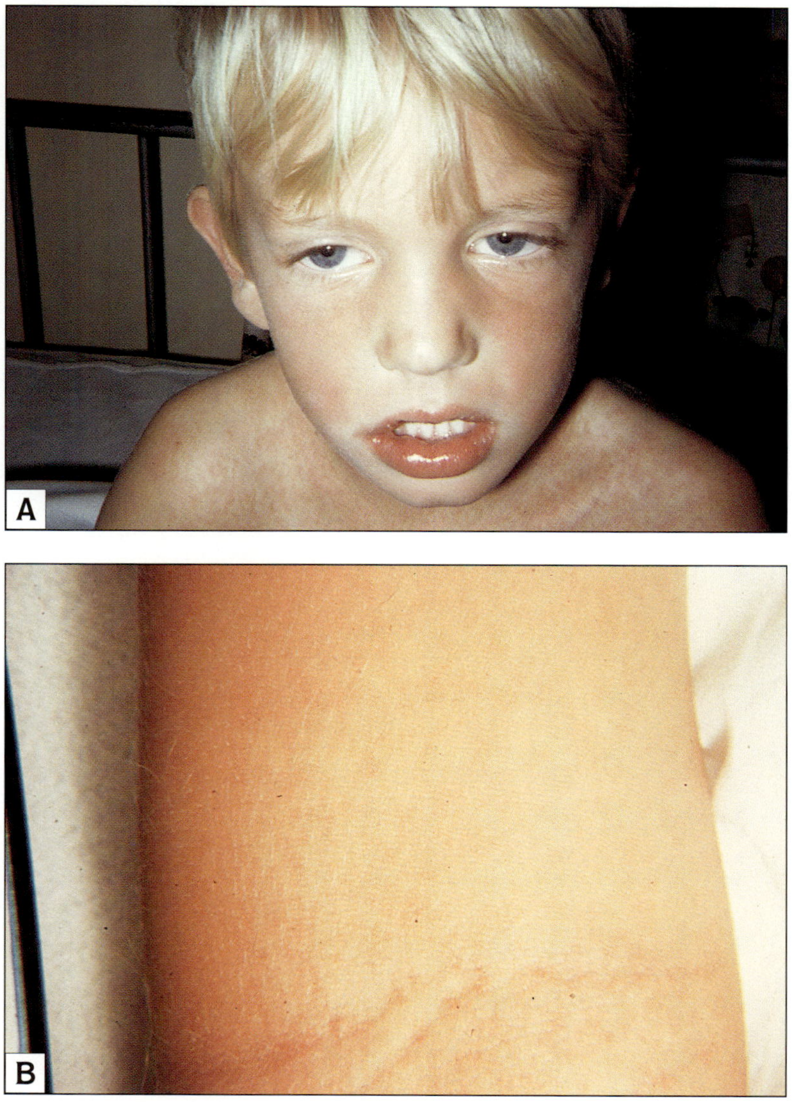

FIGURE 8-24 Staphylococcal scarlet fever secondary to an exfoliatin-producing *Staphylococcus aureus* infection in an older boy. **A,** Circumpolar pallor. **B,** Pastia's lines.

(continued on next page)

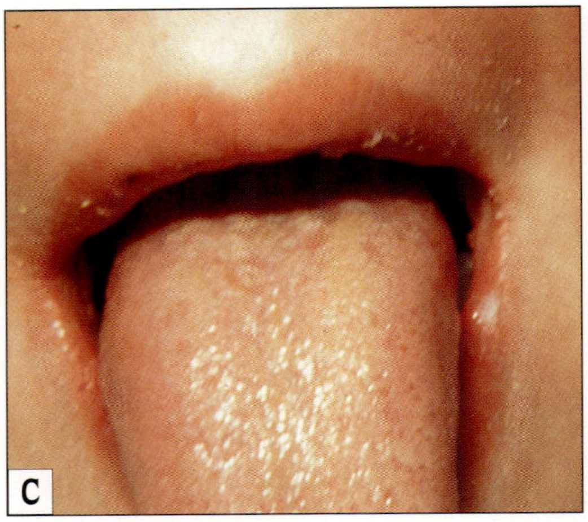

FIGURE 8-24 *(continued)* **C,** Normal tongue. These findings are consistent with classical scarlet fever caused by *Staphylococcus pyogenes*; however, the exfoliatin toxin does not cause strawberry tongue (tongue involvement is seen in scarlet fever secondary to toxic shock syndrome toxin-1–producing staphylococci and pyrogenic exotoxin–producing *S. pyogenes*).

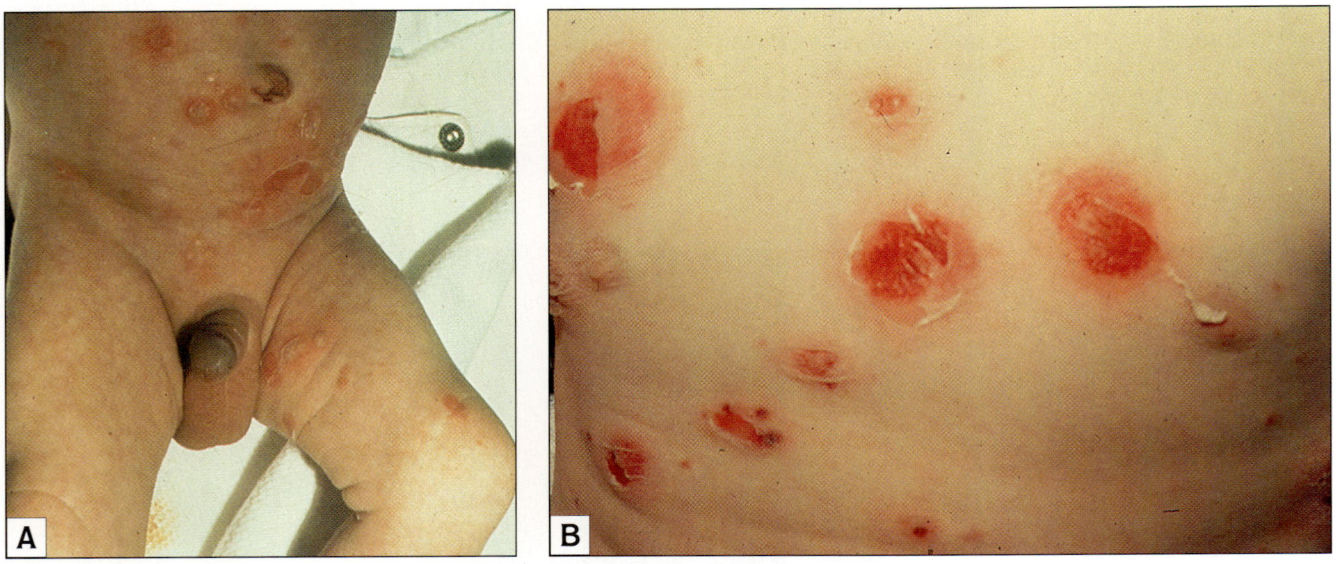

FIGURE 8-25 Bullous lesions secondary to exfoliatin-producing *Staphylococcus aureus* in children with anti-exfoliatin antibody (toxin confined to infected bullous lesions). **A,** Bullous impetigo. **B,** Bullous varicella. Patients get generalized disease caused by exfoliatin toxin if they have no antibody, but they suffer localized disease if they have preexisting antibody.

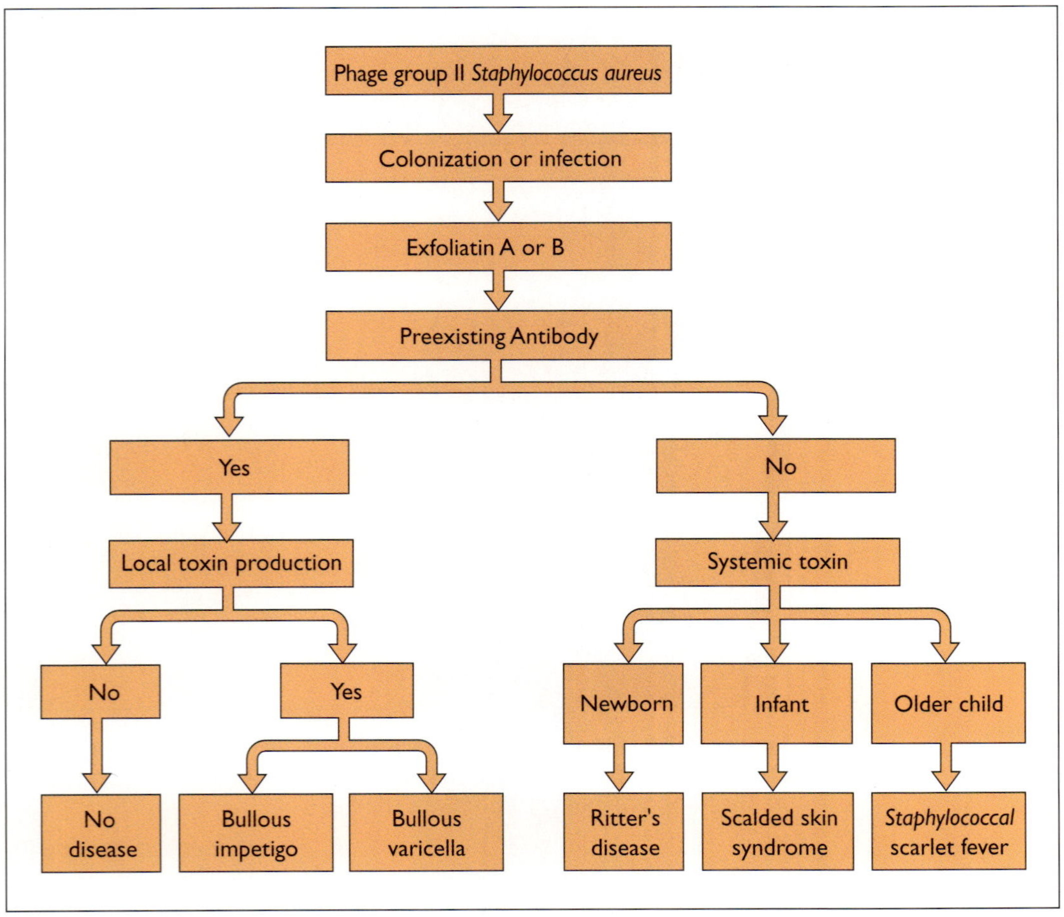

FIGURE 8-26 Pathogenesis of scalded skin syndrome. The clinical findings of exfoliatin toxin disease depend on the antibody status and age of the patient.

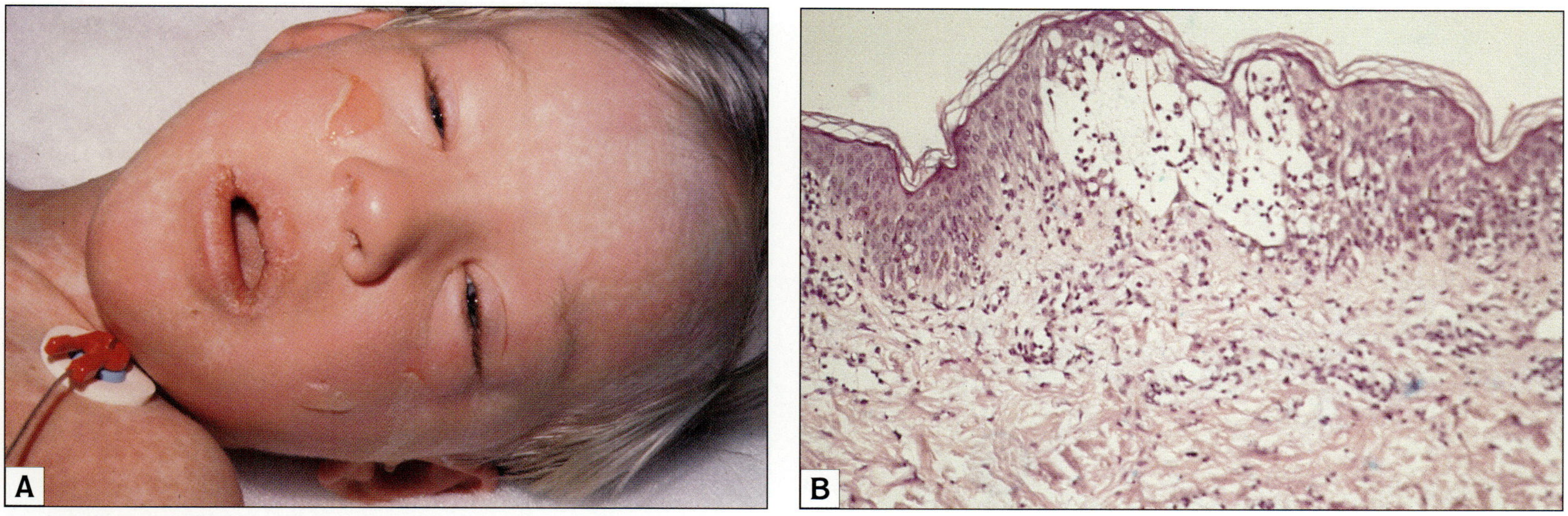

FIGURE 8-27 Drug-induced scalded skin syndrome caused by an adverse reaction to an anticonvulsant. **A,** Bullous lesions and positive Nikolsky's sign in a boy on phenobarbital. **B,** Deeper cleavage plane of epidermal necrolysis at basal cell layer. Not every case of scalded skin syndrome is caused by *Staphylococcus aureus*. A good drug-exposure history should be taken (antibiotics and anticonvulsants are often the culprit). Biopsy specimens show a deeper cleavage plane in drug-associated cases.

Differential diagnosis of scalded skin syndrome

	Staphylococcal toxin	Drug
Painful erythroderma	+	+
Nikolsky's sign	+	+
Drug exposure	+	+
Staphylococcal colonization	+	(+)
Epidermal necrolysis		
Granular layer	+	–
Basal layer	–	+

+—present; (+)—sometimes present; –—absent.

FIGURE 8-28 Differential diagnosis of scalded skin syndrome. Staphylococcal disease is associated with young age, no drug exposure, and a superficial cleavage plane.

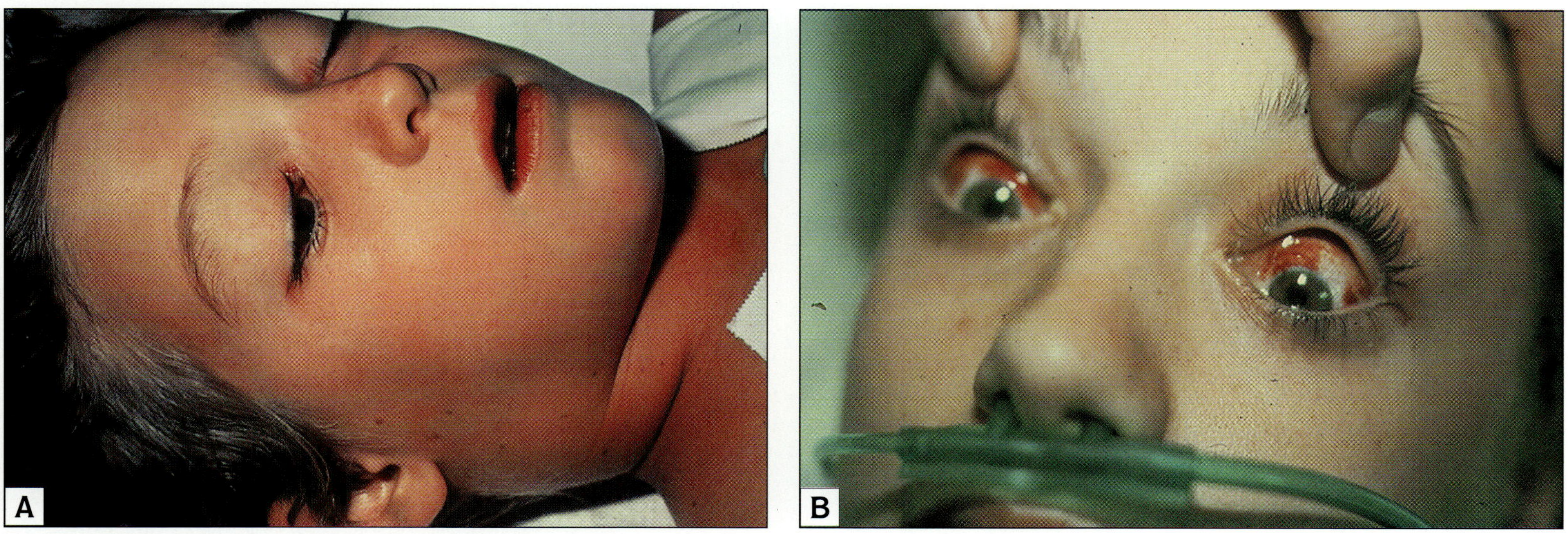

FIGURE 8-29 Toxic shock syndrome. Toxic shock syndrome is secondary to focal infections caused by toxic shock syndrome toxin-1 or enterotoxin-producing *Staphylococcus aureus*. **A,** Scarlet fever rash in a boy with suppurative lymphadenitis. **B,** Conjunctival hyperemia and subconjunctival hemorrhages in a menstruating girl using a tampon.

(continued on next page)

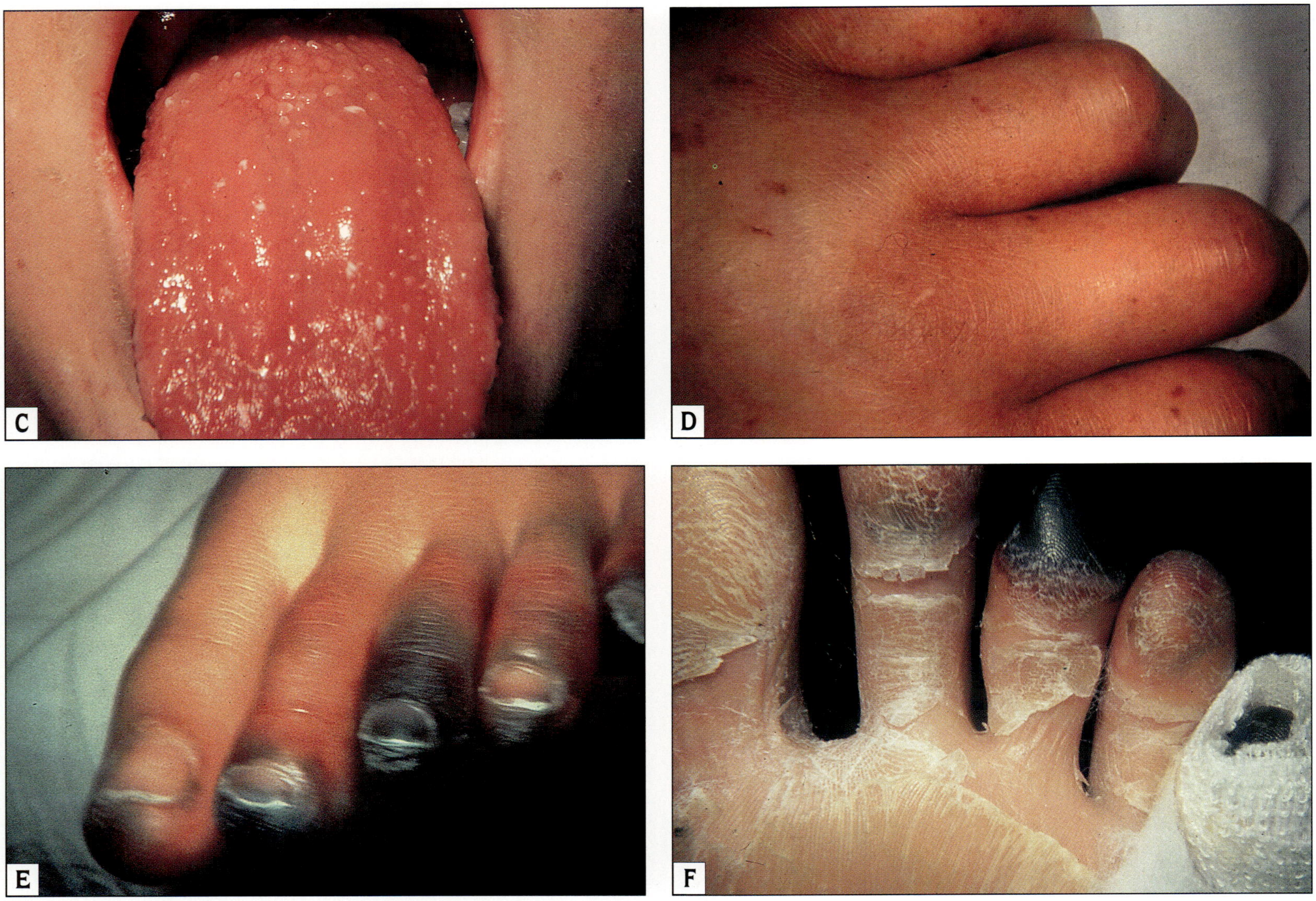

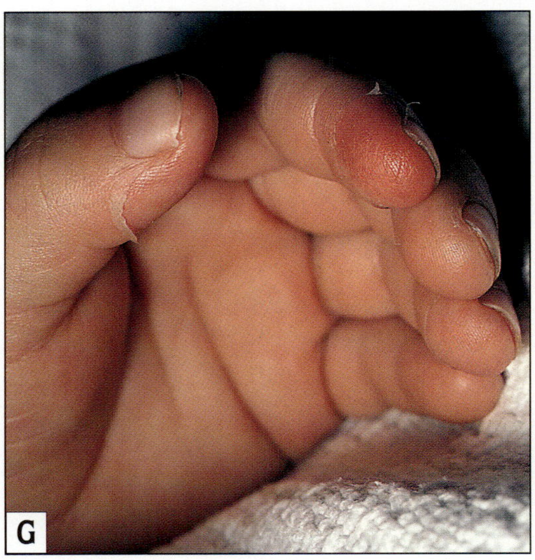

Figure 8-29 *(continued)* **C,** Strawberry tongue. **D,** Edematous hand secondary to capillary leakage. **E,** Rash and gangrene of toes secondary to shock. **F,** Desquamation of toes. **G,** Peeling of finger tips.

Criteria for toxic shock syndrome diagnosis
Acute fever >38.9°C
Erythroderma
Hypotension
Desquamation of fingers and toes (usually late)
Multiorgan system involvement (at least three)
Mucus membranes (conjunctival, oral)
Renal
Hepatic
Gastrointestinal
Hematologic
Central nervous system
Muscular
Exclusion of other diseases

Figure 8-30 Criteria for toxic shock syndrome diagnosis.

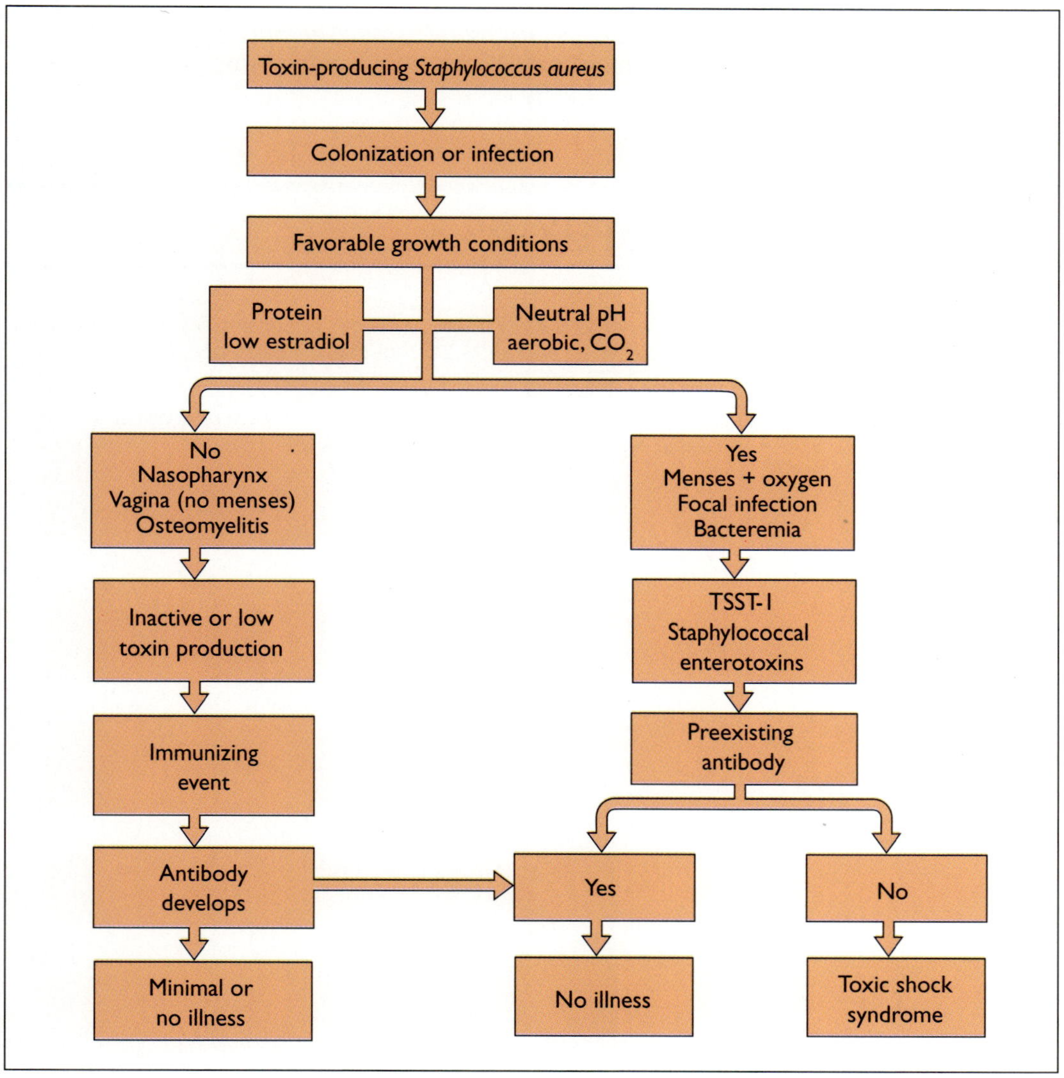

Figure 8-31 Pathogenesis of toxic shock syndrome. Toxic shock syndrome is caused by strains of *Staphylococcus aureus* that produce toxins that stimulate the production of tumor necrosis factor, which causes shock. Risk factors include growth of the organism under conditions that increase toxin production (*eg*, abscess, menstruation while using a tampon) and absence of antibody. CO_2—carbon dioxide. TSST-1—toxic shock syndrome toxin-1.

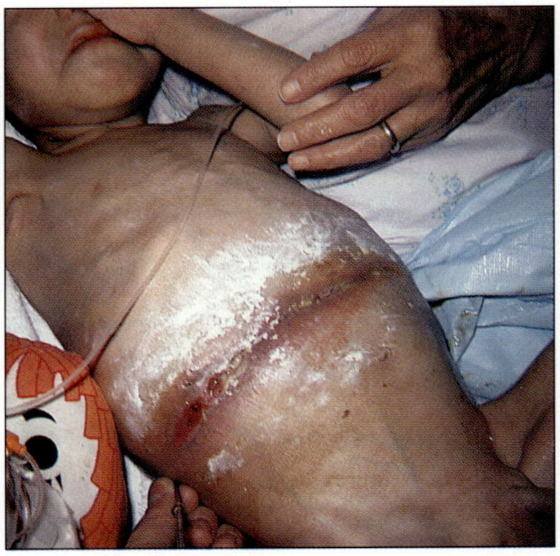

FIGURE 8-32 Chronic granulomatous disease. This child has severe infection secondary to a chronic granulomatous disease–sex-linked neutrophil defect that predisposes to infection with catalase-producing organisms like *Staphylococcus aureus*.

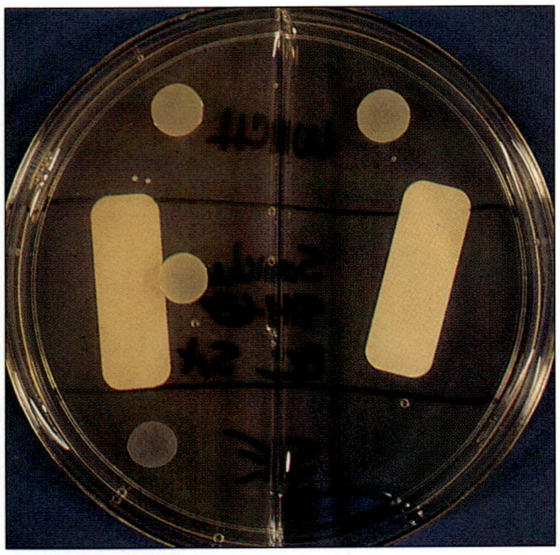

FIGURE 8-33 Methicillin-resistant *Staphylococcus aureus* (MRSA). Most strains of *S. aureus* produce a β-lactamase that makes them resistant to penicillin and ampicillin, but remain susceptible to β-lactamase–resistant penicillins such as oxacillin, nafcillin, and the cephalosporins. MRSA, which are resistant to all β-lactams, are increasing in frequency. This biplate has three organisms growing on the *left side*. The bottom two on the *right side*, which contain oxacillin, are inhibited. The organism at the *top* is an MRSA.

SELECTED BIBLIOGRAPHY

Todd JK: Staphylococcal infections. In *Rudolph's Textbook of Pediatrics*, ed 19. Edited by Rudolph AM. Stamford, CT: Appleton & Lange; 1991:601–603.

Todd JK: Staphylococcal infection. In *Current Pediatric Therapy*. Philadelphia: WB Saunders; 1993:553–557.

Todd JK: Staphylococcal scalded skin syndrome. In *Current Therapy in Pediatric Disease*. Edited by Kaplan SL. St. Louis: Mosby Year Book, Inc.; 1993:124–126.

Todd JK: Toxic shock syndrome. In *Principles and Practice of Pediatric Infectious Diseases*. New York: Churchill Livingstone; 1997:107–111.

Chapter 9

HIV and AIDS

Mark W. Kline

IMPORTANT FEATURES DISTINGUISH HIV INFECTION AND AIDS in infants and children from the disease observed in adults. Vertical transmission of HIV and the effects of the virus on an immature and naive immune system undoubtedly influence disease expression in ways that are poorly defined. Difficulties in confirming the diagnosis of HIV infection in early infancy and rapid disease progression in infants with vertically acquired infection, limit opportunities for early therapeutic intervention. In addition, HIV has important adverse effects on the developing central nervous system and normal growth. This chapter highlights some of the more characteristic or distinctive features of HIV infection in infants and children.

Epidemiology

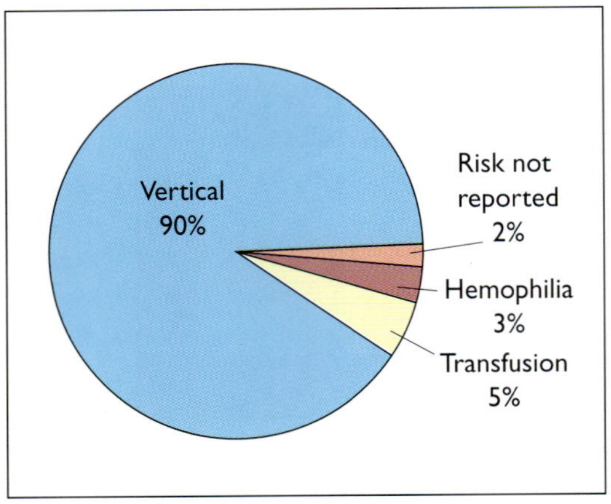

Figure 9-1 Percentage of pediatric AIDS cases by exposure category. Through December, 1996, over 7600 children younger than 13 years of age with AIDS had been reported to the U.S. Centers for Disease Control and Prevention. The predominant mode of HIV transmission to children is vertical, representing about 90% of pediatric AIDS cases [1].

Possible risk factors for HIV vertical transmission
Maternal factors
Advanced HIV disease
Low CD4+ lymphocyte count
High viral load
Obstetric factors
Prolonged rupture of membranes
?Vaginal delivery
Fetal/newborn factors
First-born twin
Prematurity
Breast-fed

Figure 9-2 Possible risk factors for HIV vertical transmission. Approximately 20% to 30% of infants born to untreated HIV-infected mothers acquire HIV infection. Transmission of infection can occur in utero, intrapartum, or postpartum via breast milk.

Pathogenesis

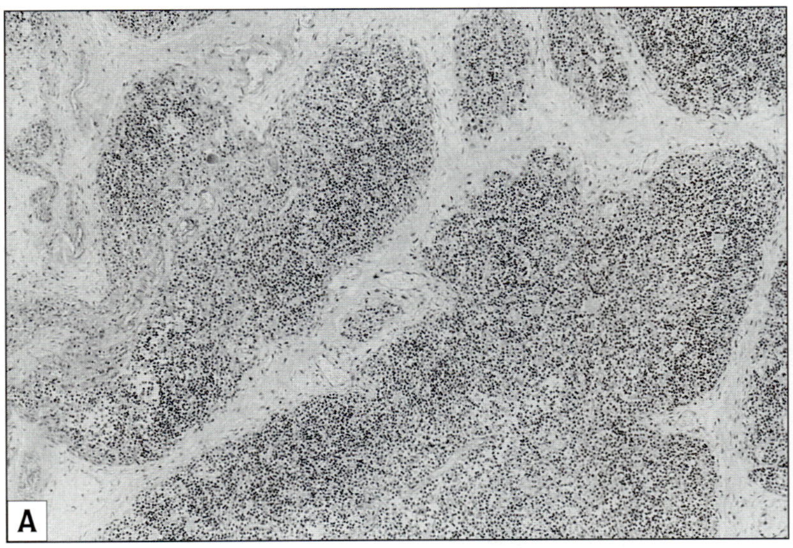

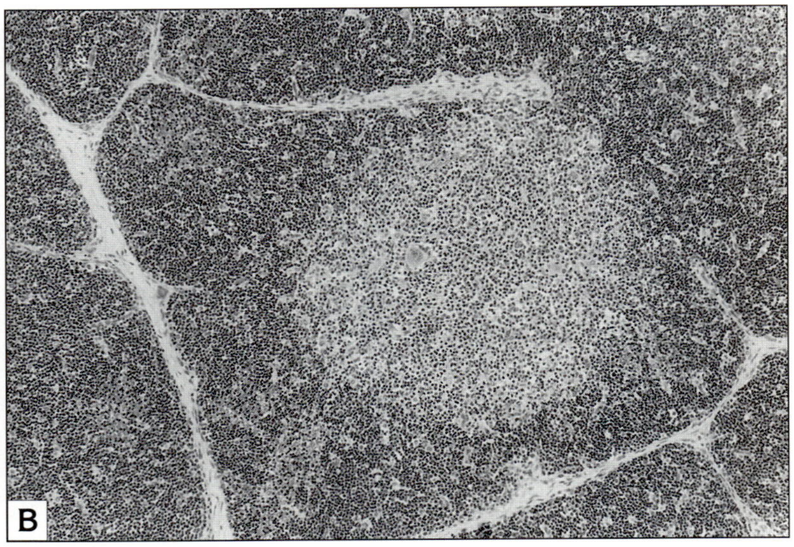

Figure 9-3 **A**, Thymus gland of midgestation fetus infected with HIV. Extensive destruction of normal thymic tissue and passenger lymphocytes is observed. **B**, Normal fetal thymus showing mature thymic cells, Hassall's corpuscles, and passenger lymphocytes. Early compromise of developing immunity in HIV-infected fetuses may lead to a greater-than-expected rate of fetal loss and severe compromise of cellular immunity in surviving infants. The naivety of the developing immune system is a possible explanation for susceptibility of the fetus and infant to rapid progression of HIV disease. (*Courtesy of* Claire Langston, Houston, TX.)

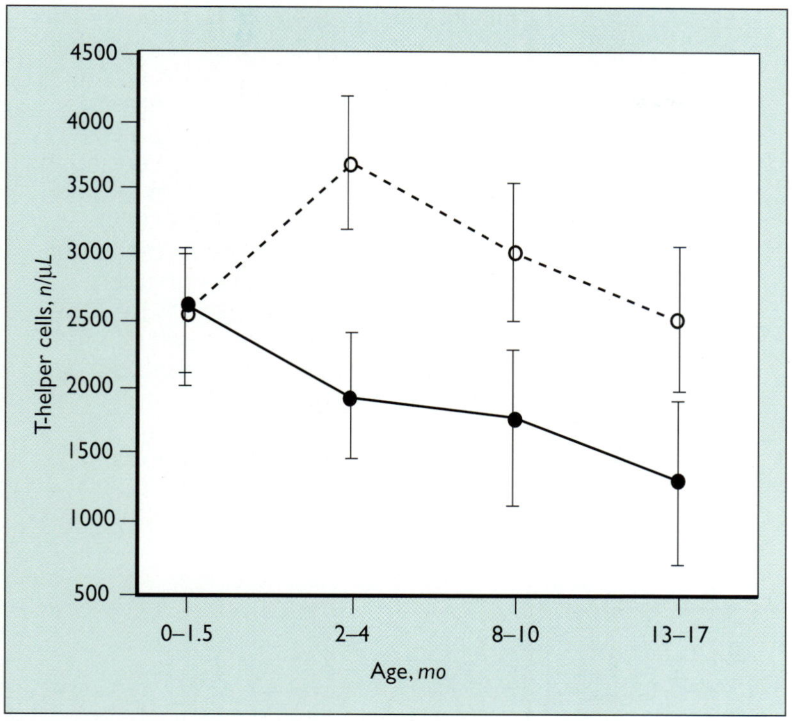

FIGURE 9-4 Sequential peripheral blood CD4+ lymphocyte counts in infants born to HIV-infected women. HIV-exposed infants who escape infection display an early rise in CD4+ lymphocyte count in the first few months of life (*dashed line*), whereas HIV-infected infants show a blunted rise and subsequent decrease in CD4+ lymphocyte count (*solid line*). The immunologic changes observed in adults and infants with HIV infection are similar, with several exceptions. Lymphopenia and CD4+ lymphocyte depletion are observed less consistently among HIV-infected infants than among adults, in part because of the relative lymphocytosis of infancy. Serious opportunistic infections occur among HIV-infected infants with adult normal CD4+ lymphocyte counts. Hyperimmunoglobulinemia is observed in almost all HIV-infected infants by 6 months of age and is thought to result from polyclonal stimulation of B lymphocytes and immune dysregulation caused by HIV. (*Adapted from* Shearer *et al.* [2].)

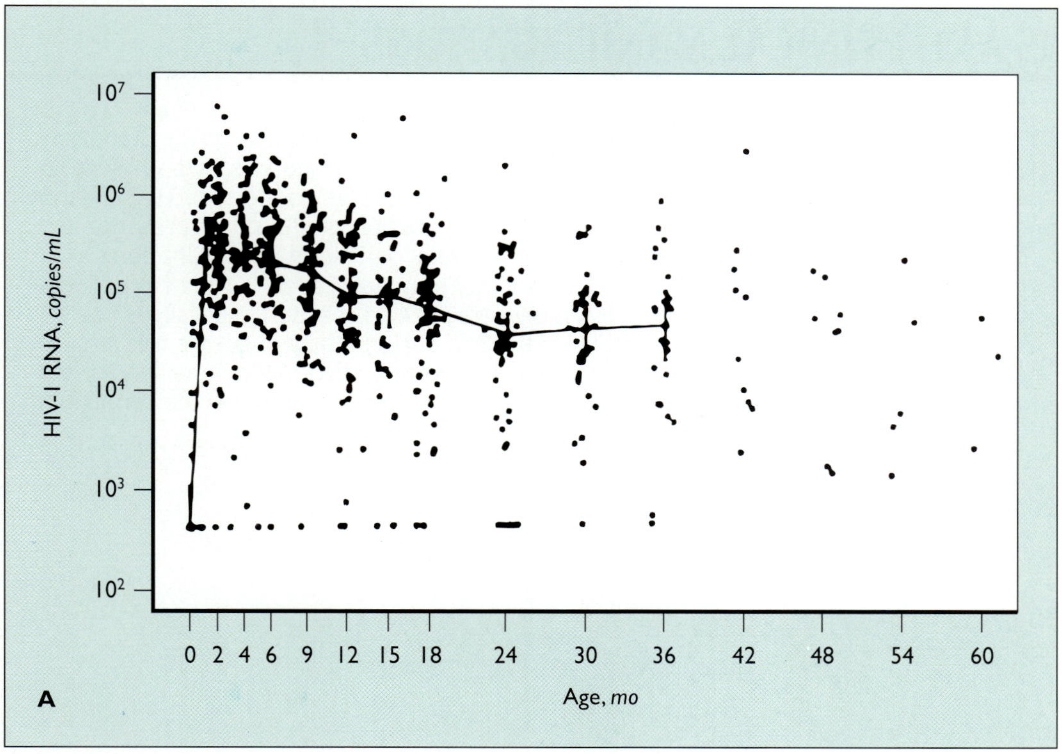

FIGURE 9-5 **A**, Plasma HIV RNA concentrations in multiple samples from 106 infants, according to age. The solid line connects the median values of the individual data points. Median RNA concentration at birth was below the level of detectability (<400 copies/mL). It rose to 318,000 and 256,000 copies/mL at 1 and 2 months of age, respectively, with a gradual decline to 34,000 copies/mL by 24 months of age. *(continued)*

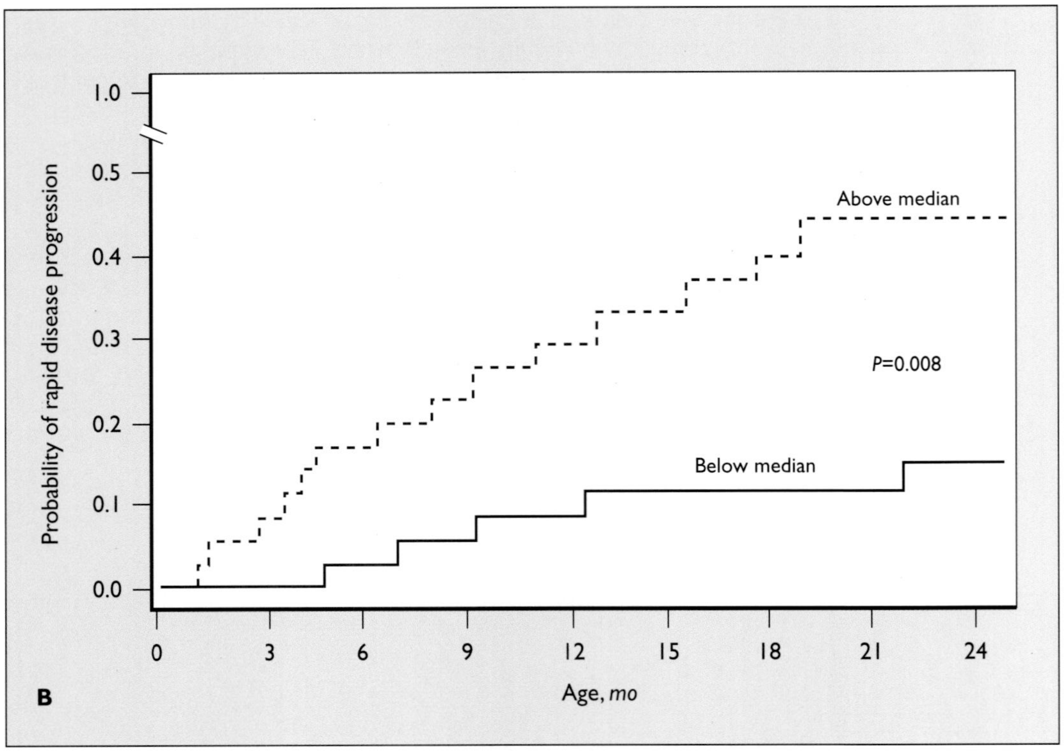

Figure 9-5 *(continued)* **B**, Kaplan–Meier estimates of the probability of disease progression (Centers for Disease Control and Prevention class C HIV disease or death by 18 months of age) by median plasma HIV RNA concentration during the first 2 months of life. A median plasma HIV RNA concentration of 299,000 copies/mL was used as the threshold for predicting rapid disease progression. Infants with very high plasma HIV RNA concentrations are at increased risk for HIV disease progression. (Adapted from Shearer et al. [3].)

Diagnosis and Clinical Manifestations

Definition of HIV infection in children

Infants and children under 18 mo of age with vertical infection

Positive results on two separate determinations (excluding cord blood) from one or more of the following HIV detection tests:

- HIV culture
- HIV polymerase chain reaction
- HIV p24 antigen

or

Meets criteria for the CDC case definition of AIDS

Older children with vertical infection and children with HIV infection acquired otherwise

Repeatedly reactive enzyme immunoassay and confirmatory tests (*eg*, Western blot or immunofluorescence assay) for anti-HIV antibody

or

Meets any of the criteria for infants and children under 18 mo of age

CDC—Centers for Disease Control and Prevention

Figure 9-6 Definition of HIV infection in children [4]. Standard HIV serologic tests, including enzyme immunoassay and Western blot immunoassay, are not useful in the diagnosis of HIV infection during infancy because of the possible confounding presence in infants' blood of transplacentally derived maternal antibody. Detectable anti-HIV antibody may persist for 18 months or longer in some cases. HIV polymerase chain reaction generally is preferred for diagnosis of HIV infection during infancy because it is less expensive and more readily available than HIV culture, and it has greater diagnostic sensitivity than HIV p24 antigen determination.

Classification of HIV infection in children

	Clinical categories			
Immunologic categories	**N (no signs or symptoms)**	**A (mild signs or symptoms)**	**B (moderate signs or symptoms)**	**C (severe signs or symptoms)**
1 (no suppression)	N1	A1	B1	C1
2 (moderate suppression)	N2	A2	B2	C2
3 (severe suppression)	N3	A3	B3	C3

FIGURE 9-7 Classification of HIV infection in children [4]. All AIDS-defining conditions with the exception of lymphoid interstitial pneumonitis/pulmonary lymphoid hyperplasia (LIP/PLH) are included in clinical category C. Degree of immunosuppression is defined on the basis of age-specific CD4+ lymphocyte counts and percentages. An infant with HIV vertical exposure and indeterminate (unconfirmed) infection status has the letter E (for vertically exposed) placed as a prefix to the appropriate classification code (*eg*, EN1).

A. Clinical categories for children with HIV: Category N

Category N (not symptomatic)

Children who have no signs or symptoms considered to be the result of HIV infection or who have only one of the conditions listed in category A

B. Clinical categories for children with HIV: Category A

Category A (mildly symptomatic)

Children with two or more of the conditions listed below but none of the conditions listed in categories B and C:
- Lymphadenopathy (>0.5 cm at more than two sites; bilateral, one site)
- Hepatomegaly
- Splenomegaly
- Dermatitis
- Parotitis
- Recurrent or persistent upper respiratory infection, sinusitis, or otitis media

C. Clinical categories for children with HIV: Category B

Category B (moderately symptomatic)

Children who have symptomatic conditions other than those listed for categories A or C that are attributed to HIV infection; examples of conditions in clinical category B include but are not limited to:
- Anemia (<8 g/dL), neutropenia (<1000/mL), or thrombocytopenia (<100,000/μL) persisting >30 d
- Bacterial meningitis, pneumonia, or sepsis (single episode)
- Candidiasis, oropharyngeal (thrush), persisting for >2 mo in children >6 mo of age
- Cardiomyopathy
- Cytomegalovirus infection, with onset before 1 mo of age
- Diarrhea, recurrent or chronic
- Hepatitis
- Herpes simplex virus (HSV) stomatitis, recurrent (more than two episodes within 1 y)
- HSV bronchitis, pneumonitis, or esophagitis with onset before 1 month of age
- Herpes zoster (shingles) involving at least two distinct episodes or more than one dermatome
- Leiomyosarcoma
- Lymphoid interstitial pneumonia (LIP) or pulmonary lymphoid hyperplasia complex
- Nephropathy
- Nocardiosis
- Persistent fever (lasting >1 mo)
- Toxoplasmosis, onset before 1 mo of age
- Varicella infection, disseminated (complicated chickenpox)

FIGURE 9-8 Clinical categories for children with HIV infection [4].

(continued on next page)

D. Clinical categories for children with HIV: Category C

Category C (severely symptomatic)

Children who have any condition listed in the 1987 surveillance case definition for AIDS, with the exception of LIP.

- Serious bacterial infections, multiple or recurrent (*ie*, any combination of at least two culture-confirmed infections within a 2-y period), of the following types:septicemia, pneumonia, meningitis, bone or joint infection, or abscess of an internal organ or body cavity (excluding otitis media, superficial skin or mucosal abscesses, and indwelling catheter-related infections)
- Candidiasis, esophageal or pulmonary (bronchi, trachea, lungs)
- Coccidioidomycosis, disseminated (at site other than or in addition to lungs or cervical or hilar lymph nodes)
- Cryptococcosis, extrapulmonary
- Cryptosporidiosis or isosporiasis with diarrhea persisting >1 mo
- Cytomegalovirus disease with onset of symptoms at >1 mo of age (at a site other than liver, spleen, or lymph nodes)
- Encephalopathy (at least one of the following progressive findings present for at least 2 mo in the absence of a concurrent illness other than HIV infection that could explain the findings:1) failure to attain or loss of development milestones or loss of intellectual ability, verified by standard developmental scale or neuropsychological tests; 2) impaired brain growth or acquired microcephaly demonstrated by head circumference measurements or brain atrophy demonstrated by computerized tomography or magnetic resonance imaging [serial imaging is required for children <2 y of age]; 3) acquired symmetric motor deficit manifested by two or more of the following:paresis, pathologic reflexes, ataxia, or gait disturbance)
- Herpes simplex virus infection, causing a mucocutaneous ulcer that persists for >1 mo; or bronchitis, pneumonitis, or esophagitis for any duration affecting a child >1 mo of age.
- Histoplasmosis, disseminated (at a site other than or in addition to lungs or cervical or hilar lymph nodes)
- Kaposi's sarcoma
- Lymphoma, primary, in brain
- Lymphoma, small, noncleaved cell (Burkitt); immunoblastic or large cell lymphoma; or B-cell or unknown immunologic phenotype
- *Mycobacterium tuberculosis*, disseminated or extrapulmonary
- *Mycobacterium avium* complex or *Mycobacterium kansasii*, disseminated (at site other than or in addition to lungs, skin, or cervical or hilar lymph nodes)
- *Pneumocystis carinii* pneumonia
- Progressive multifocal leukoencephalopathy
- *Salmonella* septicemia (nontyphoid), recurrent toxoplasmosis of the brain with onset at >1 mo of age
- Wasting syndrome in the absence of a concurrent illness other than HIV infection that could explain the following findings:1) persistent weight loss >10% of baseline, 2) downward crossing of at least two of the following percentile lines on the weight-for-age chart (*eg*, 95th, 75th, 50th 25th, 5th) in a child >1 y of age, or 3) <5th percentile on weight-for-height chart on two consecutive measurements >30 d apart plus chronic diarrhea (*ie*, at least two loose stools a day for >30 d) or documented fever (for >30 d, intermittent or constant)

FIGURE 9-8 *(continued)* Clinical categories for children with HIV infection [4].

Immunologic categories based on age-specific CD4+ T-lymphocyte counts and percentages of total lymphocytes

Immunologic category	Age-specific CD4+ T-lymphocyte counts, *cells/μL*: <12 mo of age	1–5 y of age	6–12 y of age	Percentage of total lymphocytes, %
1 (no evidence of suppression)	≥1500	≥1000	≥500	≥25
2 (evidence of moderate suppression)	750–1499	500–999	200–499	15–24
3 (severe suppression)	<750	<500	<200	<15

FIGURE 9-9 Immunologic categories based on age-specific CD4+ lymphocyte counts and percentages [4]. Absolute CD4+ lymphocyte counts decline normally over the first 5 years of life.

Common AIDS-defining conditions of children	
Condition	**Percentage of AIDS-defining events**
Definitive or presumptive *Pneumocystis carinii* pneumonia	24
Definitive or presumptive LIP/PLH	20
Multiple or recurrent bacterial infections	20
HIV encephalopathy	17
HIV wasting syndrome*	15
Definitive or presumptive Esophageal candidiasis	13

LIP/PLH—Lymphoid interstitial pneumonitis/pulmonary lymphoid hyperplasia.

*Growth failure is a manifestation of pediatric HIV infection observed far more commonly than wasting syndrome per se.

Figure 9-10 Common AIDS-defining conditions of children [1]. Each condition is expounded on in subsequent figures.

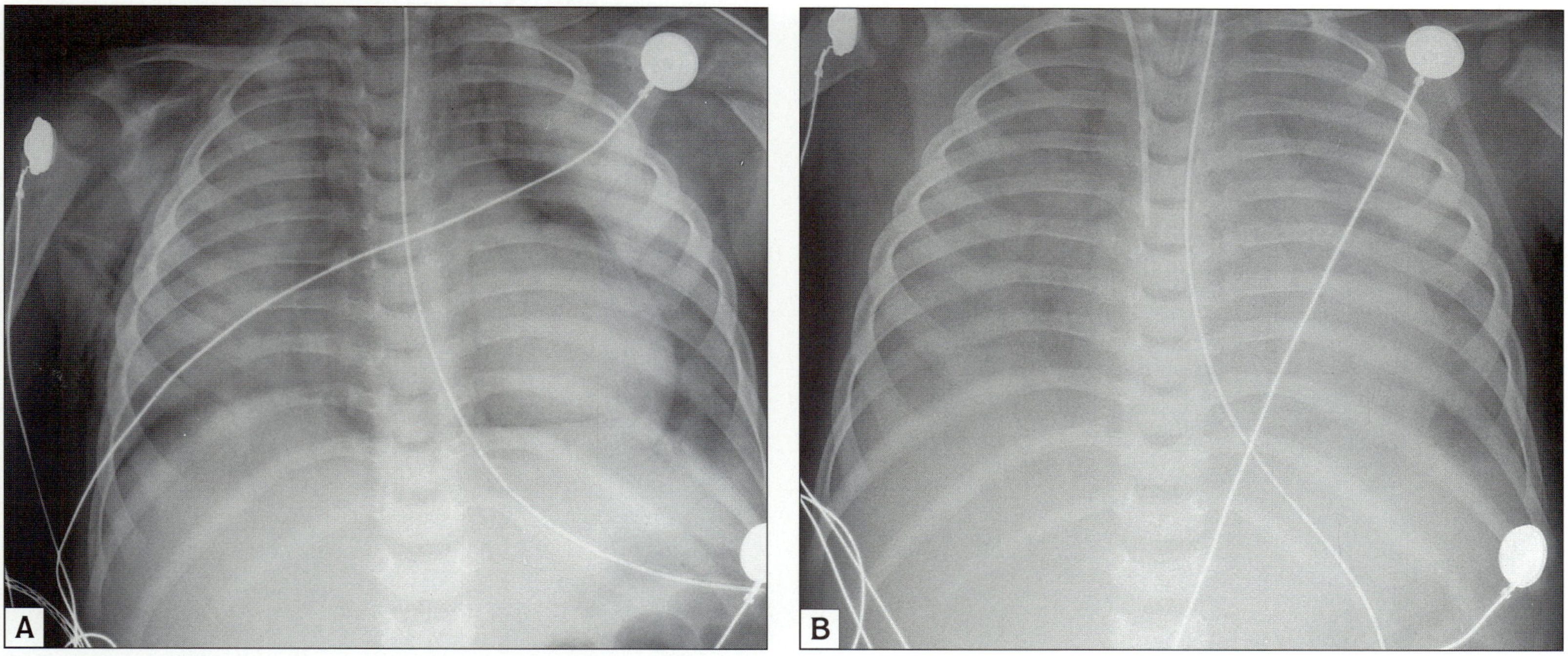

Figure 9-11 A, Chest radiograph demonstrating *Pneumocystis carinii* pneumonia in a 2-year-old boy with vertical HIV infection. Bilateral interstitial lung disease is evident. Subcutaneous emphysema and pneumomediastinum also are present. **B**, Chest radiograph of the same child performed 24 hours later, showing progression of pulmonary infiltrates despite therapy with trimethoprim-sulfamethoxazole. The child died approximately 24 hours after this radiograph was obtained.

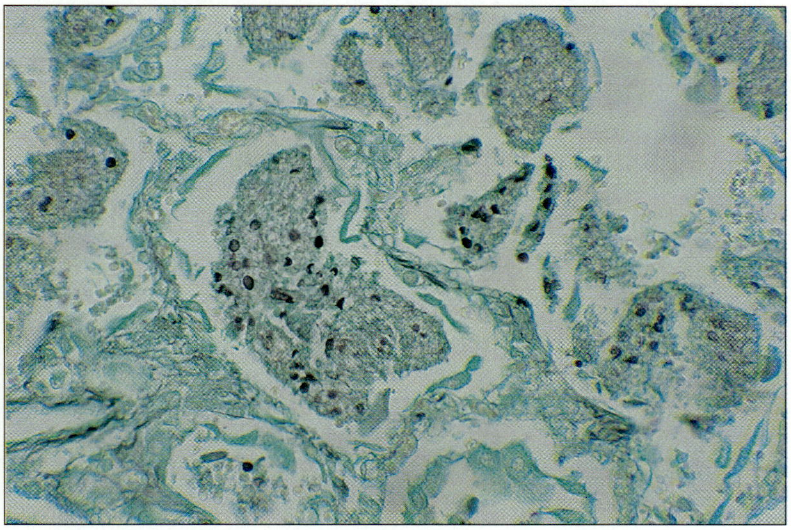

Figure 9-12 Lung biopsy specimen from a child with HIV infection and pneumonia. Gomori-methenamine silver stain shows numerous dark-staining cysts of *Pneumocystis carinii*. (*Courtesy of* Claire Langston, Houston, TX.)

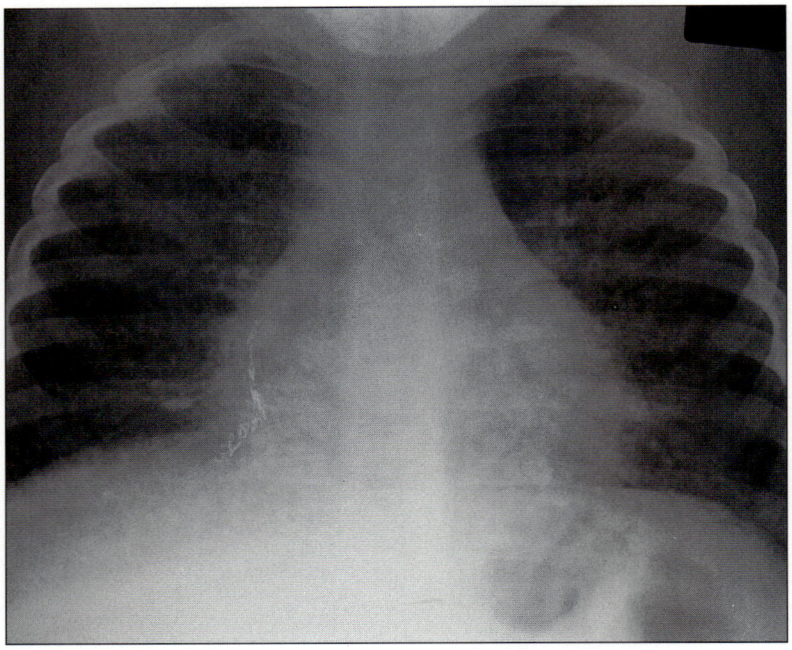

FIGURE 9-13 Chest radiograph showing bilateral reticulonodular interstitial infiltrates in a 3-year-old girl with vertical HIV infection and lymphoid interstitial pneumonitis/pulmonary lymphoid hyperplasia (LIP/PLH). Presumptive diagnosis of LIP/PLH is based on persistence for 2 months or more of characteristic radiographic features. Definitive diagnosis is made by open lung biopsy.

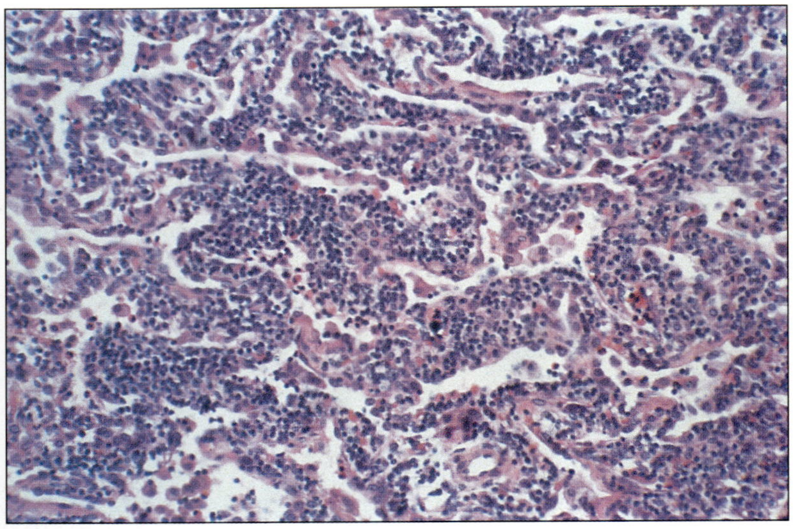

FIGURE 9-14 Lung biopsy specimen showing mononuclear interstitial infiltration in a child with vertical HIV infection and lymphoid interstitial pneumonitis/pulmonary lymphoid hyperplasia (LIP/PLH). Immunocytochemistry reveals a predominance of immunoblasts, plasma cells, and CD8+ lymphocytes in the lung interstitium of many such children with LIP/PLH. The pathogenesis of LIP/PLH is poorly understood, but Epstein–Barr virus has been implicated as a cofactor in its development. (*Courtesy of* Claire Langston, Houston, TX.)

Features useful in the differentiation of lymphoid interstitial pneumonitis/pulmonary lymphoid hyperplasia from *Pneumocystis carinii* pneumonia

Finding	LIP/PLH	PCP
Acute onset	No	Yes
Fever	No	Yes
Retractions	Late	Early
Rales	No	Yes
Hypoxia	Late	Early
Clubbing	Yes	No
Salivary enlargement	Yes	No

LIP/PLH—Lymphoid interstitial pneumonitis/pulmonary lymphoid hyperplasia; PCP—*Pneumocystis carinii* pneumonia.

FIGURE 9-15 Features useful in the differentiation of lymphoid interstitial pneumonitis/pulmonary lymphoid hyperplasia (LIP/PLH) from *Pneumocystis carinii* pneumonia (PCP). Although the radiographic features of LIP/PLH and PCP are similar, clinical features serve to differentiate the two conditions.

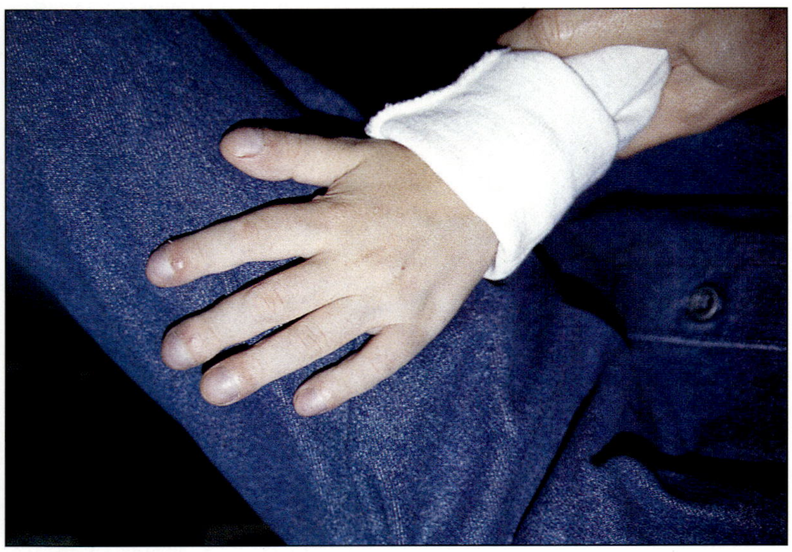

FIGURE 9-16 Digital clubbing in a child with HIV infection and lymphoid interstitial pneumonitis/pulmonary lymphoid hyperplasia (LIP/PLH). Marked generalized lymphadenopathy, hepatosplenomegaly, and salivary gland enlargement also are observed in many children with LIP/PLH. The clinical course of LIP/PLH is variable. Spontaneous clinical remission sometimes is observed. Exacerbation of signs and symptoms can occur in association with intercurrent viral respiratory illnesses. Progressive hypoxia and respiratory failure can occur in severe cases of LIP/PLH. Management is largely supportive.

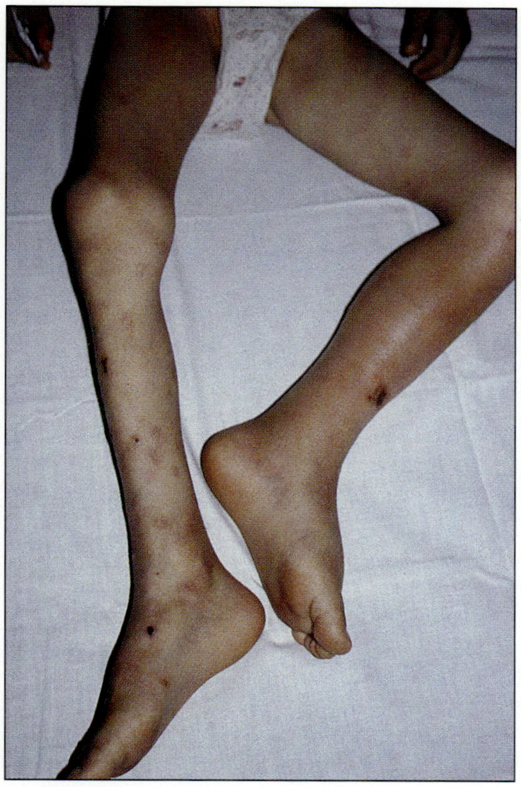

Figure 9-17 A girl with HIV-associated granulocytopenia and *Staphylococcus aureus* septicemia. Note the presence of multiple necrotic skin lesions. The left thigh is held in a position of flexion, abduction, and external rotation at the hip, indicating the presence of septic arthritis at the hip. The left calf is erythematous, swollen, and indurated secondary to bacterial myositis and cellulitis. Recognition of the frequently serious and repetitive nature of bacterial infections in HIV-infected children has led to the designation of some of these as indicator diseases for AIDS in children. Granulocytopenia is not an essential prerequisite to invasive bacterial disease in HIV-infected children, but it may increase the magnitude of the risk.

Clinical features of HIV-associated progressive encephalopathy

Impaired brain growth
Developmental delay or regression
Spastic weakness
Pathologic reflexes
Dystonia
Gait disturbance

Figure 9-18 Clinical features of HIV-associated progressive encephalopathy. There is evidence that many cases of encephalopathy result directly from HIV infection of the central nervous system, rather than from a complicating infection or malignancy. Virus has been isolated from cerebrospinal fluid, intrathecal synthesis of anti-HIV antibody has been demonstrated, and HIV nucleotide sequences have been identified in brain tissue at autopsy. Neuropathologic features noted in the brains of HIV-infected children include atrophy, subcortical inflammatory lesions, multinucleate giant cells, and vascular calcification.

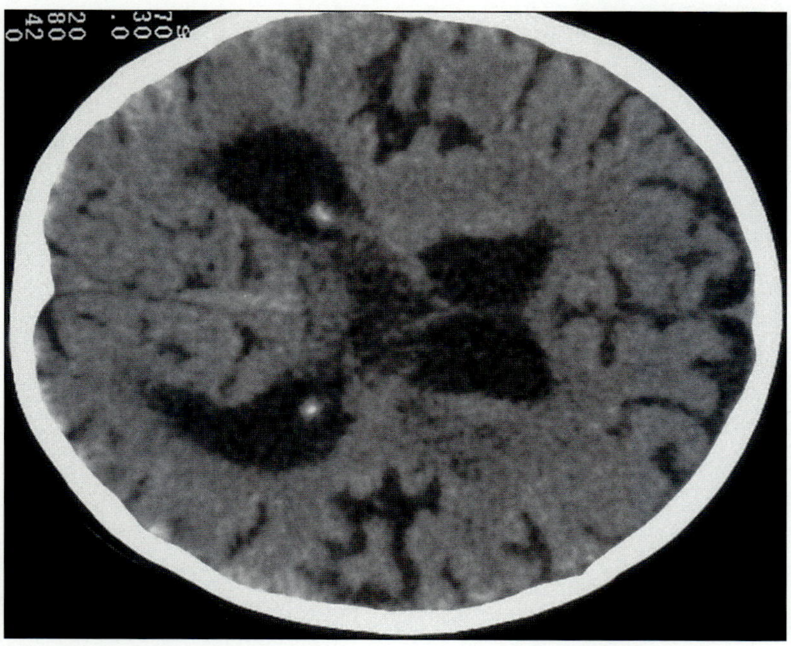

Figure 9-19 Computed tomography (CT) scan of the brain of an 8-year-old boy with HIV infection, showing marked generalized brain atrophy. Characteristic features seen on CT scans of children with HIV-associated encephalopathy include cerebral atrophy and bilateral symmetric calcification of the basal ganglia.

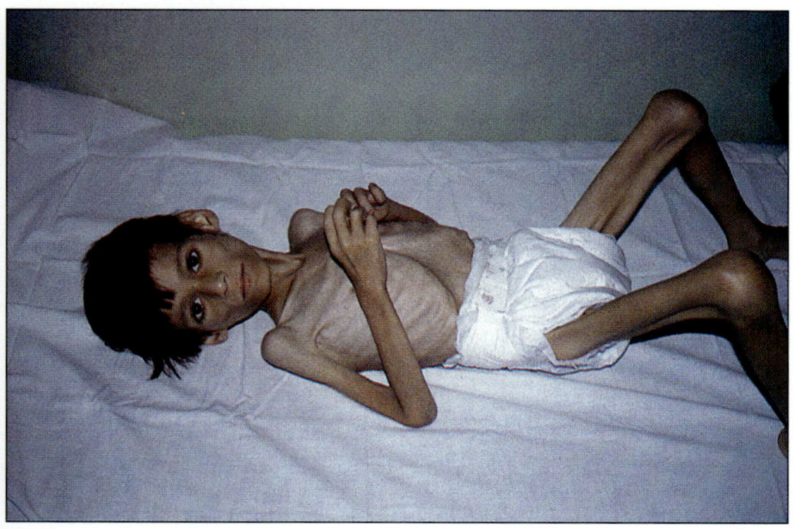

Figure 9-20 Severe wasting in an HIV-infected boy. Disturbances in growth, including growth failure and wasting, are common in pediatric HIV infection. HIV-infected children with wasting are at increased risk for early death. The pathogenesis of wasting is poorly understood.

Clinical features of esophageal candidiasis
Fever
Irritability
Odynophagia
Dysphagia

Figure 9-21 Clinical features of esophageal candidiasis. Children with esophageal candidiasis usually have concomitant oral candidiasis. Differentiation of esophageal candidiasis from other esophageal diseases (*eg*, esophagitis due to cytomegalovirus or herpes simplex virus, reflux esophagitis, lymphoma, and aphthous ulcers) can be difficult. Radiographic differentiation of various types of esophageal ulcerative disease, as well as recognition of dual infection, is impossible. Esophagoscopy with biopsy sometimes is necessary.

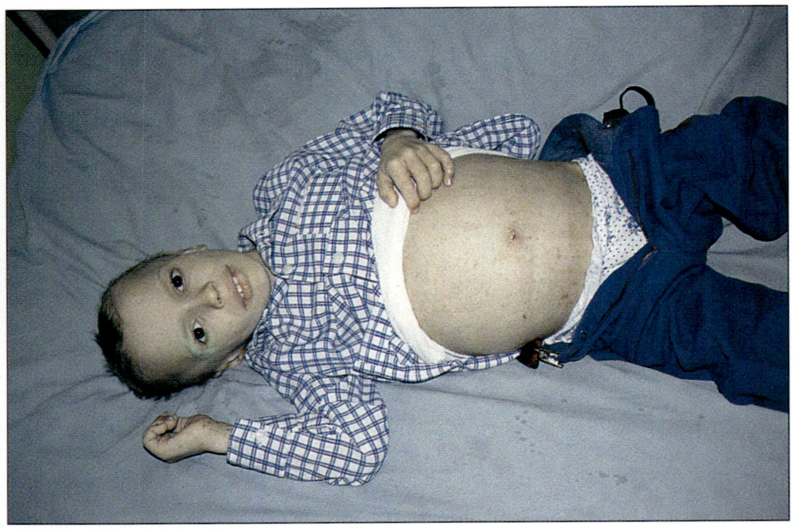

Figure 9-22 An HIV-infected boy with an abdominal lymphoma. Malignancies are uncommon among HIV-infected children, accounting for only approximately 2% of AIDS-defining illnesses reported to the Centers for Disease Control and Prevention [1]. The most common cancer of HIV-infected children is non–Hodgkin's lymphoma (Burkitt's or immunoblastic). Patients often manifest fever, weight loss, and evidence of "extranodal" disease (*eg*, hepatomegaly, jaundice, abdominal distention, and myelophthisis). Children with central nervous system lymphoma may experience cranial nerve palsies, seizures, hemiparesis, or loss of developmental milestones.

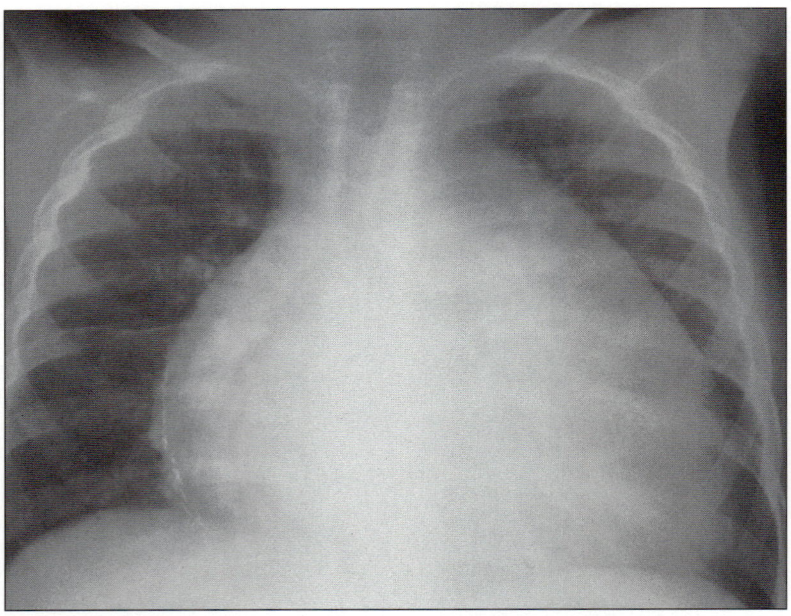

Figure 9-23 Chest radiograph showing cardiomegaly in a 5-year-old girl with vertical HIV infection, cardiomyopathy, and congestive heart failure. In one retrospective study of 81 HIV-infected children, serious dysrhythmia, congestive heart failure, and unexpected cardiac arrest occurred in 28 (35%), eight (10%), and seven (9%) patients, respectively [5]. Many HIV-infected children with congestive heart failure respond well to medical management.

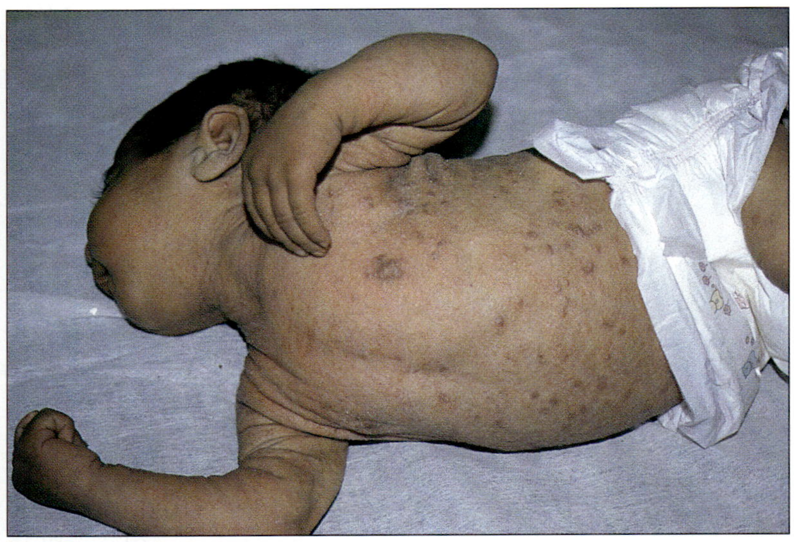

Figure 9-24 Generalized scabies in an infant with vertical HIV infection. Exaggerated scabies, with a generalized, papular pruritic eruption, has been noted in HIV-infected infants and children.

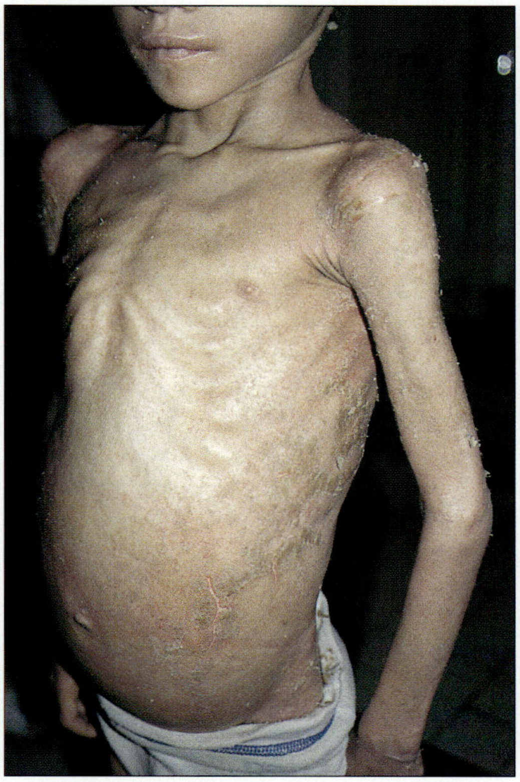

FIGURE 9-25 Norwegian (crusted) scabies in an HIV-infected boy. Generalized scaling and hyperkeratotic, crusted plaques are noted. Skin lesions of such patients harbor numerous *Sarcoptes scabiei* mites. Microscopic examination of skin scrapings to rule out scabies is recommended for any HIV-infected child with a generalized skin eruption.

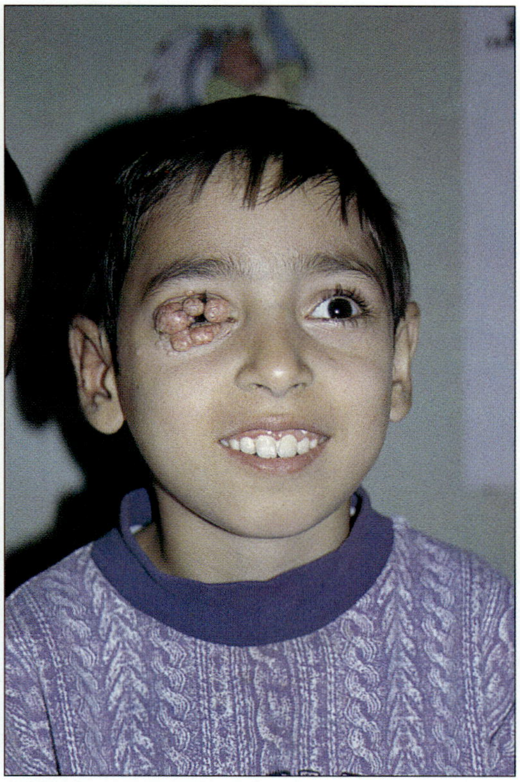

FIGURE 9-26 Severe molluscum contagiosum in an HIV-infected boy. Some HIV-infected children develop molluscum contagiosum lesions that are unusually large or widespread. Lesions involving the eyelids can obscure vision. Specific therapy for molluscum contagiosum is not currently available.

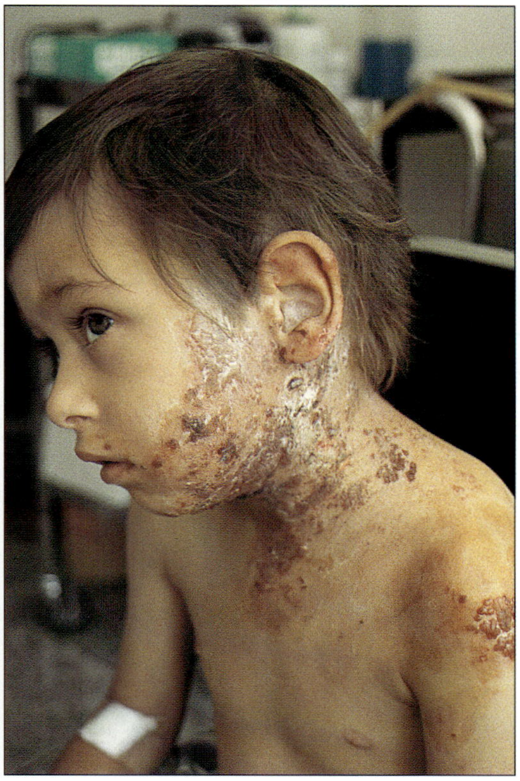

FIGURE 9-27 Uncomplicated dermatomal herpes zoster in an HIV-infected boy. Such cases can be complicated by dissemination or chronicity. Therapy with oral or intravenous acyclovir often is indicated. Postherpetic neuralgia occurs in some cases.

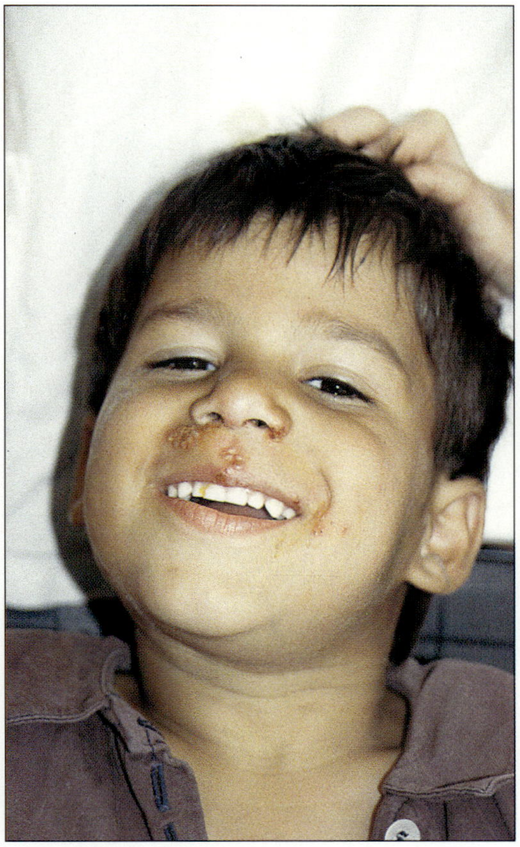

FIGURE 9-28 Herpes simplex virus infection involving the upper lip of a boy with HIV infection. Note the clustered vesicles on an erythematous base. Chronic or progressive herpetic skin lesions are observed occasionally in HIV-infected children. Frequent recurrences of lesions sometimes are amenable to chronic suppressive acyclovir therapy.

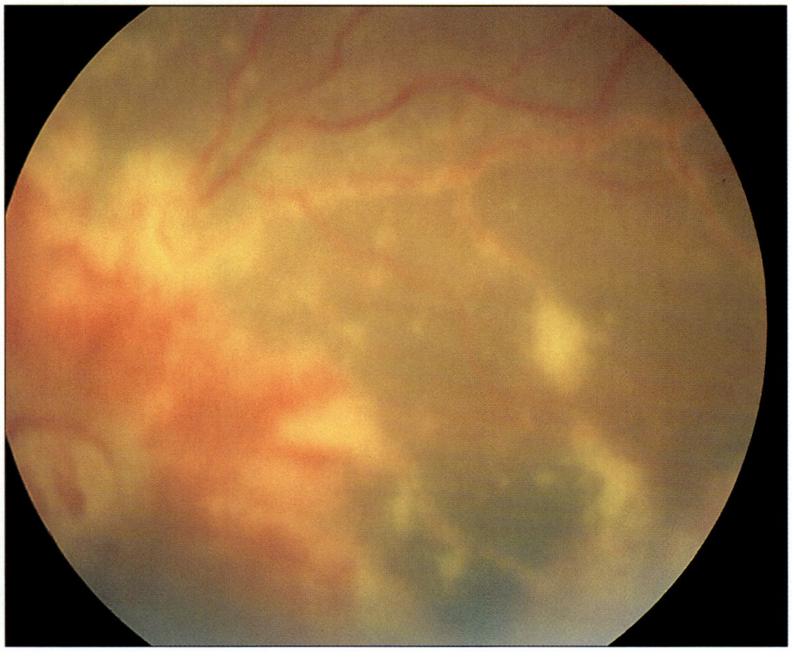

FIGURE 9-29 Funduscopic examination of a 16-year-old girl with HIV infection and cytomegalovirus retinitis. There are extensive areas of hemorrhage, with white retinal exudates. The optic nerve is pale. Children with cytomegalovirus retinitis usually present with painless visual impairment. Most cases occur in children with advanced HIV disease. (*Courtesy of* David Coats, Houston, TX.)

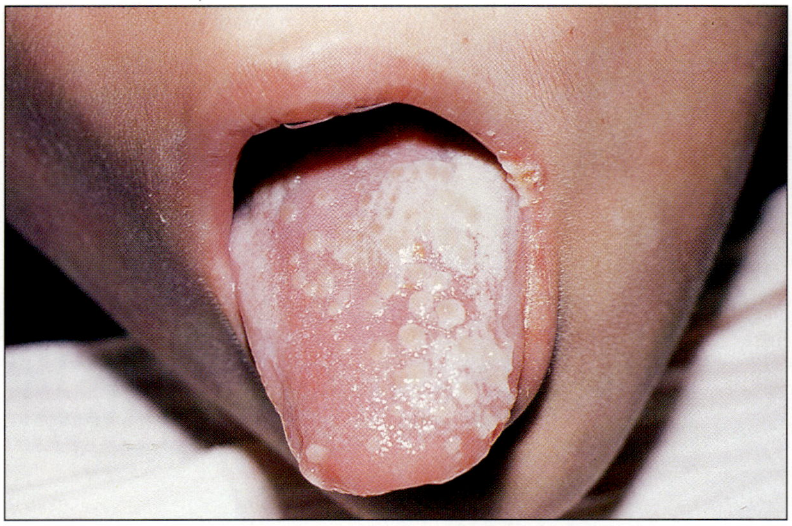

Figure 9-30 Multiple ulcers of the lips and tongue caused by herpes simplex in a child with HIV infection. Pseudomembranous candidiasis overlies many of the tongue lesions. Oral herpetic lesions may be larger and last longer than those observed in immunocompetent individuals. (*From* Kline [6]; with permission.)

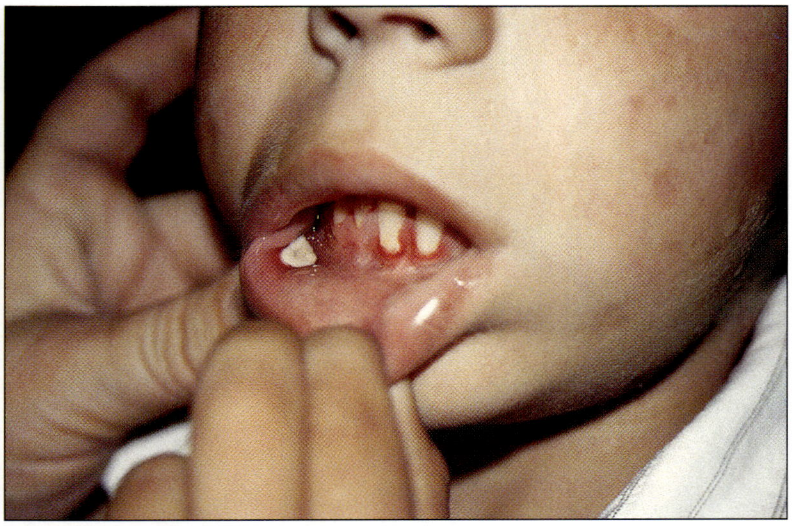

Figure 9-31 Major aphthous ulcer in an HIV-infected child. Note necrotizing ulcerative gingivitis in the area of the lower central incisors. Major aphthae are large (≥1 cm), painful ulcers that may be either solitary or multiple. They can occur anywhere in the oropharynx or in other parts of the gastrointestinal tract. Lesions may heal slowly, if at all, over a period of weeks to months.

Differential diagnosis of oral ulcers in individuals with HIV infection
Viral infections
Herpes simplex virus
Cytomegalovirus
Varicella zoster virus
Bacterial infections
Ulcerative periodontal disease (gingivitis or periodontitis)
Necrotizing ulcerative stomatitis
Mycobacterium tuberculosis
Mycobacterium avium-intracellulare complex
Fungal infections
Cryptococcus neoformans
Histoplasma capsulatum
Aspergillus sp.
Neoplastic conditions
Kaposi's sarcoma
Non–Hodgkin's lymphoma
Medications
Zalcitabine (dideoxycytidine)
Foscarnet
Other conditions
Granulocytopenia
Aphthous ulcers

Figure 9-32 Differential diagnosis of oral ulcers in individuals with HIV infection. Oral ulcers are problematic from a diagnostic standpoint because of the broad array of possible causes. These lesions can be severely debilitating because they interfere with normal speaking, chewing, and swallowing and sometimes result in weight loss, dehydration, and an inability to take oral medications.

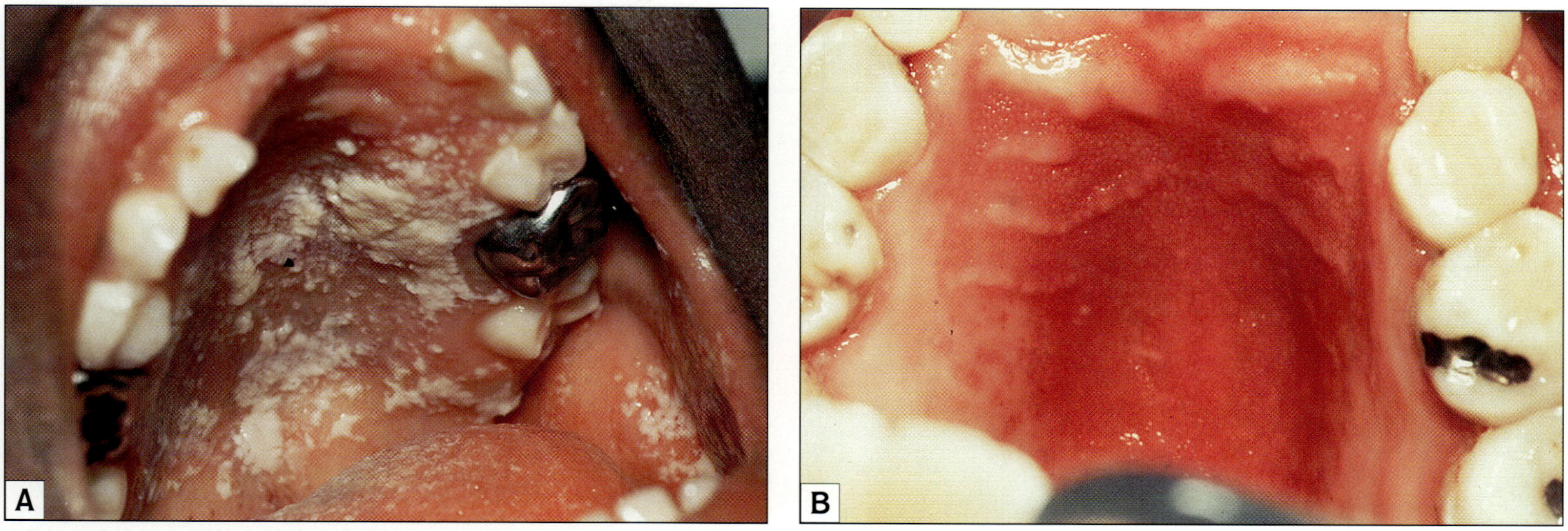

Figure 9-33 **A,** Pseudomembranous candidiasis. In pseudomembranous candidiasis, white or yellow plaques can be present on any oral mucosal surface. The pseudomembrane is removed easily, revealing erythema and, sometimes, superficial hemorrhage of underlying mucosa. **B,** Erythematous (atrophic) candidiasis. Erythematous candidiasis is characterized by the presence of often inconspicuous erythematous changes of the palate and dorsum of the tongue. Oral candidiasis is more common among children with low CD4+ lymphocyte counts or symptomatic HIV disease than among those with normal counts or no symptoms. Oral candidiasis may be a marker for rapid HIV disease progression. (*From* Kline [6]; with permission.)

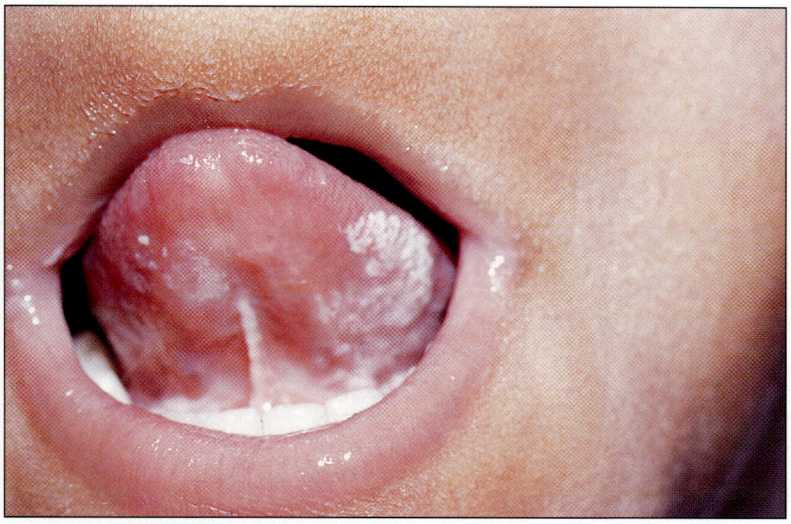

Figure 9-34 Oral hairy leukoplakia in an HIV-infected child. The typical findings of hairy leukoplakia include white or gray lesions along the lateral margins of the tongue. Lesions often have vertical corrugations and are not removable. They may appear hairy when the affected mucosa is dried. Induction of hairy leukoplakia is associated with the presence of Epstein–Barr virus within the oral mucosal epithelium of a severely immunosuppressed individual.

Prevention

Recommended regimen for interruption of HIV vertical transmission
Maternal
Antepartum ZDV: 100 mg orally five times daily
Intrapartum ZDV: 2 mg/kg intravenously over 1 h, followed by a 1 mg/kg/h intravenous infusion until delivery
Neonatal
ZDV: 2 mg/kg orally every 6 h for 6 wk

Figure 9-35 Recommended regimen for interruption of HIV vertical transmission. This regimen is based on AIDS Clinical Trials Group protocol (ACTG) 076, which showed that zidovudine (ZDV) given to HIV-infected pregnant women and their newborn infants can reduce the likelihood of HIV vertical transmission by approximately two thirds (from 25.5% to 8.3% in the study) [7]. Because of the design of the ACTG 076 trial, the findings are directly applicable only to women who initiate ZDV treatment during the pregnancy and who have baseline CD4+ lymphocyte counts greater than 200 cells/μL. Comprehensive recommendations for the use of antiretroviral drugs in HIV-infected pregnant women recently have been published [8].

Treatment

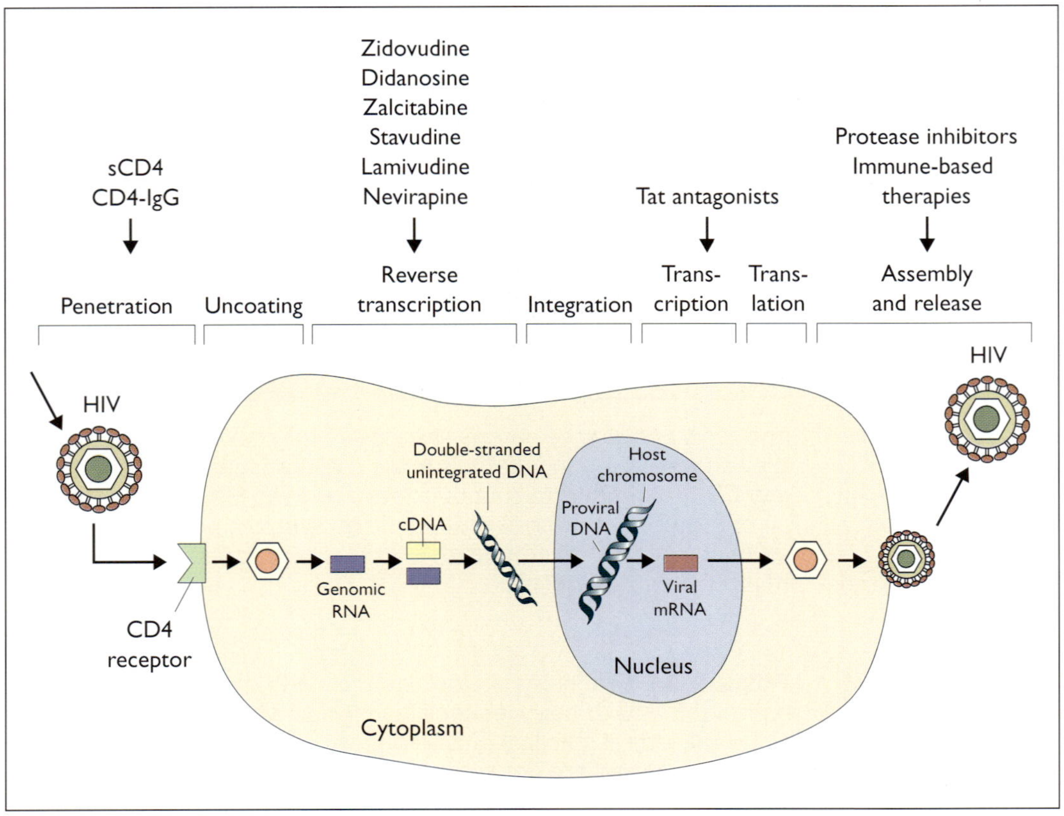

Figure 9-36 Diagrammatic representation of the HIV replicative cycle, showing sites of action of some antiretroviral agents. Using the viral envelope protein gp120, HIV attaches to the CD4 molecule on the surface of T-helper (CD4+) lymphocytes. After attachment, the virion uncoats, and viral genome is injected into the cytoplasm where, using the novel viral enzyme reverse transcriptase, viral RNA is transcribed into DNA. The proviral DNA product then moves to the cell nucleus and is integrated into the host cell genome. Viral RNA and viral proteins are produced and assembled into whole viral particles, which then bud at the cell surface and pass into the extracellular environment. The complex replicative life cycle of HIV lends itself to multiple potential sites of therapeutic attack. Most current treatment regimens combine two nucleoside analogs (which inhibit viral nucleic acid synthesis by binding preferentially to the reverse transcriptase enzyme) with a protease inhibitor (which prevents processing of viral polyproteins into smaller, functional structural and enzymatic proteins).

Antiretroviral medications

Agent	Mode of action	Common Toxicities	Comments
Zidovudine (ZDV, AZT)	NRTI	Neutropenia, anemia	—
Didanosine (ddI)	NRTI	Pancreatitis, peripheral neuropathy	Must be given on an empty stomach
Zalcitabine (ddC)	NRTI	Peripheral neuropathy, oral ulcers	No approved liquid formulation
Stavudine (d4T)	NRTI	Rarely, peripheral neuropathy	—
Lamivudine (3TC)	NRTI	Pancreatitis	—
Nevirapine	NNRTI	Rash, including Stevens–Johnson syndrome	Requires incremental dosing; no approved liquid formulation
Ritonavir	PI	Gastrointestinal intolerance or oral dysesthesia	Terrible taste; many drug interactions
Nelfinavir	PI	Diarrhea	—
Saquinavir	PI	—	No approved liquid formulation; pediatric dosing uncertain
Indinavir	PI	Nephrolithiasis, hyperbilirubinemia	No approved liquid formulation; pediatric dosing uncertain

NNRTI, non–nucleoside reverse transcriptase inhibitor; NRTI, nucleoside reverse transcriptase inhibitor; PI, protease inhibitor.

Figure 9-37 Antiretroviral medications. Agents generally are used in combination for treatment of most HIV-infected children. Most authorities recommend initial therapy with two nucleoside reverse transcriptase (RT) inhibitors (such as zidovudine or stavudine plus lamivudine or didanosine) plus a protease inhibitor (if feasible).

Laboratory findings indicating a need for antiretroviral therapy and *Pneumocystis carinii* pneumonia prophylaxis

	CD4+ lymphocyte counts, *cells/μL*	CD4+ lymphocyte percentage, *%*
Antiretroviral therapy		
1–11 mo	<1750	<30
12–23 mo	<1000	<30
24 mo–5 y	<750	<25
≥6 y	<500	<20
PCP prophylaxis		
1–11 mo	*See* legend	*See* legend
12–23 mo	<500	<15
24 mo–5 y	<500	<15
≥6 y	<200	<15

FIGURE 9-38 CD4+ lymphocyte counts and percentages indicating a need for antiretroviral therapy and *Pneumocystis carinii* pneumonia prophylaxis [9,10]. Indications for antiretroviral therapy are undergoing rapid change. Most authorities believe that antiretroviral therapy is indicated for any child with 1) clinical symptoms related to HIV infection, or 2) evidence of HIV-related immune suppression as indicated by a low CD4+ count or percentage [11]. Most authorities also recommend antiretroviral therapy for all HIV-infected infants under 12 months of age, regardless of clinical, immunologic, or virologic status. Some authorities recommend deferral of antiviral therapy for asymptomatic HIV-infected children greater than one year of age with normal immune status. Factors that should be considered in deciding to initiate therapy in such children include 1) development of HIV-related signs and symptoms, 2) rapidly declining CD4+ lymphocyte count or percentage, and 3) high or increasing plasma HIV RNA concentration.

P. carinii pneumonia prophylaxis is recommended for all HIV-exposed infants beginning at 4 to 6 weeks of age. All HIV-infected infants and those with indeterminate infection status should receive prophylactic therapy until they are at least 12 months of age. Prophylaxis should be discontinued if HIV infection has been reasonably excluded on the basis of two or more negative viral diagnostic tests (HIV culture or polymerase chain reaction), both of which are performed at or after 1 month of age, and either of which is performed at or after 4 months of age.

Regimens for *Pneumocystis carinii* pneumonia prophylaxis in children

Recommended regimen

Trimethoprim-sulfamethoxazole (TMP-SMZ): 150 mg TMP/m^2/d (750 mg SMZ/m^2/d) orally in divided doses twice daily on 3 consecutive days (*eg,* Monday, Tuesday, and Wednesday)

Alternative TMP-SMZ regimens include the same daily dose as above given orally as a single dose on 3 consecutive days per week; the same daily dose as above given orally twice daily; or the same daily dose as above given orally twice daily on 3 alternating days per week (*eg,* Monday, Wednesday, and Friday).

Alternative regimens (if TMP-SMZ is not tolerated)

Aerosolized pentamidine: 300 mg given via Respirgard II inhaler monthly (children ≥5 y)

Dapsone: 2 mg/kg (maximum dose 100 mg) given orally once every day.

Intravenous pentamidine, 4 mg/kg every 2–4 wk.

FIGURE 9-39 Regimens for *Pneumocystis carinii* pneumonia prophylaxis in children. Trimethoprim-sulfamethoxazole is preferred to any other agent for prophylaxis of *P. carinii* pneumonia.

Laboratory monitoring and immunization for the HIV-exposed infant (birth to 6 months of age)*

	Age								
	Birth	2 wk	4 wk	6 wk	2 mo	3 mo	4 mo	5 mo	6 mo
Assess risk of other diseases*	x								
Continuation of ACTG-076 regimen†	x	x	x	x					
CBC and differential leukocyte counts‡	x		x	x	x	x	x		
PCR for HIV DNA and/or viral culture for HIV§	x		x				x		
T-cell profile¶			x			x			
Quantitative immunoglobulins							x		
Initiate prophylaxis for *Pneumocystis carinii* pneumonia				x					
Immunizations									
Hepatitis B	x		x						x
Diphtheria-pertussis-tetanus					x		x		x
*Haemophilus influenzae***					x		x		x
Polio vaccine (IPV)					x		x		

ACTG-076—AIDS Clinical Trials Group Protocol-076; CBC—complete blood count; PCR— polymerase chain reaction.

* Test mother or neonate if maternal status for other infections has not been assessed.

† Zidovudine therapy to decrease the risk of HIV infection in the infant is discontinued at 6 wk of age.

‡ CBC and differential leukocyte count should continue monthly beyond 4 mo of age in the infected child and in the child whose infection status is unclear at 4 mo.

§ Repeat PCR or viral culture immediately if positive to confirm infection. If initial test is negative, repeat test at 4 wk to 2 mo. If clinical status or other laboratory parameters suggest HIV infection, repeat testing earlier than 4 mo. If at 4 mo the tests are still negative for infection, ongoing serologic follow-up is indicated.

¶ T-cell profile should be repeated at 6 mo in infected children and in those whose infection status is unclear at 6 mo.

** *Haemophilus influenzae* vaccine schedule may vary depending on which type of vaccine is used.

FIGURE 9-40 Laboratory monitoring and immunization for the HIV-exposed infant (from birth to 6 mo of age) [12].

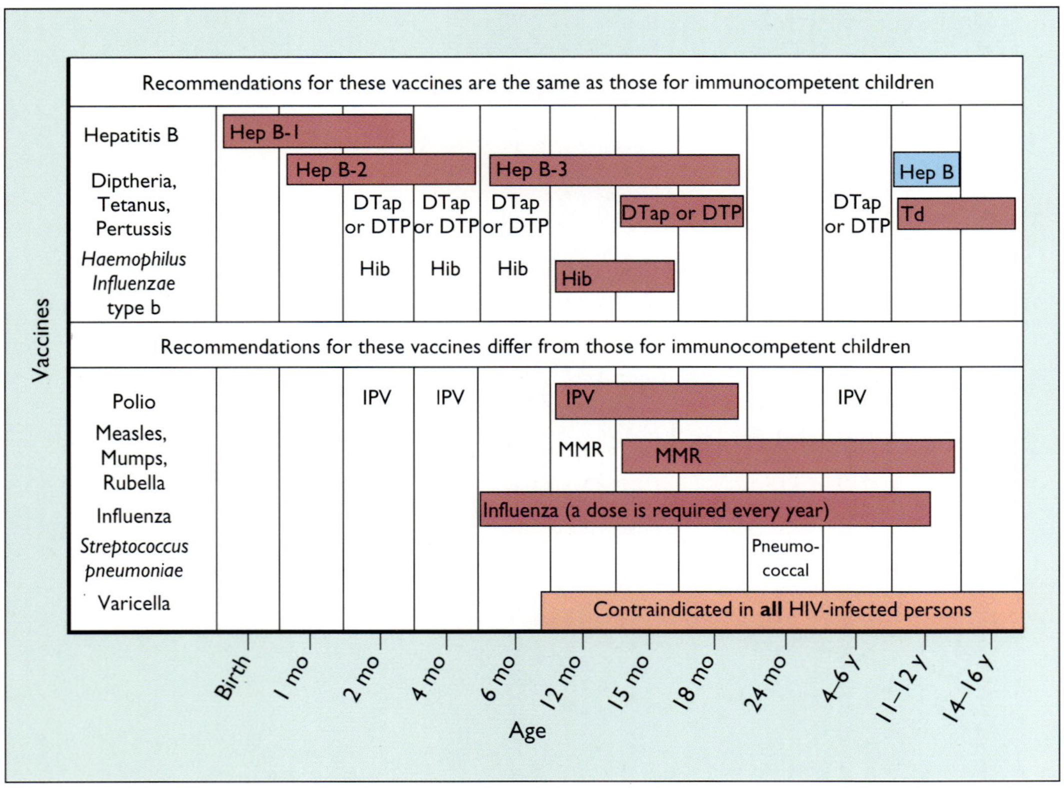

FIGURE 9-41 Recommended immunization schedule for HIV-infected children. This schedule also applies to children born to HIV-infected mothers whose HIV infection status has not been determined. Once a child is known not to be HIV infected, the schedule for immunocompetent children applies. This schedule indicates the recommended age for routine administration of currently licensed childhood vaccines. Some combination vaccines are available and may be used whenever administration of all components of the vaccine is indicated. For specific information on vaccine types and doses, please refer to the USPHS/IDSA guidelines [13].

References

1. Centers for Disease Control and Prevention. *HIV/AIDS surveillance report* 1996 (Dec).
2. Shearer WT, Rosenblatt HM, Schluchter MD, *et al.*: Immunologic targets of HIV infection: T cells. *Ann N Y Acad Sci* 1993, 693:35–51.
3. Shearer WT, Quinn TC, LaRussa P, *et al.*: Viral load and disease progression in infants infected with human immunodeficiency virus type 1. *N Engl J Med* 1997, 336:1337–1342.
4. Centers for Disease Control and Prevention: 1994 revised classification systemfor human immunodeficiency virus infection in children less than 13 years of age. *MMWR Morbidity Mortality Weekly Report* 1994, 43(RR-12):1–10.
5. Luginbuhl LM, Orav EJ, McIntosh K, Lipshultz SE: Cardiac morbidity and related mortality in children with HIV infection. *JAMA* 1993, 269:2869–2875.
6. Kline MW: Oral manifestations of pediatric human immunodeficiency virus infection: a review of the literature. *Pediatrics* 1996, 97:380–388.
7. Connor EM, Sperling RS, Gelber R, *et al.*: Reduction of maternal-infant transmission of human immunodeficiency virus type 1 with zidovudine treatment. *N Engl J Med* 1994, 331:1173–1180.
8. Centers for Disease Control and Prevention: Public Health Service Task Force recommendations for the use of antiretroviral drugs in pregnant women infected with HIV-1 for maternal health and for reducing perinatal HIV-1 transmission in the United States. *MMWR Morbidity Mortality Weekly Report* 1998, 47:1–30.
9. Working Group on Antiretroviral Therapy: Antiretroviral therapy and medical management of the human immunodeficiency virus-infected child. *Pediatr Infect Dis J* 1993, 12:513–522.
10. Centers for Disease Control: 1995 revised guidelines for prophylaxis against *Pneumocystis carinii* pneumonia for children infected with or perinatally exposed to human immunodeficiency virus. *MMWR Morbidity Mortality Weekly Report* 1995, 44(RR-4):1–11.
11. Working group on Antiretroviral Therapy and Medical Management of HIV-infected children: Guidelines for the use of antiretroviral agents in pediatric HIV infection. *MMWR Morbidity Mortality Weekly Report* 1998, 47:1–51.
12. Committee on Pediatric AIDS, American Academy of Pediatrics: Evaluation and medical treatment of the HIV-exposed infant. *Pediatrics* 1997, 99:909–917.
13. USPHS/IDSA Prevention of Opportunistic Infections Working Group: Prevention of opportunistic infections in persons infected with human immunodeficiency virus. *Clin Infect Dis* 1997, 25(suppl 3):S299—S335.

CHAPTER 10

Kawasaki Disease

Jane C. Burns
Mary P. Glode

KAWASAKI DISEASE (KD) is an acute, systemic vasculitis that affects predominantly infants and young children. The cause of this self-limited illness is unknown, although an infectious agent is strongly suspected. The inflammatory process affects the coronary arteries and other medium-sized, extraparenchymal, muscular arteries throughout the body. Coronary artery aneurysms may develop in up to 25% of untreated children. KD is now the most common cause of acquired heart disease in childhood in Japan and North America. Administration of high doses of intravenous gamma globulin (IVGG) during the first 10 days of illness, in conjunction with high-dose aspirin, markedly reduces the risk of developing coronary artery lesions.

Epidemiology

Kawasaki disease has been diagnosed in children on every continent, but Japan remains the country of highest prevalence. As of the end of 1992, 116,848 children with KD had been reported in Japan [1]. The annual incidence rate in Japan is 90 per 100,000 children younger than 5 years of age, whereas endemic rates for the United States have varied between nine and 15 per 100,000 children younger than 5 years of age. The male-to-female ratio is approximately 1.5:1. In Japan, the recurrence rate is 3% and the proportion of KD patients with affected siblings is 1%. The overall mortality from KD is less than 0.5%.

Clinical Manifestations

Kawasaki first published his series of 50 Japanese children with a new mucocutaneous inflammatory syndrome in 1968 (in Japanese) and in 1974 (in English) [2]. The current clinical criteria for establishing the diagnosis of KD are unchanged from Kawasaki's original disease description. The illness usually begins abruptly with the onset of high fever in a previously healthy child. Fever is followed by a generalized, erythematous rash, changes in the oral mucosa (including fissured lips, strawberry tongue, and pharyngeal erythema), changes in the extremities (including swollen hands and feet, red palms and soles, and periungual desquamation in the convalescent phase), bilateral nonexudative conjunctivitis, and cervical adenopathy with at least one node larger than 1.5 cm. The fever may last for up to 3 weeks in untreated patients. Associated clinical manifestations include small- and large-joint arthritis, urethritis, anterior uveitis, hydrops of the gallbladder, diarrhea, abdominal pain, and aseptic meningitis. Rarely, sensorineural hearing loss and cranial nerve palsies are noted.

Cardiac findings may include 1) tachycardia that is out of proportion to the degree of fever and anemia, and 2) a gallop rhythm. These clinical findings are most likely related to the diffuse myocarditis documented at autopsy and by endomyocardial biopsy. Pericardial effusion, valvular insufficiency, and congestive heart failure occur in a minority of patients. Coronary artery aneurysms develop in 15% to 25% of untreated children and may manifest as coronary artery insufficiency or myocardial infarction.

Laboratory Testing

Laboratory tests reveal generalized inflammation with an elevated leukocyte count with a predominance of immature forms, a nonregenerative anemia, elevated platelet count, and elevated acute-phase reactants (*eg*, erythrocyte sedimentation rate, C-reactive protein, α_1-antitrypsin) [3]. Approximately one third to one half of KD patients will have a cerebrospinal fluid (CSF) pleocytosis with mononuclear cell predominance and normal CSF glucose and protein [4]. Hepatobiliary tract inflammation is suggested by an elevated serum γ-glutamyl peptidase and alanine amino transferase. Hypoalbuminemia is common and has been correlated with the severity of inflammation.

Cardiac Evaluation

Two-dimensional echocardiography is the method of choice to follow the diameter of the coronary arteries and monitor for the development of aneurysms or ectasia. The echocardiogram should be performed prior to gamma globulin therapy to establish a baseline. Repeated studies at 7 to 10 days and again 3 to 4 weeks later are recommended to document the appearance or regression of coronary artery lesions. During the acute illness, the electrocardiogram may show mild, nonspecific ST-T wave changes and prolonged PR interval consistent with myocarditis.

Treatment

Administration of IVGG plus high-dose aspirin within the first 10 days after onset of fever reduces the risk of developing coronary artery lesions, especially giant aneurysms (aneurysms > 8 mm) [5–7]. Based on the most recent survey by the Kawasaki Disease Multicenter Study Group, new coronary artery lesions developed in only nine of 323 (2.8%) KD patients. Overall, 328 of 378 (86.8%) patients became afebrile and remained without fever 48 hours after completion of their IVGG infusion (Burns *et al.*, Unpublished data). Aspirin (80 to 100 mg/kg/d divided into four doses per day) was also administered to these patients. The independent contribution of aspirin to the cessation of inflammation has not been directly evaluated. Aspirin at low doses (3 to 5 mg/kg/d) is continued for its antiplatelet effect until the cardiac evaluation is completed. The potential role of other anti-inflammatory agents including steroids has not been specifically studied in a prospective trial. Management of children with coronary artery abnormalities must be individualized and, depending on the lesion, may include antiplatelet agents (aspirin, dipyridamole) and systemic anticoagulation with coumarin. Cardiac catheterization is recommended for the evaluation of potential stenosis in patients with aneurysms. Angioplasty, coronary artery bypass surgery, and even cardiac transplantation have been used to treat coronary artery insufficiency and myocardial infarction in this patient population.

Conclusions

Kawasaki disease is the leading cause of acquired heart disease in childhood in North America. Improved understanding of the pathogenesis must await the elucidation of the etiologic agent of this puzzling disease.

Historical Perspective

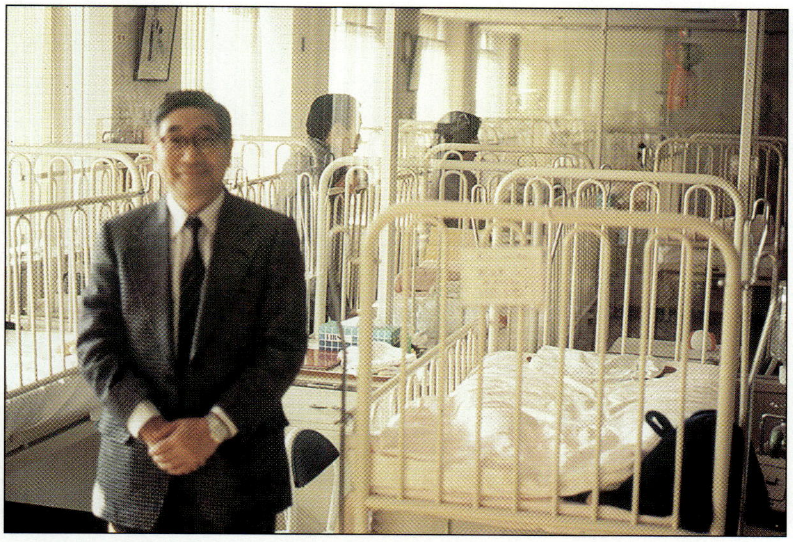

Figure 10-1 Tomisaku Kawasaki at the Red Cross Children's Hospital, Tokyo, Japan. Regarding his observation of the syndrome in January 1961, Kawasaki said that ". . . looking at him from the perspective of that time, I could not form any clear idea of the clinical process involved. The clinical chart for this child was filed under GOK (God Only Knows) without a clinical diagnosis being made."

Historical perspective of Kawasaki disease

1871: Autopsy description of coronary artery aneurysms in a boy aged 7 y at St. Bartholomew's Hospital, London

1967: Dr. Kawasaki reports (in Japanese) a series of 50 patients and establishes the clinical criteria for diagnosis

1974: First English-language report of Kawasaki disease by Dr. Kawasaki

1975: Frist series of American patients by Dr. Marian Melish, Hawaii

Figure 10-2 Historical perspective of Kawasaki disease (KD). Is KD a new disease or has this condition masqueraded in the past as atypical scarlet fever or a nonspecific viral infection? The clinical history and autopsy findings from a London teaching hospital from 1871 clearly suggest that a systemic vasculitis indistinguishable from KD has been with us for many years, albeit at a greatly reduced prevalence. Infantile polyarteritis nodosa, which has been recognized since the turn of the century, is now thought to represent a severe, usually fatal form of KD in young infants.

Epidemiology

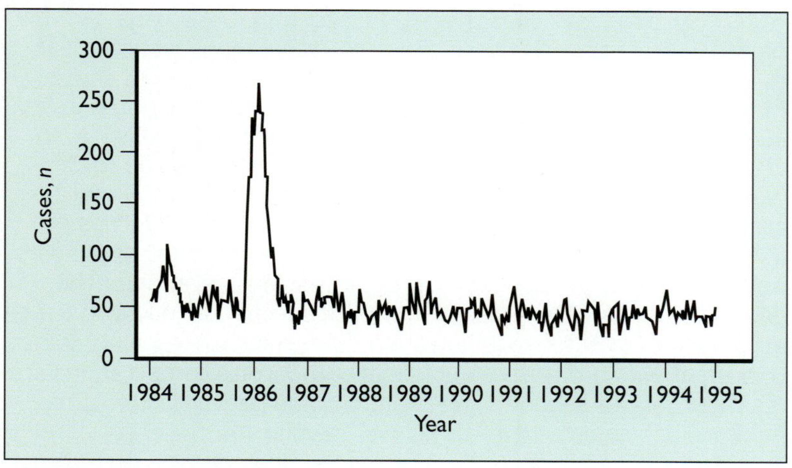

Figure 10-3 Number of Kawasaki disease (KD) patients per 10-day period in Japan between 1984 and 1994. Epidemics of KD occurred in the 1970s and 1980s in Japan but have not recurred for the past 11 years. The incidence of KD in Japan is 90 cases per 100,000 children younger than 5 years of age. The incidence in the United States has been variously reported as nine to 16 cases per 100,000 children younger than 5 years of age. (*Adapted from* Yashiro *et al.* [1]; with permission.)

Estimation of incidence of Kawasaki disease in the United States

Facts

85% of KD cases occur in children <5 y of age

18,752,000 children <5 y of age in the United States (1990 census data)

Assumptions

Endemic rate for KD in United States equals 12 cases per 100,000 children <5 y of age

Over a 1-y period, 18,752,000 children are subjected to a risk of 12 cases per 100,000; these cases represent 85% of the total number of KD cases

Final estimate

Average annual incidence: 2647 cases per year in United States

KD—Kawasaki disease

Figure 10-4 Estimated annual incidence of Kawasaki disease in the United States. Data on Kawasaki Disease are sporadically reported to the Centers for Disease Control and Prevention and, unlike Japan, no active national surveillance for the disease is performed in the United States. However, based on current estimates of attack rates in local communities, an annual incidence estimate for the United States can be calculated. This figure is likely to significantly underestimate the true burden of disease.

Clinical Presentation

Case definition of Kawasaki disease

Fever lasting at least 5 d plus 4 of the 5 following criteria:
1. Bilateral nonexudative conjunctivitis
2. Polymorphous exanthem
3. Cervical node >1.5 cm
4. Changes in the oropharynx
   a. Diffuse erythema
   b. Dry, fissured lips
   c. Strawberry tongue
5. Changes in the extremities
   a. Edema of the hands and feet
   b. Palm and sole erythema
   c. Periungal desquamation

Figure 10-5 Case definition for Kawasaki disease. The original case definition, devised by Kawasaki over 30 years ago, remains unchanged. Cervical lymphadenopathy is the least frequent clinical sign and is seen in only approximately 40% of patients. The illness usually begins with the sudden onset of high fever without a prodrome. In the 1st week following the onset of fever, the rash and mucocutaneous signs appear. (*Adapted from* Kawasaki *et al.* [2].)

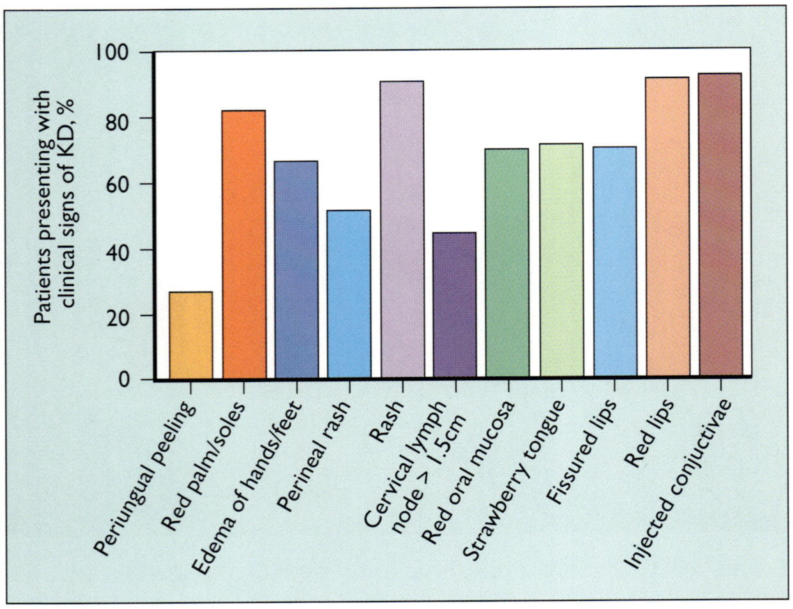

Figure 10-6 Prevalence of clinical signs and symptoms at presentation during the first 10 days of illness. Rash, red eyes, and red lips are the most common triad that lead to the diagnosis of Kawasaki disease (KD). Cervical adenopathy is the least reliable physical finding. Periungual desquamation is common in the second to third week of illness, but is usually not apparent at the time of initial presentation. (*Data from* Burns *et al.* [3]; with permission.)

Associated clinical features of Kawasaki disease

Urethritis with sterile pyuria (mononuclear cells)
Arthralgia and arthritis
Gastrointestinal: diarrhea, abdominal pain, obstructive jaundice, hepatitis, hydrops of the gall bladder
Central nervous system: cerebral spinal fluid pleocytosis, diffuse slowing on electroencephalogram
Cardiac: pericardial effusion, myocarditis, valvulitis, myocardial infarction, sudden death

Figure 10-7 Associated clinical features of Kawasaki disease (KD). KD is a systemic vasculitis that may affect multiple organs. Urethritis with a sterile pyuria consisting predominantly of mononuclear cells may be seen during the acute inflammatory phase of the disease. Arthritis is common, with small-joint arthritis noted in 15% of patients during the acute illness followed by axial arthropathy in up to one third of patients during the 2nd to 3rd week of the illness. Gastrointestinal manifestations of KD may be confused with viral hepatitis or bacterial cholangitis. Hydrops of the gallbladder may occur transiently in up to one third of patients. This clinical finding should provoke careful consideration of the diagnosis of KD. The presence of aseptic meningitis may lead to the misdiagnosis of enteroviral infection. The electroencephalogram is consistent with a diffuse encephalopathy. Cardiac complications are the most serious sequelae of KD and include pericardial effusion, myocarditis, congestive heart failure, valvular insufficiency, myocardial ischemia and infarction, and sudden death.

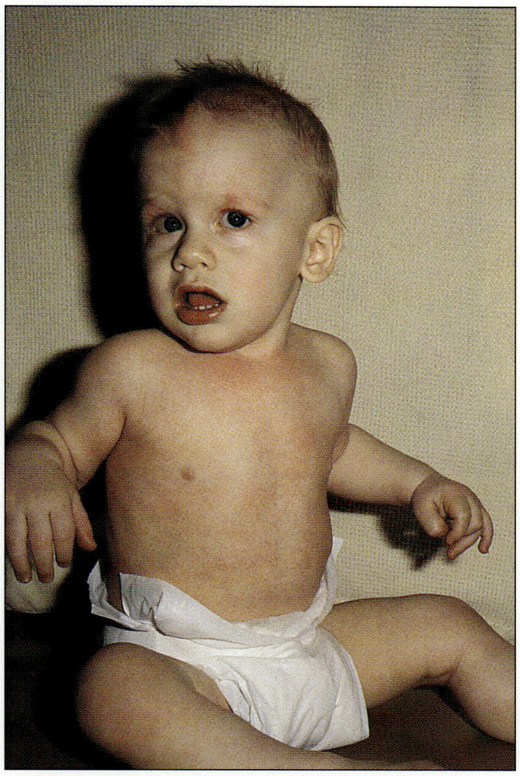

FIGURE 10-8 Two-year-old male infant with acute Kawasaki disease. Note apprehensive appearance of patient. Patients with Kawasaki disease are frequently extremely irritable and difficult to console. The patient has painful fusiform swelling of the digits that cause him to hold his hands in the air without touching anything. Note the faint maculopapular rash over the trunk.

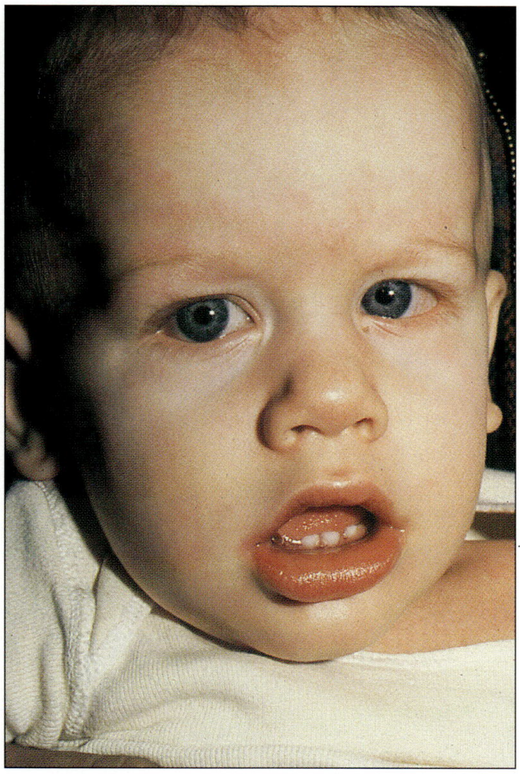

FIGURE 10-9 Close-up of patient seen in Figure 10-8. Note bilateral, nonexudative conjunctivitis and cherry-red color of the lips.

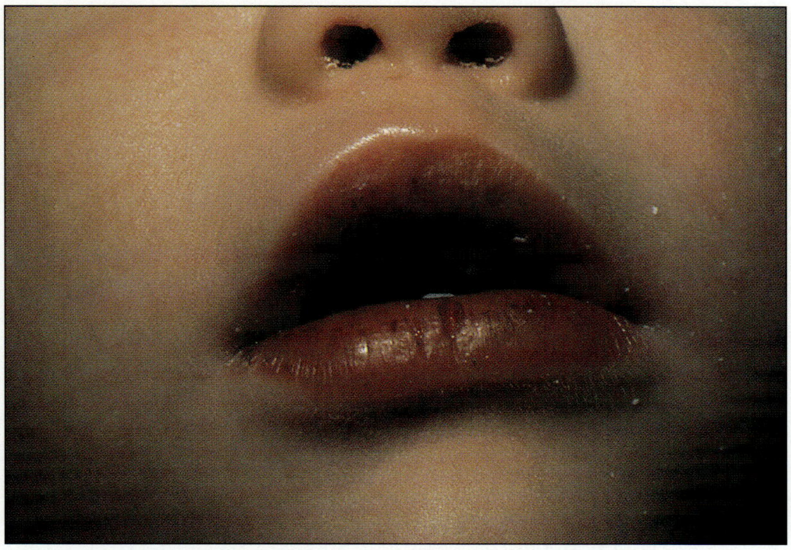

FIGURE 10-10 Close-up of lips showing fissuring in the center of the upper and lower vermillion border. Peeling and bleeding of the lips is common. This clinical finding is uncommon in other rash or fever syndromes in the pediatric age group.

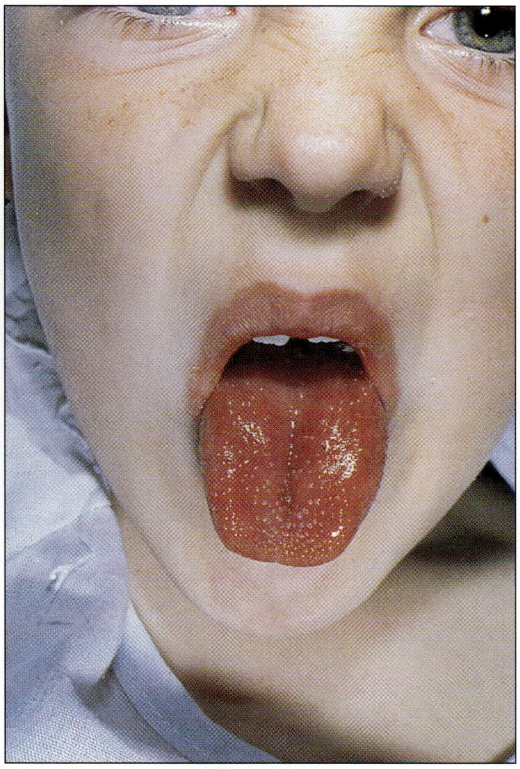

FIGURE 10-11 Characteristic "strawberry tongue" of Kawasaki disease. The essential components of a strawberry tongue are 1) the sloughing of the filiform papillae due to the systemic inflammatory process, and 2) persistence of the fungiform papillae, which form the "seeds" of the strawberry. The strawberry tongue is also associated with both streptococcal and staphylococcal toxin–mediated disease and is not specific to Kawasaki disease.

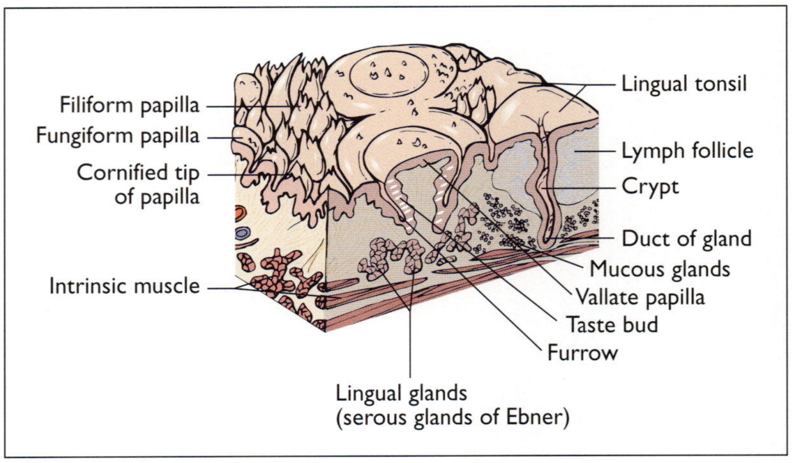

Figure 10-12 Gross anatomy of the tongue showing the different papillae. In acute Kawasaki disease, the cornified tips of the filiform papillae slough off to reveal a diffusely red, glossy surface.

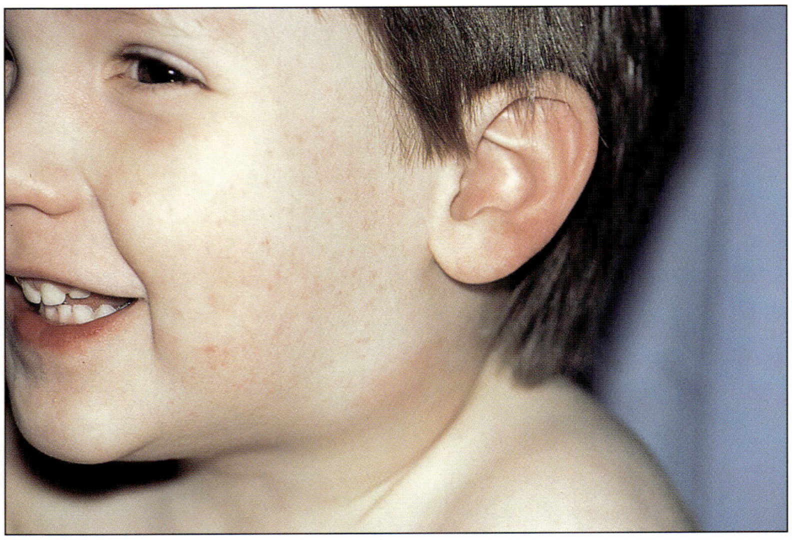

Figure 10-13 Characteristic cervical lymphadenopathy associated with Kawasaki disease (KD). A cervical node larger than 1.5 cm in diameter is noted in approximately 40% of patients with acute KD. The adenopathy is often unilateral and the jugulodigastric node is most frequently involved. However, the adenopathy may be bilateral and may involve the posterior cervical chain. Biopsy of enlarged nodes reveals only reactive hyperplasia. The adenopathy is more frequently seen in older patients and may delay the diagnosis of KD because antibiotics are prescribed for presumptive bacterial adenitis. If the KD rash appears after the initiation of antibiotic therapy, a presumptive diagnosis of "drug rash" may delay the diagnosis further.

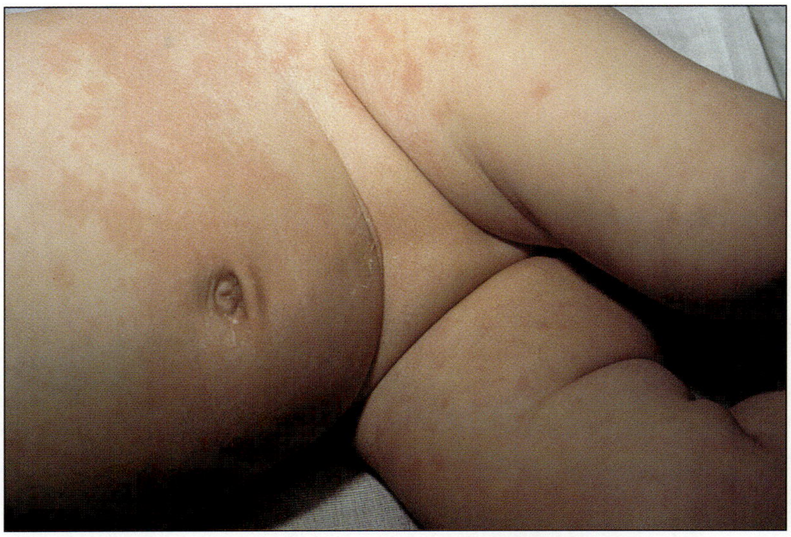

Figure 10-14 The maculopapular rash of Kawasaki disease (KD). The rash of KD may take many forms. There is no typical distribution and the rash is variably present over the trunk, face, and extremities. The rash may be macular, maculopapular, or micropustular. Target-like lesions and urticaria may occur. True vesicles or bullae are never seen. Petechiae may occur with the micropustular form of the rash. Erythroderma is rare and its presence should prompt investigation of bacterial toxin–mediated illness. The rash of KD is generally not pruritic. Biopsy of the rash is surprisingly unrevealing, although vasculitis of deeper dermal vessels with a round cell infiltrate may be seen.

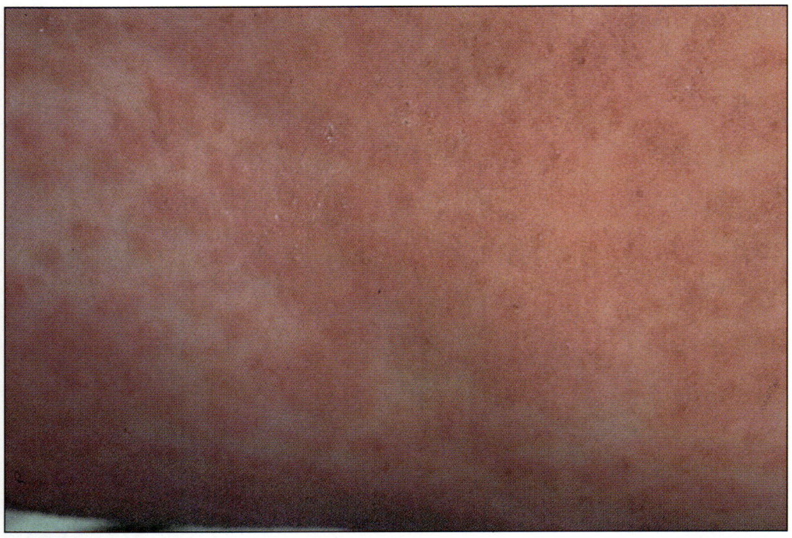

Figure 10-15 Micropustular rash of Kawasaki disease with petechiae. This unusual rash is uncommon but is quite specific for Kawasaki disease. Tiny micropustules can be see when a beam of light is shined tangentially across the skin.

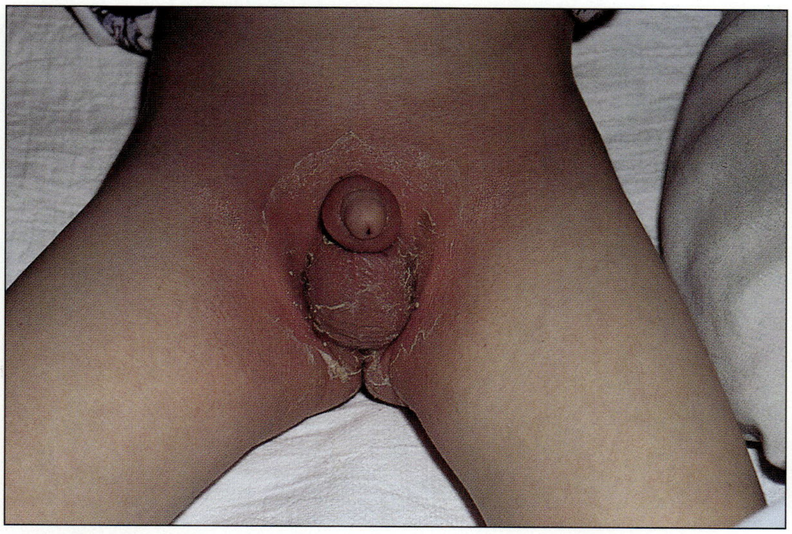

FIGURE 10-16 Accentuated groin rash in a circumcised male patient. Note the erythema of the urethral meatus and desquamation of the scrotum. Accentuation of the rash in the groin is seen during the acute phase in 50% of Kawasaki disease patients. This groin accentuation is also typical of scarlet fever and toxic shock. Peeling of the rash in the groin may be marked during the 1st week of illness and precedes the periungual peeling of the digits.

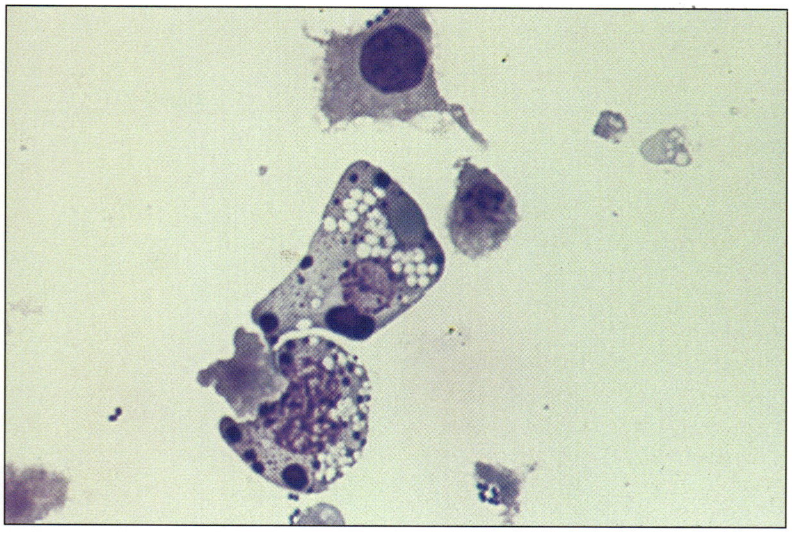

FIGURE 10-17 Papanicolaou stain of cells in a voided urine specimen. Mononuclear cells with unusual inclusions may be abundant in the urine during the acute phase of Kawasaki disease. These cells apparently originate in the urethra, because suprapubic aspiration and catheterization of the urinary bladder rarely demonstrate the sterile pyuria associated with this disease.

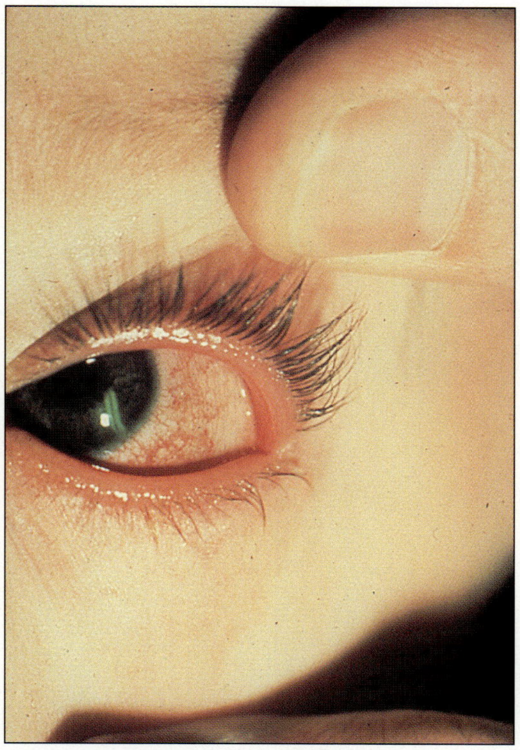

FIGURE 10-18 Characteristic bilateral, nonexudative conjunctivitis associated with Kawasaki disease. Note the perilimbal sparing with a halo of white around the iris. Conjunctival biopsy in these patients reveals surprisingly little inflammation and no cellular response in the epithelium. Keratitis is seen in the minority of patients. The dry conjunctivitis of Kawasaki disease is virtually pathognomonic for this systemic vasculitis. The conjunctivitis is distinguished from viral conjunctivitis caused by enterovirus, measles, and adenovirus by the lack of exudate, absence of keratitis, and absence of keratitic precipitates. (*See* Smith *et al.* [8].) (*From* Smith and Burns [9]; with permission.)

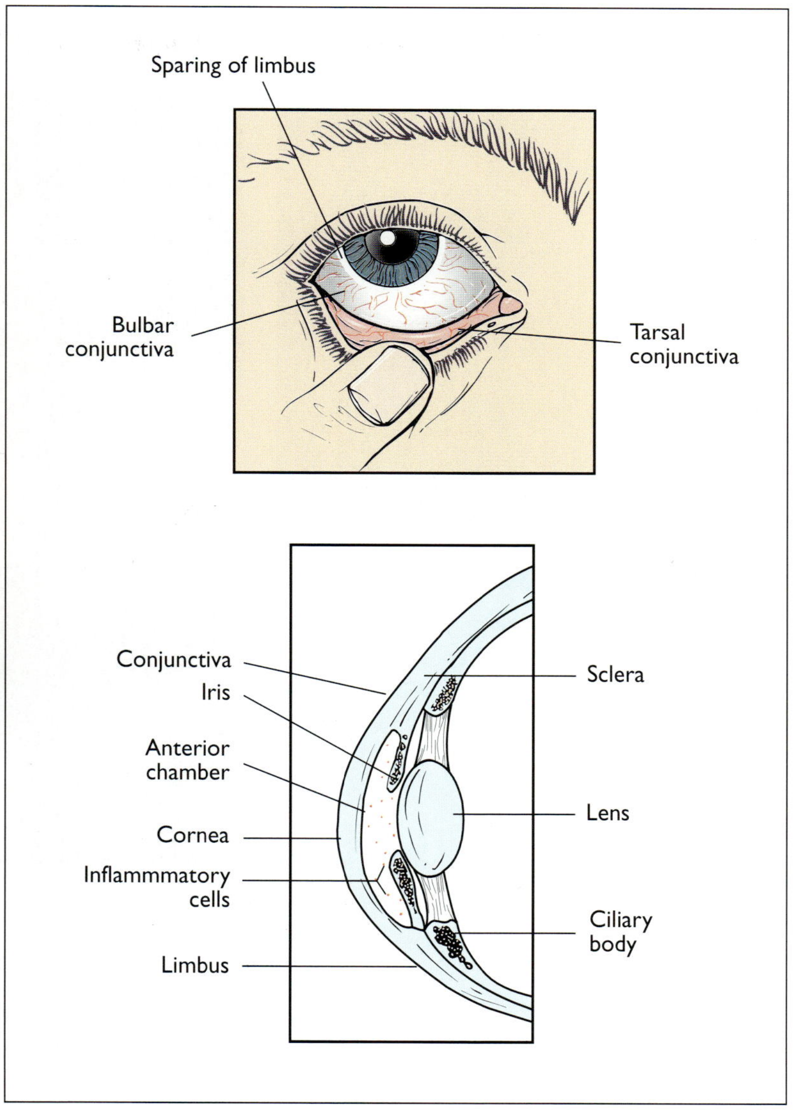

FIGURE 10-19 Conjunctival injection and anterior uveitis in Kawasaki disease. Mild anterior uveitis is present in more than 80% of patients examined by slit lamp during their 1st week of illness. Consultation with an experienced pediatric ophthalmologist may be helpful to rule out other lookalike diseases in the pediatric age group that are associated with fever, rash, and conjunctivitis. (*Adapted from* Smith *et al.* [4].)

Differential diagnosis of conjunctivitis in the pediatric patient with prolonged fever and rash
Kawasaki disease*
Streptococcal and staphylococcal toxin-mediated diseases (scarlet fever, toxic shock syndrome)
Adenovirus and other viral infections (enterovirus, measles*)
Drug reactions or Stevens–Johnson syndrome*
Leptospirosis*
Yersinia pseudotuberculosis infection
Rickettsial infection
Reiter's syndrome*
Inflammatory bowel disease*
Postinfectious immune complex disease* (*eg*, postmeningococcemia)
Sarcoidosis*
Systemic lupus erythematosus*
Behçet's syndrome*
*May have evidence of anterior uveitis on slit-lamp examination.

Figure 10-20 Differential diagnosis of conjunctivitis in the pediatric patient with prolonged fever and rash. Many of these infections are rare or restricted to certain geographical regions of the United States.

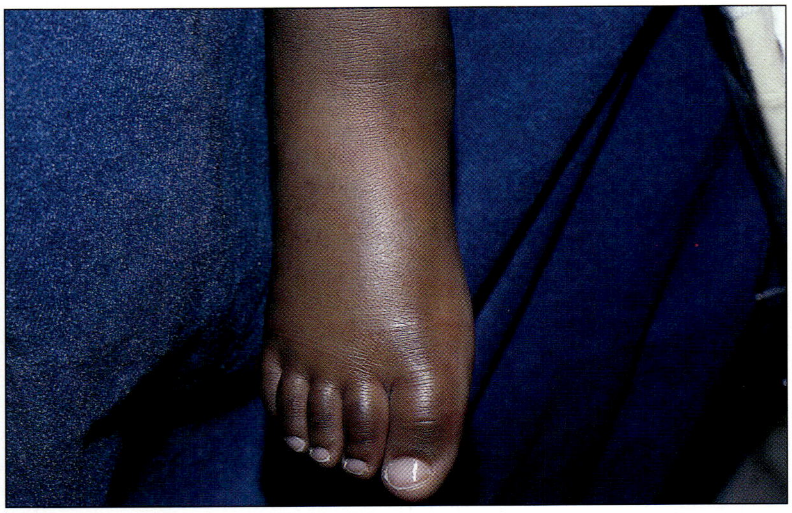

Figure 10-21 Changes in the extremities. Note the diffuse, nonpitting edema of the dorsum of the foot. This swelling is uncomfortable and patients will refuse to walk. Arthritis in the hip and knee joints may also contribute to stiffness and a reluctance to bear weight.

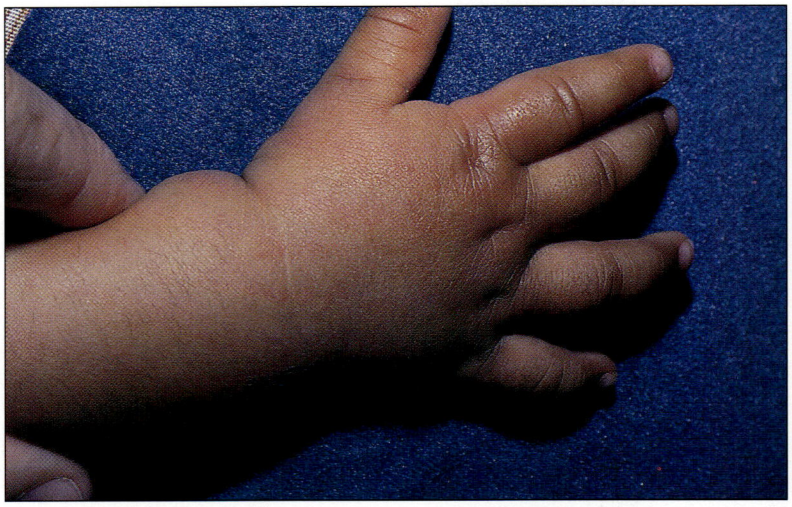

Figure 10-22 Swelling of the dorsum of the hand associated with fusiform swelling of the digits. Erythema of the proximal and distal interphalangeal joints suggests small-joint arthritis.

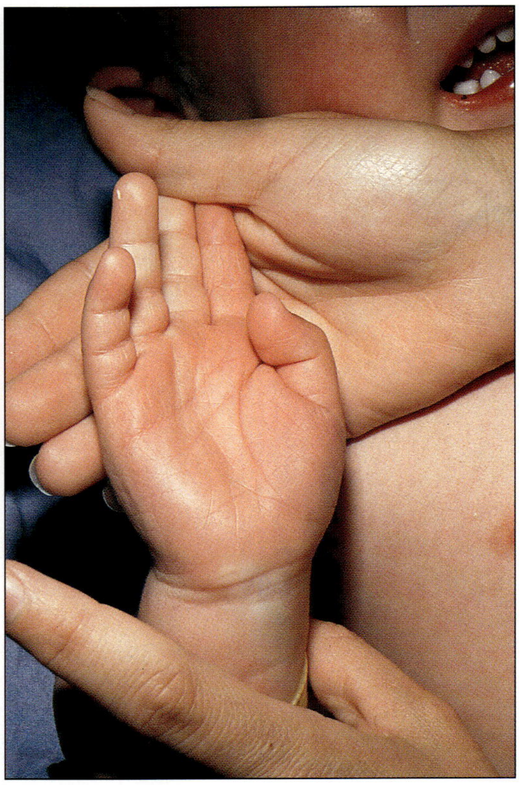

Figure 10-23 Diffuse erythema of the palm. This finding is usually bilateral and may fluctuate in intensity with the height of the fever. Unlike the rash on other parts of the body, there is no pattern to the erythema.

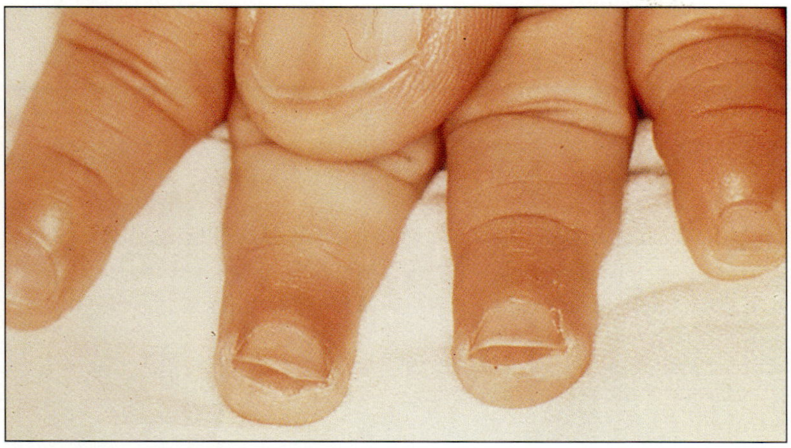

FIGURE 10-24 Periungual desquamation during the convalescent phase of Kawasaki disease. The peeling is usually noted after the acute signs and symptoms of inflammation have subsided in the 2nd to 3rd week of the illness.

Kawasaki disease in infants less than 6 months of age
Atypical presentation
High morbidity and mortality
Consider the diagnosis of Kawasaki disease in any young infant with unexplained fever lasting > 1 wk and signs of mucocutaneous inflammation
Echocardiography and slit-lamp examination may be helpful in establishing the diagnosis

FIGURE 10-25 Kawasaki disease in infants younger than 6 months of age. The signs and symptoms of Kawasaki disease may be more subtle in this group of infants. A high index of suspicion is necessary to establish the diagnosis in this age group. Any infant with prolonged, unexplained fever should undergo an echocardiogram and slit-lamp examination to seek confirmatory evidence of systemic vasculitis.

LABORATORY EVALUATION

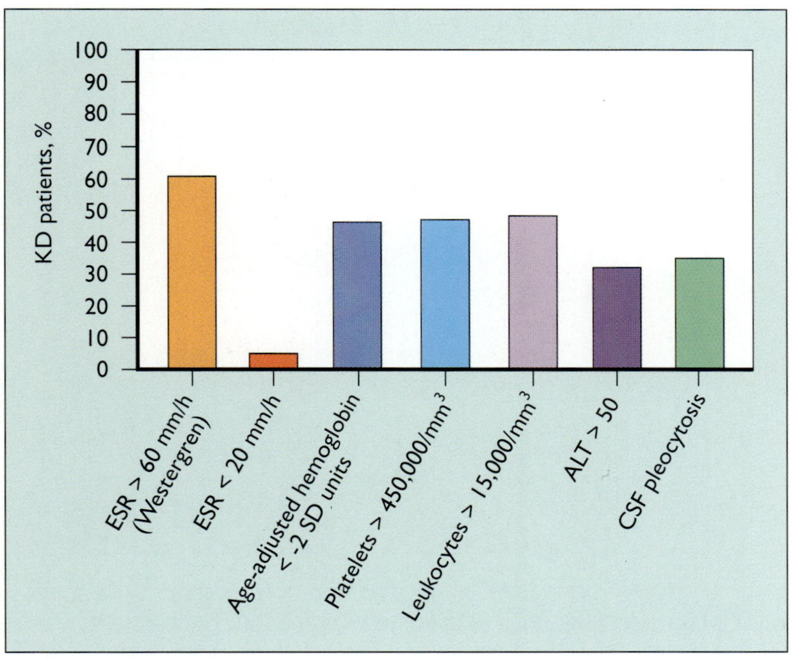

FIGURE 10-26 Common laboratory findings in acute Kawasaki disease (KD) during the first 10 days of illness. No laboratory tests can definitively establish the diagnosis of KD. There is a generalized, acute inflammatory response characterized by an elevated leukocyte count with predominance of immature forms, a nonregenerative anemia, elevated erythrocyte sedimentation rate (ESR), and other acute-phase reactants. The elevated ESR persists for weeks after the resolution of fever and may be a helpful clue to the presence of systemic vasculitis in a patient who presents during the subacute phase after the fever has subsided. The platelet count usually rises during the 2nd to 3rd week of the illness. ALT—alanine aminotransferase; CSF—cerebrospinal fluid. (*Adapted from* Burns *et al.* [3] and Dengler *et al.* [4].)

Cerebrospinal fluid abnormalities in patients with acute Kawasaki disease

CSF parameter	Patients, *n (%)**
CSF pleocytosis (>10 leukocytes per mm^3)	17 (34.7)
CSF glucose <45 mg/dL	1 (2.0)†
CSF protein >45 mg/dL	7 (14.3)

*Total, 49

†CSF glucose level, 44mg/dL

FIGURE 10-27 Cerebrospinal fluid (CSF) findings in acute Kawasaki disease (KD). CSF pleocytosis has been reported in up to 60% of unselected Japanese KD patients who were evaluated by lumbar puncture during their acute illness as part of a prospective study. In this American series, 49 patients who were subsequently diagnosed with KD underwent lumbar puncture to rule out bacterial meningitis. Approximately one third had CSF pleocytosis. All had a normal CSF glucose level, and elevated CSF protein was uncommon. (*Adapted from* Dengler *et al.* [4].)

Pathology

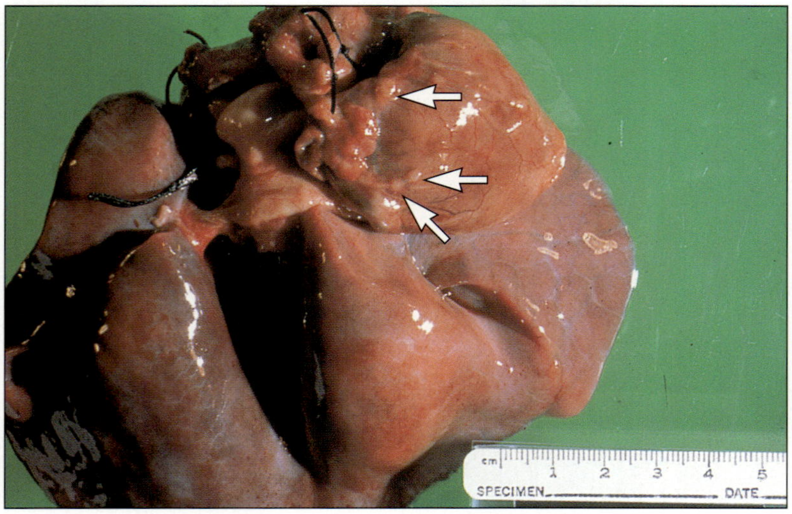

Figure 10-28 Heart and lung block. This postmortem specimen came from a 3-month-old female infant who died on day 21 of Kawasaki disease. Note the beaded appearance of the coronary arteries (*arrows*). This is the external appearance of the coronary artery aneurysm seen on transverse section in Figure 10-32.

Histologic progression of vascular lessions in Kawasaki disease

Intimal mononuclear cell accumulation with intimal thickening
Mixed inflammatory cell infiltration of outer adventitial sites
Lymphocytic infiltration of luminal side of intima
Progressive transluminal medial disruption with a mixed inflammatory infiltrate and edema
Intimal fibrinoid necrosis
Luminal thrombosis and aneurysmal dilatation

Figure 10-29 Histologic progression of vascular lesions in Kawasaki disease. Most information regarding the evolution of the patterned vasculopathy in Kawasaki disease is derived from autopsy material. One hallmark of the disease is that vascular lesions in all stages of evolution may be seen in tissues from a single point in time. The inflammatory response predominantly involves medium-sized extraparenchymal muscular arteries.

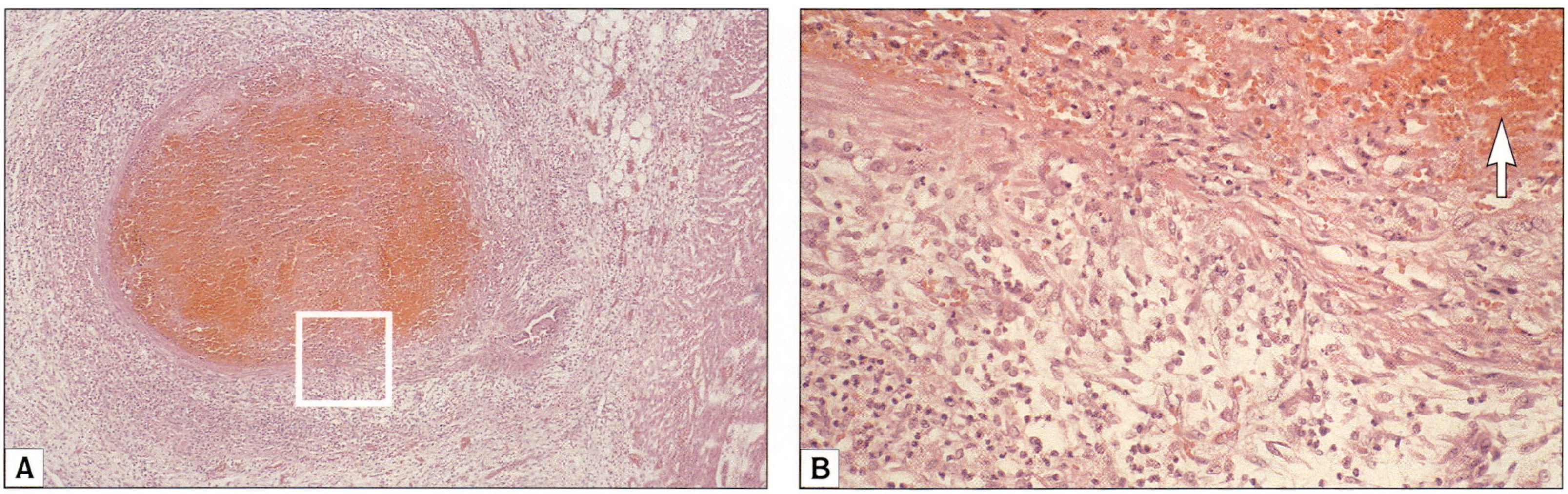

Figure 10-30 Transverse section of coronary artery aneurysm from autopsy specimen shown in Figure 10-30. **A,** This transverse section of the right coronary artery demonstrates transmural infiltration by lymphocytes and neutrophils. The inflammatory infiltrate is associated with disruption of the vessel's muscularis and intima. **B,** Higher magnification of *boxed section*. Destruction of the vessel wall's structural integrity predisposes to aneurysm formation. Concomitant destruction of the intima has lead to early thrombus formation (*arrow*). Coronary artery thrombosis associated with these aneurysms is the most common cause of death in patients with Kawasaki disease.

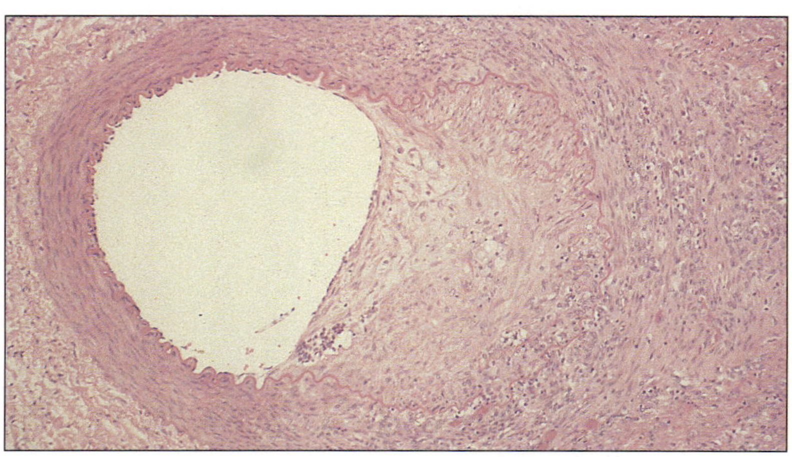

Figure 10-31 Transverse section of the axillary artery from a 4-month-old female infant 6 weeks after the onset of acute Kawasaki disease. Acute inflammatory lesions of the vessel wall heal by medial fibrosis and intimal thickening. These processes may lead to luminal narrowing or stenosis as seen in this artery.

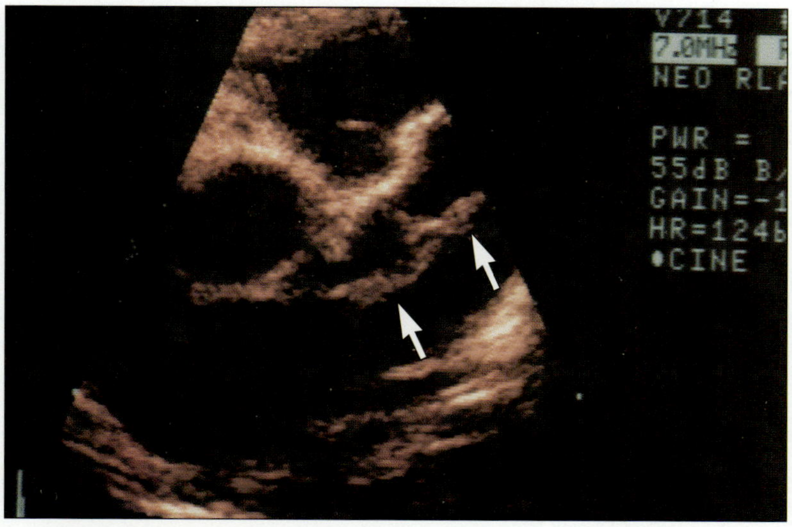

FIGURE 10-32 Echocardiogram of a 2 month-old male infant with 6-mm aneurysms of the left coronary artery. Fortunately, most pediatric patients can be evaluated initially and followed by noninvasive imaging of the coronary arteries. Echocardiography is a very sensitive and specific method to detect coronary artery dilatation and aneurysms. The technique is less sensitive for the detection of stenotic lesions that may occur as part of the healing process in large aneurysms. *Arrows* indicate two regions of focal dilatation in the left coronary artery.

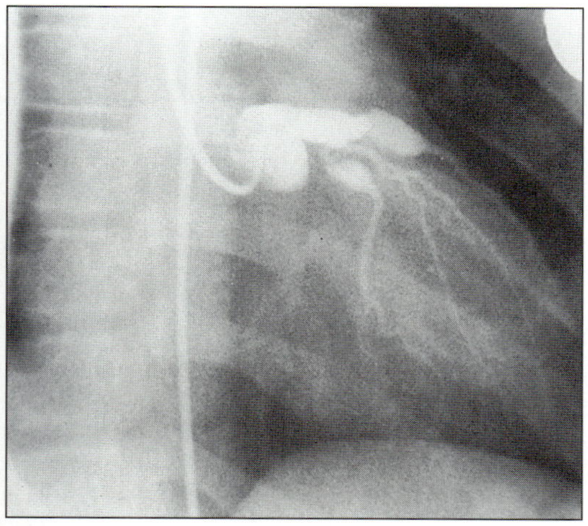

FIGURE 10-33 Selective injection of the left coronary artery demonstrating two large, saccular aneurysms in the proximal left anterior descending and circumflex coronary arteries. This 12 year-old boy had chest pain and electrocardiographic findings consistent with acute ischemia 8 months following Kawasaki disease (KD). Coronary artery aneurysms may develop in 15% to 25% of untreated KD patients as a result of the severe inflammatory destruction and weakening of the vessel wall. Thrombus formation in these aneurysms is the most serious complication of KD. Stenosis at the outlet of the aneurysm is a risk factor for thrombus formation.

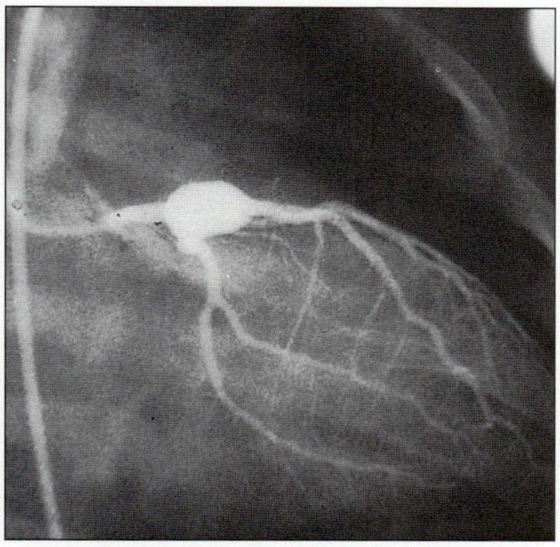

FIGURE 10-34 Selective injection of the left coronary artery demonstrating a single, saccular aneurysm at the bifurcation of the circumflex and left anterior descending arteries. Angiography is recommended for all patients who have aneurysms detected by echocardiogram in order to more precisely define the anatomy of the lesions and to detect stenosis associated with the outflow tract of the aneurysm.

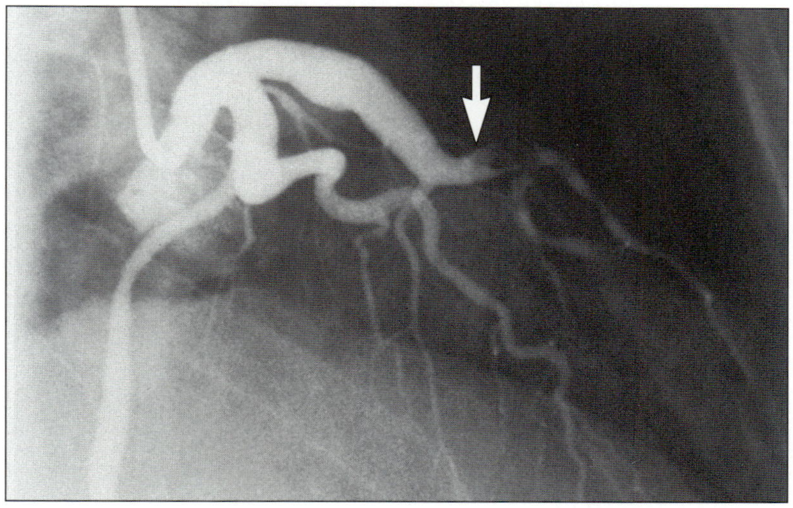

FIGURE 10-35 Selective injection of the left coronary artery in a 42-year-old man who suffered a massive anterior myocardial infarction when thrombus formed and occluded the left anterior descending artery (*arrow*). The patient had a history of "atypical scarlet fever" at 5 years of age (10 years before Kawasaki described his first 50 cases in Japanese). (*From* Burns *et al.* [10]; with permission.)

Management

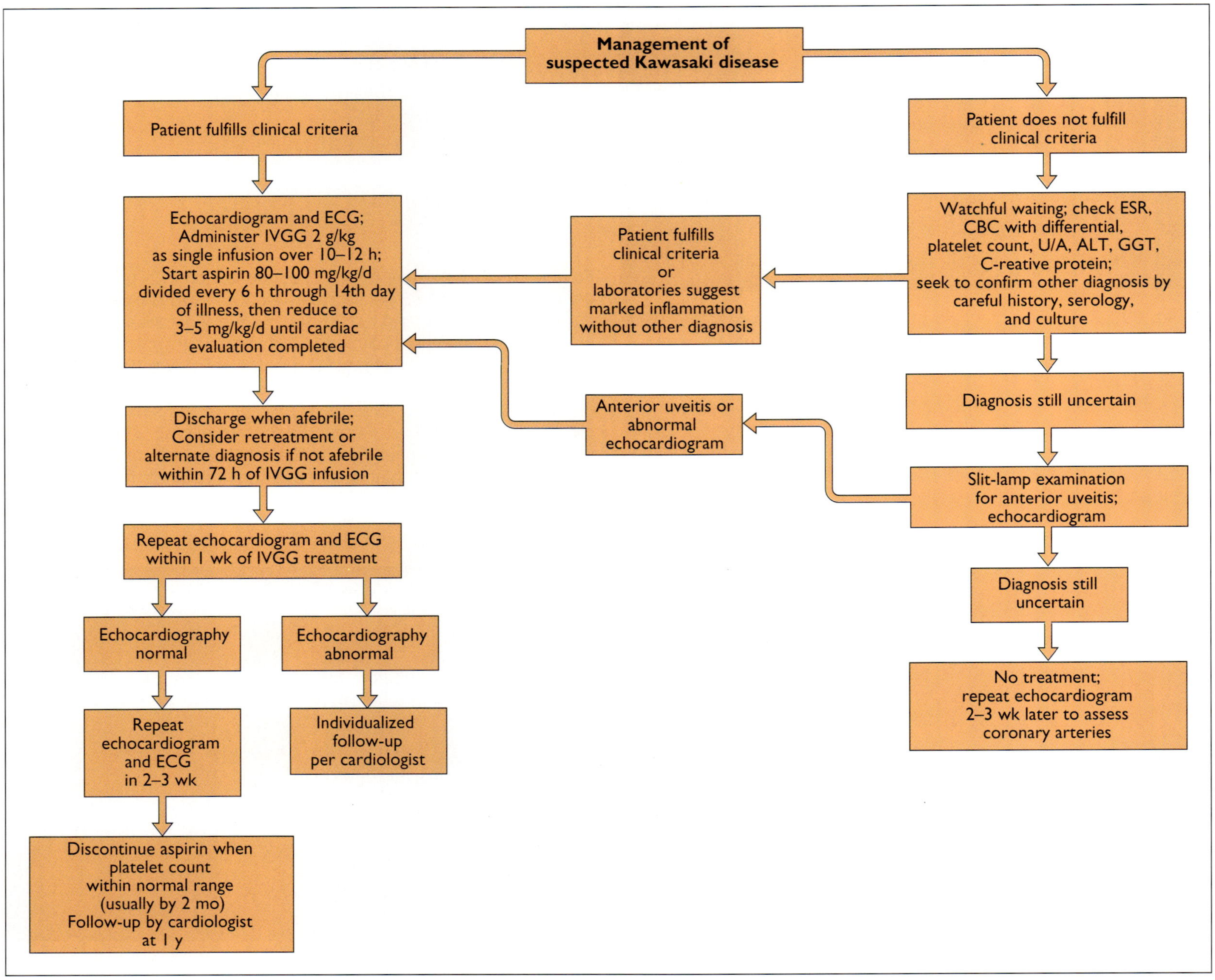

Figure 10-36 Algorithm for management of patients with suspected Kawasaki disease. The current recommended therapy for patients with Kawasaki disease who present within the first 10 days of illness is intravenous gamma globulin (IVGG), 2 g/kg as a single infusion over 10 to 12 hours, in conjunction with aspirin (80 to 100 mg/kg/d divided into four doses through illness day 14, then 3 to 5 mg/kg/d until cardiac evaluation is completed). The mechanism of action of IVGG has not been elucidated, although downregulation of the inflammatory response after treatment has clearly been demonstrated. ALT—alanine aminotransferase; CBC—complete blood count; ECG—electrocardiogram; ESR—erythrocyte sedimentation rate; GGT—γ-glutamyl transferase; U/A—urinalysis. (*See* Newburger *et al.* [5,6] and Dajani *et al.* [7].)

Prevalence of aneurysms in patients treated with intravenous gamma globulin	
Characteristic	**Patients with aneurysms/ total patients, *n (%)***†**
Age at onset	
< 1 y	10/97 (10.3)
≥ 1 y	21/500 (4.2)
Gender	
Male	28/354 (6.5)
Female	8/243 (3.3)
Age and gender	
Male < 1 y	8/58 (13.8)
Female < 1 y	2/35 (5.7)

*Excluding patients with coronary artery abnormality before intravenous gamma globulin treatment.

†Total, 597

FIGURE 10-37 The prevalence of coronary artery aneurysms in prospectively studied Kawasaki disease patients stratified by age and gender. Data from 597 prospectively studied Kawasaki disease patients enrolled in trials of different dosage regimens of intravenous gamma globulin (400 mg/kg/d for 4 d vs 2 g/kg/d) suggest that the treatment is least effective in male infants less than 1 year of age. (*Adapted from* Newburger *et al.* [5,6].)

ETIOLOGY

Paradigms for the cause of Kawasaki disease or syndrome
Single etiologic agent
Uncommon agent that immunologically cross-reacts with common agent
Common agent with unusual host response
Multiple etiologic agents with final common pathway
Common agents with unusual host response

FIGURE 10-38 Paradigms for the cause of Kawasaki disease or syndrome. Debate continues as to whether Kawasaki disease is caused by a single etiologic agent ("disease") or by multiple different agents that result in a stereotyped host response ("syndrome").

Etiology of Kawasaki disease
Clues from the epidemiology
Seasonality: Winter–Spring disease
Epidemic and endemic pattern of disease
Disease rare in infants < 3 mo of age and in adults
Association with higher socioeconomic status, carpet cleaning, and residence near body of water
Clues from the clinical illness
Acute, self-limited inflammatory process
Clinical syndrome mimics other infectious diseases: bacterial toxin–mediated diseases, viral infection, rickettsial infections
Clues from the therapy
Administration of high doses of IVIG plus aspirin reduces fever and inflammatory signs
IVIG contains antibodies to infectious agents, bacterial toxins, idiotypes, and cytokines
Plasmin-treated IVIG (Fc portion of the immunoglobulin molecule) is effective in reducing inflammation

IVIG—intravenous immunoglobulin.

FIGURE 10-39 Clues to the cause of Kawasaki disease (KD) from the epidemiology, clinical illness, and response to therapy. Several lines of evidence suggest that KD is an infectious disease. However, exhaustive attempts to isolate a novel agent have failed. Conflicting evidence surrounds the theory that KD may be caused by a bacterial toxin acting as a superantigen. IVIG—intravenous immunoglobulin.

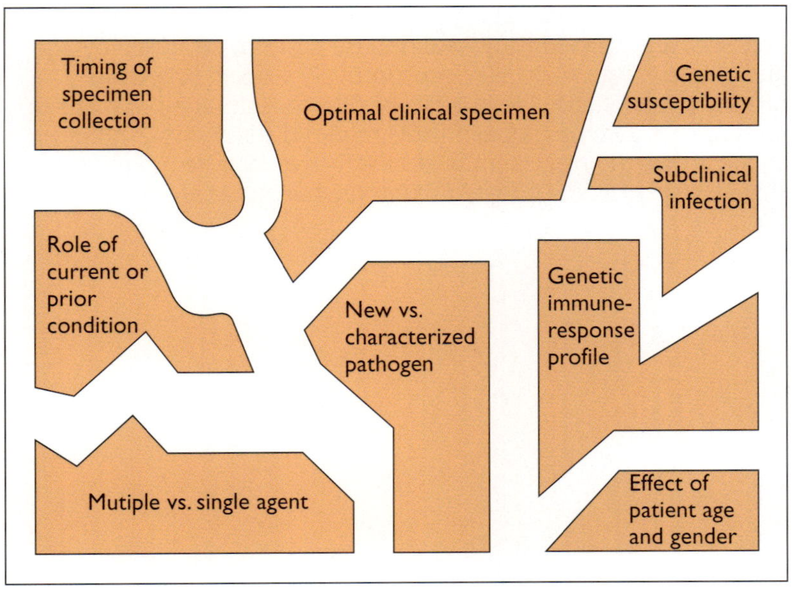

FIGURE 10-40 The puzzle of Kawasaki disease (KD). Multiple factors may be hindering the identification of the etiologic agent of KD. Epidemiologic data suggests that there is a potent effect of genetic susceptibility in that Japanese Americans have a two- to threefold increased relative risk of KD as compared with white Americans. Genetic polymorphisms that determine the magnitude of the immune response may play a role in the manifestation of clinically apparent disease. The limited availability of tissues from affected sites has hampered investigation. Most autopsy material is from the subacute phase of the illness (3rd–5th wk) when the agent may no longer be present in the tissues. In the search for the etiologic agent, it is unclear which body fluids or cells should be collected and examined for a potential pathogen. All of these factors contribute to the unsolved puzzle of KD.

ACKNOWLEDGMENTS

We thank William Weston (Department of Dermatology, University of Colorado), who took many of the clinical photographs; Harry Wilson (University of Colorado), who took many of the pathology photographs; and Glenn F. Billman and Abraham Rothman for helpful discussion.

REFERENCES

1. Yashiro M, Nakamura Y, Hirose K, Yanagawa H: Surveillance of Kawasaki Disease in Japan, 1984–1994. In *Kawasaki Disease: Proceedings of the 5th International KD Symposium, Fukuoa, Japan, May 1995*. Edited by Kato H. Amsterdam: Elsevier Press; 1995:15–21.
2. Kawasaki T, Kosaki F, Okawa S, *et al.* A new infantile acute febrile mucocutaneous lymph node syndrome (MCLNS) prevailing in Japan. *Pediatrics* 1974, 54:271–276.
3. Burns JC, Mason WH, Glode MP, *et al.*, and the U.S. Multicenter Kawasaki Study Group: Clinical and epidemiological characteristics of patients referred for evaluation of possible KD. *J Pediatr* 1991, 118:680–686.
4. Dengler LD, Capparelli EV, Bastian JF, *et al.*: Cerebrospinal fluid profile in patients with acute Kawasaki disease. *Ped Infect Dis J* 1998, in press.
5. Newburger JW, Takahashi M, Beiser AS, *et al.*: Single infusion of intravenous gamma globulin compared to four daily doses in the treatment of acute Kawasaki Syndrome. *N Engl J Med* 1991, 324:1633–1639.
6. Newburger JW, Takahashi M, Burns JC, *et al.*: Treatment of Kawasaki Syndrome with intravenous gammaglobulin. *N Engl J Med* 1986, 315:341–347.
7. Dajani AS, Taubert KA, Gerber MA, *et al.*: Diagnosis and therapy of Kawasaki disease in children. *Circulation* 1993, 87:1776–1780.
8. Smith LS, Newburger JW, Burns JC: Kawasaki disease and the eye. *Pediatr Infect Dis J* 1989, 8:116–118.
9. Smith LEH, Burns JC: Kawasaki disease and the eye. *Resident Staff Physician* 1988, 34:48–52.
10. Burns JC, Shike H, Gordon JB, *et al.*: Sequelae of Kawasaki disease in adolescents and young adults. *J Am Coll Cardiol* 1996, 28:253–257.

CHAPTER 11

Central Nervous System Infections

Kenji M. Cunnion
Kenneth A. Alexander

THE MANAGEMENT OF central nervous system (CNS) infections remains a therapeutic challenge for primary care and subspecialty physicians. CNS infections continue to have high mortality and morbidity despite improved antibiotic regimens and diagnostic techniques. This problem is due at least in part to the emergence of antimicrobial resistance in common CNS pathogens as well as to increases in the number and types of at-risk patients, especially those with primary or secondary immunodeficiencies. A high index of suspicion for CNS infection and early initiation of definitive therapy, particularly in patients with immunodeficiencies, is essential for successful treatment.

The continued emergence of antimicrobial-resistant bacteria strains continues to complicate the medical care of all patients, especially those with CNS infections. Intermediate- and high-level penicillin-resistant strains of *Streptococcus pneumoniae* are now common in most areas of the United States and Canada, often necessitating the empiric use of third-generation cephalosporins and vancomycin for suspected gram-positive meningitis. *Staphylococcus aureus* is now commonly resistant to methicillin, whereas some coagulase-negative staphylococci are resistant even to vancomycin. Vancomycin-resistant enterococci are now common in most tertiary referral centers, and are, for several reasons, associated with high patient mortality. Similarly, increasing resistance of gram-negative infections provides a continued threat to hospitalized patients and a therapeutic challenge to physicians.

Improved success in the management of AIDS with multidrug regimens has led to an increase in the numbers of severely immunocompromised HIV-infected individuals. As the size of this profoundly immunosuppressed population continues to increase, HIV "survivor's infections" (*eg*, ocular and central nervous system toxoplasmosis and cytomegalovirus disease) have become commonplace. Similarly, continued improvement in the care of preterm neonates has advanced the beginning of extrauterine viability to approximately 23 weeks gestation. The additional support required for such extremely premature infants is complicated by a substantial rate of CNS infections and complications. The improved survival of other immunodeficient patients, ranging from bone marrow transplant recipients to children with severe combined immune deficiency syndrome, has also led to an increase in both common and unusual CNS infections.

The marked decrease in the rate of invasive *Haemophilus influenzae* infections due to universal administration of *H. influenza* conjugate vaccine has been reflected by the virtual disappearance of *H. influenzae* meningitis. Few new practitioners and physicians in training have cared for children with *H. influenza* meningitis or epiglottitis, and fewer still have been called on to tap the subdural effusions so commonly seen only a few years ago. It is hoped that similar benefit will be obtained by widespread administration of pneumococcal conjugate vaccine.

Fortunately, significant improvements in imaging modalities and laboratory methods for the diagnosis of CNS infections has permitted earlier and more definitive identification of the cause and extent of infection. The resolution of clinically available magnetic resonance imaging and computed tomography scans far exceeds that which was obtainable even 5 years ago. The now common addition of polymerase chain reaction–based diagnosis in the microbiology laboratory allows rapid and definitive diagnosis of many pathogens, most notably for CNS viral infections. Continued improvements in both diagnostic imaging and laboratory diagnosis will no doubt continue at an increasing pace.

Normal cerebrospinal fluid findings by age

Age Group	Leukocyte count (mean), *leukocytes/μL*	PMNs, %	Protein concentration (mean), *mg/dL*	Glucose Concentration (mean), *mg/dL*	Opening Pressure (mean), *mm H_2O*
Preterm infant	9.0 (0–25.4)	57	115 (65–150)	24–63 (50)	—
Term infant	8.2 (0–22.4)	61	90 (20–170)	34–119 (52)	80–110 (<110)
Child	0–7	0	5–40 (lumbar) 5–15 (ventricular) 5–25 (cisternal)	40–80	<200 (lateral recumbent)

PMN—polymorphonuclear lymphocyte.

Figure 11-1 Normal cerebrospinal fluid (CSF) findings by age. CSF composition varies with patient age. Normal neonates typically have higher numbers of nucleated cells and higher CSF protein concentrations than do older children. The CSF protein concentration is also determined in part by the site from which the specimen is obtained. The CSF glucose concentration in preterm and term neonates is typically lower than in older children; however, the ratio of CSF glucose concentration to serum glucose concentration is typically higher in preterm and term neonates than it is in older children. PMNs—polymorphonuclear neutrophil leukocytes. (*Adapted from* Harriet Line Handbook [1]; with permission; *additional data from* Sarff *et al.* [2].)

A. Common causes for bacterial infections of the central nervous system

	Bacterial
Meningitis	*Streptococcus pneumoniae* *Haemophilus influenzae* *Neisseria meningitidis* Gram-negative rods Group B streptococci (neonates) *Listeria monocytogenes* (neonates) *Mycobacterium tuberculosis* *T. pallidum* *Borrelia burgdorferi* *B. henselae*
Brain abscess	*Streptococcus pyogenes* *Streptococcus milleri* or *intermedius* *Staphylococcus aureus* Anaerobes Enterobacteriaceae *Nocardia* spp
Spinal subdural abscess	S. aureus Enterobacteriaceae *S. pyogenes* *S. milleri* or *intermedius* Enterobacteriaceae Anaerobes
Cranial epidural abscess	*S. pyogenes* *S. milleri* or *intermedius* *S. aureus* Anaerobes Enterobacteriaceae
Subdural empyema	*S. pneumoniae* *H. influenzae* *S. pyogenes* *S. milleri* or *intermedius* *S. aureus*
Encephalitis	*B. burgdorferi* *B. henselae* *M. pneumoniae* *L. monocytogenes* (neonates) Group B streptococci (neonates) Enterobacteriaceae (neonates)
Transverse myelitis	*M. pneumoniae* *B. henselae*
Postinfectious encephalopathy	*M. pneumoniae*
Toxic encephalopathy	*B. pertussis* *Shigella* spp *Campylobacter jejuni* *Salmonella* spp
Congenital infections	*T. pallidum*
Catheter-associated infections	Coagulase-negative staphylococci *S. aureus* *S. pneumoniae* Diphtheroids

FIGURE 11-2 Common causes of central nervous system (CNS) infections. **A** and **B**, Summarized in the table are common bacterial (*panel A*),

(continued on next page)

B. Common causes for nonbacterial infections of the central nervous system

	Fungal	Parasitic or protozoal	Viral	Other
Meningitis	*Cryptococcus neoformans* *Candida* spp	*T. solium* *Trichinella apiralis*	Enteroviruses Arboviruses Mumps Herpes simplex Epstein–Barr virus HIV-1 Lymphocytic choriomeningitis	*Rickettsia* spp
Brain abscess	*Candida* spp *Aspergillus* spp *C. neoformans*	*Entamoeba* *Acanthamoeba*		
Encephalitis			Enteroviruses Herpes simplex Arboviruses Cytomegalovirus Epstein–Barr virus Adenovirus	*Rickettsia* spp
Transverse myelitis				Herpes simplex Respiratory viruses (postinfectious) Varicella-zoster Cytomegalovirus Mumps
Postinfectious encephalopathy				Varicella-zoster Mumps Measles Rubella Influenza
Congenital infections		Toxoplasma		Cytomegalovirus Herpes simplex Varicella zoster Enteroviruses Rubella
Catheter-associated infections	*Candida* spp *Aspergillus* spp			

Figure 11-2 *(continued)* fungal, protozoal, viral, and miscellaneous causes (*panel B*) of specific CNS infections. Also listed are organisms associated with postinfectious and toxic encephalopathies and with catheter-associated CNS infections.

Differential diagnosis of ring-enhancing lesions on computed tomograph or magnetic resonance image

	Study
Primary or metastatic brain neoplasms	Bargallo *et al.* [3], Rabin *et al.* [4], Remick *et al.* [5]
Post-radiosurgery	De Salles *et al.* [6]
Intracerebral hematoma	Salzman and Tuazon [7]
Brain abscess (numerous causes)	Schielke [8], Woods [9]
Cerebral toxoplasmosis	Bertoli *et al.* [10]
Amebic encephalitis	Zagardo *et al.* [11]
Neurocysticercosis	Kramer *et al.* [12], Nagayama *et al.* [13]
Central nervous system tuberculosis	Kim *et al.* [14]
Multiple sclerosis and other demyelinating disorders	Masdeu *et al.* [15]
Neurosyphilis	Fred and Dunn [16]

Figure 11-3 Differential diagnosis of ring-enhancing lesions on brain computed tomography or magnetic resonance imaging scans. Ring enhancement on computed tomography or magnetic resonance imaging scans result from areas of inflammation encircling sites of infection or tumor in the brain. This table outlines the common causes, along with summary causes from numerous case reports.

Recommended empirical antimicrobial therapies for common central nervous system infections*

Infection type	Historical and clinical data	Recommended empirical therapy
Meningitis	Unknown; presumed bacterial	(Ceftriaxone or cefotaxime) + vancomycin
	Gram-positive cocci	(Ceftriaxone or cefotaxime) + vancomycin
	Gram-negative rods	(Ceftriaxone or cefotaxime)† + (gentamicin or tobramycin)
	Neonatal	(Ampicillin + gentamicin) or (ampicillin + cefotaxime)
	Gram-positive rods (neonatal)	Ampicillin + gentamicin
	Acid-fast bacilli	Isoniazid + rifampin + pyrazinamide + streptomycin‡ (+ folinic acid)
	Lyme disease	Ceftriaxone
	Syphilis	Penicillin G
	Fungal	Amphotericin B ± flucytosine ± fluconazole
Brain abscess§	Unknown; presumed bacterial	Vancomycin + (ceftriaxone or cefotaxime)† + chloramphenicol
	Congenital cyanotic heart disease	Vancomycin + chloramphenicol
	Sinusitis or head/facial trauma	Vancomycin + (ceftriaxone or cefotaxime)† + chloramphenicol
	Otitis or mastoiditis	Vancomycin + (ceftriaxone or cefotaxime)† + chloramphenicol
	Fungal	Amphotericin B ± flucytosine ± fluconazole
Epidural abscess§	Unknown; presumed bacterial	(Ceftriaxone or cefotaxime)¶ + vancomycin
	Gram-positive cocci	(Ceftriaxone or cefotaxime)¶ + vancomycin
	Gram-negative rods	(Ceftriaxone or cefotaxime)¶ + (gentamicin or tobramycin)
Subdural abscess§	Unknown; presumed	(Ceftriaxone or cefotaxime)¶ + vancomycin
	Gram-positive cocci	(Ceftriaxone or cefotaxime)¶ + vancomycin
	Gram-negative rods	(Ceftriaxone or cefotaxime)¶ + (gentamicin or tobramycin)
Encephalitis	Unknown	Acyclovir
	Cat scratch disease	Doxycycline or trimethoprim-sulfamethoxazole
	Herpes simplex	Acyclovir
	Rocky Mountain spotted fever	Doxycycline or chloramphenicol
	Malaria	Quinine + doxycycline
Congenital infections	Syphilis	Penicillin G
	Toxoplasmosis	Pyrimethamine and sulfadiazine (+ folinic acid)
	Enteroviruses	Pleconaril**
	Herpes simplex	Acyclovir
Catheter-associated infections††	Presumed bacterial	Vancomycin + ceftazidime
	Fungal	Amphotericin B ± flucytosine ± fluconazole

* Therapeutic recommendations presume significant rates of penicillin-resistant *Streptococcous pneumoniae* and methicillin-resistant *Staphlyococcus aureus*. These drug combinations are recommended for empirical therapy. Adjustments to therapy must be made in light of culture and other clinical data. Infectious diseases subspecialty consultation is indicated.

† Ceftazidime should be substituted if there is significant concern for *Pseudomonas aeruginosa* infection.

‡ Additional agents should be considered in areas with significant rates of drug-resistant *Mycobacterium tuberculosis*.

§ Surgical drainage of abscesses is strongly advised whenever possible.

¶ Ampicillin-sulbactam, ticarcillin-clavulanic acid, or piperacillin-tazobactam may be substituted.

** Available on compassionate release from ViroPharma Pharmaceuticals, Malvern, PA.

†† Infected central nervous system catheters must be removed immediately.

Figure 11-4 Recommended empirical antimicrobial therapies for common central nervous system infections. Because effective antimicrobial therapy must be initiated prior to definitive identification and antimicrobial susceptibility determination of pathogens, empirical therapy must be initiated on the basis of predicted cause and sensitivity. Appropriate narrowing of antimicrobial coverage should be made on the basis of culture and antibiotic susceptibility data from the clinical laboratory.

Because of the increasing prevalence of antibiotic-resistant pneumococci, empiric therapy for gram-positive meningitis should generally include vancomycin. Similarly, empiric therapy for nosocomial gram-negative meningitis should include both a third-generation cephalosporin and an aminoglycoside. Empirical therapy for neonatal meningitis should include ampicillin for coverage of *Listeria*. There are a variety of appropriate empirical antimicrobial therapies for brain abscesses because the bacterial causes of brain abscesses vary according to patients' predisposing conditions.

Selection of empirical therapies for encephalitis and congenital infection is complicated, because diverse causes of infection often present with similar clinical pictures. In addition, the long periods of time required for completion of laboratory studies often necessitates empiric therapy for several potential pathogens. Definitive management of catheter-associated infections often requires removal or externalization of hardware, and frequent hardware replacement through the course of therapy. In all cases of suspected central nervous system infection, infectious diseases subspecialty consultation should be sought. (*Adapted from* Woods [9]; with permission.)

Clinical evaluation of meningitis
Clinical suspicion
Irritability, lethargy, emesis, anorexia, fever (may be absent in neonates), nuchal rigidity (>4 mo of age), headache (if verbal), confusion, seizures, photophobia
Evaluation
Neurologic examination
Funduscopic examination
Assess for Brudzinski's and Kernig's signs
Check for history of recent antibiotic exposure
Review immunization record
Lumbar puncture: opening pressure, cell count, protein, glucose, Gram stain, bacterial culture (consider: VDRL, cryptococcal antigen, mycobacterial culture, fungal stain and culture, cytology; bacterial antigen testing may be unhelpful or misleading)
Blood culture
Complete blood count, serum electrolytes, serum osmolality
Audiology or evoked potentials
Consider: coagulation times, purified protein derivative (may be negative in *Mycobacterium tuberculosis* meningitis), HIV ELISA/Western blot, rapid plasma reagin, viral culture of nasopharynx and stool, blood smears for malaria (if appropriate travel history)
ELISA—enzyme-linked immunosorbent assay; VDRL—Veneral Disease Research Laboratory (test).

FIGURE 11-5 Clinical evaluation of meningitis. Successful diagnosis and treatment of meningitis requires a high level of clinical suspicion, an aggressive approach to establishing the diagnosis, and early treatment with appropriate antimicrobial agents. Meningitis symptoms in infants may be subtle, presenting only with irritability, lethargy, or poor feeding. The classical physical findings of meningitis (nuchal rigidity and Brudzinski's and Kernig's signs) are often absent in young children. Fever, although common in children with meningitis, is not always present. Because of the potentially devastating consequences of untreated purulent meningitis, a definitive diagnosis should be sought as soon as reasonable clinical suspicion arises.

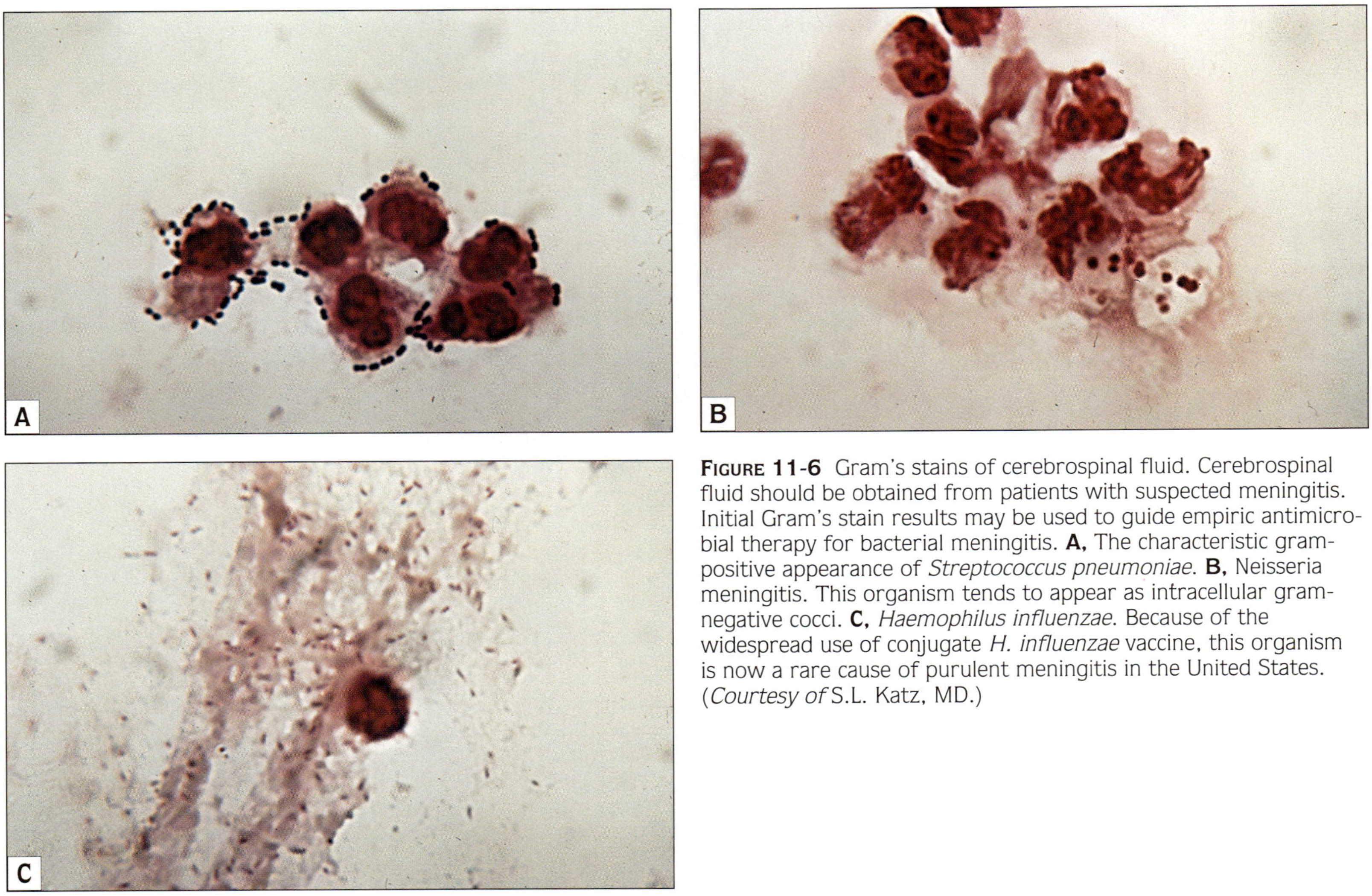

FIGURE 11-6 Gram's stains of cerebrospinal fluid. Cerebrospinal fluid should be obtained from patients with suspected meningitis. Initial Gram's stain results may be used to guide empiric antimicrobial therapy for bacterial meningitis. **A**, The characteristic gram-positive appearance of *Streptococcus pneumoniae*. **B**, Neisseria meningitis. This organism tends to appear as intracellular gram-negative cocci. **C**, *Haemophilus influenzae*. Because of the widespread use of conjugate *H. influenzae* vaccine, this organism is now a rare cause of purulent meningitis in the United States. (*Courtesy of* S.L. Katz, MD.)

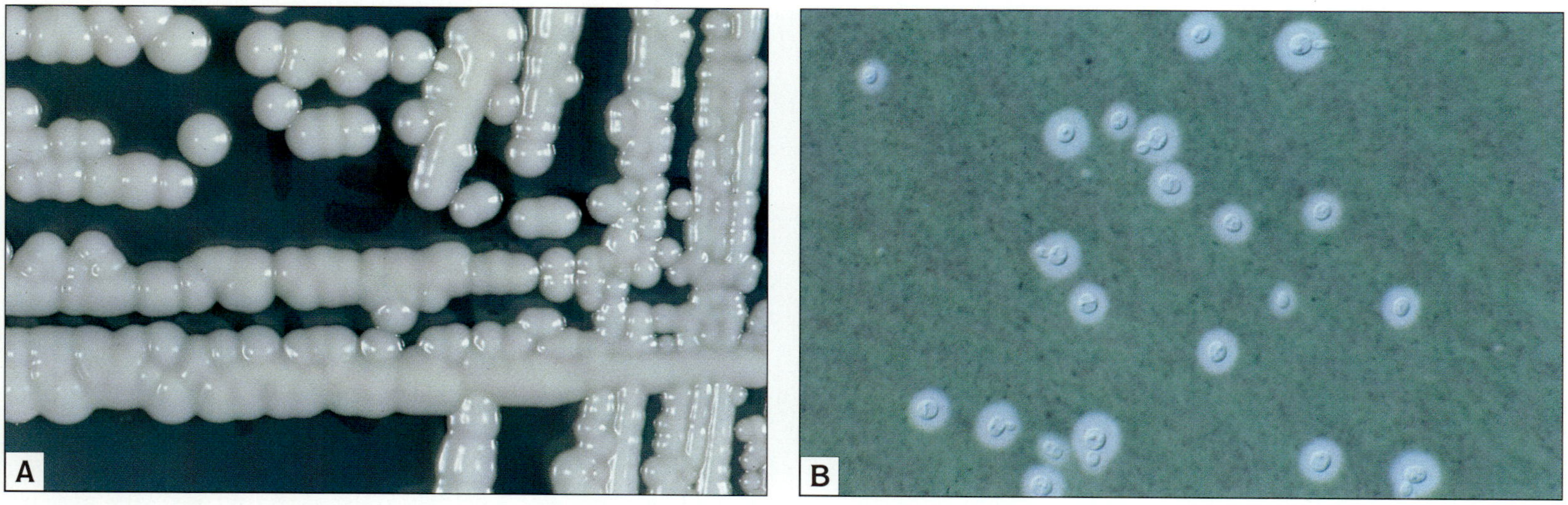

Figure 11-7 Culture and India ink preparations of *Cryptococcus neoformans*. **A,** Plate cultures of cryptococci are notable for the pearly appearance of colonies. **B,** India ink preparations of cerebrospinal fluid in patients with cryptococcal infections reveal a characteristic halo caused by the mucopolysaccharide capsule. Quantitative latex agglutination tests of cerebrospinal fluid and serum are useful and rapid diagnostic tools.

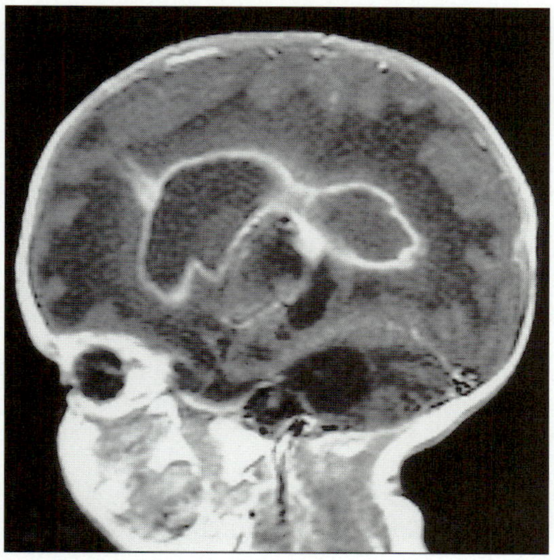

Figure 11-8 Purulent ventriculitis. This contrast head computed tomographic image of a 3-week-old infant with fever, lethargy, and bulging fontanel shows hydrocephalus and severe ventriculitis. The clinical and radiographic findings are consistent with a suppurative perinatal meningitis that has progressed to ventriculitis. Likely bacterial pathogens include group B streptococci, enteric gram-negative rods, and *Listeria*. This condition warrants emergency management, including external ventriculostomy and antibiotic therapy with ampicillin and gentamicin. Neonatal meningitis that has progressed to this stage is most often fatal. Survivors are likely to suffer permanent cognitive damage, deafness, and noncommunicating hydrocephalus.

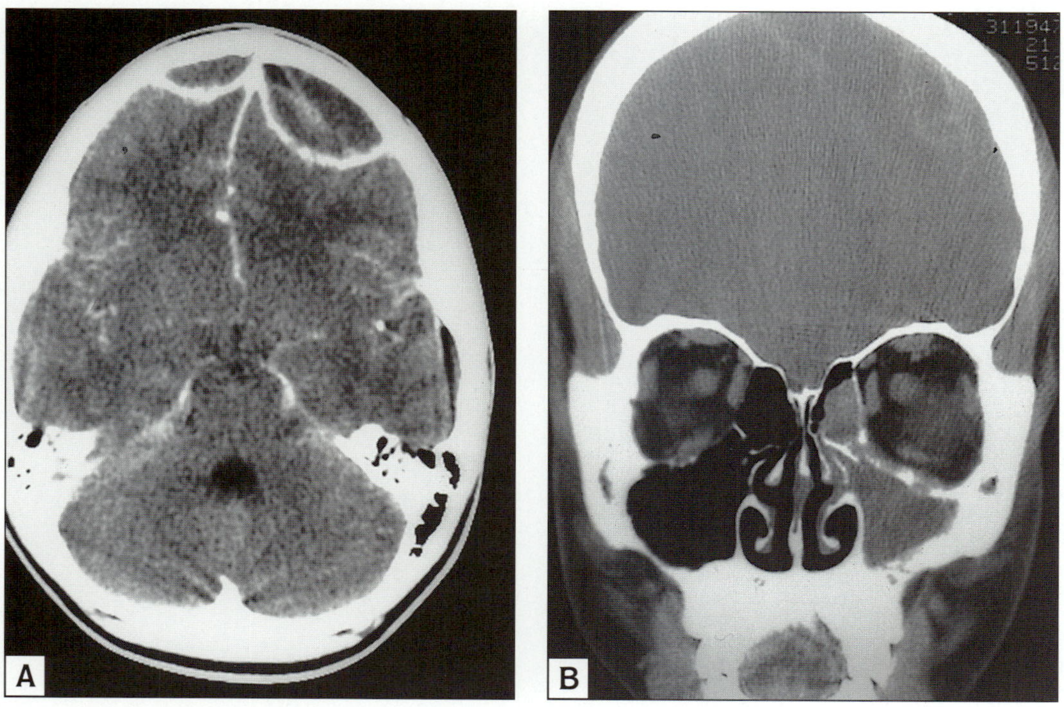

Figure 11-9 Bilateral epidural abscesses. This contrast head computed tomographic image was taken of a 13-year-old child with a 10-day history of headache and fever. **A,** The axial image shows bilateral frontal epidural abscesses. **B,** The coronal image demonstrates left ethmoid and maxillary sinusitis. Frontal epidural abscesses are usually complications of suppurative sinusitis. The organisms include pneumococci, streptococci, staphylococci, and mixed anaerobe infections. Management includes surgical drainage of the abscesses and involved sinuses, and empiric antibiotics with ceftriaxone or cefotaxime, vancomycin, and chloramphenicol. Recovery is likely to be complete, but a 4- to 6-week course of antibiotics is warranted.

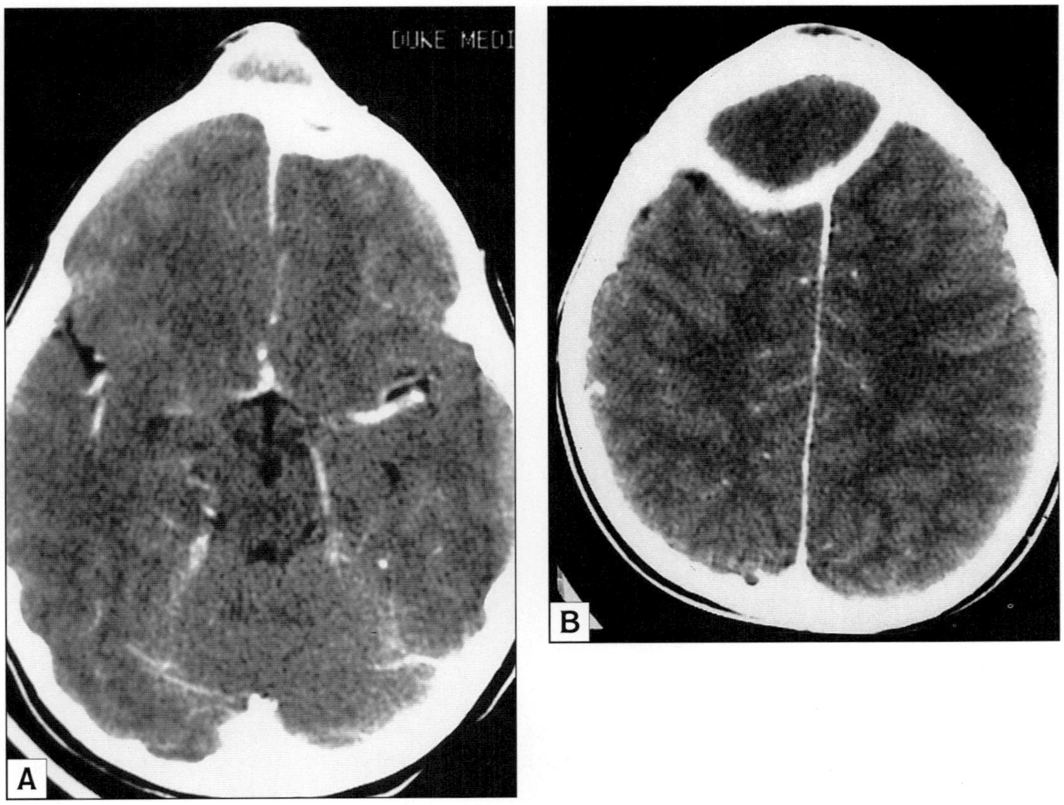

FIGURE 11-10 Epidural abscess with Pott's puffy tumor. This contrast head computed tomographic image was taken of a 5-year-old child with a 1-week history of enlarging mass in the middle of the forehead, headache, and fever. **A,** Axial image shows a subperiosteal abscess protruding from the forehead and frontal epidural abscess. These abscesses generally arise from frontal or ethmoid sinusitis; however, careful evaluation for trauma leading to skull fracture and laceration of the dura is warranted. **B,** Coronal image shows significant ethmoid and frontal sinusitis. The infected ethmoid sinus is the likely source of this subperiosteal abscess. Urgent surgical drainage and debridement of necrotic bone and sinuses should be performed. In addition to epidural abscess, patients with Pott's puffy tumor have osteomyelitis, which merits a lengthy antibiotic course.

Clinical evaluation of epidural empyema

Clinical suspicion

Headache, fever, symptoms of increased intracranial pressure, focal neurologic findings, symptoms of mastoiditis, frontal sinusitis, or chronic otitis

Evaluation

Neurologic examination

Funduscopic examination

Lumbar puncture: opening pressure, cell count, protein, glucose, Gram's stain, bacterial culture

Head magnetic resonance imaging scan (preferred) or head computed tomography scan with contrast

Surgical drainage: Gram's stain and aerobic and anaerobic bacterial culture

FIGURE 11-11 Clinical evaluation of epidural empyema. Diagnosis of epidural empyema is often difficult. Patients often present with nonspecific symptoms such as malaise, fever, or headache. The clinical course may be prolonged. Pain complaints are often nonfocal, and physical findings may be unremarkable. Lumbar puncture typically reveals sterile cerebrospinal fluid with variable degrees of reactive pleocytosis. Epidural empyema may also follow as a complication of trauma or other medical condition. Patients with onset of headache who have histories of head and neck trauma, sinusitis, otitis, mastoiditis, septicemia, or endocarditis should be evaluated for epidural empyema. Imaging studies such as computed tomography or magnetic resonance imaging scanning are often required to evaluate the suspicion of epidural empyema.

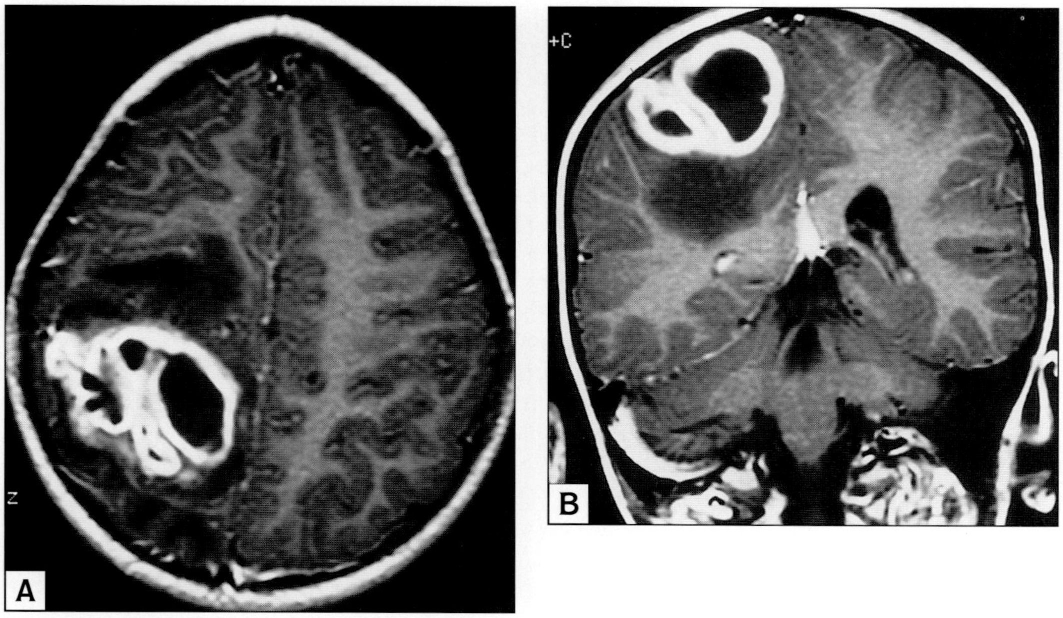

FIGURE 11-12 Parenchymal brain abscess. This contrast head magnetic resonance image was taken of a 5-year-old child with a 2-week history of emesis and headaches, but no focal neurologic signs. The axial (**A**) and coronal (**B**) images show a large loculated right parietal abscess. Likely bacterial sources include suppurative sinusitis, dental caries, and hematogenous dissemination in cyanotic heart disease. The most common bacterial causes of parenchymal brain abscesses include pneumococci, streptococci, staphylococci, and mixed anaerobic infections. Management includes surgical drainage of the abscesses, treatment of the anatomic source of infection (if identified), and empiric antibiotic therapy with vancomycin and either ceftriaxone or cefotaxime and chloramphenicol. Recovery is likely to be complete, but a 4- to 6-week course of antibiotics is warranted.

Clinical evaluation of brain abscess

Clinical suspicion

Onset is usually insidious; fever, headache, symptoms of increased intracranial pressure, seizures, focal neurologic symptoms, history of congenital heart disease (with right-to-left shunt), history of head or facial trauma

Evaluation

- Neurologic examination
- Funduscopic examination
- Dental examination
- Head magnetic resonance imaging or head computed tomography scan with contrast (include sinuses)
- Blood culture
- Complete blood cell count
- Surgical drainage: Gram's stain, aerobic and anaerobic bacterial cultures, mycobacterial stain and culture, fungal stain and culture, histology
- Consider: lumbar puncture, electroencephalogram, echocardiogram, surgical drainage of sinuses if sinusitis is present

FIGURE 11-13 Clinical evaluation of brain abscess. As with the diagnosis of other CNS infections, the diagnosis of brain abscess is often difficult and requires a high degree of clinical suspicion for patients at risk. Patients may be asymptomatic or may present with nonspecific symptoms, such as malaise, fever, or headache. Pain complaints are often nonfocal, and physical findings may be unremarkable. Neurologic findings (*eg*, behavioral changes, aphasia, hemianopsia, and paralysis) may occur. Brain abscesses in infants may become very large prior to diagnosis. The clinical course of brain abscesses may be prolonged. Lumbar puncture typically reveals sterile cerebrospinal fluid with variable degrees of reactive pleocytosis. Occasionally, brain abscesses rupture into the intraventricular or subarachnoid spaces. In such events, patients have acute onset of meningitis-like symptoms; clinical outcome is often poor.

Brain abscesses result either from extension of infection from contiguous structures or from hematogenous dissemination from a distant body site. Patients with onset of headache who have histories of head and neck trauma, dental infection, extensive dental treatment, sinusitis, otitis, mastoiditis, septicemia, endocarditis, or significant structural heart disease with right-to-left shunt should be evaluated for epidural brain abscess. Computed tomography or magnetic resonance imaging scanning are often required to evaluate patients with suspected brain abscesses.

Clinical evaluation of subdural empyema

Clinical suspicion

- Headache, fever, symptoms of increased intracranial pressure, suppurative bacterial meningitis (most commonly *Streptococcus pneumoniae* or *Haemophilus influenzae*), chronic sinusitis, otitis, or mastoiditis

Evaluation

- Neurologic examination
- Funduscopic examination
- Lumbar puncture: opening pressure, cell count, protein, glucose, Gram stain, bacterial culture
- Head magnetic resonance imaging scan (preferred) or head computed tomography scan with contrast
- Surgical drainage: Gram stain aerobic and anaerobic bacterial culture

Figure 11-14 Clinical evaluation of subdural empyema. Subdural empyemas are uncommon in children. Many such infections appear as complications of bacterial meningitis, whereas the etiology of other cases is never determined. In older children, subdural empyema may result from either the extension of infection from contiguous structures or, rarely, from hematogenous dissemination from a distant body site.

Patients with subdural empyema may be asymptomatic or may present with headache, fever, and signs of meningeal irritation. Neurologic signs (most notably seizure) may occur. Infants may present with somnolence, irritability, vomiting, or increased or fullness of the fontanelles. Rarely, epidural empyema occurs as a consequence of trauma or surgery. Computed tomography or magnetic resonance imaging scanning are often required to evaluate the suspicion of subdural empyema.

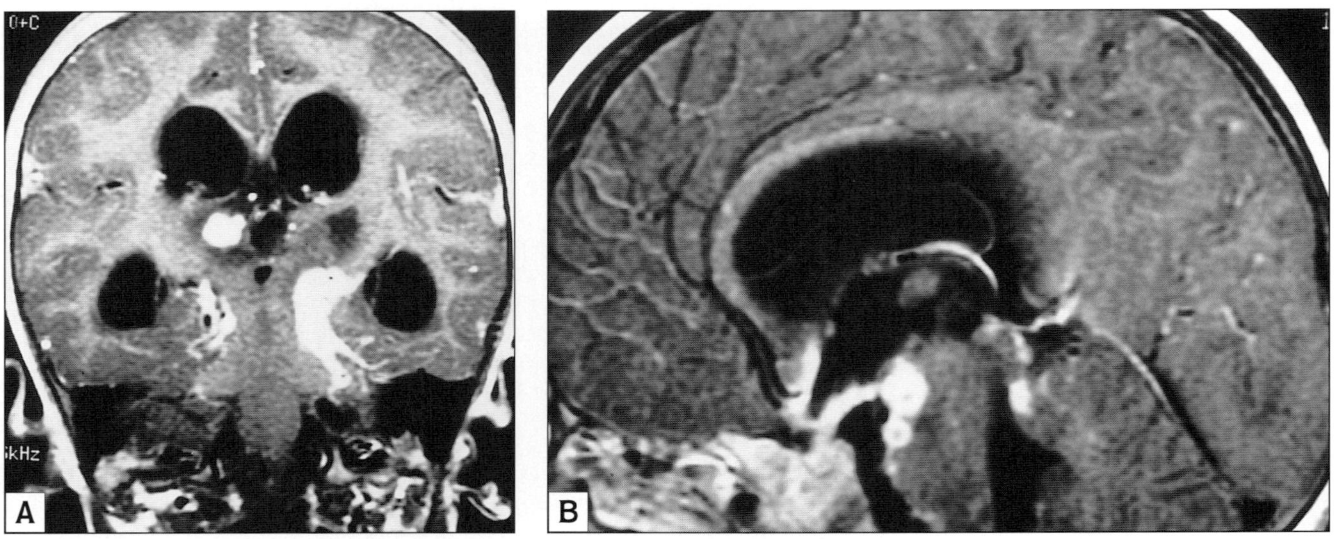

Figure 11-15 Cerebral *Mycobacterium tuberculosis* infection. **A** and **B**, These contrast head magnetic resonance images were taken of a 15-month-old child with fever, headaches, cranial nerve deficits, and gait disturbance. The sagittal (*panel A*) and coronal (*panel B*) images show communicating hydrocephalus and multiple enhancing parenchymal tuberculomas predominantly involving the brain stem. The clinical history and radiographic findings are typical for tuberculosis of the central nervous system. Management of suspected central nervous system tuberculosis must be aggressive, with immediate empirical initiation of therapy with isoniazid, rifampin, streptomycin, and pyrazinamide. Additional agents may be required in locations with significant rates of multidrug-resistant *M. tuberculosis*.

Because mycobacterial cultures of cerebrospinal fluid are typically of low yield, even in severe disease, the infecting isolate should be vigorously sought by obtaining several early morning gastric aspirates or bronchoscopic isolates from the patient. Additionally, sputum specimens from the likely adult source should be obtained and sent for mycobacterial stain and culture. Positive cultures should be forwarded to an experienced laboratory for antimycobacterial susceptibility testing.

Communicating hydrocephalus is a common complication thought to be caused by infection-induced dysfunction of the choroid plexus, and often requires placement of a permanent ventricular drain. Complications of tuberculous cerebritis and meningitis include death, deafness, cognitive impairment, cranial nerve deficits, and impairment of coordination.

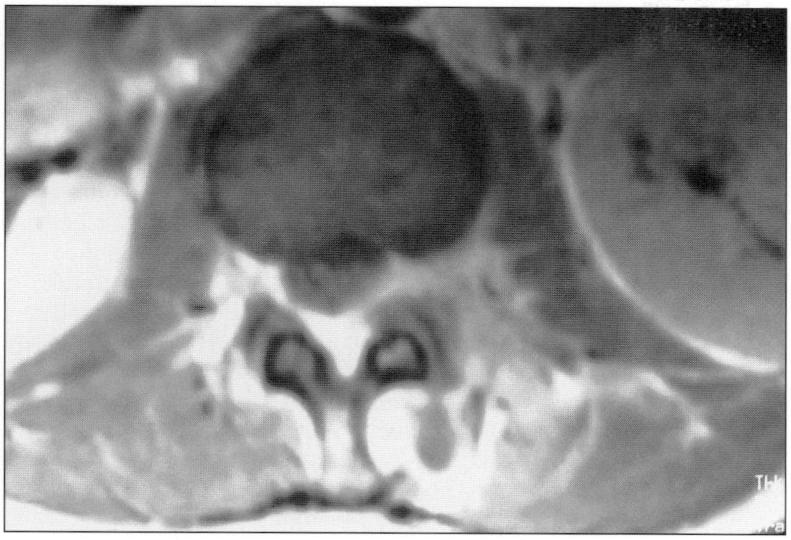

FIGURE 11-16 Paraspinous abscess. This contrast magnetic resonance image was taken of a 16-year-old patient with fever, back pain, and gait disturbance. The image shows a paraspinous abscess at the T1-T2 level involving the left paraspinous muscles with vertebral erosion, and displacement of the spinal cord. The most likely infecting organisms are *Staphylococcus aureus*, streptococci, gram-negative rods, and anaerobes. Appropriate management includes immediate surgical or computed tomography–guided drainage of the abscess, and empiric initiation of vancomycin and either cefotaxime or ceftriaxone. A 4- to 6-week course of antibiotics is warranted following surgical drainage. Recovery is likely to be complete if the spinal cord does not suffer ischemic damage prior to drainage of the abscess.

Clinical evaluation of paraspinous abscess

Clinical suspicion

Fever, spinal pain (increases with motion), nuchal rigidity, paresthesias, decreased deep tendon reflexes, weakness, paralysis, vertebral tenderness

Evaluation

- Neurologic examination (motor neuron weakness or loss of bladder or bowel control should be considered neurosurgical emergencies)
- Check for Brudzinski's and Kernig's signs
- Spinal magnetic resonance imaging or computed tomography scan with contrast
- Blood culture
- Complete blood cell count
- Surgical drainage: Gram's stain, aerobic and anaerobic bacterial cultures, mycobacterial stain and culture, fungal stain and culture, histology
- Consider: echocardiogram or bone scan if suspicious for multifocal osteomyelitis

FIGURE 11-17 Clinical evaluation of spinal epidural abscess. Patients with spinal epidural abscesses often present with nonspecific symptoms, such as malaise, fever, or backache. This condition is rare in children. Infections may be acute or chronic, and the clinical course may be prolonged. Fever is common in patients with spinal epidural abscesses, whereas weakness and paralysis occur in cases of advanced infection. Pain complaints are often nonfocal, and local tenderness is often absent. Patients with evidence of cord compression should be evaluated and treated immediately. Surgical drainage followed by antibiotic therapy are the mainstays of therapy.

Lumbar puncture is essential for diagnosis. In cases of spinal epidural abscess, purulent material may be encountered prior to the needle entering the thecal sac. Cerebrospinal fluid often contains a moderate amount of nucleated white cells with lymphocytes predominating. Bacterial cultures are often negative. Spinal imaging studies such as computed tomography or magnetic resonance image scanning are often required to evaluate the suspicion of spinal epidural abscess.

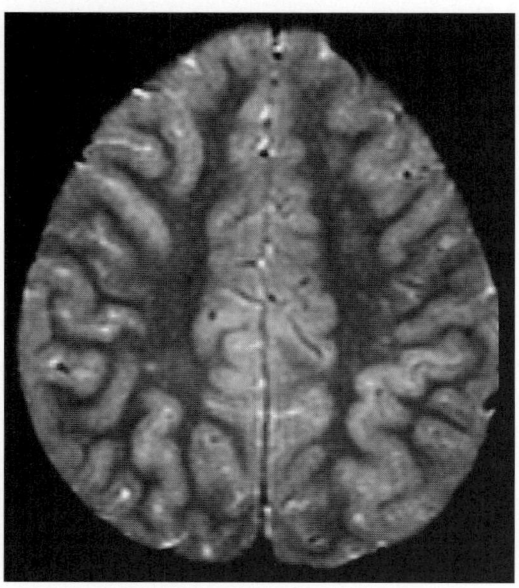

FIGURE 11-18 California encephalitis. This head magnetic resonance image was taken from a 7-year-old child with acute onset of headache, fever, emesis, confusion, and a left-sided focal motor seizure. The image shows multiple scattered low attenuation lesions primarily involving the white matter. This nonspecific pattern for encephalitis may be due to a variety of causes. Testing should be directed by demographic and travel information, and by exposure history to ticks, mosquitoes, other animals, and ill humans. Treatment and outcome depend on the cause.

Clinical evaluation of encephalitis

Clinical suspicion

Fever, alteration in consciousness, seizures, no symptoms of meningeal irritation

Evaluation

Check exposure history: sick contacts, animals, ticks, mosquitoes, travel

Check immunization record

Neurologic examination

Funduscopic examination

Lumbar puncture: opening pressure, cell count, protein, glucose, Gram's stain, bacterial culture, HSV polymerase chain reaction, viral culture

Consider: VDRL, cryptococcal antigen, mycobacterial culture, fungal stain and culture, enterovirus polymerase chain reaction, arbovirus polymerase chain reaction, cytology

Head magnetic resonance imaging scan or head computed tomography scan with contrast

Complete blood cell count, serum electrolytes

Brain biopsy of local lesions: Gram's stain, aerobic and anaerobic bacterial cultures, mycobacterial stain and culture, fungal stain and culture, histology

Consider serum titers for syphilis, HIV, cat scratch disease, Rocky Mountain spotted fever, arboviruses, enteroviruses, Epstein–Barr virus, measles, lymphocytic choriomeningitis, leptospirosis, toxoplasmosis, hepatitis (A, B, and C), Lyme disease, human herpesvirus 6 and 7, mumps, dengue (if appropriate travel history)

Consider coagulation times, liver enzymes, purified protein derivative, viral culture of nasopharynx and stool, blood smears for malaria (if appropriate travel history)

Consider noninfectious causes: toxins, metabolic disorders, trauma, neoplasm, autoimmune vasculitis, Reye's syndrome, acute demyelinating encephalomyelitis or multiple sclerosis, intracranial hemorrhage

VDRL—Veneral Disease Research Laboratory (test).

Figure 11-19 The clinical evaluation of encephalitis. The clinical evaluation of encephalitis is among the most difficult challenges facing the infectious diseases consultant. Although the spectrum of infectious agents that cause encephalitis is broad, there are often few specific clinical findings to direct the clinician to a singular diagnosis. Because there are many noninfectious causes of encephalopathy that may mimic infectious encephalitis, consultations with a radiologist and a neurologist should also be sought. Clinical guidance from a genetics and metabolism specialist may also be useful in evaluating encephalopathy in young children. Consultation from a rheumatologist should be sought if there is concern for a systemic inflammatory process.

For the diagnostic assessment of encephalitis, obtaining detailed historical information is especially important. A careful travel history and a summary of recent animal exposures may provide insight. The clinician must also be aware of local epidemiologic trends because forms of encephalitis may be vector-borne or may occur seasonally.

Because herpes simplex virus infection figures prominently in the list of treatable causes of encephalitis, early empiric therapy with high-dose intravenous acyclovir should be initiated in all patients with suspected encephalitis, especially those with fevers and new onset of seizures or mental status changes.

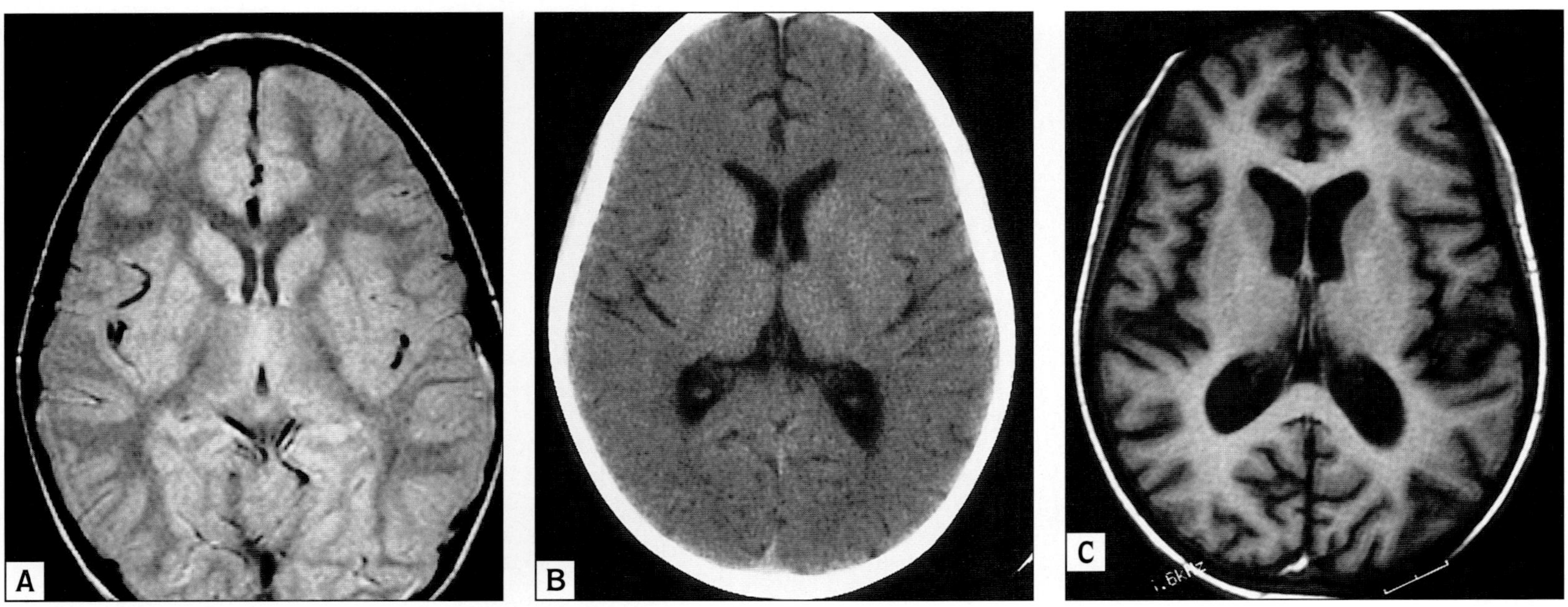

Figure 11-20 HIV-related brain atrophy. These axial images taken at approximately the same plane of section allow comparison of anatomy. **A**, This image of a 6-year-old child with congenital HIV shows normal parenchymal anatomy with slit-sized ventricles and sulci. **B**, An image of the same child at 9 years of age shows marked ventricular enlargement indicative of hydrocephalus ex vacuo. **C**, An image taken at 11 years of age shows progressive ventriculomegaly and greatly enlarged sulci consistent with massive parenchymal loss. HIV encephalopathy is associated with poor cognitive development. Marked immunosuppression generally precedes the development of demonstrable cerebral atrophy.

Assessment of suspected congenital infection involving the central nervous system

	Most common perinatal clinical findings	Initial diagnostic assessment
HSV*	Lethargy	HSV culture of blood, surface swabs, conjunctiva, rectum
	Irritability	Tzanck preparation, direct fluorescence and culture of vesicular lesions
	Fever	Complete blood count with differential
	Seizures	Liver function tests, PT/PTT, bilirubin
	Sepsis syndrome	Lumbar puncture with viral culture and HSV PCR
	Vesicular rash	Cranial contrast CT or MRI
	Conjunctivitis	Ophthalmologic examination
	Bleeding	Electroencephalography
	Hepatosplenomegaly, jaundice, hepatitis	Brain biopsy (rarely needed)
CMV	Purpuric or petechial rash	Complete blood count with differential
	Hepatosplenomegaly, jaundice, hepatitis	Liver function tests, PT/PTT, bilirubin
	Small for gestational age	Viral culture of blood and urine
	Microcephaly	Ophthalmologic examination
	Chorioretinitis	Cranial contrast CT or MRI
		Audiologic assessment/auditory evoked potentials
Neonatal VZV*	Perinatal maternal varicella (onset of maternal rash 5 d before to 2 d after delivery)	VZV culture of blood, nasopharynx, conjunctiva; Tzanck preparation, direct fluorescence and culture of vesicular lesions
	Vesicular rash	Complete blood count with differential
	Pneumonitis	Liver function tests, PT/PTT, bilirubin
	Hepatosplenomegaly, jaundice, hepatitis	
	Meningoencephalitis	
Enteroviruses†	Fever	Complete blood count with differential
	Sepsis-like syndrome	Liver function tests, PT/PTT, bilirubin
	Lethargy	Lumbar puncture with viral culture and enterovirus PCR
	Rash	Viral cultures of stool, urine and blood
	Seizures	Electroencephalogram
	Myocardiopathy	Cardiologic assessment
	Hepatosplenomegaly, jaundice, hepatitis	
	Aseptic meningitis, encephalitis	
Rubella	Maternal history of rubella during pregnancy	Viral culture of nasopharynx, oropharynx, blood, and CSF
	Intrauterine growth retardation	Complete blood count with differential
	Cataracts	Liver function tests, PT/PTT, bilirubin
	Chorioretinitis	Ophthalmologic examination
	Hepatosplenomegaly, jaundice, hepatitis	Cardiologic evaluation
	Meningoencephalitis	Audiologic assessment, auditory evoked potentials
	Purpuric rash	Long bone radiographs
		Cranial contrast CT or MRI
Syphilis*	Hepatosplenomegaly, jaundice, hepatitis	Complete blood count with differential
	Small for gestational age	Serum RPR or VDRL
	Desquamating or erythematous rash	Lumbar puncture (include CSF VDRL)
	Fever	Ophthalmologic examination
	Extremity edema, pain or paralysis	Long bone plane films (optional)
	Rhinitis	Dark field examination of nasal discharge or rash
	Pneumonia	HIV serology (ELISA and Western blot)
	Chorioretinitis	
Toxoplasmosis*	Fever	Complete blood count with differential
	Hepatosplenomegaly, jaundice, hepatitis	Toxoplasma serologies (IgG and IgM)‡
	Microcephaly or hydrocephalus	Cranial contrast CT or MRI
	Intrauterine growth retardation	Ophthalmologic examination
	Seizures	Electroencephalogram

* Presumptive therapy should be initiated when diagnosis is first suspected.

† Specific antienteroviral therapy (Plecaonaril; ViroPharma, Inc., Malvern, PA) is available through compassionate release.

‡ Specimen referral to an experienced reference laboratory is strongly recommended.

CMV—Cytomegalovirus; CSF—cerebrospinal fluid; CT—computed tomography; ELISA—enzyme-linked immunosorbent assay; HSV—herpes simplex virus; MRI—magnetic resonance imaging; PCR—polymerase chain reaction; PT—prothrombin time; PTT—partial thromboplastin time; RPR—rapid plasma reagin; VDRL—Venereal Disease Research Laboratory (test); VZV—varicella-zoster virus.

FIGURE 11-21 Assessment of suspected congenital infection involving the central nervous system. Congenital infections in infants may be difficult to recognize and present with varying degrees of severity, ranging from asymptomatic infection through devastating systemic disease and still birth. Historical findings suggestive of possible congenital infection include inadequate prenatal care, maternal substance abuse, maternal history of sexually transmitted infection, and maternal illness. Neonatal physical findings common to many infants with congenital infection include microcephaly, small gestational size, hepatosplenomegaly, anemia, thrombocytopenia, leukopenia, congenital cataracts, rash, seizures, and fever. Radiologic findings include intracranial calcifications, brain inflammation,

(legend continued on next page)

Figure 11-21 *(continued)* or atrophy. Because of the high potential for significant morbidity or mortality, infants suspected of having congenital infections should be evaluated aggressively. Furthermore, specific antimicrobial therapy, when available, should not await definitive diagnosis; rather, early presumptive therapy should be initiated while a diagnosis is sought. Infants diagnosed with congenital infection due to syphilis or Herpes simplex virus should also be evaluated for possible chlamydia and HIV infection. Appropriate management of HIV-exposed infants is detailed elsewhere in this text (*see* Chapter 9). Infants with congenital infections are at high risk for a variety of developmental disabilities. Infants identified as infected require comprehensive, longitudinal follow-up that should begin in the neonatal period. Studies should include sensory, developmental, and neuromotor assessments and radiological imaging. Regular reassessments of general development, sensory function, neuromotor abilities, and language should be performed, with cognitive, academic, and language skills assessed during the preschool years.

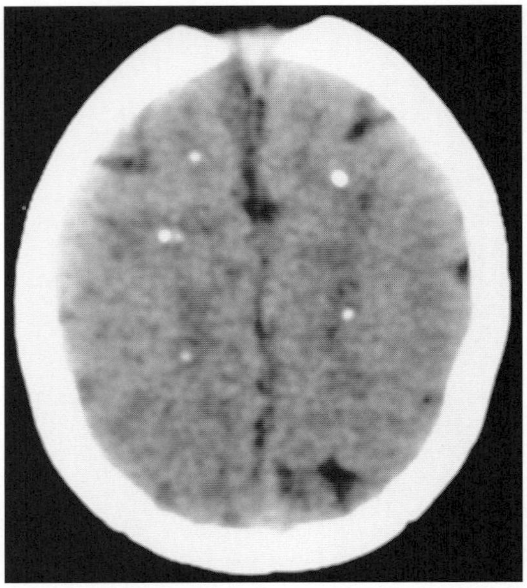

Figure 11-22 Congenital toxoplasmosis. This axial noncontrast head computed tomographic image of a 7-month-old child with microcephaly shows multiple scattered areas of calcification. The slowed cranial growth and parenchymal calcifications suggest the diagnosis of a congenital central nervous system infection. The scattered nonlocalizing pattern of the lesions is consistent with congenital toxoplasmosis. Diagnosis may be confirmed by serum titers for toxoplasma IgM, IgA, or by a fourfold rise in toxoplasma IgG. Treatment for congenital toxoplasmosis is with pyrimethamine and sulfadiazine for 3 to 6 weeks. Complications may include seizure, learning disabilities, mental retardation, and visual impairment.

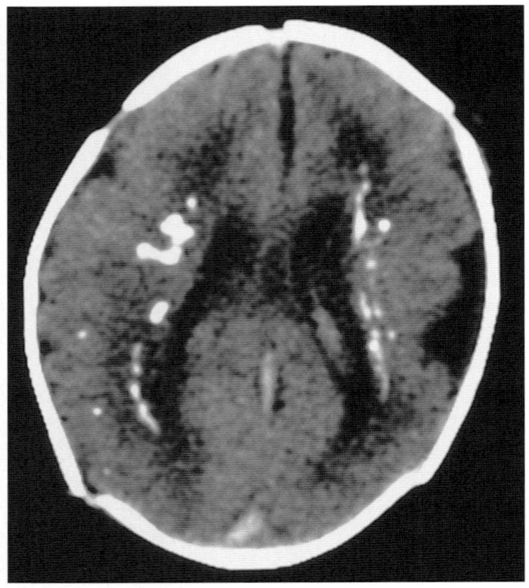

Figure 11-23 Congenital cytomegalovirus infection. This axial noncontrast head computed tomographic image of a full-term neonate with poor suck reflex and severe extremity clonus shows severe intracranial calcifications that are predominantly periventricular. This pattern of periventricular parenchymal calcifications is most commonly seen in congenital cytomegalovirus (CMV). The diagnosis may be confirmed by CMV culture of the infant's urine, saliva, or blood. Treatment with ganciclovir is controversial because of the insufficient efficacy data. Complications may include mental retardation and deafness.

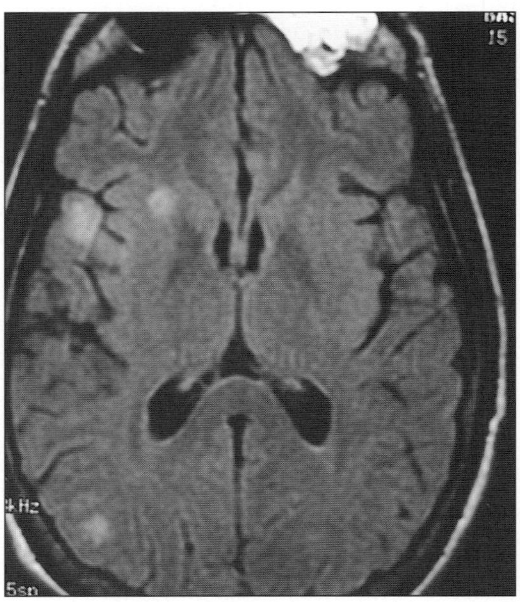

Figure 11-24 Acute demyelinating encephalomyelitis (ADE). This axial head magnetic resonance image of a 15-year-old patient with a 1-week history of fever, sore throat, and rhinorrhea followed by acute onset of dysarthria, diplopia, and nystagmus shows multiple scattered low attenuation areas involving both white and gray matter. ADE is usually preceded by a nonspecific viral illness and likely represents a postinfectious immune-mediated event. ADE is a diagnosis is of exclusion; treatable infectious causes, most notably herpes meningoencephalitis, should be sought aggressively. ADE may present with signs and symptoms similar to those of an initial multiple sclerosis attack; however, oligoclonal bands will be absent from the cerebrospinal fluid, and ADE should not be recurrent. The efficacy of steroids in this condition is controversial.

A. Acute management and evaluation for possible rabies exposure*

- Aggressive wound decontamination and debridement are probably the most important factors in postexposure management of rabies
- Tetanus toxoid should be administered to individuals without recent booster immunization
- Antibacterial prophylaxis may be considered for puncture wounds that cannot be decontaminated adequately
- Consult with local health authorities regarding potential rabies exposure
- Notify animal control officials of possible exposure, providing the following information:
  - Name, age, address of patient
  - Location of injuries
  - Nature of injuries (bites, scratches)
  - Location of attack or exposure
  - Species of attacking animal
  - Location of attacking animal
  - Circumstances of attack or exposure (*eg*, provoked vs unprovoked)
- Prophylaxis decisions following face or neck injuries are especially urgent

* Appropriate management of potential rabies exposures requires consultation with local animal control and public health authorities.

B. Guidelines for rabies postexposure management and prophylaxis*

Animal type	Evaluation and dispensation of animal	Postexposure prophylaxis recommendations
Dogs, cats	Healthy and available for observation by licensed veterinarian or animal control officials; period of observation is dictated by local animal control authorities	Provide prophylaxis and immunization only if animal develops signs of rabies
	Rabid or suspected rabid	Initiate rabies vaccination and prophylaxis; discontinue if laboratory tests for rabies are negative
	Unknown or escaped	Consult local health authorities
Raccoons, foxes, skunks, most other carnivores, woodchucks†	Regard as rabid unless geographic area is known to be rabies-free or until animal is demonstrated uninfected by euthanasia and testing	Initiate rabies vaccination and prophylaxis; discontinue if laboratory tests for rabies are negative
Bats‡	Regard as rabid unless geographic area is known to be rabies-free or until animal is demonstrated uninfected by euthanasia and testing	Initiate rabies vaccination and prophylaxis; discontinue if laboratory tests for rabies are negative
Livestock, ferrets, rodents, lagomorphs	Consult with animal control officials	Consult local health authorities
Exotic species§	Consult with animal control officials	Consult local health authorities

* Appropriate management of potential rabies exposures requires consultation with local animal control and public health authorities.

† These animals should be euthanized and tested as soon as possible. Holding for rabies observation is not recommended as symptoms of rabies may not be recognized in wild animals.

‡ Rabies prophylaxis may be indicated following bat exposures even in the absence of bites or scratches (*eg*, bat found in room of sleeping person). Contact local health officials.

FIGURE 11-25 Recommendations for rabies postmanagement and prophylaxis. The prevalence of animal rabies continues to increase through many regions of the United States and Canada. Attendant with this increase in sylvatic rabies is an increase in the number of human rabies exposures. **A,** Summarized are recommendations for evaluation and management of rabies exposure. It should be reemphasized that aggressive wound decontamination and debridement are of paramount importance to successful postexposure treatment. **B,** Rabies prophylaxis decisions are based on the risk of rabies infection in the exposing animal. Because of the devastating and usually fatal course of rabies and the substantial expense of rabies prophylaxis, medical management and rabies prophylaxis decisions should be made in conjunction with local animal control and public health authorities. (*Adapted from* 1997 Red Book [17]; with permission.)

REFERENCES

1. Barone MA (ed):Diagnostic tests. In *The Harriet Lane Handbook*, ed 13. St. Louis:Mosby; 1996:115–126.
2. Sarff LD, Platt LH, McCracken GH Jr:Cerebrospinal fluid evaluationin neonates:comparison of high-risk infants with and without meningitis. *J Pediatr* 1976, 88:473-477.
3. Bargallo J, Berenguer J, Garcia-Barrionuevo J, *et al.*:The "target sign":is it a specific sign of CNS tuberculoma? *Neuroradiology* 1996, 38:547–550.
4. Rabin BM, Meyer JR, Berlin JW, *et al.*:Radiation-induced changes in the central nervous system and head and neck. *Radiographics* 1996, 16:1055–1072.
5. Remick SC, Diamond C, Migliozzi JA, *et al.*:Primary central nervous system lymphoma in patients with and without the acquired immune deficiency syndrome:a retrospective analysis and review. *Medicine* 1990, 69:345–360.
6. De Salles AA, Brekhus SD, De Souza EC, *et al.*:Early postoperative appearance of radiofrequency lesions on magnetic resonance imaging. *Neurosurgery* 1995, 36:932–936.
7. Salzman C, Tuazon CU:Value of the ring-enhancing sign in differentiating intracerebral hematomas and brain abscesses. *Arch Intern Med* 1987, 147:951–952.
8. Schielke E:Der bakterielle hirnabszess [Bacterial brain abscess]. *Nervenarzt* 1995, 66:745–753.
9. Woods CR Jr.:Brain abscesses and other intracranial suppurative complications. *Adv Pediatr Infect Dis* 1995, 10:41–79.
10. Bertoli F, Espino M, Arosemena JR 5th, *et al.*:A spectrum in the pathology of toxoplasmosis in patients with acquired immunodeficiency syndrome. *Arch Pathol Lab Med* 1995, 119:214–224.
11. Zagardo MT, Castellani RJ, Zoarski GH, Bauserman SC:Granulomatous amebic encephalitis caused by leptomyxid amebae in an HIV-infected patient. *AJNR Am J Neuroradiol* 1997, 18:903–908.
12. Kramer LD, Locke GE, Byrd SE, Daryabagi J:Cerebral cysticercosis:documentation of natural history with CT. *Radiology* 1989, 171:459–462.
13. Nagayama M, Shinohara Y, Nagakura K, *et al.*:Distinctive serial magnetic resonance changes in a young woman with rapidly evolved neurocysticercosis, with positron emission tomography results. *J Neuroimag* 1996, 6:198–201.
14. Kim TK, Chang KH, Kim CJ, *et al.*:Intracranial tuberculoma:comparison of MR with pathologic findings. *AJNR Am J Neuroradiol* 1995, 16:1903–1908.
15. Masdeu JC, Moreira J, Trasi S, *et al.*:The open ring:a new imaging sign in demyelinating disease. *J Neuroimag* 1996. 6:104–107.
16. Fred HL, Dunn K:A ring-enhancing parietal lobe lesion in an HIV-positive man. *Hosp Prac (Off Ed)* 1995, 30:66–68.
17. American Academy of Pediatrics:*1997 Red Book Report of the Committee on Infectious Diseases*, ed 24. Elk Grove Village, IL:American Academy of Pediatrics; 1997.

SELECTED BIBLIOGRAPHY

Feigin RD:Bacterial meningitis beyond the neonatal period. In *Textbook of Pediatric Infectious Diseases.* Edited by Feigin RD, Cherry JD. Philadelphia:WB Saunders; 1992:401–428.

Oski FA:Laboratory values. In *Principles and Practice of Pediatrics*, ed 2. Philadelphia:JB Lippincott; 1994:2196–2169.

CHAPTER 12

Congenital and Perinatal Infections

Gail J. Demmler

CONGENITAL AND PERINATAL INFECTIONS are infections of the fetus and newborn. They may be acquired in utero, during delivery, or during the immediate postpartum period. They may be asymptomatic, cause overt disease at birth, cause long-term or late sequelae, or even result in death. The pathogenesis and disease expression of congenital and perinatal infections depends on the type and pathogenicity of the infectious organism as well as the stage of development of the fetus or newborn when the infection occurred.

A wide variety of organisms (*eg*, viruses, bacteria, parasites, and fungi) may produce congenital and perinatal infection and disease. Many of these organisms produce similar clinical manifestations, so it is important to search for diagnostic clues in the history and physical examination. A specific laboratory diagnosis, however, is the best approach and leads to correct management and appropriate therapy when available. Because long-term sequelae of the nervous system often occurs, long-term follow-up of sensory, motor, and cognitive development also is important for the infant who is diagnosed with a congenital or perinatal infection.

Definitions relevant to congenital and perinatal infections

Term	Definition
Natal	Acquired during delivery
Prenatal	Acquired before delivery
Postnatal	Acquired after delivery
Perinatal	Acquired around delivery; the perinatal period also may refer to the time from 28 wk gestation to 7 d of postnatal life
Neonatal–newborn	Refers to the first month or the first 28 d of postnatal life
Congenital	Acquired at or before birth; may be acquired prenatally or natally, but often remains active postnatally
Vertical transmission	An infection of the fetus or newborn that is acquired from the mother during pregnancy or at the time of delivery; almost all congenital or perinatal infections are vertically transmitted
Horizontal transmission	An infection of the newborn that is acquired from a person other than the mother; may be caused by infectious agents that also cause congenital or perinatal infection
Infection	Entry of an infectious agent into the body; usually accompanied by a host immune response and isolation of the infectious agent; may or may not be associated with symptoms or signs of disease in congenital or perinatal infections
Disease	An infectious agent causes damage to tissue that produces signs or symptoms; disease may or may not be present in congenital or perinatal infections
IgG	Antibody made at or soon after the time of infection; usually persists; may be transferred transplacentally from mother to fetus and may persist in the infant for months postnatally
IgM	Antibody made at the time of infection; does not persist for long periods; is not transferred transplacentally from mother to fetus

FIGURE 12-1 Definitions relevant to the study of congenital and perinatal infections. The 10-month period from conception to the end of the first month of life is a unique period. Susceptibility to infection is greater because the maternal immune system is suppressed and the fetal and neonatal immune system is immature, with specific defects in function. Intrauterine protection of the fetus is accomplished physically by the fetal membranes and placenta, which act as barriers, and functionally by passive transfer of maternal IgG. Passive immunity by transplacental transfer of IgG persists for months postnatally, and breast milk provides additional protection against infection. The fetus and newborn also are uniquely vulnerable to damage, especially permanent damage to the central nervous system, because cell growth and organ differentiation occur at high rates during this period.

For these and many other reasons, an understanding of the terms commonly used when discussing congenital and perinatally acquired infections is helpful to understand these unique concepts of pathogenesis, clinical presentation, and interpretation of diagnostic tests. Further, all congenital infections present in live-born infants are neonatal, by definition, but not all neonatal infections are congenital. Also, some infections that can cause congenital infections (*eg*, cytomegalovirus and herpes simplex virus) also may cause perinatal infections. Finally, the distinction between infection and disease should be clearly understood, because not all congenital or perinatal infections produce disease.

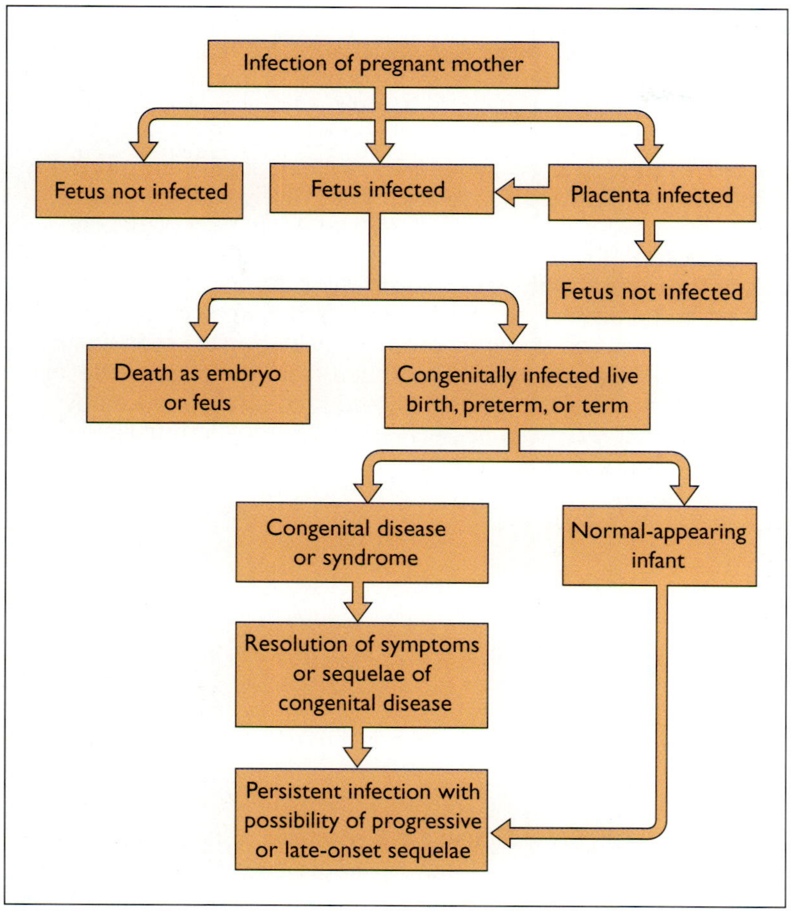

FIGURE 12-2 Possible consequences of infection of a pregnant mother. If a pregnant mother acquires an infection, she may or may not transmit the infection to her fetus. Transmission depends on many factors, such as the infecting agent and the time of gestation. The outcome of an infection in the embryo or fetus may be embryonic death, spontaneous abortion or stillbirth, premature birth, or a congenital disease or syndrome, often accompanied by intrauterine growth retardation, low birth weight, or developmental anomalies due to teratogenesis. It also is possible that a normal-appearing infant may be born that is congenitally infected, but not damaged or diseased. Infections of the fetus also may persist postnatally for months, even years, and produce late sequelae. For example, progressive hearing loss is commonly seen in congenital cytomegalovirus infection, and deterioration in motor and mental skills has been documented in older children born with congenital rubella syndrome.

Signs, symptoms, and laboratory findings commonly associated with congenital infections

Intrauterine growth retardation
Jaundice at birth
Hepatosplenomegaly
Hepatitis (elevated transaminases, direct and indirect hyperbilirubinemia)
Skin lesions (petechiae, purpura, vesicles, maculopapular rash, scars)
Hematologic abnormality (thrombocytopenia, anemia, lymphopenia, neutropenia)
Generalized adenopathy
Pneumonitis
Cardiac lesions (myocarditis, congenital defects)
Bone lesions
Eye lesions (glaucoma, chorioretinitis, retinopathy, cataracts, optic atrophy)
Microphthalmia, uveitis, keratoconjunctivitis
Sensorineural hearing loss
Central nervous disease (microcephaly, meningoencephalitis, ventriculomegaly, hydrocephalus, intracranial calcifications)

FIGURE 12-3 Signs, symptoms, and laboratory findings commonly associated with congenital infections. A variety of clinical manifestations at birth commonly are associated with congenital infection and disease. Most congenitally infected infants will exhibit nonspecific signs that a congenital infection is present, such as growth retardation or hepatosplenomegaly, but each agent also may have a unique effect on the fetus, such as the presence of patent ductus arteriosus and cataracts in congenital rubella syndrome. These clinical clues in the patient point to the specific etiologic agent causing the congenital disease.

Viruses that may cause congenital or perinatally acquired infection or disease

DNA viruses
Cytomegalovirus
Herpes simplex virus types 1 and 2
Varicella-zoster virus
Human parvovirus B19
Hepatitis B virus
Variola virus (smallpox virus)
Human papillomaviruses

RNA viruses
Rubella virus
Mumps virus
Measles virus
Enteroviruses (coxsackievirus, echovirus, polioviruses)
Hepatitis C virus
Lymphocytic choriomeningitis virus
HIV

FIGURE 12-4 Viruses that may cause congenitally or perinatally acquired infection or disease. A variety of DNA and RNA viruses have been documented to cause congenital or perinatally acquired infections or disease. Currently, the virus most commonly associated with congenital and perinatal infections is cytomegalovirus. Herpes simplex virus also continues to cause significant morbidity and mortality. Conversely, measles virus rarely has been documented to produce congenital or perinatal infection or disease. The incidence of congenital rubella syndrome and perinatally acquired hepatitis B infection has dramatically decreased since routine immunization has been implemented, and congenital or perinatally acquired smallpox probably will never be seen again because this illness has been eradicated from the planet. The incidence of congenital and perinatally acquired disease caused by varicella-zoster virus can be decreased if routine immunization with varicella vaccine is implemented.

Bacteria, fungi, and parasites that may have been associated with congenital or perinatally acquired infection or disease

Bacteria
Listeria monocytogenes (listeriosis)
Group A and B streptococci
α-Hemolytic streptococci
Neisseria gonorrhoeae (gonococcus)
Enterococci
Escherichia coli
Proteus spp.
Klebsiella spp.
Pseudomonas spp.
Salmonella spp.
Shigella spp.
Haemophilus influenzae and parainfluenza
Anaerobic bacteria
Mycobacterium tuberculosis (tuberculosis)
Trepanema pallidum (syphilis)
Borrelia burgdorferi (Lyme disease)

Fungi
Candida albicans
Coccidioides immitis
Cryptococcus neoformans
Blastomyces dermatitidis

Mycoplasma and chlamydia
Mycoplasma hominis
Ureaplasma urealyticum
Chlamydia trachomatis

Parasites and protozoa
Toxoplasmosis gondii (toxoplasmosis)
Plasmodium vivax, P. falciparum, P. malariae, P. ovale (malaria)
Trypanosoma cruzi (Chagas' disease)
Trypanosoma brucei (African sleeping sickness)
Ascaris lumbricoides
Trichinella spiralis (trichinosis)

FIGURE 12-5 Bacteria, fungi, and parasites that may be associated with congenital or perinatally acquired infection or disease. A variety of bacteria, fungi, and parasites may cause congenital or perinatally acquired infection or disease. Some agents, such as group B streptococci and *Trepanema pallidum*, are relatively common in the United States, whereas other agents, such as *Trypanosoma cruzi* in Central and South America and *Toxoplasma gondii* in France, are a significant problem in other parts of the world. Congenital infection with other agents, such as *Mycobacterium tuberculosis* and the fungi, are exceedingly rare in all parts of the world.

Noninfectious conditions that may mimic congenital infections

Genetic	Hematologic
Aicardi's syndrome Walker–Warburg syndrome Miller–Dieker syndrome Tuberous sclerosis Incontinentia pigmenti	Congenital leukemia Erythroblastosis fetalis Absent radius/ thrombocytopenia syndrome
Metabolic	**Other conditions**
Congenital hyperthyroidism (neonatal Graves' disease) α_1-Antitrypsin deficiency Galactogenia Zellweger syndrome Neonatal adrenoleukodystrophy Infantile Refsum's disease Urea cycle enzyme deficiencies Organic acidemias Liposomal storage disorders Dihydropteridine reductase deficiency	Maternal conditions (sensitization to platelet antigens, idiopathic thrombocytopenic purpura, drug therapy, placental insufficiency) Toxins Retinoic acid embryopathy Fetal alcohol syndrome Cocaine abuse during pregnancy Neonatal calcium administration Pre- or postnatal ischemia

FIGURE 12-6 Noninfectious conditions that may mimic congenital infections. Some noninfectious disorders may produce symptoms or signs similar to those seen in infants with congenital infections. These disorders may be caused by genetic, metabolic, hematologic, or toxic conditions. For example, the microcephaly, seizures, mental retardation, and retinopathy seen in infants with the genetically determined Aicardi's syndrome may mimic congenital toxoplasmosis or congenital cytomegalovirus disease. Similarly, the intracranial calcifications that may occur in tuberous sclerosis appear similar to calcifications seen in congenital toxoplasmosis or cytomegalovirus, and the papulovesicular skin lesions and seizures seen in newborns with the neurocutaneous syndrome incontinentia pigmenti can appear similar to the vesicular skin lesions and meningoencephalitis caused by herpes simplex virus. Infants with metabolic diseases, such as galactosemia or congenital hyperthyroidism, may present with jaundice, hyperbilirubinemia, hepatosplenomegaly, and thrombocytopenia. Cataracts, although associated with congenital rubella syndrome, also may be seen in certain metabolic and genetic disorders. In infants who appear to have a congenital infection, but in whom an infectious agent cannot be detected, noninfectious disorders should be considered and the appropriate tests performed.

Evaluation of the newborn suspected to have a congenital infection

Maternal history	Physical examination
Results of prenatal serology screens Exposure history Significant maternal illness Abnormal fetal growth or development	Birth measurements Skin color or lesions Hepatosplenomegaly Funduscopic examination
	Laboratory evaluation
	Viral and bacterial cultures Specific serologies Histopathology on tissue

FIGURE 12-7 Evaluation of a newborn suspected to have a congenital infection. The suggested evaluation of a newborn suspected to have a congenital infection should focus on expeditiously identifying a specific infectious agent. Consultation with a pediatric infectious diseases specialist may be extremely helpful. A thorough maternal history should be taken and particular attention should be given to the results of the prenatal serologic screens routinely performed for syphilis, rubella, hepatitis B, and HIV. For example, a woman noted to be rubella-nonimmune would be at risk for having an infant with congenital rubella syndrome. The mother also may have had serologic tests for other infections such as cytomegalovirus (CMV) or toxoplasmosis, which would be helpful in documenting the presence or absence of a specific seroconversion during pregnancy. A maternal exposure history should include travel history; exposure to unusual, raw, or undercooked foods; animal exposure; care of young children; or a sexual partner known to have a sexually transmitted disease. For example, travel to France, eating undercooked meat, or exposure to cats and kittens pose a risk for toxoplasmosis; exposure to contaminated dairy products has been linked to listeriosis. Many maternal infections that produce congenital infections are trivial or asymptomatic in the mother, however, a significant maternal illness, such as prolonged fever or a mononucleosis syndrome, suggest CMV or toxoplasmosis. Similarly, a maculopapular rash in a rubella-nonimmune pregnant mother exposed to young children suggests congenital rubella syndrome. Maternal syphilis or HIV infection, especially if the mother was not treated during pregnancy, has serious implications for the fetus. Abnormal fetal growth or development noted during prenatal visits or ultrasound examinations also may provide clues that an intrauterine infection is present.

The physical examination of a newborn suspected to have a congenital infection should pay particular attention to growth measurements, because many of these infants suffer from intrauterine growth retardation. It is particularly important to notice the presence or absence of microcephaly. Jaundice at birth is abnormal, signifying presence of disease; the skin may have generalized petechiae or purpura. Hepatosplenomegaly also is noted, often to a significant degree. A careful funduscopic examination, performed by an ophthalmologist, may reveal chorioretinitis. The laboratory evaluation of a newborn suspected to have a congenital infection should follow the clinical clues gleaned from the maternal history and newborn physical examination. Whenever possible, specific identification of the infectious agent suspected to be causing the congenital infection should be sought. The indiscriminate use of TORCH (toxoplasmosis, other infections, rubella, CMV, and herpes simplex) titer panels should be discouraged because they often merely reflect transplacental transmission of maternal antibody. Further, the routine use of skull and long-bone radiographs provides very little information about the specific cause of most congenital infections. Therefore, if a viral cause is suspected, appropriate viral cultures, antigen, or nucleic acid detection tests should be obtained, similar to what is routinely done when a bacterial illness is suspected to be the cause of a congenital or perinatal infection. For example, CMV is best isolated from the urine, whereas herpes simplex virus may be isolated from mucocutaneous sites. A serologic approach to the diagnosis of congenital syphilis, toxoplasmosis, or lymphocytic choriomeningitis virus, however, is still appropriate in most cases.

Evaluation of the newborn proven to have a congenital infection
Complete blood count Liver function tests Lumbar puncture Neurologic examination Imaging studies Ophthalmologic examination Audiologic evaluation

Figure 12-8 Evaluation of the newborn proven to have a congenital infection. The suggested evaluation of these newborns includes a complete blood count, with differential and platelet count. Infants with congenital infections commonly have thrombocytopenia, which may be severe or prolonged. They also may have lymphocytosis, neutropenia, or anemia, and eosinophilia may occur in infants with congenital toxoplasmosis. Because hepatitis also may occur, transaminase and bilirubin levels should be monitored. It is especially important to thoroughly evaluate the neurologic status of the infant, because congenital infections commonly involve the central nervous system. It should be determined whether the patient has feeding or swallowing problems, or has experienced episodes of seizure activity. The infant's muscle tone, reflexes, motor patterns, and response to stimuli should be noted. The head size should be measured and recorded; overriding sutures and scalp rugae suggest extreme microcephaly with severe underlying brain abnormalities. A lumbar puncture should be performed in most infants, if clinical condition and platelet count deem the procedure safe, and the cerebrospinal fluid sent for routine studies as well as appropriate special studies. For most infants with a congenital infection, and especially those with congenital cytomegalovirus and toxoplasmosis, an unenhanced cranial computed tomographic (CT) scan is the most appropriate study, because it will show ventricular size, calcifications, and abnormal structural patterns or lucencies in the brain. Cranial ultrasound, commonly performed in newborns to monitor for intraventricular hemorrhage and ventricular size, provides incomplete information, and plain skull radiographs are even less useful. In infants with herpes simplex virus infection or unusual findings, an enhanced CT scan or a magnetic resonance imaging scan may be needed. An ophthalmologic examination should be performed to determine if there are abnormalities that could affect vision, such as microphthalmia, cataracts, glaucoma, keratoconjunctivitis, or chorioretinitis. Visual evoked responses may be indicated in unusual cases. An audiologic evaluation also should be performed to determine if a hearing loss is present. In some congenital infections, especially congenital cytomegalovirus infection, the sensorineural hearing loss may be progressive; therefore serial hearing tests should be performed.

Evaluation of the infant with signs of a congenital infection but in whom an infectious agent is not identified
Maternal history Family history Physical and neurologic examination Lumbar puncture Imaging studies Ophthalmologic examination Audiologic examination Laboratory evaluation (complete blood count; Coombs' test; arterial pH; serum ammonia and lactate levels; urine-reducing substances and organic acids; drug screen; chromosomal analysis)

Figure 12-9 Evaluation of the infant with signs of a congenital infection but in whom an infectious agent is not identified. The evaluation of these newborns should focus on identifying a possible genetic, metabolic, or hematologic disorder, or a condition produced by an *in utero* exposure to a drug or toxin. Consultation with a pediatric neurologist or geneticist can be extremely helpful. A maternal history of the use of isotretinoin, alcohol or cocaine, or exposure to toxins would be significant. A thorough family history should be obtained, with special emphasis on consanguinity, infant deaths, and inherited neurologic conditions. A physical examination, noting dysmorphic features or skin lesions, as well as a careful neurologic examination should be performed. A lumbar puncture to obtain cerebrospinal fluid for routine studies, as well as special studies (*eg*, lactate levels), should be considered. Imaging studies of the brain, either computed tomographic scan or magnetic resonance imaging, also should be performed to determine if structural or developmental abnormalities are present. An ophthalmologic examination is important to identify abnormalities of the eye and retina. Both an otologic examination to detect any structural anomalies of the ear and an audiologic evaluation, including brain stem–evoked responses, should be performed to determine if deafness is present. The laboratory evaluation of these infants should include a complete blood count and differential if congenital leukemia is suspected, and a Coombs' test if anemia or hemolysis is present. Arterial pH for metabolic acidosis, serum ammonia and lactate levels, urinary reducing substances, and organic acids also may be indicated. Rarely, plasma amino acids or very long chain fatty acid determinations may be indicated. Genetic disorders may be identified by chromosomal analysis and a drug screen may reveal maternal cocaine or alcohol use.

Suggested long-term neurodevelopmental follow-up of infants with a congenital infection

Age	Assessments
Neonatal period	Neurodevelopmental Vision and hearing Brain imaging
4–6 mo	Neurodevelopmental
9–12 mo	Neurodevelopmental Vision and hearing
18–24 mo	Neurodevelopmental Language Vision and hearing
3–5 y	Neurodevelopmental Vision and hearing Language School readiness
School age	Cognitive Language Learning differences Academic performance Vision and hearing
Adolescence	Cognitive Learning differences Academic performance Vision and hearing

FIGURE 12-10 Suggested long-term neurodevelopmental follow-up of infants with a congenital infection. An infant born with a congenital infection is at high risk for developmental disabilities, including visual problems, hearing loss, and motor problems, as well as cognitive, language, attention, and academic difficulties. The clinical management of a congenitally infected infant therefore must include careful, multidisciplinary longitudinal follow-up to detect disabilities that are age-specific in their presentation, as well as those problems that may be progressive and cause deterioration in function. For example, progressive hearing loss or deterioration of vision may occur in infants born with congenital cytomegalovirus infection, rubella, toxoplasmosis, or syphilis, whereas a progressive encephalopathy may occur in congenital HIV infection. Consultation with a developmental pediatrician is recommended.

During the neonatal period, baseline sensory function (hearing, vision, tactile), neurodevelopmental status (assessed by physical and neurological examination), and neuroanatomic findings (detected by brain imaging) should be carefully noted. If initial problems are noted, such as hearing loss or active retinitis, then follow-up during the first weeks and months of life should be arranged, dictated by the needs of each patient. At 4 to 6 months of age, routine assessment of the infant's tone, reflexes, neuromotor function, and developmental milestones should be performed. Infants who are severely affected neurologically will display abnormalities at this early age. At 9 to 12 months of age, developmental milestones and neuromotor function should be assessed, as well as vision and hearing. At 18 to 24 months of age, in addition to developmental milestones, the physician should carefully evaluate language skills. Some congenital infections, such as cytomegalovirus, also warrant a repeat evaluation of hearing, whereas others, such as toxoplasmosis, warrant a repeat ophthalmologic examination. During the infancy and toddler period, most cases of severe disability will be detected, including cerebral palsy, mental retardation, deafness, and significant visual impairment, and the appropriate interventions should be initiated. At 3 years of age, developmental milestones, including motor function and expressive and receptive language skills, should once again be assessed; most cases of moderate retardation will be identified at this age.

Readiness for preschool and kindergarten should be assessed. The congenitally infected child who enters the school-age years without significant developmental disabilities still may experience mild cognitive, language, or motor problems or have a specific learning disability or difference, such as dyslexia, dysgraphia, attention-deficit hyperactivity disorder, or higher level language disorders, which can only be identified with certainty when a child is 6 years of age or older. It also is helpful to perform a comprehensive neurodevelopmental and academic assessment at the end of first grade to monitor academic performance. If problems are identified, then periodic follow-up every 2 to 3 years is necessary to document progress and determine the need for intervention. It also is important to continue to assess the child through adolescence. Progressive disease has been documented in teenagers born with congenital rubella and toxoplasmosis, and may occur in teenagers born with other congenital infections.

Congenital toxoplasmosis

Organism
Toxoplasmosis gondii

Mode of transmission
Mother acquires primary infection from oocysts present in undercooked meat or contaminated soil or litter

Clinical signs
Small for gestational age
Hepatosplenomegaly
Petechiae
Microcephaly
Scattered intracranial calcifications
Hydrocephalus
Chorioretinitis (focal), microphthalmia

Laboratory diagnosis
Serology
IgG by Sabin-Feldman dye test (preferred); IgG by IHA, IFA, EIA, or ISAGA (acceptable alternatives) IgM by ISAGA (preferred method); IFA or DS-EIA (acceptable alternatives) IGA by EIA
Isolation
Inoculate body fluids or tissue into mice or tissue culture
Histology
Demonstrate tachyzoites in tissue or body fluids
Detection
PCR of blood, CSF, amniotic fluid, tissue

Treatment
Pyrimethamine plus sulfadiazine plus folinic acid; consider corticosteroids if active chorioretinitis or high CSF protein

CSF—cerebrospinal fluid; DS-EIA—double sandwich enzyme immunoassay; EIA—enzyme immunoassay; IFA—indirect fluorescent antibody immunofluorescence assay; IHA—hemagglutination assay; ISAGA—immunosorbent agglutination assay; PCR—polymerase chain reaction.

FIGURE 12-11 Congenital toxoplasmosis. Congenital toxoplasmosis is caused by the parasite *Toxoplasmosis gondii.* It is acquired in utero by transplacental transmission from the mother. Infants born with congenital toxoplasmosis may have abnormal growth, hepatosplenomegaly, petechiae, and central nervous system involvement, with microcephaly or hydrocephalus, intracranial calcifications, and focal chorioretinitis. The diagnosis is the best made by specific serology performed in experienced reference laboratories. Specific detection of the infecting parasite also may be made by histopathology, culture, or DNA detection using polymerase chain reaction. A prompt and accurate diagnosis is important because specific therapy is available.

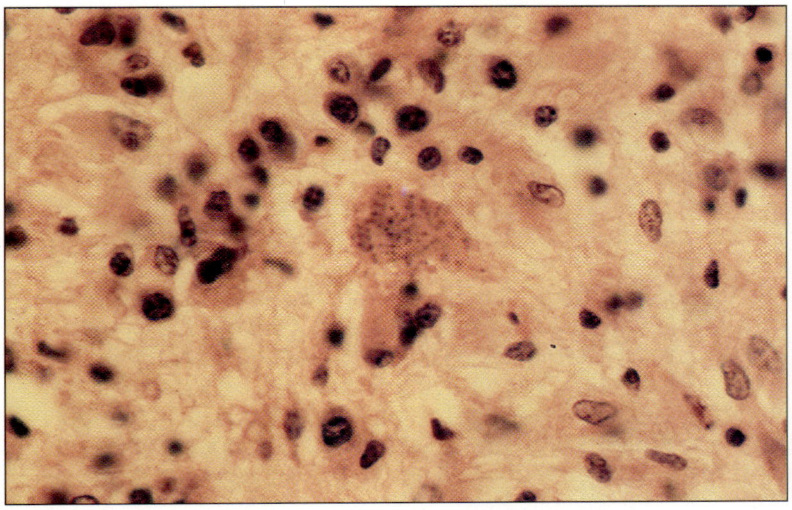

FIGURE 12-12 *Toxoplasma gondii* tachyzoites in neuron of cerebral cortex from an infant who died of congenital toxoplasmosis. Tachyzoites are crescent or oval in shape and stain well with Wright's or Giemsa stain. They occur within a well-defined space or vacuole of the host cell and are seen during the acute stage of infection.

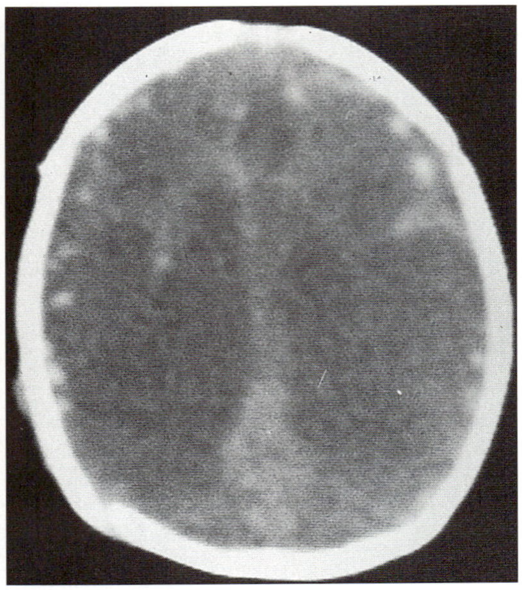

FIGURE 12-13 Computed tomographic scan of brain of infant with fatal congenital toxoplasmosis. There is near-total destruction of the cortex and brain, accompanied by massive hydrocephalus and marked, diffuse cerebral calcifications.

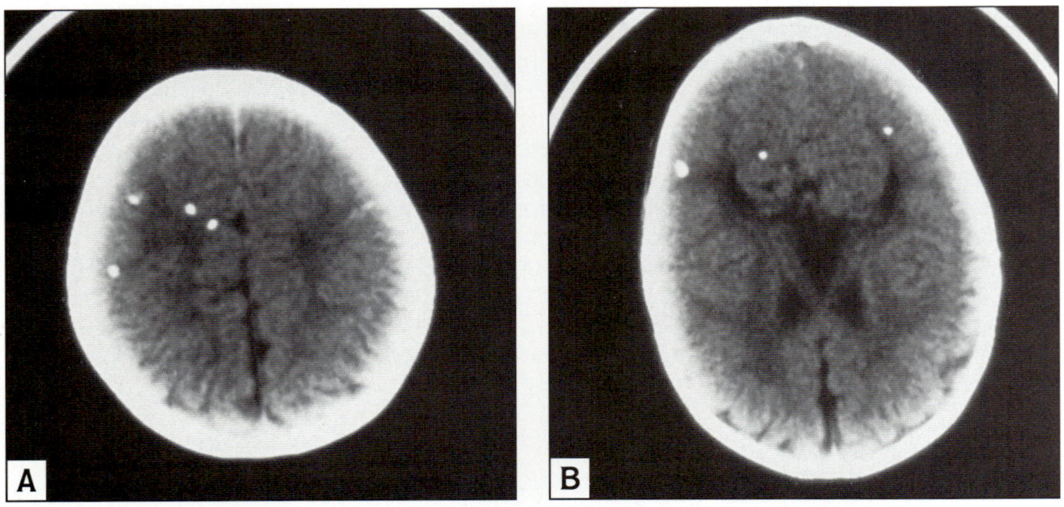

FIGURE 12-14 Cranial computed tomographic scans of a child with asymptomatic congenital toxoplasmosis who presented with strabismus due to vision loss in infancy. Scattered intracranial calcifications are visible.

Congenital rubella syndrome

Organism
Rubella virus

Mode of transmission
Mother acquires primary infection from another person, usually a child, with rubella

Clinical signs
Small for gestational age
Hepatosplenomegaly
Petechiae
Patent ductus arteriosus
Microcephaly
Chorioretinitis (pigmentary), cataracts, glaucoma
Deafness

Laboratory diagnosis
Virus isolation from nasal and throat washes, urine, blood, CSF
Serology for rubella-specific IgG and IgM by EIA, LA, or HAI

Treatment
Supportive; no specific antiviral therapy available

CSF—cerebrospinal fluid; EIA—enzyme immunoassay; HAI—hemagglutination inhibition assay; LA—latex agglutination.

FIGURE 12-15 Congenital rubella syndrome. Congenital rubella syndrome is caused by rubella virus, an RNA virus that is a member of the *Togaviridae* family. It is passed transplacentally from the mother to the fetus. Although the fetus may be susceptible to infection during any stage of development, the greatest risk for transmission and overt disease appears to be during the first trimester. Clinical manifestations at birth include abnormal growth, heart defect, hepatosplenomegaly, petechiae and purpura, and central nervous system involvement (*eg*, meningoencephalitis, microcephaly, diffuse chorioretinitis, and sensorineural hearing loss. The diagnosis may be made serologically or by isolation of the virus from body fluids. There is no specific antiviral therapy available, but the disease is preventable by appropriate immunization.

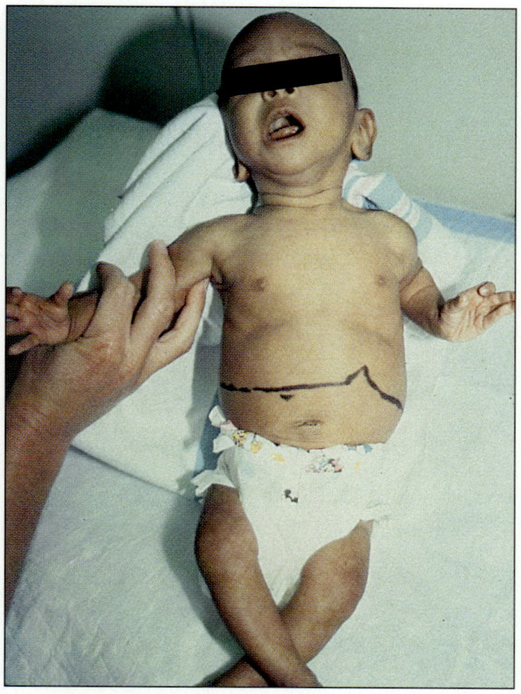

Figure 12-16 A 2-month-old infant born with congenital rubella syndrome. Clinical manifestations includehepatosplenomegaly, patent ductus arteriosus, and chronic-meningoencephalitis that produced neurologic sequelae.

Congenital cytomegalovirus infection and disease

Organism
Cytomegalovirus

Mode of transmission
Mother acquires primary infection from another person with whom she is in close contact, usually a child or sexual partner; recurrent infection in mother also may produce a congenitally infected newborn

Clinical signs
Asymptomatic infection common
Small for gestational age
Hepatosplenomegaly
Petechiae
Microcephaly
Periventricular intracranial calcifications
Chorioretinitis (focal)
Deafness (progressive)

Laboratory diagnosis
Virus isolation from body fluid, usually urine, obtained in first 21 d of life
Serology for cytomegalovirus-specific IgG and IgM by EIA or IFA.

Treatment
Supportive; experimental antiviral treatment with ganciclovir

EIA—enzyme immunoassay; IFA—indirect fluorescent antibody immunofluorescence assay.

Figure 12-17 Congenital cytomegalovirus infection and disease.

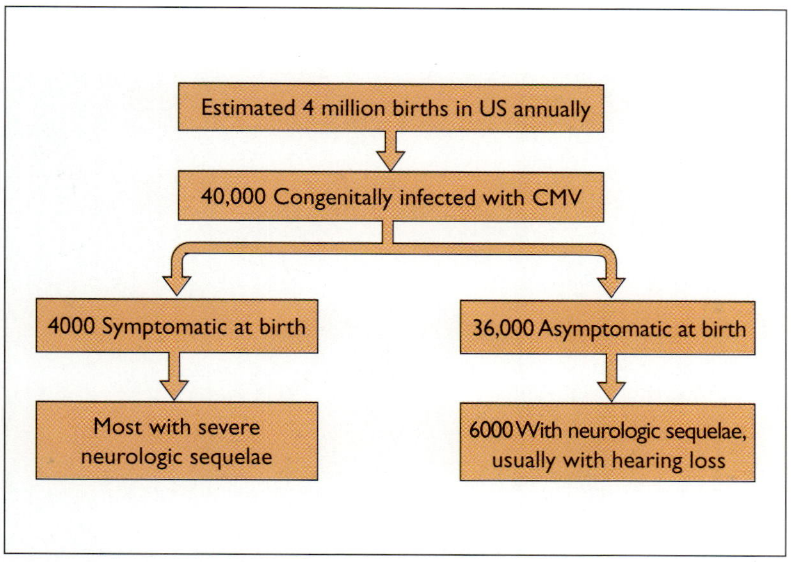

Figure 12-18 The public health impact of congenital cytomegalovirus (CMV) infection. One percent of all infants in the United States are born congenitally infected with CMV, making it the most common congenital infection in humans. Approximately 10% of congenitally infected newborns will be symptomatic at birth, and many will suffer permanent neurologic sequelae. The majority of infants with congenital CMV infection are asymptomatic at birth, yet approximately 15% of these "silently" infected infants also will experience neurologic sequelae, most often progressive hearing loss.

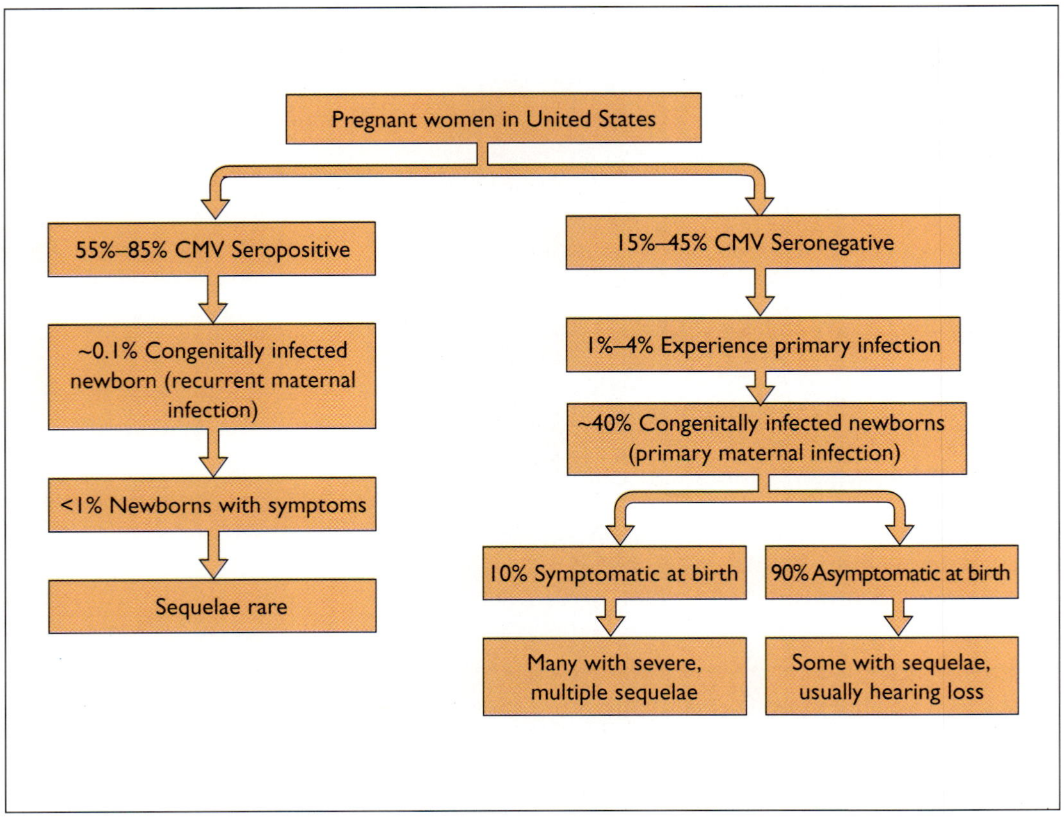

Figure 12-19 The epidemiology of cytomegalovirus (CMV) transmission in the pregnant woman and her infant. The epidemiology of this group is complex because both primary and recurrent maternal infections can produce congenital infection, even sequelae, in the infant. Because CMV is ubiquitous, most women of child-bearing age will have already experienced a CMV infection and will have detectable cytomegalovirus-specific antibody as a marker of this past infection. During pregnancy, these seropositive mothers rarely may experience a recurrent infection and transmit the virus to the infant, producing a congenitally infected newborn. Almost always, the infant is asymptomatic at birth and sequelae are unusual. However, rare reports of infants with symptomatic congenital infection from maternal recurrent infection do exist, especially if the mother is immune-compromised during pregnancy.

Between 15% and 45% of women of child-bearing age will be antibody-negative for cytomegalovirus and therefore susceptible to acquiring the virus for the first time during pregnancy and experiencing a primary infection. Approximately 40% of the time, the virus will be transmitted to the fetus, producing a congenitally infected newborn. Although most infants will be asymptomatic, even if they are born to a mother with a primary infection, there is a significant risk for sequelae (primarily hearing loss). Approximately 10% percent of newborns born from women who had primary infection during pregnancy will be symptomatic at birth, and many of these infants will experience multiple, severe neurologic sequelae, especially if there is evidence of neurologic involvement with the virus at birth.

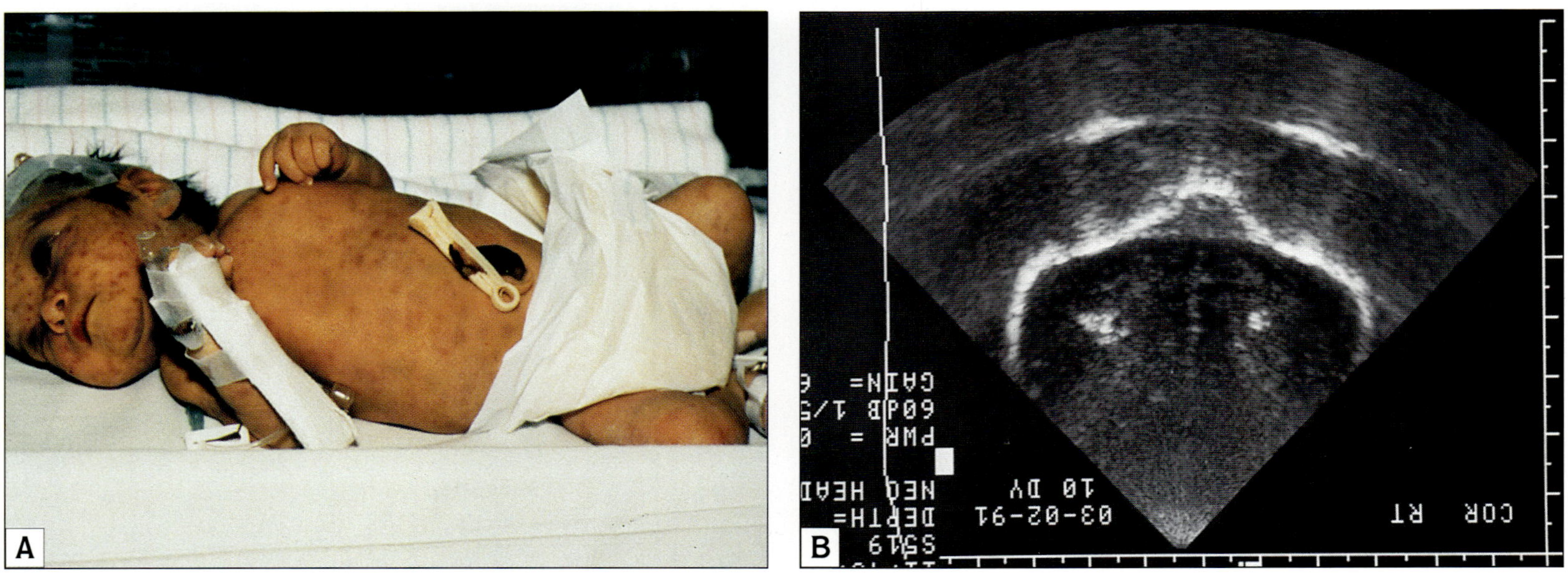

Figure 12-20 Newborn with symptomatic congenital cytomegalovirus (CMV) infection. **A,** This 3-day-old infant was born with hepatosplenomegaly and jaundice, and with ecchymosis, petechiae, and purpuric skin lesions. Laboratory evaluation revealed a platelet count of 22,000/µL, total bilirubin level of 36.5 mg/dL, and alanine aminotransferase level of 266 IU/L. CMV was isolated from his urine and blood. Clinical evaluation of this newborn's central nervous system revealed microcephaly, bilateral severe sensorineural hearing loss, and peripheral retinal hemorrhages and exudates consistent with active chorioretinitis.

(continued on next page)

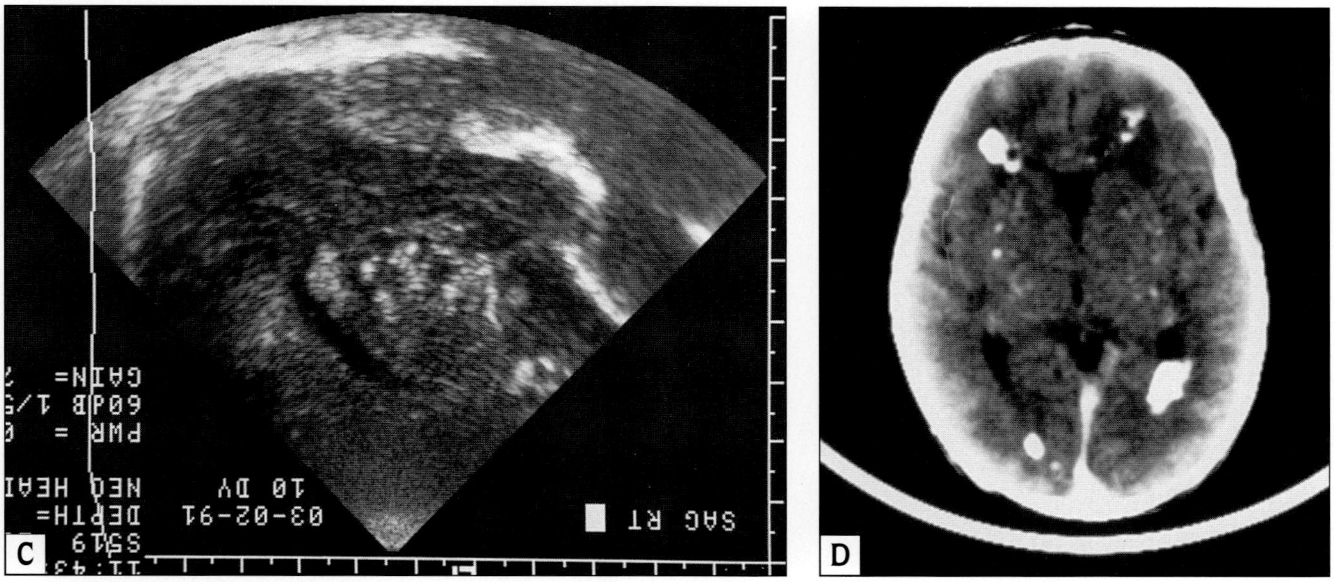

Figure 12-20 (*continued*) **B–D.** Diagnostic imaging of the head using ultrasound (*panels B and C*) and computed tomography (*panel D*). These images reveal multiple intracranial calcifications, mostly periventricular in distribution, but also involving vascular structures of the brain.

Neonatal herpes simplex virus disease	
Organism Herpes simplex virus, types 1 and 2 (type 2 more common) **Mode of transmission** Vertical; prenatal or perinatal horizontal; neonatal **Clinical signs** Vesicles (skin and mucous membranes) Meningoencephalitis Hepatosplenomegaly Petechiae Eye disease	**Laboratory diagnosis** Viral isolation Viral DNA detection by PCR in CSF **Treatment** Acyclovir

CSF—cerebrospinal fluid; PCR—polymerase chain reaction.

Figure 12-21 Neonatal herpes simplex virus infection. Neonatal herpes simplex virus infection may be acquired congenitally, perinatally, or postnatally. It is most commonly caused by herpes simplex virus type 2, but type 1 also causes disease in the newborn. Clinical manifestations include skin lesions, hepatosplenomegaly, and central nervous system involvement (*eg*, meningoencephalitis and eye disease). The diagnosis is best made by isolation of the virus from skin lesions or body fluids, and the virus is best detected in the cerebrospinal fluid using polymerase chain reaction–based DNA detection methods performed in experienced reference laboratories. A prompt diagnosis is important because specific antiviral therapy can decrease morbidity and mortality.

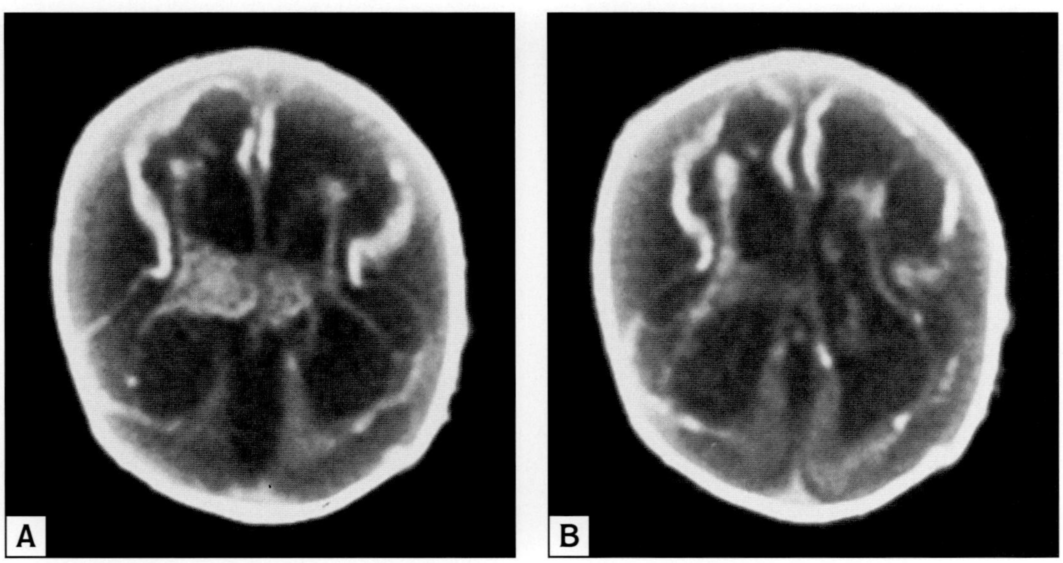

Figure 12-22 Computed tomographic image showing severe destruction of the brain in a newborn with congenital herpes simplex virus (HSV) infection. Intrauterine or congenital HSV infection occurs through *in utero* vertical transmission from mother to fetus. Although this disease is the rarest form of neonatal HSV infection, it is also the most devastating from a neurologic perspective. The disease involves the classic triad of skin vesicles or scarring at birth, eye disease such as chorioretinitis, and severe neurologic damage that includes microcephaly, hydranencephaly, or intracranial calcifications.

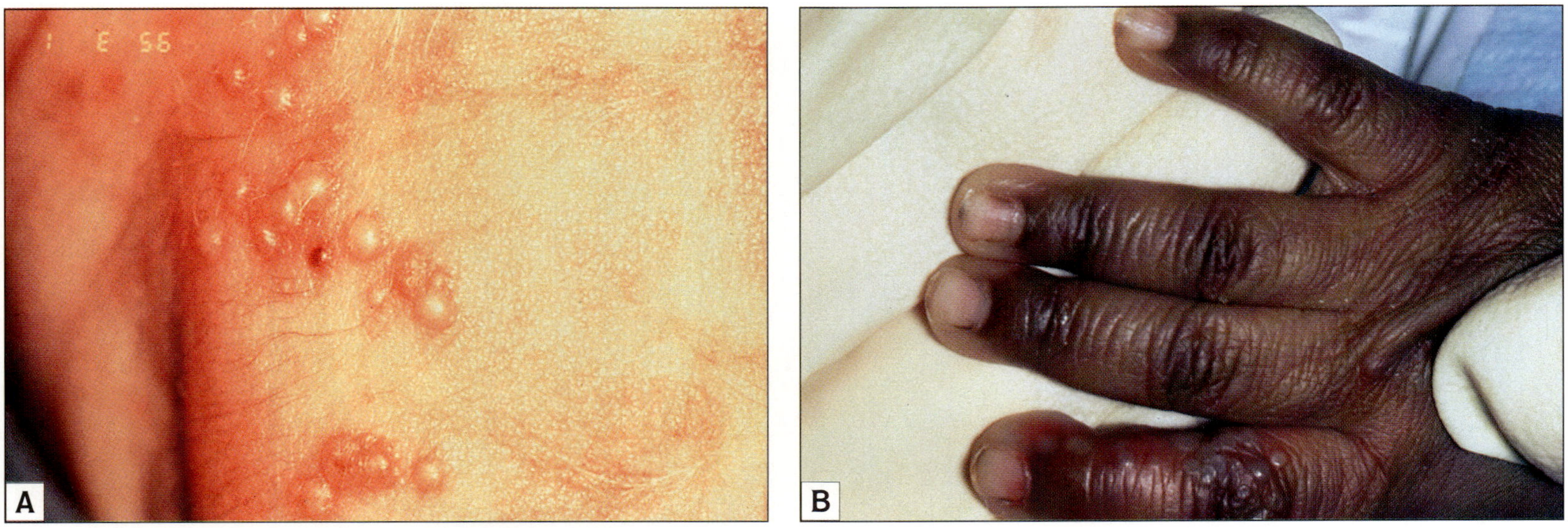

Figure 12-23 Peri- and postnatally acquired neonatal herpes simplex virus (HSV) infection. **A,** Neonatal HSV infection acquired perinatally can cause localized disease of the skin, eye, or mouth. Clusters of vesicles on an erythematous base are characteristic, and may be seen on almost any part of the body. This form of neonatal HSV infection is most commonly acquired perinatally through vertical transmission from a mother shedding HSV from the genital tract. **B,** Mucocutaneous neonatal HSV infection also may be acquired postnatally by horizontal transmission from a close family member. The vesicles on the finger of this newborn developed after exposure to an older sibling with primary herpetic gingivostomatitis, who liked to suck on his baby brother's fingers as a form of sibling play. Prompt antiviral treatment is indicated, not only to treat the skin vesicles, but also to prevent central nervous system disease, which appears to develop in approximately 30% of newborns with mucocutaneous disease.

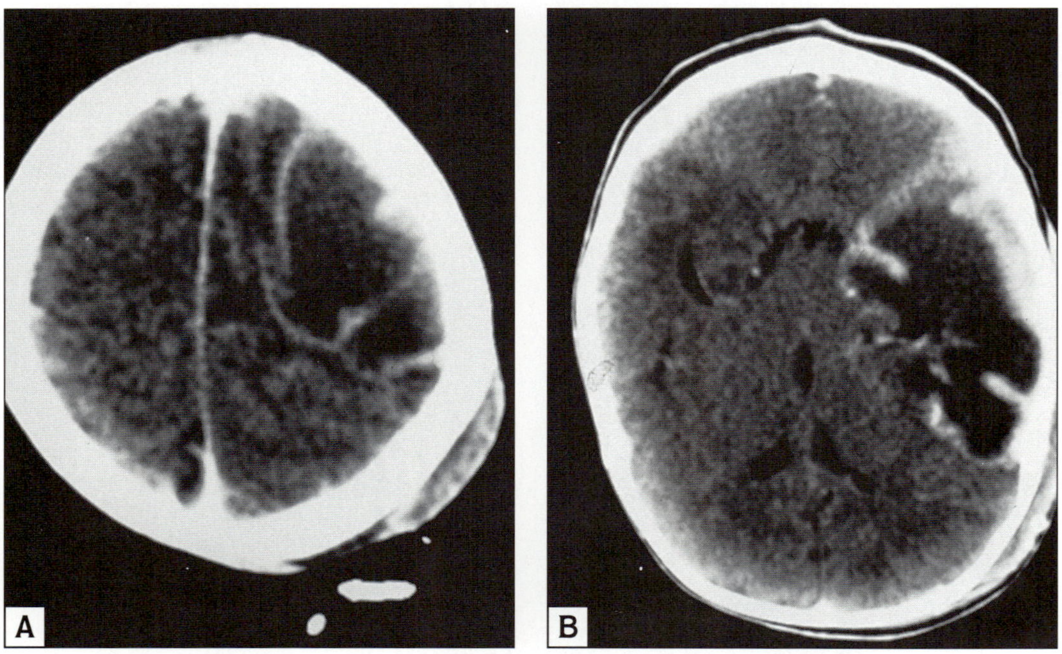

Figure 12-24 Computed tomographic image of the brain of an infant with neonatal herpes encephalitis showing extensive destruction of the temporal lobe. Infection of the central nervous system with herpes simplex virus (HSV) may occur alone or in combination with disseminated disease or mucocutaneous disease in newborns. Approximately 30% of newborns with neonatal HSV infection will have isolated central nervous system disease, and its diagnosis should be suspected in any newborn with aseptic meningitis. Clinical manifestations include seizures, lethargy, and irritability, and pleocytosis and proteinosis can be seen on cerebrospinal fluid examination.

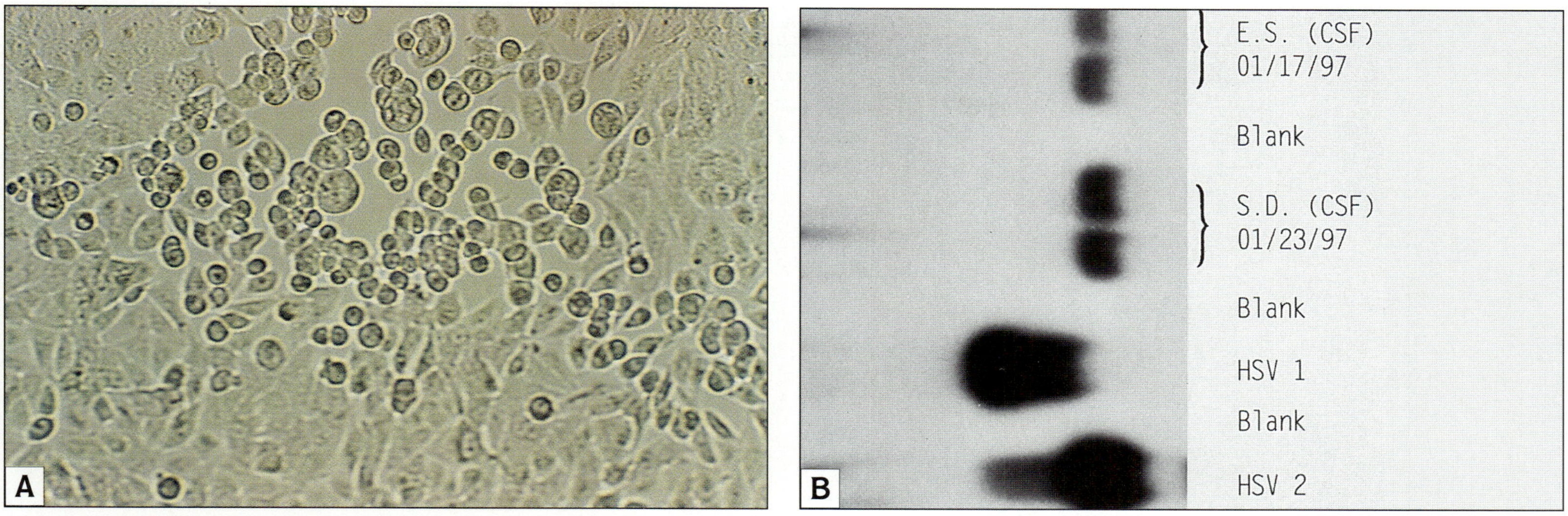

FIGURE 12-25 Detection of neonatal herpes simplex virus (HSV) infection. **A**, Typical HSV cytopathic effect on A549 cell line. The diagnosis of neonatal HSV infection can be made by isolating the virus in cell culture in samples obtained from skin vesicles, mucous membranes, tissue, or cerebrospinal fluid. The virus usually grows within 1 to 3 days on a variety of cell-culture lines. **B**, Herpes simplex virus type 2 DNA in the cerebrospinal fluid of two patients with encephalitis caused by HSV. The virus also may be detected by polymerase chain reaction–based methods that detect viral DNA in clinical samples. This method is particularly useful in the diagnosis of herpes encephalitis, because it is difficult to grow the virus from cerebrospinal fluid.

Congenital syphilis

Organism
Trepanema pallidum (spirochete)

Mode of transmission
Prenatal, vertical from mother with syphilis

Clinical signs
Hepatosplenomegaly
Pneumonia
Ascites
Skin lesions
Long bone abnormalities
CNS disease
Late sequelae

Laboratory diagnosis
Nonspecific screening tests: VDRL, RPR, ART
Specific treponemal tests: FTA-ABS, MHA-TA
Quantitative nonspecific tests can be used to assess adequate therapy or detect reinfection or relapse
CSF VDRL detects neurosyphilis

Treatment
Penicillin

ART—automated reagin test; CNS—central nervous system; CSF—cerebrospinal fluid; FTA-ABS—fluorescent treponemal antibody absorption; MHA-TA—microhemagglutination test for *T. pallidum*; RPR—rapid plasma reagin; VDRL—Venereal Disease Research Laboratory (test).

FIGURE 12-26 Congenital syphilis. Congenital syphilis is caused by the spirochete *Trepanema pallidum*. The infection is transmitted prenatally from the mother to the fetus and produces a variety of clinical manifestations, including abnormal growth, hepatosplenomegaly, petechiae and purpura, pneumonia, bone lesions, and central nervous system disease. The diagnosis is best made serologically by specific treponemal tests. Accurate diagnosis is important because specific and appropriate therapy with penicillin is curative.

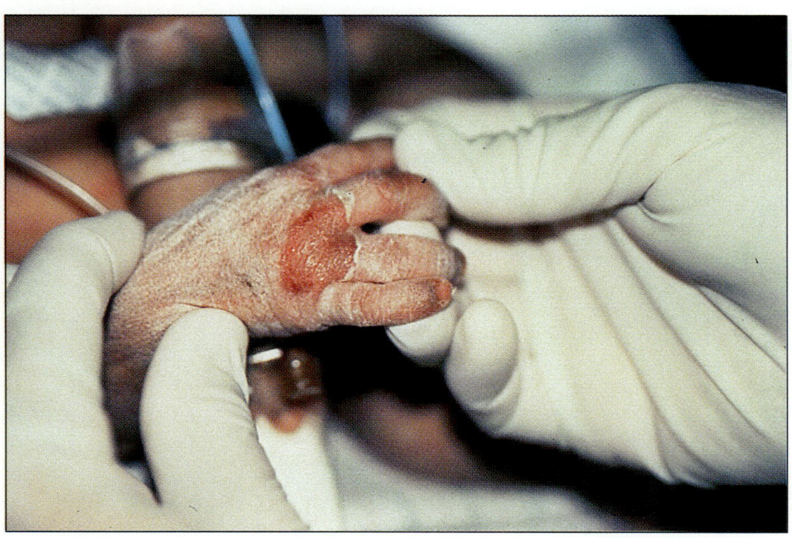

FIGURE 12-27 Skin manifestations of congenital syphilis. Newborns with congenital syphilis may have a variety of skin manifestations, including petechiae, edema, jaundice, oral maculopapular lesions, and vesiculobullous lesions. This infant had a disseminated vesiculobullous eruption that involved the palms and soles. These lesions contain infectious spirochetes.

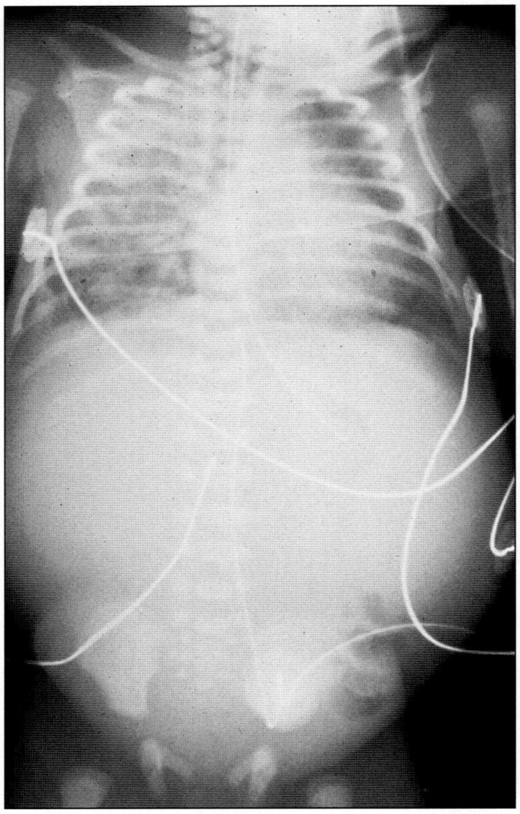

FIGURE 12-28 Common manifestations of congenital syphilis. This newborn had generalized edema, ascites, and hepatosplenomegaly. Bone lesions also are common and usually appear as a periosteitis or osteochondritis. Bone lesions usually are asymptomatic, but they may be painful and produce a pseudoparalysis in the infant. Pneumonia also can be a very serious manifestation of congenital syphilis and usually is called "pneumonia alba."

SELECTED BIBLIOGRAPHY

Remington JS, Klein JO (eds):*Infectious Diseases of the Fetus and Newborn Infant*, ed 4. Philadelphia:WB Saunders Co.; 1995.

Semin Pediatr Dis 1995, 5.

Demmler GJ:Summary of a workshop on surveillance for congenital cytomegalovirus disease. *Rev Infect Dis* 1991, 13:315–329.

Istas A, Demmler GJ, Dobbins J, *et al.*:Surveillance for congenital cytomegalovirus disease:a report from the national congenital cytomegalovirus disease registry. *Clin Infect Dis* 1995, 20:665–670.

Whitley RJ, Arvin A, Prober C, *et al.*:A controlled trial comparing vidarabine with acyclovir in neonatal herpes simplex virus infection. *N Engl J Med* 1991, 324:444–449.

Whitley RJ, Arvin A, Prober C, *et al.*:Predictions of morbidity and mortality in neonates with herpes simplex virus infection. *N Engl J Med* 1991, 324:450–454.

Ikeda MK, Jenson HB:Evaluation and treatment of congenital syphilis. *J Pediatr* 1990, 117:843–852.

Roizen N, Swisher C, Stein M, *et al.*:Neurologic and developmental outcome in treated congenital toxoplasmosis. *Pediatrics* 1995, 95:11–20.

Centers for Disease Control:Rubella and congenital rubella:United States, January 1, 1997 to May 7, 1994. *MMWR Morbidity Mortality Weekly Report* 1994, 43:391–401.

Chapter 13

Tuberculosis

Richard F. Jacobs

THIS CHAPTER CONTAINS epidemiologic maps, graphic data, clinical presentations, photographs, and radiographic representation of numerous presentations of tuberculosis (TB). It also includes interesting diseases included in the differential diagnosis of tuberculosis and appropriate cases of extrapulmonary TB. The current recommendations by the American Academy of Pediatrics Committee on Infectious Diseases relate to 1) new tuberculin skin-test guidelines and interpretation guidelines and 2) treatment guidelines and tabular representation of antituberculous medications. Specific photographs and radiographs have been included for HIV/AIDS with TB coinfection and bacille Calmette–Guérin (BCG) immunization.

The number of TB cases in the United States has declined from 1993 (25,287 cases reported to the Centers for Disease Control and Prevention [CDC]) to 1996 (21,337 cases reported to the CDC). However, these figures represent only cases of tuberculous disease; there are still no accurate records in the United States for TB infection in asymptomatic patients that have a tuberculin skin-test conversion and a normal chest radiograph. In 1996, the rate of TB in the United States was 8:100,000, representing a 6.7% decline from 1995. The regional distribution and endemic areas for increased risk of TB are included in this chapter, and the importance of TB cases in foreign-born persons is also highlighted. Of the 21,337 cases of tuberculous disease reported in 1996, 7704 cases among all ages occurred in foreign-born persons. This included 103 cases in patients under 5 years of age, 209 cases in patients aged 5 to 14 years, and 1042 cases in patients aged 15 to 24 years. Immigrants, migrant workers, refugees, persons with a history of international travel, and internationally adopted children are targeted groups for selective tuberculin skin testing due to the increased identification of foreign-born persons with tuberculosis in the United States.

The recommendation for tuberculin skin testing has moved away from screening mass populations. The new skin-test guidelines highlight those children who require immediate, periodic, or annual skin testing. The new recommendations have reduced the number of children who require annual skin testing to only those with HIV/AIDS infection and children, adolescents, and young adults who have been incarcerated.

A major change in the new recommendations for the treatment of TB includes the consideration that 6 months of preventive therapy in an asymptomatic tuberculin skin-test converter with a normal chest radiograph is adequate for effective treatment. The recommendation for intermittent therapy for treatment of TB infection and pulmonary disease is provided as an alternative to ensure adherence. Directly observed therapy should be the accepted gold standard for the treatment of tuberculous disease.

The clinician must first consider TB in order to effectively diagnose it. A hallmark in the identification of TB in children is the contact investigation. When an adult patient is diagnosed with TB, assessment and tuberculin skin testing of all contacts is mandatory and should be investigated in an aggressive and expedient manner. This chapter provides several radiographic presentations of children and adolescents with pulmonary and extrapulmonary TB. The clinical pictures and radiographs include infants with pulmonary TB and children and adolescents with pulmonary TB (including hilar adenopathy), lobar pneumonia, collapse-consolidation lesions, and cavitary lesions (including lung abscess). The manifestations of extrapulmonary TB include cervical lymphadenopathy, bone and joint TB, and tuberculous meningitis. A section addresses TB disease in HIV-infected children and the manifestations of cutaneous and disseminated BCG in HIV-infected children. The author hopes that this representation promotes proper use of tuberculin skin testing, encourages adherence to diagnostic and treatment guidelines, and provides the clinician with the incentive to include TB in appropriate differential diagnoses.

Tuberculosis in the United States: Epidemiologic Considerations

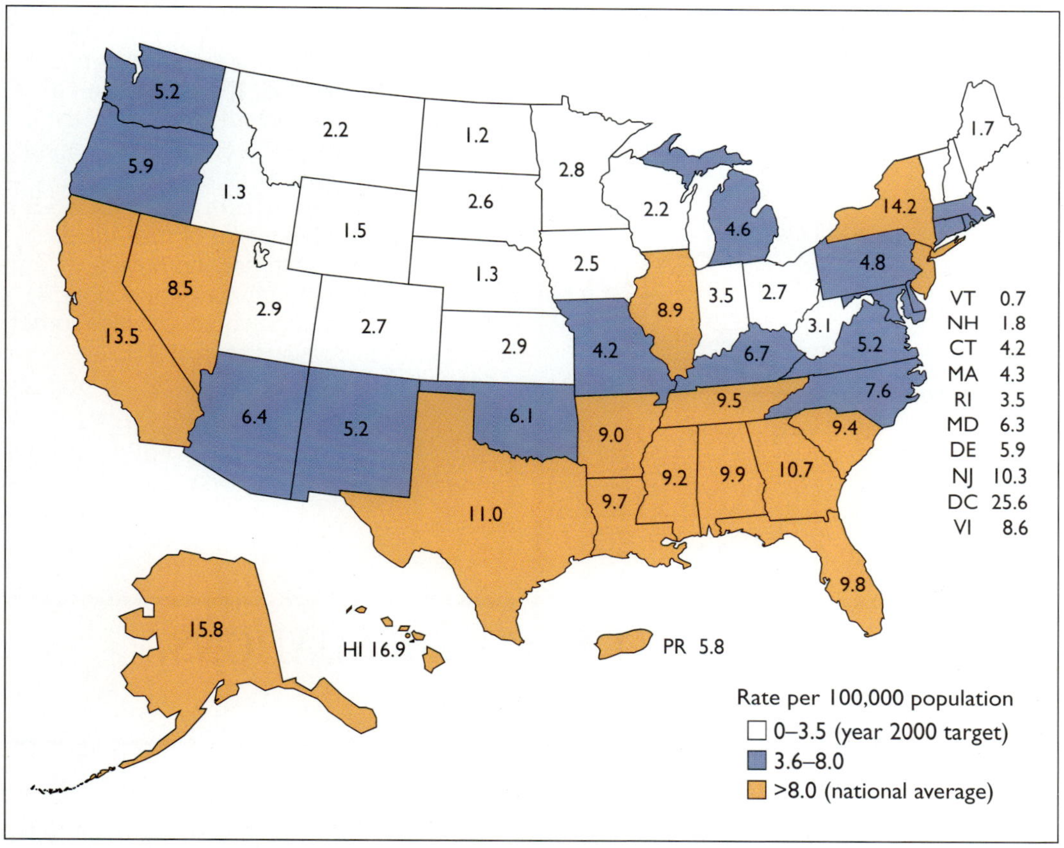

Figure 13-1 Tuberculosis (TB) case rates by state in the United States in 1996. The rates of reported cases of TB in the United States in 1996 per 100,000 population is depicted in this map. The states with higher case rates of TB include those areas 1) with larger metropolitan inter-city populations, 2) with a higher incidence of HIV/AIDS cases, 3) with a higher number of foreign-born individuals, and 4) that share borders or immigration patterns with areas that have increased rates of TB. (*Adapted from* U.S. Department of Health and Human Services, Public Health Service, Centers for Disease Control and Prevention [1]; with permission.)

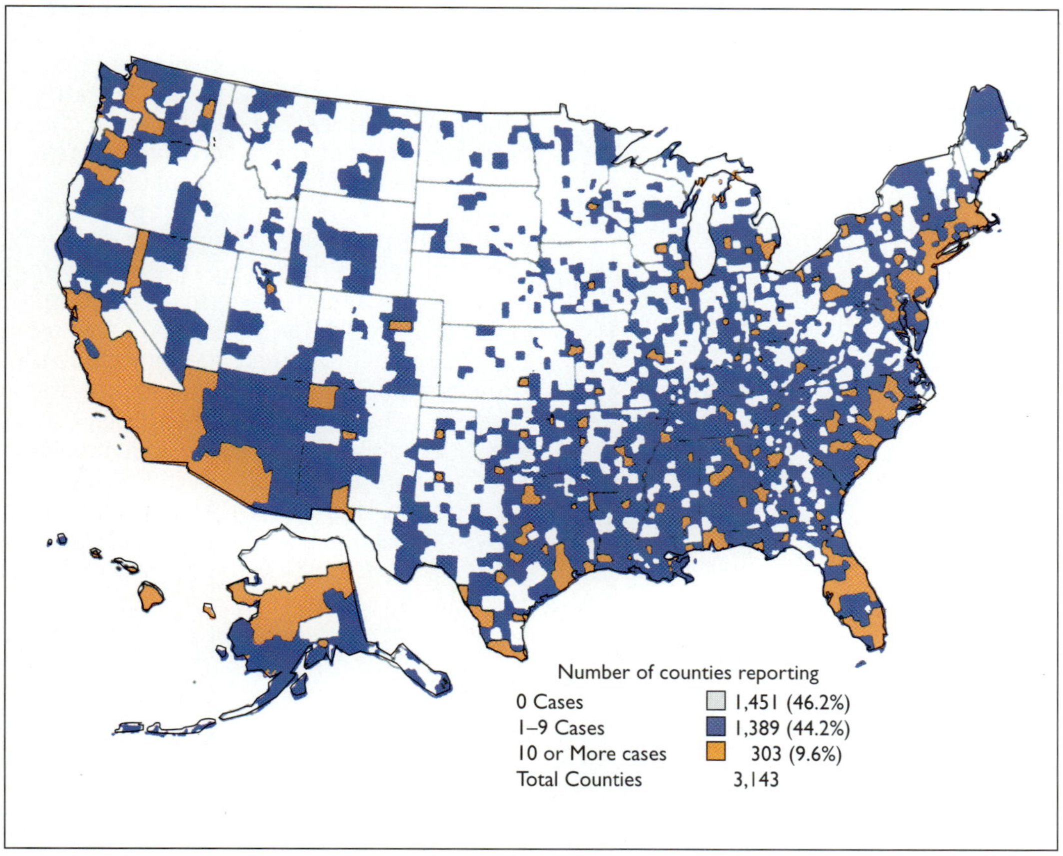

Figure 13-2 Tuberculosis (TB) cases reported by county of residence in the United States in 1996. Although Fig. 13-1 gives TB case rates by state, this graphic representation depicts reported cases of tuberculous disease by county of residence. The highest incidence of disease is localized in areas of increased population, coinciding with counties that 1) have the highest reported case rates of HIV/AIDS, 2) have a higher number of immigrant or foreign-born individuals, 3) are contiguous to areas with increased rates of TB, or 4) have any combination of the three. (*Adapted from* U.S. Department of Health and Human Services, Public Health Service, Centers for Disease Control and Prevention [1]; with permission.)

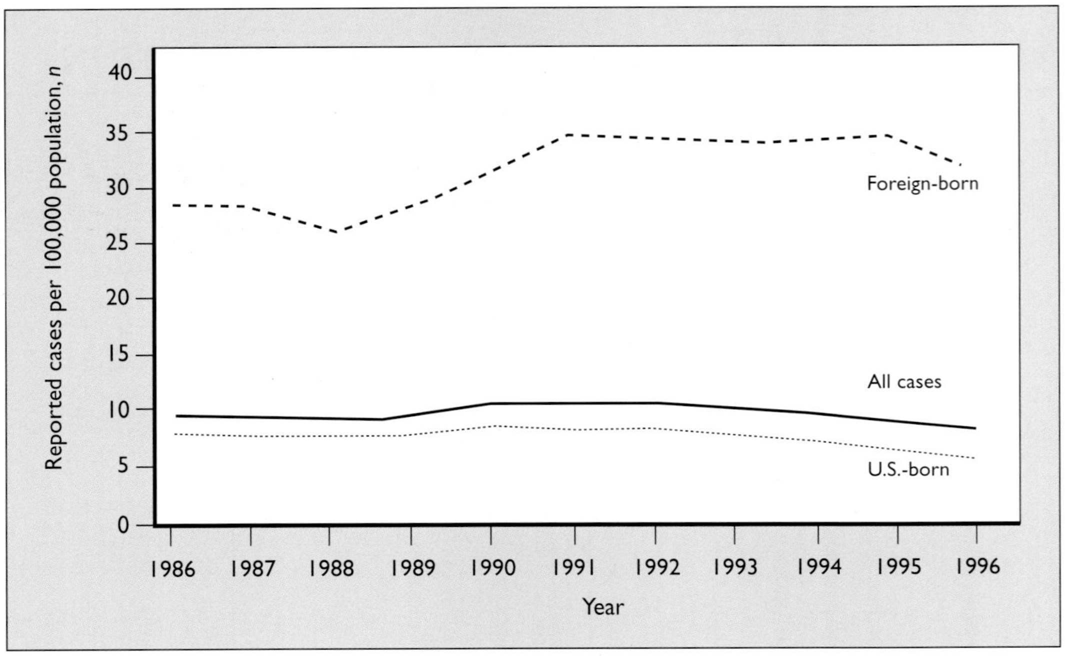

FIGURE 13-3 Tuberculosis (TB) case rates by origin in the United States from 1986 to 1996. This graph shows the reported cases per 100,000 population per year in the United States. Although these graphs show continued reporting between 8 and 10 cases per 100,000 population over the decade 1986 to 1996, there has been a slight decline in reported cases of TB in people born in the United States. Of importance is the increase in cases of TB in foreign-born persons from 1988 to 1995. Clinicians should be aware of individuals who are foreign born or who have a history of international travel and significant contact with indigenous people from a region with increased rates of TB.

TUBERCULIN SKIN TESTING, TREATMENT RECOMMENDATIONS, AND ANTITUBERCULOUS MEDICATIONS

Definitions of positive Mantoux skin test results in children*

Induration ≥5 mm

Close contact with known or suspected infectious cases of tuberculosis (TB):

- Children who live in a household with a person or persons who have (or have previously had) tuberculous disease for which 1) treatment cannot be verified as adequate before exposure, 2) treatment was initiated after the child's contact, or 3) reactivation is suspected

Suspected TB:

- Children with a chest radiograph consistent with active or previously active TB
- Children with clinical evidence of TB on physical examination or laboratory assessment that would include TB in the working diagnosis (*eg*, meningitis)

Immunosuppression:

- Children receiving immunosuppressive therapy (*eg*, immunosuppressive doses of corticosteroids) or who have immunosuppressive conditions (*eg*, HIV infection)

Induration ≥10 mm

Increased risk of disseminated disease:

- Young children (<4 y)
- Children with other medical risk factors (*eg*, Hodgkin's disease, lymphoma, diabetes mellitus, chronic renal failure, or malnutrition).

Increased environmental exposure to TB:

- Children who travel to, were born in, or have parents who were born in high-prevalence regions of the world
- Children who are frequently exposed to adults who are HIV-infected, homeless, incarcerated, institutionalized, users of illicit drugs, residents of nursing homes, or migrant farm workers

Induration ≥15 mm

Children ≥4 y of age without risk factors

*Mantoux skin test dosage is 5 TU of tuberculin; tests should be read at 48 to 72 hours after tuberculin placement; these definitions apply regardless of previous Bacille Calmette–Guérin vaccination.

FIGURE 13-4 Definitions for a positive tuberculin skin test. The Mantoux intracutaneous skin test is now recommended as the only tuberculin skin test to be used in children. This test should be read at 48 to 72 hours and induration recorded in millimeters of diameter; they should no longer be read as "positive" or "negative." The change in recommendations for the interpretation of the tuberculin skin test as positive now includes diameters of induration of greater than or equal to 5, 10, or 15 mm. All of these determinations should be made regardless of previous bacille Calmette–Guérin vaccination. Follow-up to the determination of a positive tuberculin skin test should include the immediate initiation of a contact investigation, a chest radiograph, and the consideration for antituberculous medication for infection or disease following appropriate appraisal of symptoms and physical examination findings. (*Adapted from* Jacobs *et al.* [2]; with permission.)

Tuberculin skin-test recommendations*

Immediate testing is indicated for:

Contacts of persons with confirmed or suspected infectious tuberculosis (TB) via contact investigation, including children identified as contacts of family members or associates in jail or prison in the last 5 y

Children with radiographic or clinical findings suggesting TB

Children emigrating from endemic countries (*eg*, Asia, Middle East, Africa, Latin America)

Children with a history of travel to endemic countries, significant contact with indigenous persons from such countries, or both

Annual testing for TB is indicated for:†

Children infected with HIV or living in a household with HIV-infected persons

Incarcerated adolescents

Testing every 2–3 y is indicated for:†

Children exposed to the following individuals: HIV-infected, homeless, nursing home residents, illicit-drug users, institutionalized or incarcerated adolescents or adults, and migrant farm workers

Foster children with exposure to adults in the high-risk groups above

Testing at ages 4–6 y and 11–16 y is indicated for:

Children of parents with unknown tuberculin skin-test status who emigrated from regions of the world that have a high prevalence of TB; continued potential exposure by travel to the endemic areas and household contact with persons (whose tuberculin skin-test status is unknown) from the endemic areas should be an indication for repeat tuberculin skin testing

Children without specific risk factors who reside in high-prevalence areas; in general, a high-risk neighborhood or community does not mean an entire city is at high risk; rates in any area of the city may vary by neighborhood or even from block to bloc; physicians should be aware of these patterns in determining the likelihood of exposure; public health officials or local TB experts should help clinicians identify areas that have appreciable TB rates.

Those with increased risk of progression of infection to disease include:

Those with other medical risk factors, including diabetes mellitus, chronic renal failure, malnutrition, and congenital or acquired immunodeficiencies deserve special consideration; without recent exposure, these persons are not at increased risk of acquiring TB infection; underlying immune deficiencies associated with these conditions theoretically would enhance the possibility for progression to severe disease; initial histories of potential exposure to TB should be included for all of these patients; if these histories or local epidemiologic factors suggest a possibility of exposure, immediate and periodic tuberculin skin testing should be considered; an initial Mantoux tuberculin skin test should be performed before initiation of immunosuppressive therapy in any child with an underlying condition that necessitates immunosuppressive therapy.

* Bacille Calmette–Guérin immunization is not a contraindication to tuberculin skin testing.

† Initial tuberculin skin testing is performed at the time of diagnosis or circumstance, beginning as early as 3 mo of age.

FIGURE 13-5 Tuberculin skin-test recommendations. This table outlines recommendations for tuberculin skin testing in infants, children, and adolescents. The recommendations highlight those children for whom immediate skin testing is indicated. This would include any child who is a contact of a person with confirmed or suspected infectious tuberculosis (classic contact investigations). Recommendations are also provided for those children who should be skin tested annually or every 2 to 3 years and those who should be considered for testing at ages 4 to 6 years and 11 to 16 years during the preschool and adolescent health visits. These recommendations replace the consideration of mass-population screenings and the determination of annual skin testing in high-risk infants. (*Adapted from* Jacobs *et al.* [2]; with permission.)

Recommended treatment regimens for drug-susceptible tuberculosis in infants, children, and adolescents

Infection or disease category	Regimen*	Remarks
Asymptomatic†		
Isoniazid-susceptible	6–9 mo of isoniazid once daily	If daily therapy is not possible, therapy twice weekly may be used for 6–9 mo. HIV-infected children should be treated for 12 mo.
Isoniazid-resistant	6–9 mo of rifampin once daily	
Isoniazid- and rifampin-resistant4	Consult a tuberculosis specialist	
Pulmonary	6-monthly regimens	
	2 mo of isoniazid, rifampin, and pyrazinamide once daily, followed by 4 mo of isoniazid and rifampin once daily	If possible drug resistance is a concern, another drug (ethambutol or streptomycin) is added to the initial three-drug therapy until drug susceptibilities are determined
	or	
	2 mo of isoniazid, rifampin, and pyrazinamide daily, followed by 4 mo of isoniazid and rifampin twice weekly	If nonadherence is likely, drugs can be given two or three times weekly under direct observation in the initial phase.
	9-monthly alternative regimens (for hilar adenopathy only)	
	9 mo of isoniazid and rifampin once daily	Regimens consisting of either 6 mo of isoniazid and rifampin once daily and 1 mo of isoniazid and rifampin once daily, followed by 5 mo of isoniazid and rifampin twice weekly, have been successful in patients living in areas where drug resistance is rare.
	or	
	1 mo of isoniazid and rifampin once daily, followed by 8 mo of isoniazid and rifampin twice weekly.	
Extrapulmonary ‡	12-monthly regimens	
	2 mo of isoniazid, rifampin, pyrazinamide, and streptomycin once daily, followed by 10 mo of isoniazid and rifampin once daily	Streptomycin is given with initial therapy until drug susceptibility is known.
	or	
	2 mo of isoniazid, rifampin, pyrazinamide, and streptomycin once a day, followed by 10 mo of isoniazid and rifampin twice weekly	For patients who may have acquired tuberculosis in geographic areas where resistance to streptomycin is common, capreomycin (15–30 mg/kg/d) or kanamycin (15–30 mg/kg/d) may be used instead of streptomycin.
Other (*eg*, cervical lymphadenopathy)	*See* Pulmonary category	*See* Pulmonary category

* Duration of therapy is longer in HIV-infected persons and additional drugs may be indicated

† Positive skin test, no disease.

‡ Meningitis, disseminated (miliary) tuberculosis, bone and joint disease

Figure 13-6 Treatment regimens for tuberculosis (TB) in infants, children, and adolescents. This table gives the recommendations for the treatment of infants, children, and adolescents who have asymptomatic infection or a Mantoux tuberculin skin-test conversion, a normal chest radiograph, and the absence of clinical symptoms or signs of extrapulmonary TB. Of importance is the new recommendation that 6 months of isoniazid once daily is adequate for the treatment of asymptomatic infection. In pulmonary TB, the 6-month regimen of multiple-drug therapy continues to represent the official recommendation for appropriate treatment. For specific cases of extrapulmonary TB (*eg*, meningitis, miliary TB, and bone and joint disease), an extended treatment duration of 12 months is still recommended due to the lack of data for shorter-course therapy. All other types of extrapulmonary TB (*eg*, cervical lymphadenitis) are treated for 6 months. (*Adapted from* Jacobs *et al.* [2]; with permission.)

Commonly used drugs for the treatment of tuberculosis in infants, children, and adolescents

Drug	Dose forms	Daily dosage, *mg/kg/d*	Twice-weekly dosage, *mg/kg/dose*	Maximum dose	Adverse reactions
Ethambutol	Tablets (100 mg, 400 mg)	15–25	50	2.5 g	Optic neuritis (usually reversible), decreased visual acuity and red-green color discrimination, gastrointestinal disturbances, hypersensitivity
Isoniazid*	Scored tablets (100 mg, 300 mg) Syrup (10 mg/mL)	10–15†	20–30	300 mg (daily) 900 mg (twice weekly)	Mild hepatic enzyme elevation, hepatitis†, peripheral neuritis, hypersensitivity
Pyrazinamide*	Scored tablets (500 mg)	20–40	50	2 g	Hepatotoxicity, hyperuricemia
Rifampin*	Capsules (150 mg, 300 mg) Syrup (formulated from capsules)	10–20	10–20	600 mg	Orange discoloration of secretions/urine, staining contact lenses, vomiting, hepatitis, flu-like reaction, and thrombocytopenia; may render birth-control pills ineffective
Streptomycin‡	Vials (1 g, 4 g)	20–40	20–40	1 g	Auditory and vestibular toxicity, nephrotoxicity, rash

* Rifamate is a capsule containing 150 mg of isoniazid and 300 mg of rifampin; two capsules provide the average adult (>50 kg body weight) daily doses of each drug. Rifater is a capsule containing 50 mg of isoniazid, 120 mg of rifampin, and 300 mg of pyrazinamide.

† When more than 10 mg/kg/d of isoniazid is used in combination with rifampin, the incidence of hepatotoxicity may be increased.

‡ Administered intramuscularly.

FIGURE 13-7 Commonly used drugs for the treatment of tuberculosis in infants, children, and adolescents. This table gives the first-line therapeutic agents for the treatment of tuberculosis. It represents primarily bacteriocidal agents with their dose forms and formulations, daily dosages, twice-weekly dosages, maximum doses, and adverse reactions. It also describes combination medications that can be used in capsule form only. Specific recommendations for dosing of isoniazid in relationship to the instance of hepatotoxicity (primarily in adolescents and adults) is provided. (*Adapted from* Jacobs *et al.* [2]; with permission.)

Less commonly used drugs for treatment of drug-resistant tuberculosis in infants, children, and adolescents*

Drug	Dose forms	Dosage, *mg/kg/d*	Maximum dose	Adverse reactions
Capreomycin†	Vials (1 g)	15–30	1.0 g	Ototoxicity, nephrotoxicity
Ciprofloxacin‡	Tablets (250 mg, 500 mg, 750 mg)	500–1500 (in two divided doses)	1.5 g	Theoretical effect on growing cartilage, gastrointestinal tract disturbances, rash, headache
Cycloserine	Capsules (250 mg)	10–20	1.0 g	Psychosis, personality changes, convulsions, rash
Ethionamide	Tablets (250 mg)	15–20 (in two or three divided doses)	1.0 g	Gastrointestinal tract disturbances, hepatotoxicity, hypersensitive reactions
Kanamycin†	Vials (75 mg/2 mL, 500 mg/2 mL, 1 g/3 mL)	15–30	1.0 g	Auditory toxicity, nephrotoxicity, vestibular toxicity
Ofloxacin‡	Tablets (200 mg, 300 mg, 400 mg)	400–800 (in two divided doses)	0.8 g	Theoretical effect on growing cartilage, gastrointestinal tract disturbances, rash, headache
Para-amino salicylic acid	Tablets (500 mg)	200–300 (three or four times daily)	10.0 g	Gastrointestinal tract disturbances, hypersensitivity, hepatotoxicity

* These drugs should be used in consultation with a tuberculosis specialist.

† Administered intramuscularly.

‡ Fluoroquinolones are not currently approved for use in persons younger than 18 y; their use in younger patients necessitates assessment of the potential risks and benefits.

FIGURE 13-8 Less commonly used drugs for the treatment of drug-resistant tuberculosis (TB) in infants, children, and adolescents. These less commonly used drugs should be used in consultation with a TB expert. The use of these antituberculous agents may be considered in areas in which multiple-drug-resistant TB is confirmed by contact investigation or is prevalent within a specific epidemiologic focus. The consideration for drug-resistant TB is also highlighted when the contact investigation yields an individual who has been previously and only partially treated for TB. The importance of organism isolation and drug-susceptibility testing warrants the aggressive pursuit of culture specimens in all patients with suspect TB. (*Adapted from* Jacobs *et al.* [2]; with permission.)

Tuberculin Skin Testing: Application and Measurement

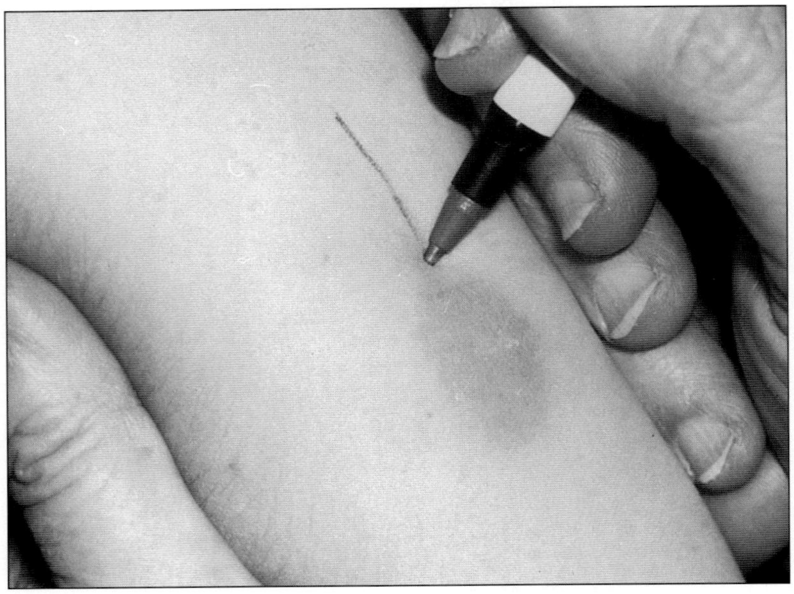

Figure 13-9 The ballpoint-pen technique for interpretation of the tuberculin skin-test reaction. The ballpoint-pen technique has been repeatedly demonstrated to be the most accurate method for measurement of the diameter of induration from a tuberculin skin test. The arm is held firmly, drawing the skin tight, while the ballpoint pen is dragged in four quadrants directed toward the area of induration. When the pen meets resistance or when blanching of the area of induration is seen, this represents the border of the area of induration. After completion of the ballpoint pen method, the area of induration can then be measured more accurately. The tuberculin skin test should be read at 48 to 72 hours by a trained healthcare professional. There is no current data to validate that parents or nonhealthcare professionals can accurately measure and interpret tuberculin skin-test reactions. Following the placement of the lines using the ballpoint-pen method, a ruler can be used to measure the diameter of induration in its single, longest axis. The exact millimeters of diameter of the tuberculin skin-test reaction should be recorded in the patient's permanent medical record. Recommended guidelines for the interpretation of the diameter of induration can then be followed, using the 5-, 10-, and 15-mm categories.

Pulmonary Tuberculosis in Infants

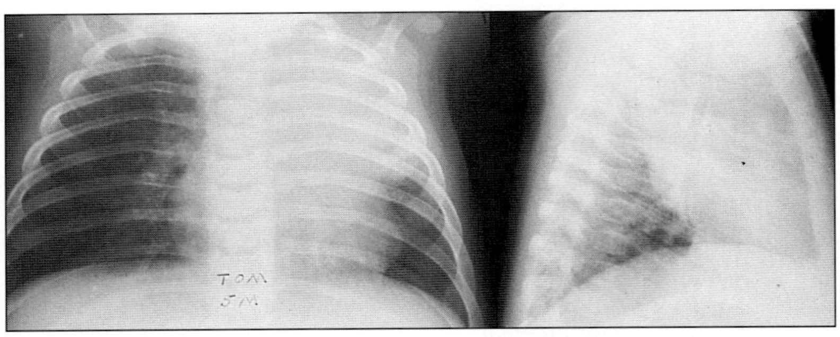

Figure 13-10 Pulmonary tuberculosis (TB) in a 3-month-old infant. This 3-month-old infant presented with fever, tachypnea, cough, and diminished breath sounds in the left upper lobe, posteriorly, on physical examination. She had been treated for lobar pneumonia with multiple β-lactam antibiotics without clinical response for 2 weeks. Pneumonia that is unresponsive to β-lactam antibiotics is a typical presentation for pulmonary TB in infants. On further investigation of historical information, it was found that the maternal aunt, who also was the primary caretaker for this infant, had cough, occasional fever, some night sweats, and a 15-lb weight loss over the previous 3 months. Her chest radiograph showed pneumonia in the right upper lobe, and her sputum revealed 3+ acid-fast bacilli, subsequently growing *Mycobacterium tuberculosis*. This infant was treated with a combination of isoniazid, rifampin, and pyrazinamide for 2 months of daily therapy followed by an intermittent therapy of isoniazid and rifampin twice weekly for an additional 4 months. The aunt's culture of *Mycobacterium tuberculosis* revealed a sensitive organism.

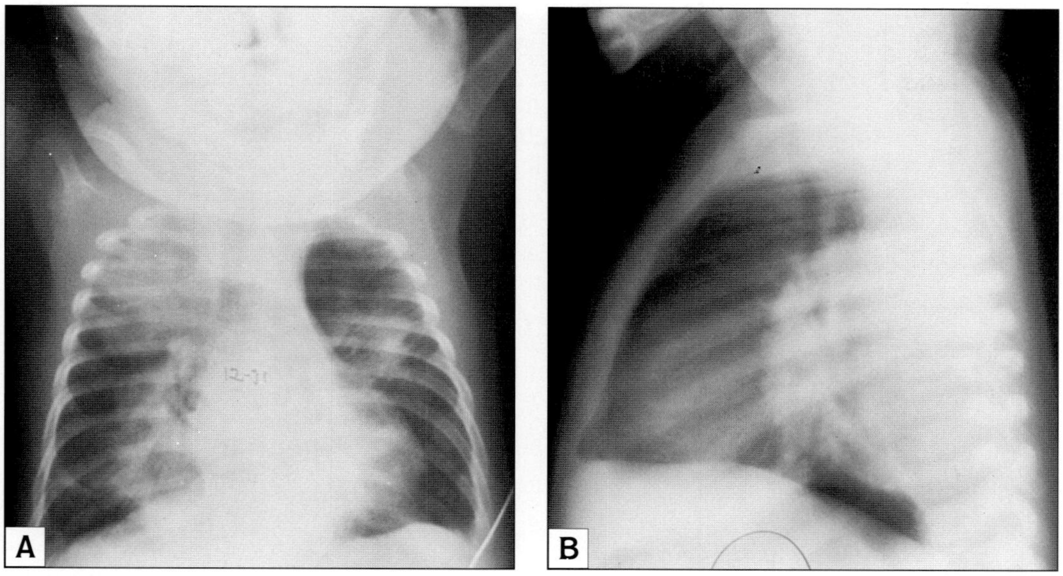

FIGURE 13-11 Chest radiographs of a 3 month-old infant with a right upper lobe mass. This 3 month-old infant presented with fever, cough, and a right upper lobe rounded-mass lesion depicted in these posteroanterior (*panel A*) and lateral (*panel B*) chest radiographs. Because this patient presented before the advent of computerized tomographic imaging, the initial referral was for neuroblastoma with the opinion that the mass was in the posterior mediastinum. However, prior to the consideration of biopsy with surgical resection, an additional history revealed two individuals in the immediate family (the child's mother and maternal grandmother) who experienced cough, fever, night sweats, and weight loss (the maternal grandmother also had a history of hemoptysis). Both the mother's and the maternal grandmother's sputum tested positive for acid-fast bacilli and grew *Mycobacterium tuberculosis* sensitive to all antituberculous drugs. The infant's early morning gastric aspirate also grew *Mycobacterium tuberculosis* sensitive to all antituberculous drugs. Thus, instead of having to undergo surgical exploration with resection, the infant (who was treated in an era when 12 months of antituberculous medication was recommended for infants with pulmonary disease) was discharged on isoniazid and rifampin for 2 months of daily therapy, followed by 10 months of isoniazid and rifampin given twice weekly. Although the infant responded clinically to this treatment and did not develop evidence of disseminated disease, today the infant would have only received 6 months of antituberculous medications (isoniazid, rifampin, and pyrazinamide given daily for 1 to 2 months, followed by 4 to 5 months of intermittent, directly-observed therapy).

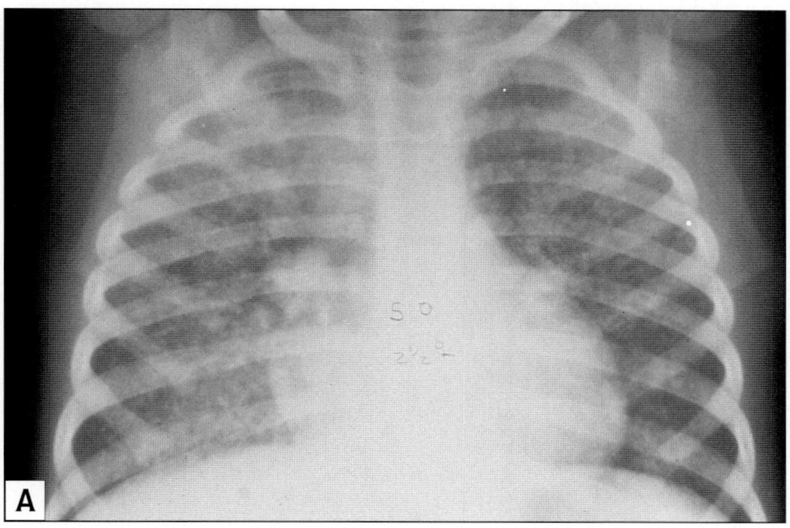

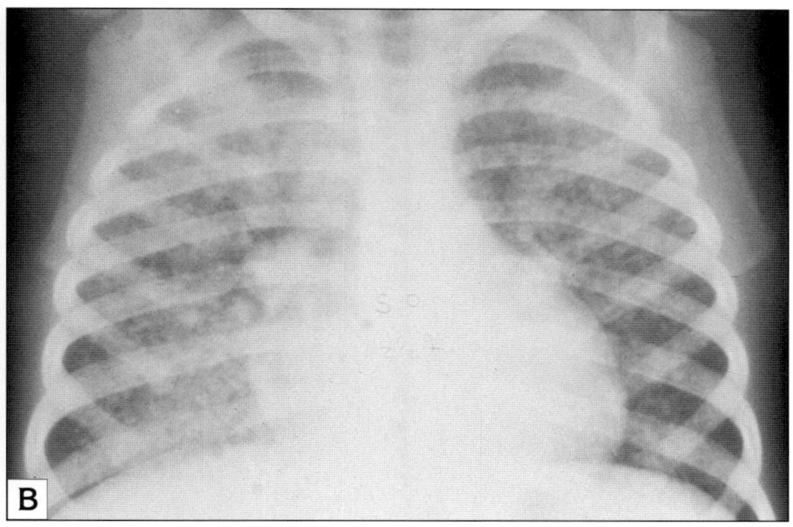

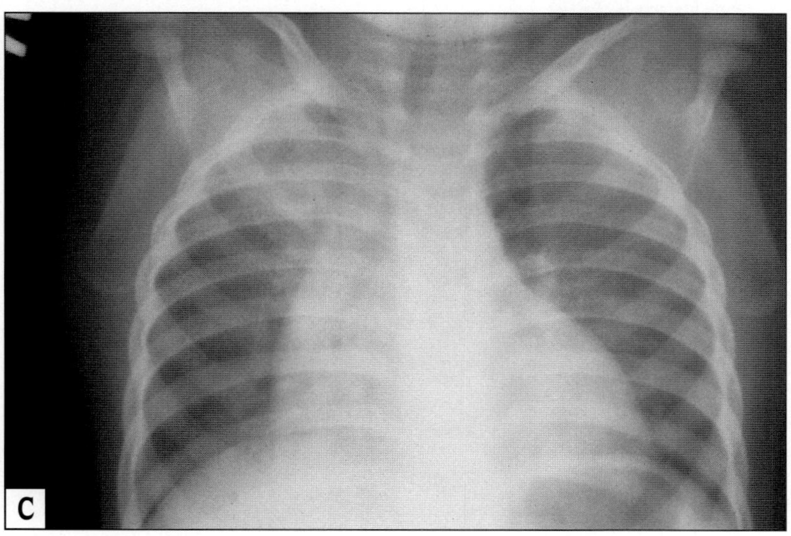

FIGURE 13-12 Radiographic presentation of miliary tuberculosis (TB). **A,** This chest radiograph of a 6-month-old infant (who presented initially with fever, tachypnea, respiratory distress, and hypoxia) shows the classic reticular nodules and multi-lobed alveolar infiltrates consistent with miliary TB (the infant also had right paratracheal and peribronchial adenopathy). Contact investigation revealed a maternal grandfather whose chest radiograph indicated right upper lobe pneumonia. Although no organism was isolated from the infant's early morning gastric aspirate, the grandfather's sputum grew *Mycobacterium tuberculosis* sensitive to all antituberculous drugs. The infant was treated initially with isoniazid, rifampin, and pyrazinamide; her hypoxia and necessity for supplemental oxygen therapy was resolved over a period of 7 days. **B,** A follow-up radiograph, taken two months later, demonstrates the slow resolution of pulmonary TB in children. **C,** This radiograph taken after 1 year shows resolution of the infant's miliary alveolar pattern of pulmonary TB. Follow-up chest radiographs for children with hilar adenopathy do not show resolution for up to 12 to 18 months. For pulmonary parenchymal disease, 6 to 12 months may be required for normalization of the chest radiograph; however, the appearance of the chest radiograph alone is not an indication for continuation of antituberculous medications.

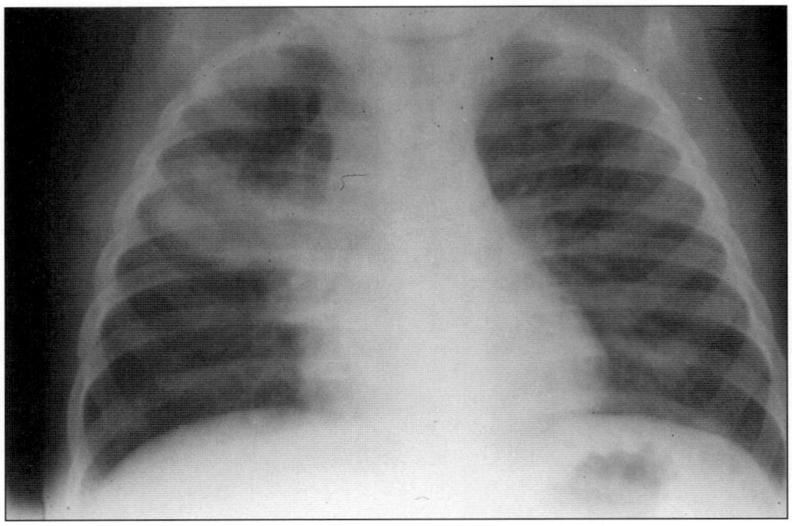

FIGURE 13-13 Collapse-consolidation pulmonary tuberculosis (TB). This posteroanterior chest radiograph demonstrates the findings of a right upper lobe collapse-consolidation area of pulmonary TB. The infant was initially diagnosed with pulmonary TB following examination for a right upper lobe pneumonia with hilar adenopathy. Following clinical response over a period of 6 weeks with antituberculous medication, the infant returned with worsening cough but with an afebrile clinical course. The chest radiograph demonstrates a linear density that represents atelectasis and persistent pulmonary infiltrate in an area distal to hilar adenopathy in the right paratracheal and peribronchial region. However, this is not an indication of a treatment failure or a lack of clinical response in the treatment of pulmonary TB in infants.

PULMONARY TUBERCULOSIS IN CHILDREN, ADOLESCENTS, AND YOUNG ADULTS

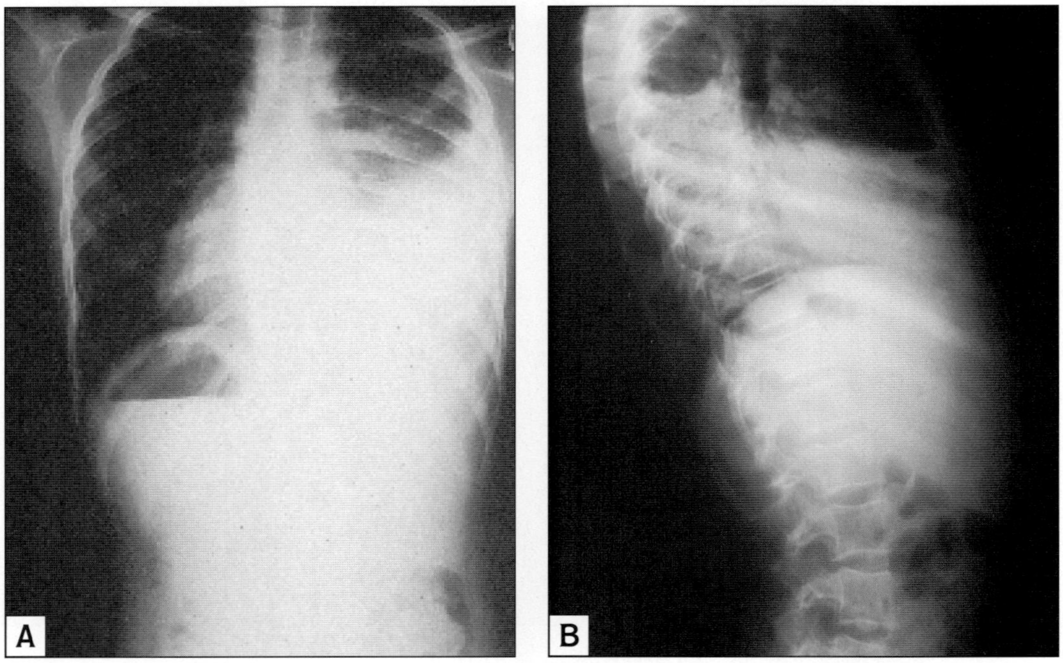

FIGURE 13-14 Pulmonary tuberculosis with pleural effusion. This 10-year-old black boy presented with fever, cough, tachypnea, dyspnea, and intercostal retractions. He had a previous history of 10 days of intermittent fever and cough that had been treated with successive courses of amoxicillin, erythromycin, and, finally, ceftriaxone intravenous therapy at a referring hospital. The posteroanterior (**A**) and lateral (**B**) chest radiographs demonstrate a left lower lobe pneumonia with large pleural effusion. Following ultrasound evaluation of the pleural effusion, which demonstrated no loculations, a diagnostic thoracentesis was performed. The fluid revealed a pH of 7.26 and 350 white blood cells with 75% lymphocytes. Acid-fast staining of the pleural effusion did not reveal organisms. Subsequent Gram stain and culture for bacterial pathogens were negative. The contact investigation of the immediate family did not reveal any individuals with a positive tuberculin skin test. This patient's tuberculin skin test elicited 15 × 20 mm of induration. No sputum could be effectively obtained, and the patient was initiated on isoniazid, rifampin, and pyrazinamide therapy. Subsequent culture of the pleural fluid grew *Mycobacterium tuberculosis* sensitive to all antituberculous drugs. Over a period of 18 months, the pleural effusion resolved and the left lower lobe normalized on chest radiograph.

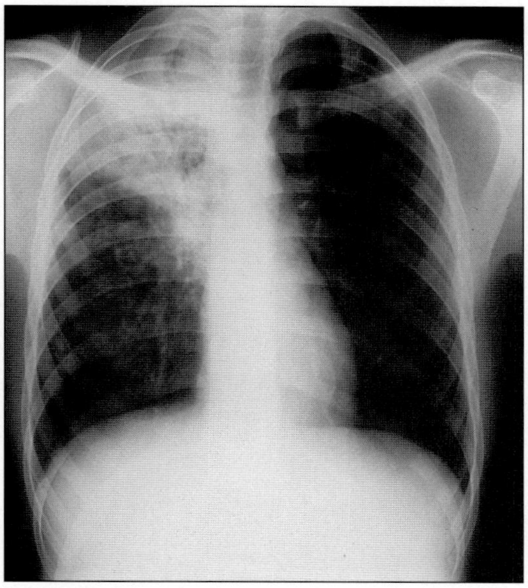

FIGURE 13-15 Pulmonary tuberculosis (TB) presenting as a right upper lobe infiltrate. This 16-year-old white boy presented with fever, cough, and a 15-lb weight loss over the previous 3 months. He had returned to the United States 2 weeks prior to this evaluation, following 1 year of providing missionary work with his family in Honduras. His tuberculin skin test status prior to leaving the United States had been negative. When performed again, the skin test revealed an induration of 20 × 25 mm. The tuberculin skin tests performed on his family were all negative. This posteroanterior radiograph demonstrates a right upper lobe consolidated infiltrate representative of pulmonary TB. Due to the negative contact investigation and lack of a clinical isolate from an area of known drug-resistant *Mycobacterium tuberculosis*, the patient underwent flexible bronchoscopy with bronchoalveolar lavage. Initially, he was started on daily therapy of isoniazid, rifampin, pyrazinamide, and ethambutol. Six weeks into his daily therapy, the culture from his bronchoalveolar lavage grew *Mycobacterium tuberculosis* sensitive to all antituberculous medications. Subsequently, he was placed on intermittent, directly observed therapy with isoniazid and rifampin and exhibited good clinical response. The aggressive diagnostic approach in this patient was warranted due to the concern over drug-resistant TB and the necessity for attempts at culture confirmation and identification of organism for susceptibility testing.

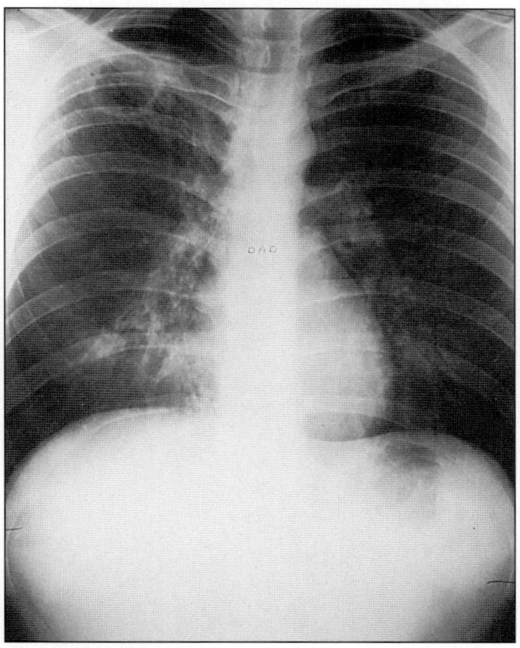

FIGURE 13-16 Cavitary tuberculosis (TB) in an adolescent. This 18-year-old black man presented to his primary care physician with a 3-week history of cough, chills, and occasional night sweats. He denied persistent fever, but stated that he had intermittent mild headaches and myalgias (no documented temperatures were provided). With the history of cough and possible weight loss, this posteroanterior chest radiograph was obtained, demonstrating a right upper lobe cavitary lesion with peribronchial infiltrates in the right middle and right lower lobes. The radiograph was interpreted as being consistent with pulmonary TB, and a tuberculin skin test elicited an induration of 20 × 30 mm. A contact investigation and subsequent tuberculin skin tests revealed eight immediate and extended family members with induration diameters greater than 15 mm. The source case was felt to be the maternal grandfather who had right upper lobe cavitary pulmonary TB caused by an organism sensitive to all antituberculous medications. The 18-year-old man was treated with isoniazid and rifampin daily therapy for 2 months with intermittent, directly observed therapy for an additional 4 months.

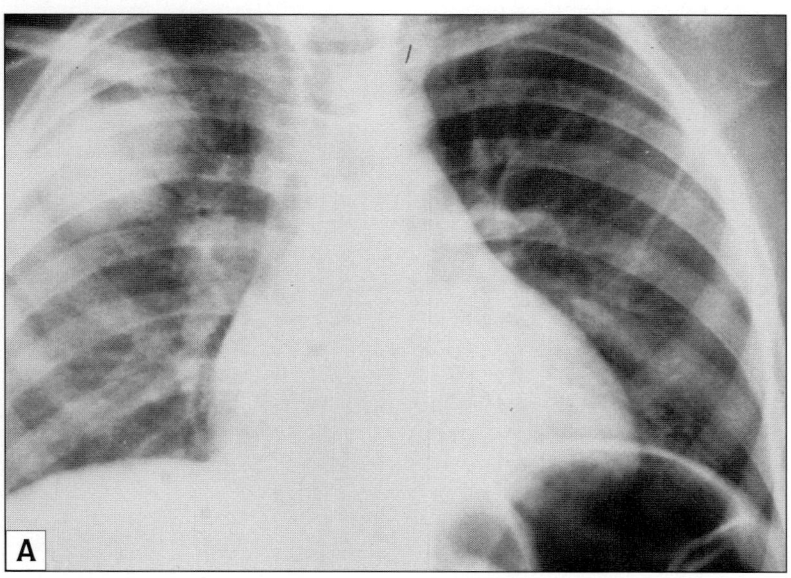

FIGURE 13-17 Pulmonary tuberculosis (TB) presenting as a lung abscess. This 8-year-old black boy presented to his local physician with an acute onset of 3 days of fever, cough, and chest pain. On physical examination, he was found to have diminished breath sounds in his right upper lobe, anteriorly and laterally. **A,** A chest radiograph demonstrated a right upper lobe round infiltrate with a potential air-fluid level in the apex.

(continued on next page)

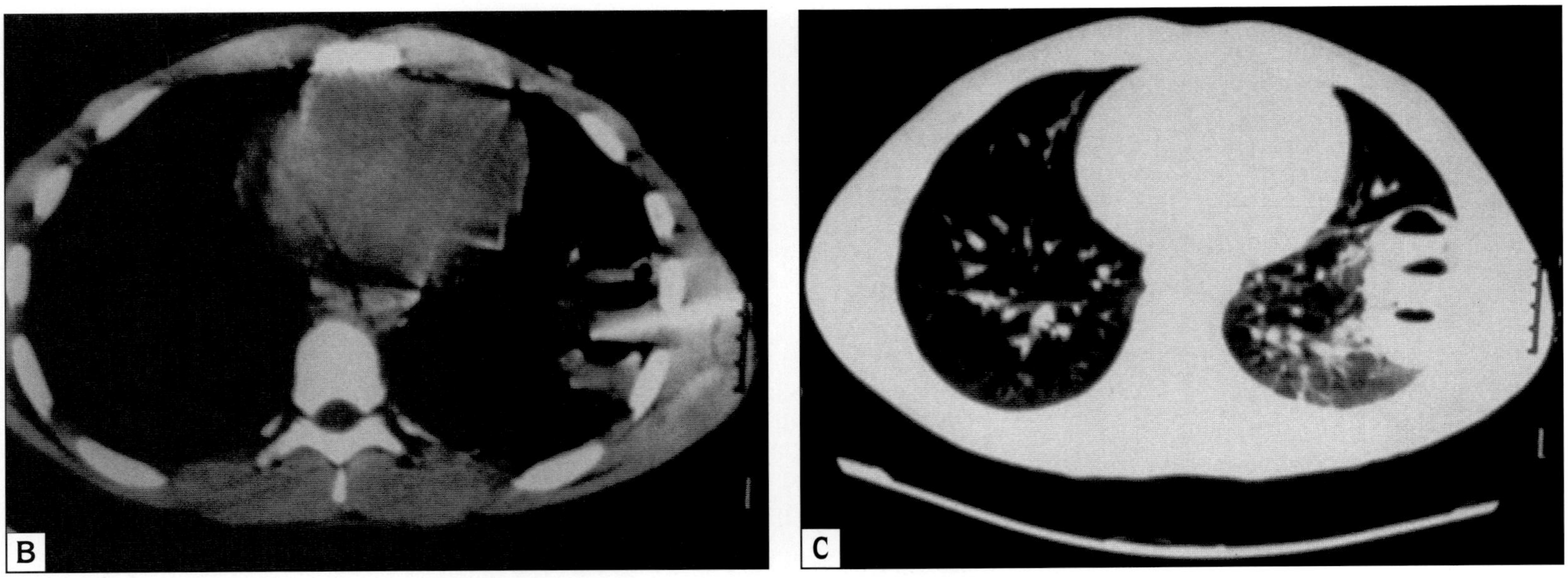

Figure 13-17 *(continued)* **B** and **C**, A subsequent chest computerized tomographic image revealed a rounded lobar infiltrate with multiple air-fluid levels. Initially, pulmonary TB was considered due to the high incidence of TB in the patient's place of residence and known contact with a person previously diagnosed with pulmonary TB. A tuberculin skin test was placed and at 48 hours revealed an induration 20 × 25 mm. Bronchoalveolar lavage via flexible bronchoscopy was performed, but the acid-fast bacillus smears and subsequent cultures were negative. The patient was placed on isoniazid, rifampin, and pyrazinamide therapy. The source cases in the contact investigation had previously yielded organisms sensitive to all antituberculous medications. No surgical intervention was performed, and the patient responded clinically over 3 weeks of daily therapy. The patient was then treated successfully with 2 months of daily therapy, followed by 4 months of intermittent therapy. A chest radiograph taken 12 months after the initiation of therapy showed marked resolution of the infiltrate with no residual cavity.

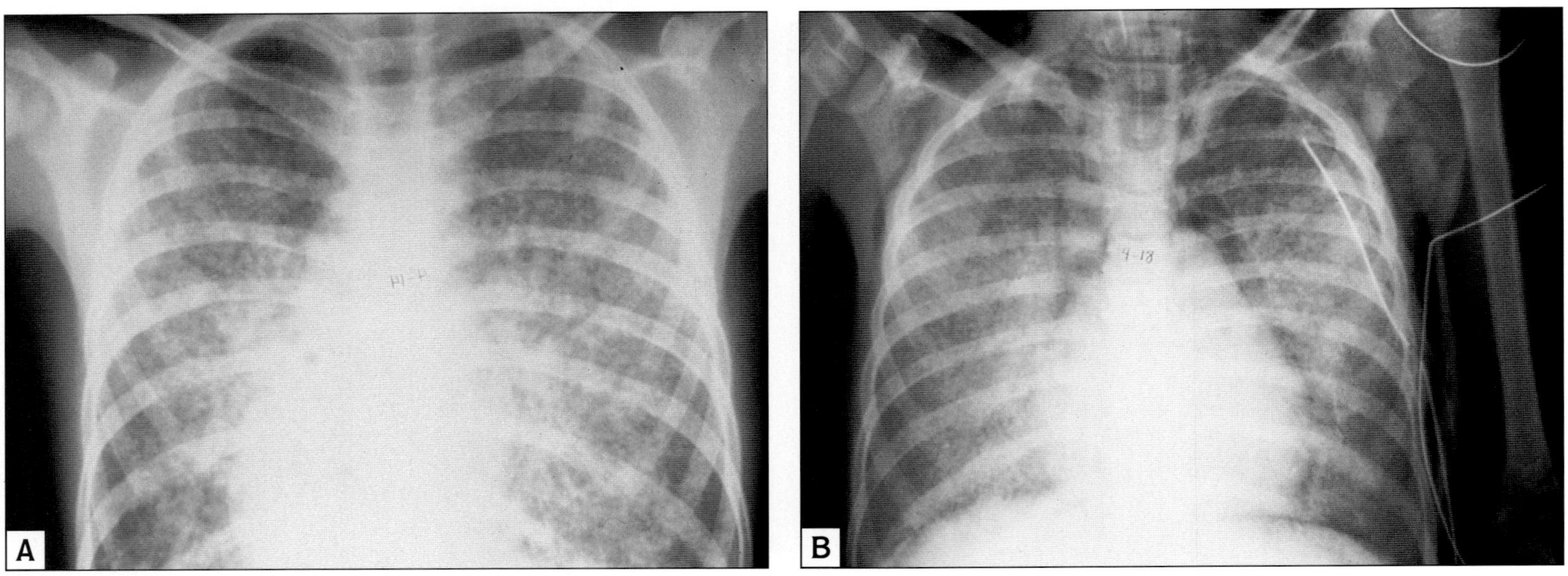

Figures 13-18 Progressive pulmonary tuberculosis (TB) in an immunocompromised adolescent. A 15-year-old black boy, who was receiving immunosuppressive therapy for a renal transplant, presented with fever, marked tachypnea, hypoxia, and a posteroanterior chest radiograph (**A**) that demonstrated diffuse nodular infiltrates and peribronchial infiltrates. Due to his presentation as an immunocompromised patient with diffuse pneumonitis, *Pneumocystis carinii* pneumonia was suspected, and the patient was placed on therapeutic doses of trimethoprim-sulfamethoxazole. Flexible bronchoscopy with bronchoalveolar lavage was performed, and direct florescent antibody was negative for *Pneumocystis carinii*. The patient deteriorated with continued hypoxia and subsequent assisted ventilation; however, bacterial cultures, Gram stain, and stains and smears for fungi and acid-fast bacillus were all negative. During his hospitalization, the patient had been placed on multiple antibiotic regimens and had received 5 days of intravenous acyclovir for the possibility of herpes simplex virus pneumonitis. He subsequently developed adult respiratory distress syndrome (ARDS), and a second chest radiograph (**B**) revealed diffuse parenchymal involvement with pneumothorax of the left lung, requiring closed chest-tube placement. The patient eventually died due to ARDS and multiple-organ failure.

(continued on next page)

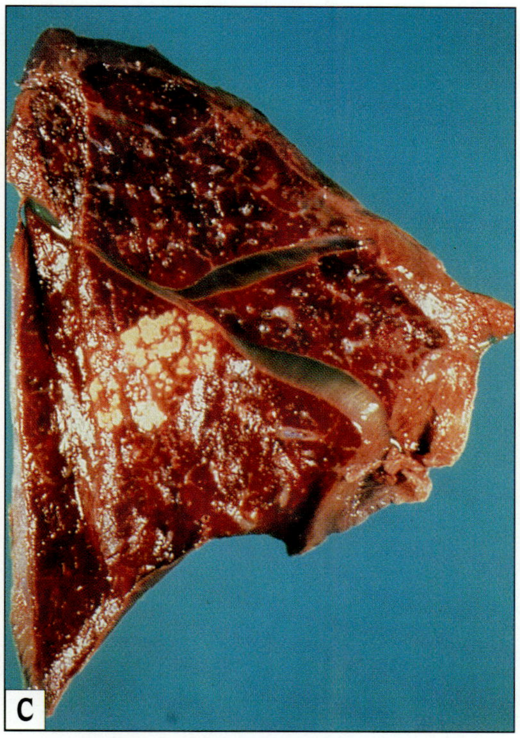

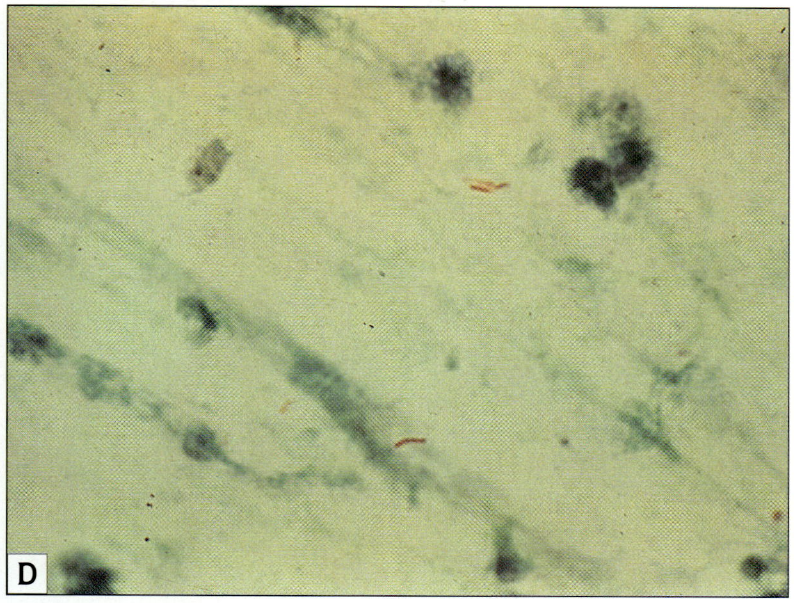

FIGURES 13-18 *(continued)* The representation of his gross pulmonary pathology (**C**) shows the lung specimen with areas of caseating granulomatous infiltration and diffuse peribronchial inflammation. A smear from the area of caseating granuloma (**D**) reveals acid-fast bacilli. Postmortem cultures grew *Mycobacterium tuberculosis* that was sensitive to all antituberculous medications. On identification of the postmortem diagnosis of progressive pulmonary TB, a maternal grandmother was identified with chronic cough, left upper lobe infiltrate, and a tuberculin skin-test induration of 20 × 30 mm in diameter. She was subsequently diagnosed and treated for pulmonary TB.

TUBERCULOSIS COINFECTION WITH HIV/AIDS IN CHILDREN

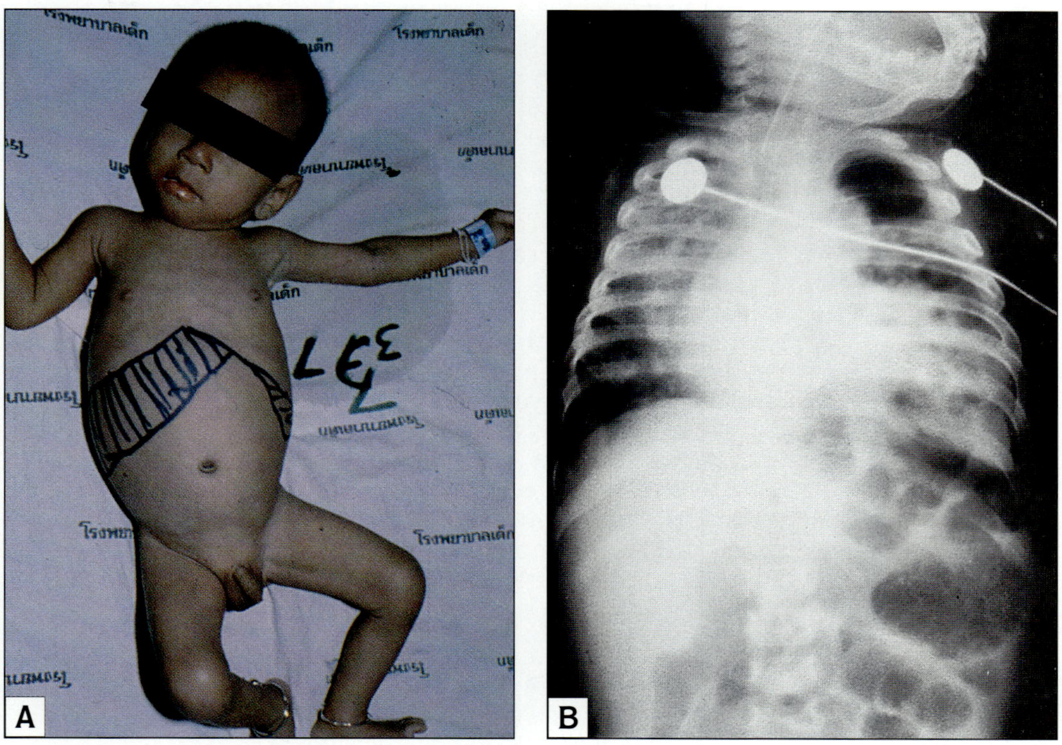

FIGURE 13-19 Infant with HIV/AIDS and pulmonary tuberculosis (TB) coinfection. **A,** This 3-month-old infant from Thailand with hepatosplenomegaly due to HIV infection presented with fever, respiratory distress, and tachypnea. **B,** The posteroanterior chest radiograph shows right upper lobe and left lower lobe pulmonary parenchymal involvement. His mother was a known contact with a tuberculin skin test induration of 20 × 25 mm in diameter, a right middle lobe infiltrate, and a sputum smear positive for acid-fast bacilli. A tuberculin skin test placed on this infant showed no induration. The mother was subsequently diagnosed with pulmonary TB, and was initiated on isoniazid, rifampin, and ethambutol therapy. The infant was placed on isoniazid, rifampin, and ethambutol with the intended treatment duration of 12 months. The diagnosis of TB in an infant should prompt the inclusion of HIV serology in the initial work up. An infant with known HIV infection and pneumonia should prompt the initial evaluation for TB.

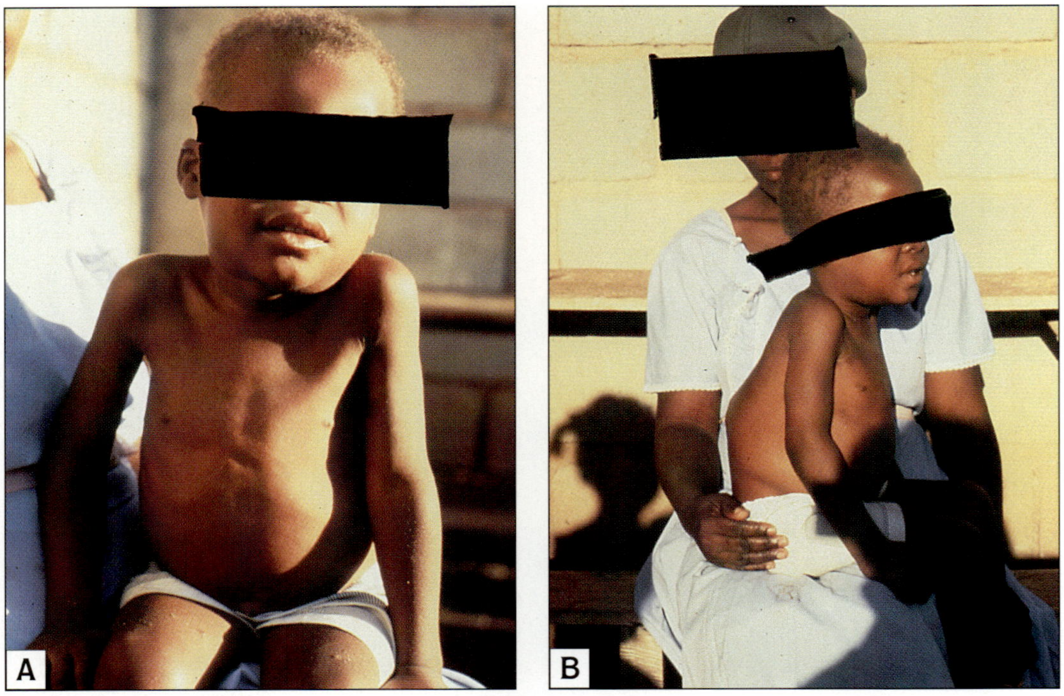

Figure 13-20 Extrapulmonary tuberculosis (TB) in a child with AIDS. **A,** This is an 18-month-old African boy with obvious kyphoscoliosis due to extrapulmonary TB. He was infected with HIV and presented to the clinic with the obvious skeletal deformity in the thoracic vertebral region. **B,** The patient on physical examination had kyphoscoliosis of the thoracic vertebra, but no radiographic capability was available. The child was a known contact to several source cases of TB, and had previously been diagnosed with HIV infection. The patient was placed on isoniazid, rifampin, and ethambutol therapy with no further follow-up available.

Extrapulmonary Tuberculosis in Children

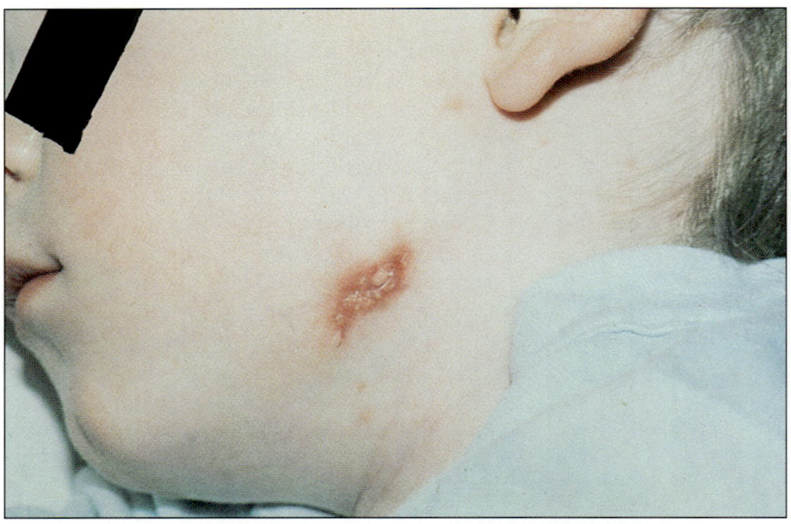

Figure 13-21 Cervical lymphadenitis. This 3-year-old white girl presented to her local physician with chronic cervical lymphadenopathy of 3.5-weeks' duration. The lymph node measured 2 ×14 3 cm in size and was thought to have some evidence of fluctuance. An incision and drainage procedure was performed with subsequent Gram stain, revealing no organisms; a culture grew no bacterial pathogens. Over the ensuing 2 weeks, the patient continued to have fever and presented with a chronic draining sinus tract in the left submandibular region. Further contact investigation revealed that the paternal grandfather had a history of fever, chills, and weight loss. His tuberculin skin-test induration was 20 × 15 25 mm, and chest radiograph showed right upper lobe infiltrate. Reexploration, excisional biopsy, and two-step cosmetic-repair procedures were performed. Subsequent resection of residual submandibular lymph nodes revealed caseating granuloma and acid-fast bacilli. Both the culture from the grandfather's sputum and from the cervical lymph node grew *Mycobacterium tuberculosis* sensitive to all antituberculous medications. The patient was treated with isoniazid, rifampin, and pyrazinamide for 1 month, with an additional 5 months of intermittent, directly observed therapy of isoniazid and rifampin.

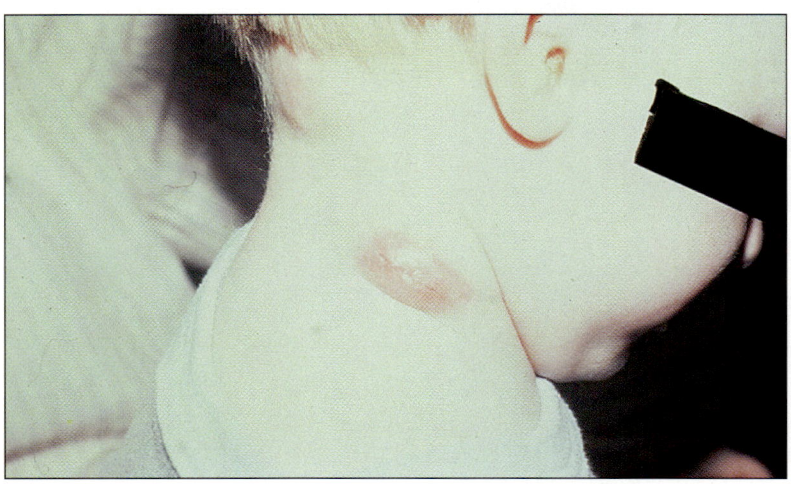

Figure 13-22 Cervical lymphadenitis. This 18-month-old white boy presented to a primary care physician with posterior and occipital subacute cervical lymphadenitis. The lymph nodes had been present for approximately 2 weeks, and the patient was found to have a history of intermittent fever, irritability, and slowly increasing neck size. The patient had a positive exposure for ticks, kittens, and cats, and lived in the Southeastern United States. Therefore, the differential diagnosis included tularemia, cat-scratch disease, nontuberculous mycobacteria, and *Mycobacterium tuberculosis.* A tuberculin skin test was placed and yielded an induration of 10 × 10 mm. A chest radiograph was normal, and an investigation of the family revealed no contacts with a positive tuberculin skin test or symptoms. An excisional biopsy of the occipital node and drainage of the posterior cervical node revealed acid-fast bacilli on smear. Subsequent cultures from the lymph node material grew *Mycobacterium kansasii.* No antituberculous medication was prescribed.

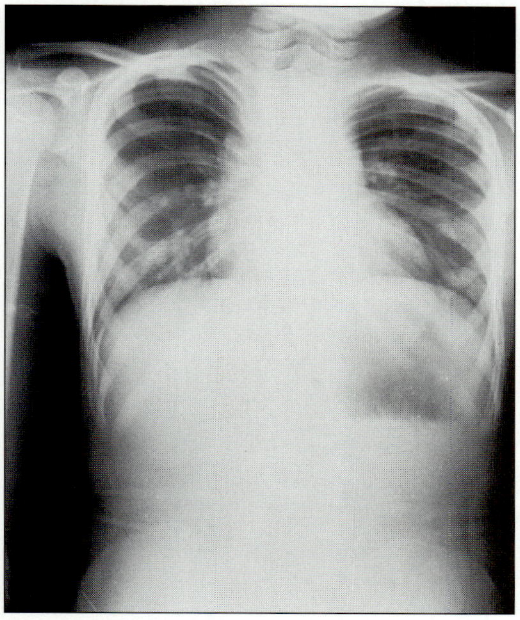

FIGURE 13-23 Tuberculous peritonitis. A 16-year-old black boy presented to the primary care physician with abdominal pain, fever, anorexia, and a 12-lb weight loss. He was a known contact of two family members with positive tuberculin skin tests, abnormal chest radiographs, and sputum smear positive for acid-fast bacilli. The chest and abdominal radiograph shown here revealed questionable peribronchial infiltrates, a possible right lower lobe infiltrate, but absence of bowel gas in the small and large intestine. Abdominal examination revealed diffuse tenderness without guarding, diminished bowel sounds, and a slightly rigid abdomen. A tuberculin skin test was placed and revealed an induration of 20 × 25 mm. A peritoneocentesis revealed serosanguineous fluid with lymphocytic infiltration, slightly elevated protein, but no organisms seen on Gram, fungal, or acid-fast stains. Due to the positive tuberculin skin test, the patient was placed on isoniazid, rifampin, and pyrazinamide therapy. Subsequent cultures of the peritoneal fluid grew *Mycobacterium tuberculosis.*

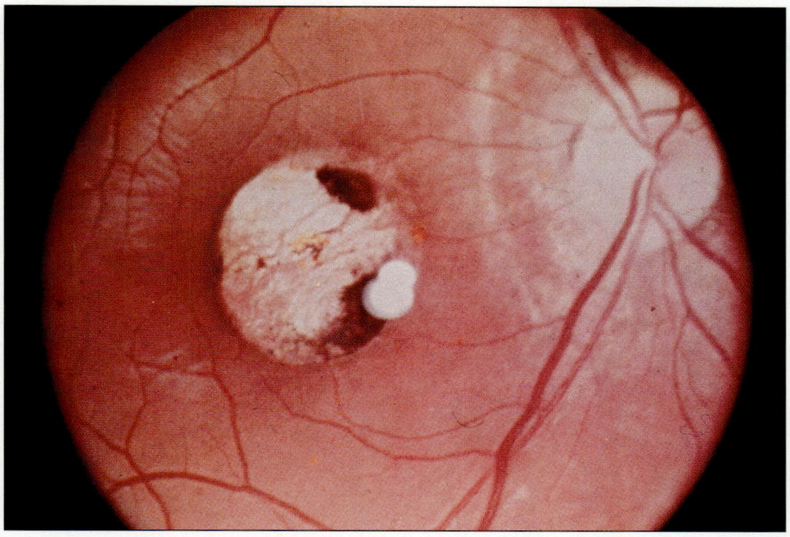

FIGURE 13-24 Tuberculous chorioretinitis. The funduscopic presentation of tuberculous chorioretinitis in a patient with disseminated tuberculosis on immunosuppressive therapy can be seen here as a localized retinal lesion with some hemorrhage and exudate.

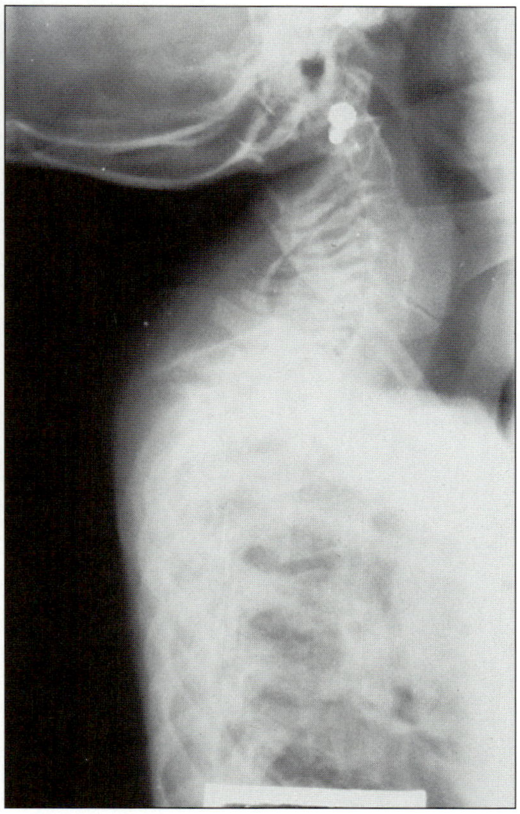

FIGURE 13-25 Vertebral osteomyelitis secondary to tuberculosis. This lateral neck radiograph shows cervical vertebral destruction with obvious kyphosis deformity secondary to the bony destruction of Pott's disease with vertebral osteomyelitis caused by *Mycobacterium tuberculosis*. The patient had a tuberculin skin-test induration of 30 × 40 mm and was a known contact of several adults with pulmonary tuberculosis. The patient received 12 months therapy of isoniazid, rifampin, and pyrazinamide given daily, followed by intermittent therapy.

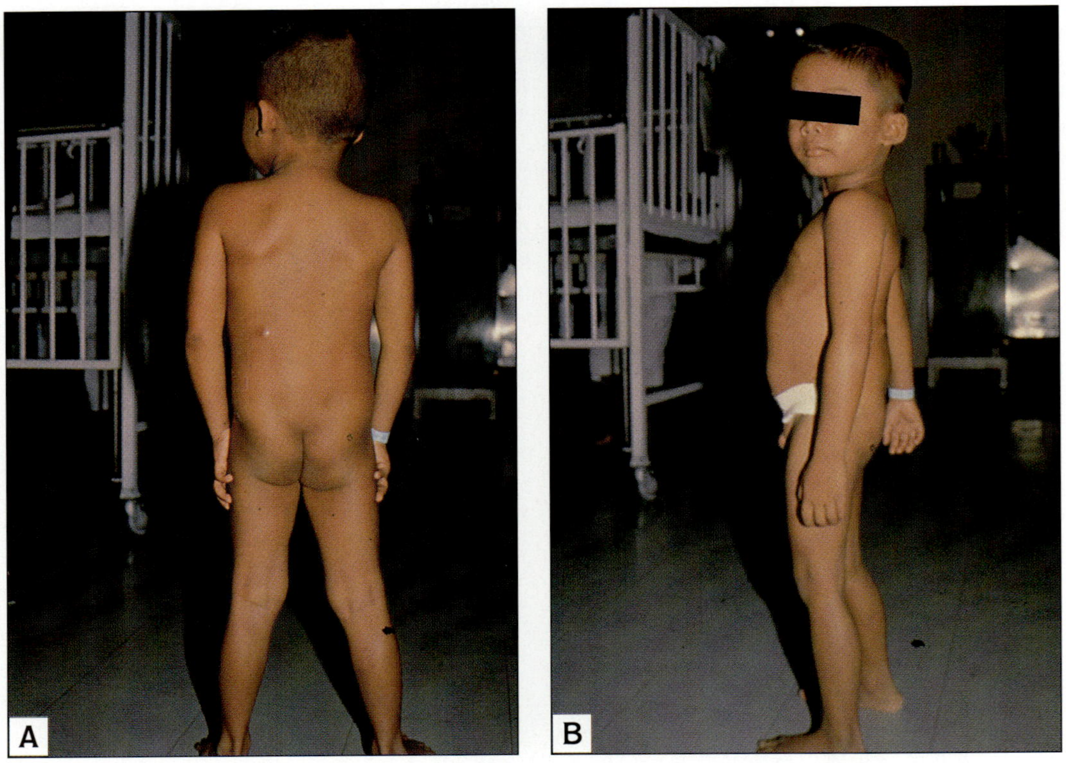

Figure 13-26 Vertebral osteomyelitis secondary to *Mycobacterium tuberculosis*. **A** and **B**, This 3-year-old boy from Thailand presented to the physician with obvious scoliosis. Radiographs demonstrated multiple lytic lesions in the thoracic and lumbar vertebral bodies. He is the known contact of several individuals with pulmonary tuberculosis. His tuberculin skin-test induration was 20 × 22 mm, and the diagnosis of Pott's disease or vertebral osteomyelitis secondary to *Mycobacterium tuberculosis* was made. He was placed on isoniazid, rifampin, and ethambutol for 12 months.

Bacille Calmette–Guérin Vaccine in Children

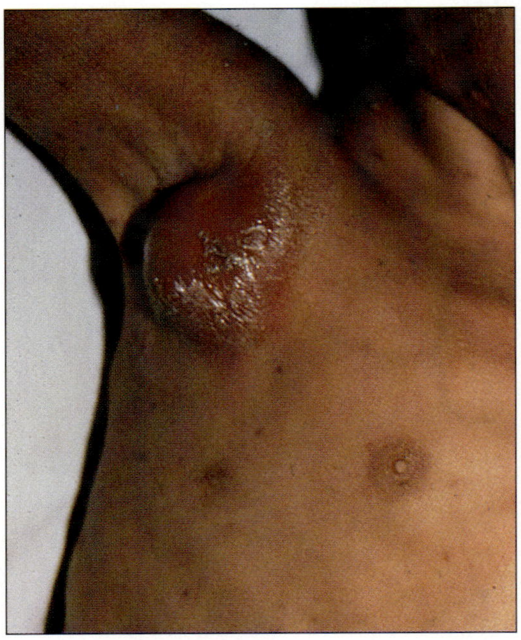

Figure 13-27 Osteomyelitis, lymphadenitis, and chronic cutaneous ulcer secondary to bacille Calmette–Guérin (BCG) immunization. This 14-month-old infant from Thailand was immunized at 1 year of age with BCG vaccine. Over the ensuing 2 months, a chronic axillary ulcerative lesion with underlying lymphadenitis had rapidly progressed to the lesion depicted here. The infant was a known HIV-infected patient due to perinatal transmission. BCG immunization was given at 1 year of age due to continued exposure to family and close contacts with pulmonary tuberculosis. The infant was also found to have an osteolytic humeral lesion and was diagnosed with disseminated BCG-osis.

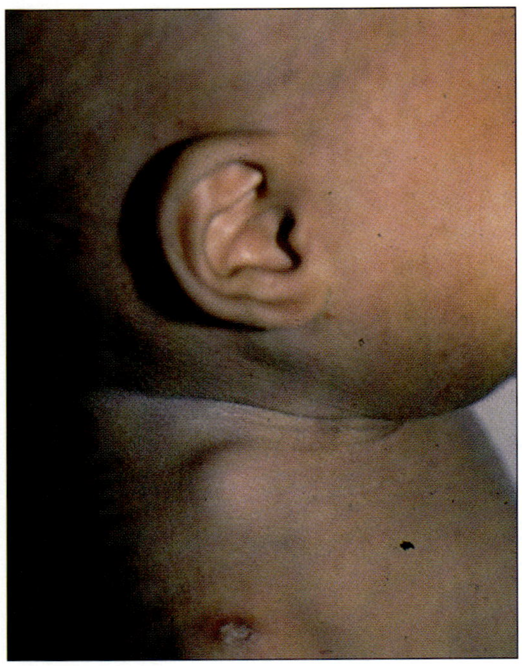

Figure 13-28 Chronic ulcer and lymphadenopathy secondary to bacille Calmette–Guérin (BCG) vaccine. This 14-month-old infant from Thailand was immunized at 1 year of age with BCG vaccine in the right deltoid region. Over the ensuing 2 months, a chronic ulcer developed, and a supraclavicular mass was noted. The supraclavicular area was thought to represent lymphadenopathy secondary to spread of the BCG organism. This infant was HIV seronegative but still manifested the finding of BCG lymphadenitis and chronic ulcers secondary to immunization at 1 year of age.

Tuberculous Meningitis

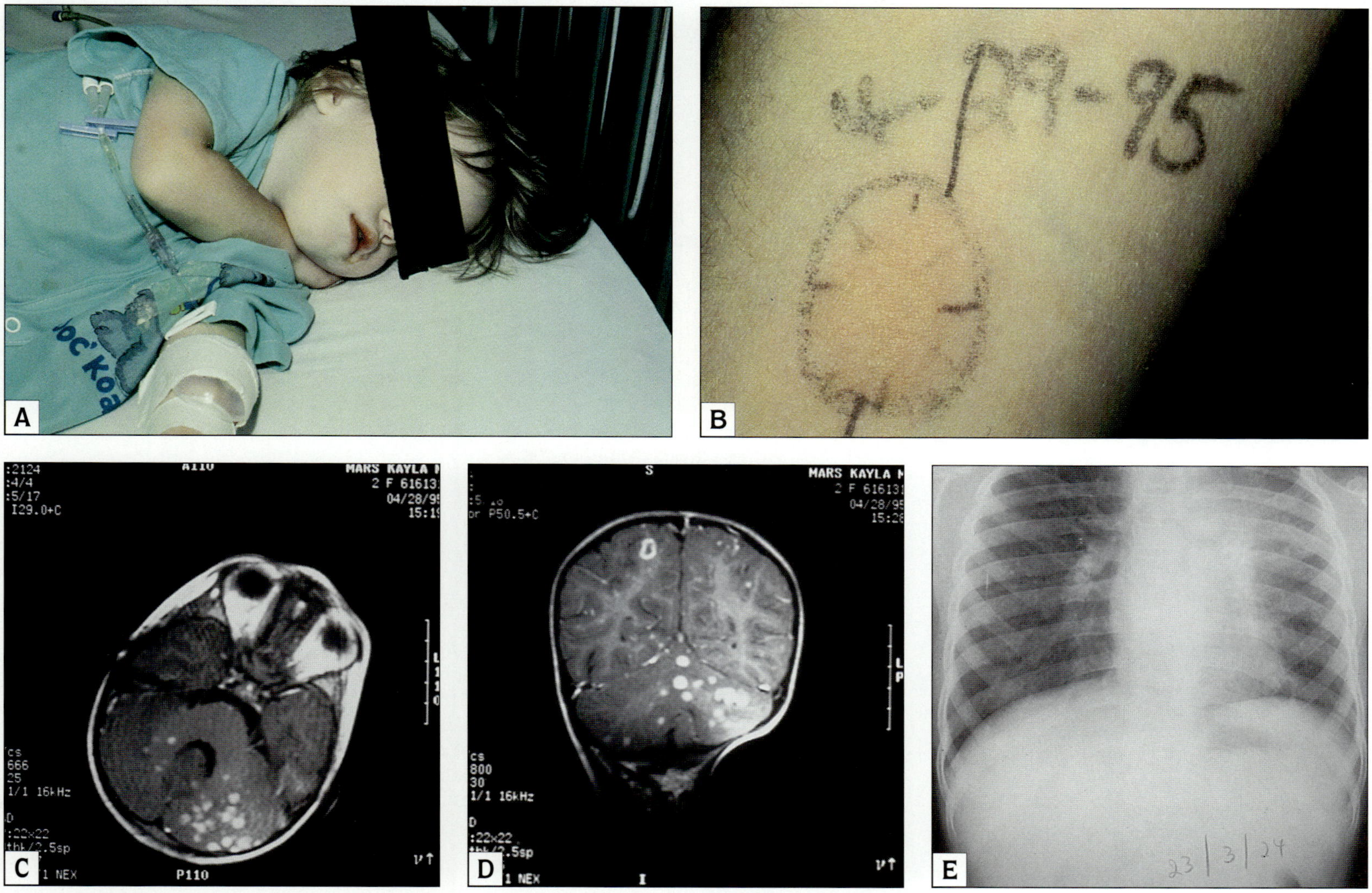

Figure 13-29 Tuberculous meningitis. **A,** This 5-year-old white girl presented with fever, obtundation, and cranial nerve palsy of the left VI cranial nerve. She had obvious meningeal signs and symptoms with nuchal rigidity. A lumbar puncture was performed, revealing cerebrospinal fluid with 357 white blood cells/mm^3 and a differential of 87% lymphocytes, 5% monocytes, and 8% neutrophils; protein, 130 mg/mL; and glucose, 20 mg/mL. *Panel A* reveals the clinical appearance of obtundation. **B,** The patient's tuberculin skin-test induration was 15 × 10 mm. **C** and **D,** the cranial computerized tomographs with contrast show multiple nodular lesions consistent with tuberculomas localized in the cerebral cortex as well as in the mid-brain and basilar areas of the cerebrum. Cerebellar lesions were also identified. She was treated initially with isoniazid, rifampin, pyrazinamide, and ethambutol plus corticosteroids. She completed a 12-month course of antituberculous therapy, and recovered without residua. On initial history during her evaluation, the paternal grandfather was present and had a chronic cough. In the examination room, it was found that he had hemoptysis and a history of night sweats, chills, and weight loss of approximately 2-months' duration. **E,** His posteroanterior chest radiograph shows left upper lobe pneumonia, and a subsequent tuberculin skin test was 30 × 35 millimeters diameter induration. His sputum revealed 3+ acid-fast bacilli, and subsequently grew *Mycobacterium tuberculosis* sensitive to all antituberculous drugs.

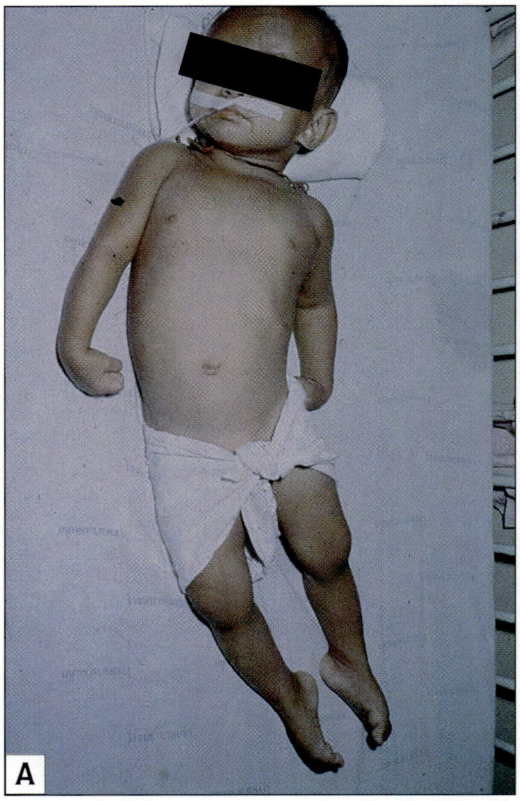

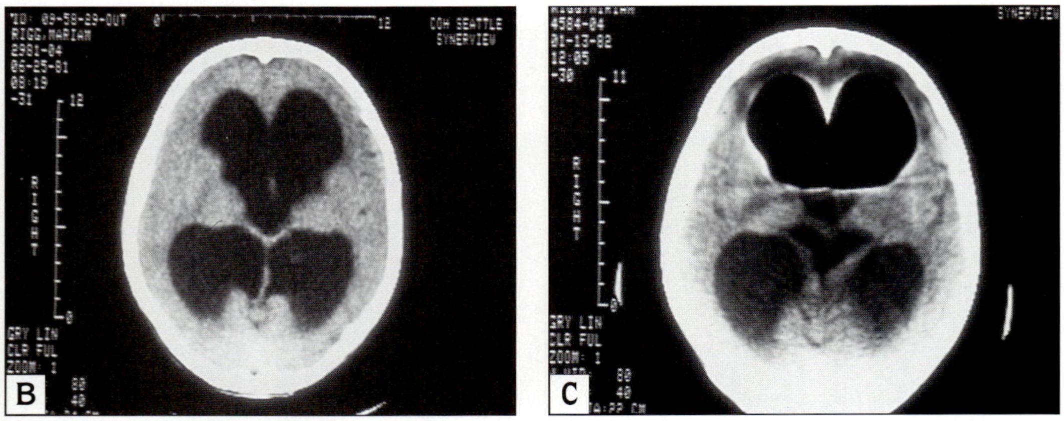

Figure 13-30 Stage IV tuberculous meningitis. **A**, This 18 month-old boy from Thailand presented with obtundation, generalized seizures, eye deviation to the right, and obvious posturing with stage-four tuberculous meningitis. **B** and **C**, In these computerized tomography scans, acute onset of hydrocephalus with obvious tuberculoma is found. The acute presentation of tuberculoma with hydrocephalus and the stage-four manifestations of tuberculous meningitis are all poor prognostic features. The patient subsequently died, and at postmortem was found (through evaluation of the cerebrospinal fluid) to have *Mycobacterium tuberculosis* with evidence of meningitis.

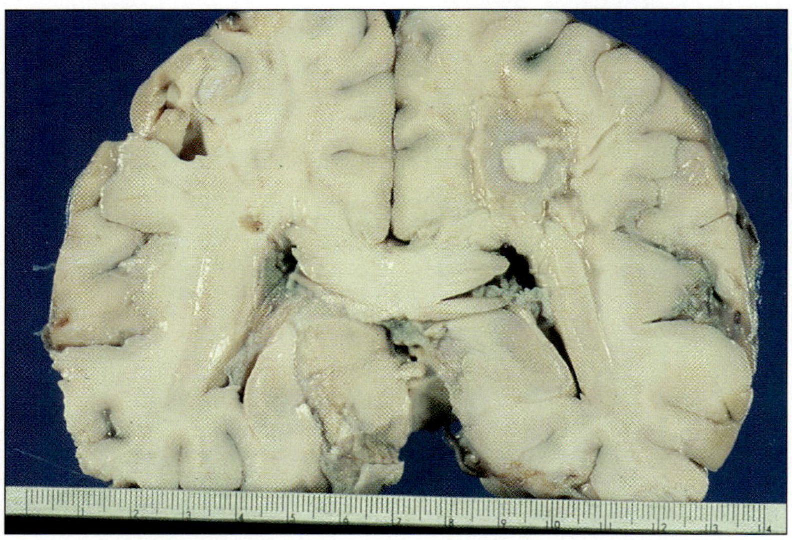

Figure 13-31 Tuberculoma. The gross finding in the left cerebral hemisphere of a focal nodular lesion is consistent with a tuberculoma. This is the postmortem specimen of the patient who presented with stage-four tuberculous meningitis, and subsequently died. On microscopic examination, the lesion was found to have caseating granulomas but did not show evidence of acid-fast bacilli on histopathologic staining.

References

1. U.S. Department of Health and Human Services, Public Health Service, Centers for Disease Control and Prevention: *Reported Tuberculosis in the United States* 1996.
2. American Academy of Pediatrics: Tuberculosis. In *1997 Red Book: Report of the Committee on Infectious Diseases*, ed 24. Edited by Peter G. Elk Grove Village, IL: American Academy of Pediatrics; 1997:541–562.

CHAPTER 14

Ehrlichiosis, Babesiosis, Rocky Mountain Spotted Fever, and Lyme Disease

David H. Spach

TICK-BORNE DISEASES have clearly become the most common vector-borne diseases in the United States. During the past 20 years, tick-borne diseases have become more common as a result of the increase in human encroachment into rural areas and greater recreational outdoor activity in areas not typically inhabited by humans. Ticks can harbor and transmit an array of infectious pathogens, including bacteria, rickettsia, viruses, and protozoa. All ticks belong to the class Arachnida, which also includes spiders, mites, and scorpions. Two major tick families contain species capable of transmitting infectious pathogens to humans: the Ixodidae, or hard ticks, and the Argasidae, or soft ticks. In the United States, the most important hard tick species that cause human disease are *Amblyomma, Dermacentor*, and *Ixodes*. Hard ticks derive their name from the hard, dorsal shield known as the dorsal scutum. Ornithodoros ticks are the most important soft tick related to human disease and are the vector for tick-borne relapsing fever. Hard ticks generally partake in long blood meals, often feeding for several days. Soft ticks have a leathery integument, but do not have a dorsal scutum. The soft ticks generally feed for brief periods (usually <30 min).

In the United States, ticks cause eight important human diseases: ehrlichiosis, babesiosis, Rocky Mountain spotted fever (RMSF), Lyme disease, relapsing fever, tularemia, Colorado tick fever, and tick paralysis. These diseases generally occur in specific geographic regions that correspond with the location of the tick vector and reservoir. Most, but not all, tick-borne diseases occur in late spring and summer during the time of active tick feeding. In recent years, investigators have made significant advances in our understanding of the biology, epidemiology, clinical features, diagnosis, and treatment of tick-borne diseases. This chapter focuses on four important tick-borne diseases: ehrlichiosis, babesiosis, RMSF, and Lyme disease.

Background on Ticks

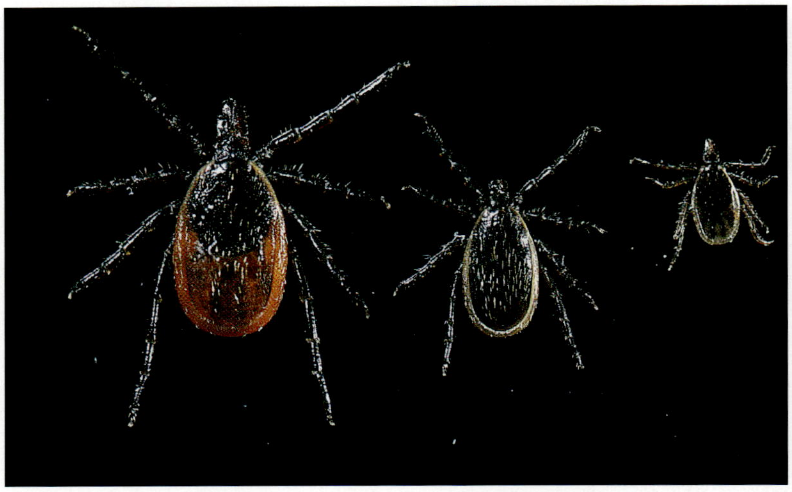

Figure 14-1 *Ixodes scapularis* ticks. Two major *Ixodes* species cause human disease in the United States: *I. scapularis* (formerly known as *Ixodes dammini*; commonly known as the deer tick) and *Ixodes pacificus* (commonly referred to as the western black-legged tick). Both of these *Ixodes* species have a characteristic tan–brown color. The *I. scapularis* female (*left*) generally is significantly larger than the adult male (*middle*). Both have a prominent dorsal scutum. This structure limits the quantity of blood ingested, and because the female ticks have a smaller dorsal scutum than that of male ticks, they can engorge to larger dimensions and thus take a bigger blood meal. The immature nymphal tick (*right*) is significantly smaller than either of the adults. *I. pacificus* ticks look similar to the *I. scapularis* tick. In the United States, ixodid ticks are the vector for multiple tick-borne diseases, including Lyme disease, babesiosis, and human granulocytic ehrlichiosis.

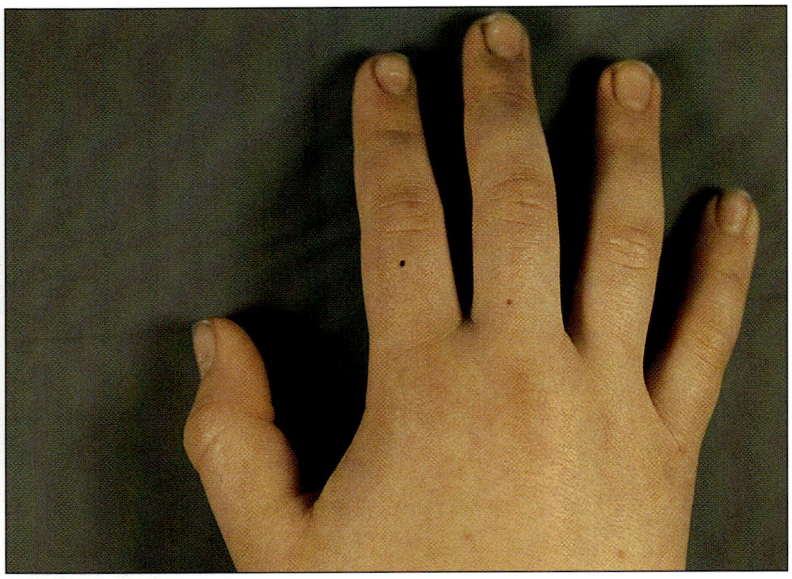

Figure 14-2 Ixodid nymphal tick on the hand of a child. Detecting a feeding ixodid nymphal tick can be difficult because of the relatively small size of these ticks. The nonengorged ixodid nymphal tick shown here on the index finger of a child is similar in size to the freckle on the third finger. Once these nymphal ticks engorge, they are easier to detect, but still remain relatively small in size. The nymphal ticks are responsible for most cases of *Ixodes*-related tick-borne diseases.

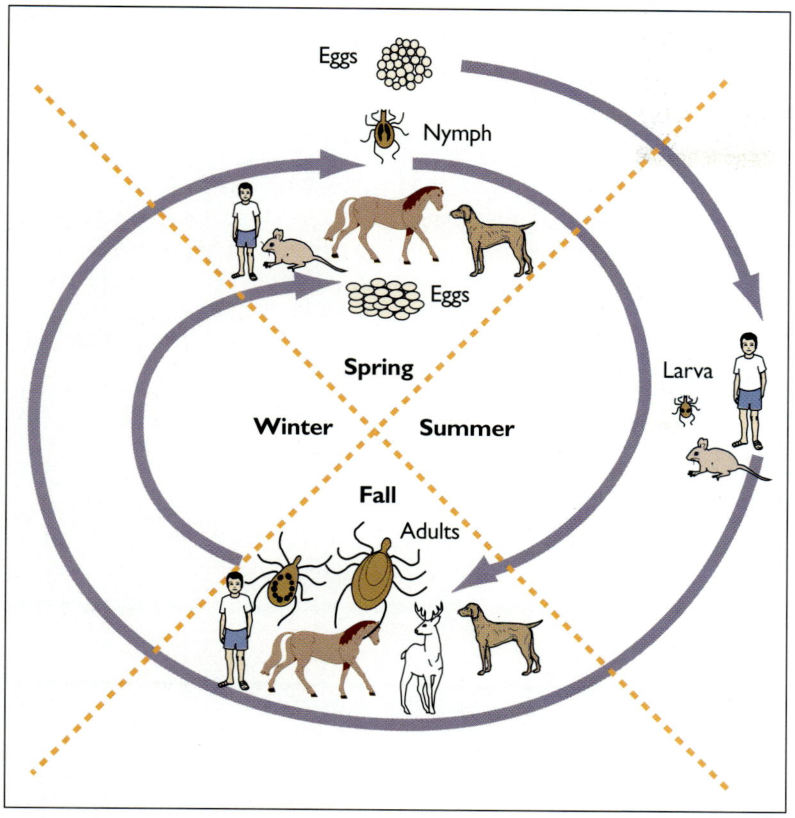

FIGURE 14-3 The life cycle of *Ixodes scapularis*. The life cycle of ixodid ticks typically spans 2 years and includes three blood meals. In the spring, the adult female tick releases her eggs, which hatch as six-legged larvae; during the summer, the larvae take a blood meal that lasts approximately 2 days. Subsequently, the larval ticks enter a dormant phase as the cooler fall weather sets in. The ticks then molt in the spring, entering the second phase of their life cycle as eight-legged nymphal ticks. In the late spring or summer, the nymphal ticks take a blood meal that typically lasts for 2 to 3 days. The nymphal ticks then molt as eight-legged adults in the fall. The adults mate on white-tailed deer; after mating, the male dies, but the female takes one more blood meal before she lays her eggs and dies. Larvae and nymphal ticks can feed on a variety of hosts, but most often on the white-footed mouse (*Peromyscus leucopus*); this mouse serves as the reservoir for *Borrelia burgdorferi* (the organism that causes Lyme disease). Although ticks at any of the stages of development can infect humans, most cases of Lyme disease result from the nymphal ticks. (*Adapted from* Habicht *et al.* [1]; with permission.)

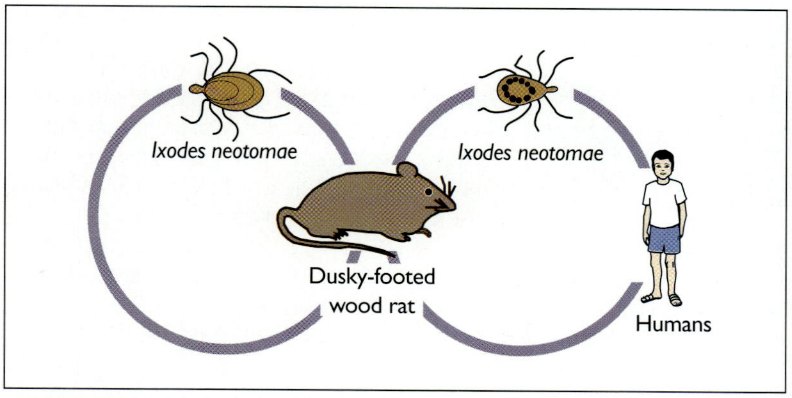

FIGURE 14-4 Enzootic transmission cycle of *Borrelia burgdorferi* in California (the California "bi-cycle"). In the western United States, the *Ixodes pacificus* tick is the major vector for transmission of *B. burgdorferi*. In California, Brown and Lane [2] recently showed that two distinct ixodid ticks and the dusky-footed wood rat sustain the disease in that region. The dusky-footed wood rat serves as the reservoir for *B. burgdorferi*, and *I. pacificus* ticks become infected when feeding on these rodents. Subsequently, these *I. pacificus* ticks can then transmit *B. burgdorferi* to humans. The *Ixodes neotomae* also become infected when feeding on the wood rat, but these ticks do not feed on humans. They do, however, appear to play a very important role in infecting other dusky-footed wood rats and thus serve as the source to infect the reservoir. In essence, the dusky-footed wood rat occupies the central place in a two-cycle pattern, with one cycle involving *I. pacificus* and the other *I. neotomae*. (*Adapted from* Barinaga [3]; with permission.)

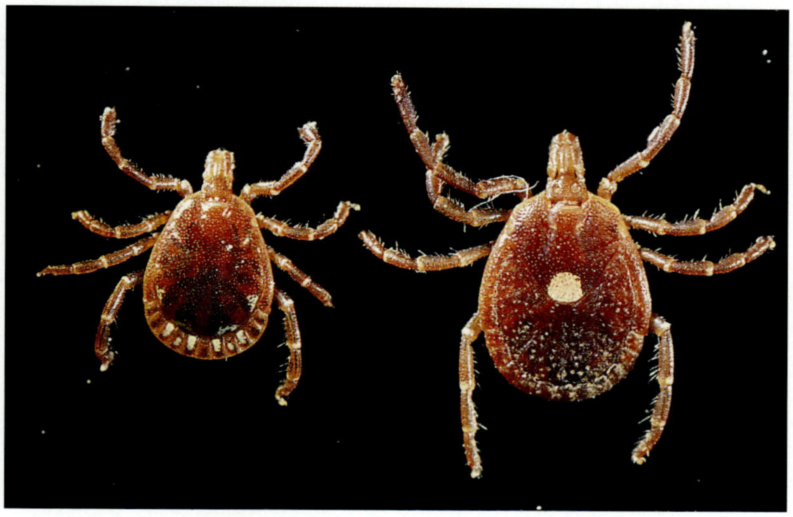

FIGURE 14-5 *Amblyomma americanum* ticks. *A. americanum*, also known as the Lone Star tick, can feed on livestock, dogs, deer, and humans. In the United States, the geographic distribution of *A. americanum* ticks includes the southern, southeastern, and central regions, as well as part of Texas. These ticks are the vector for *Ehrlichia chaffeensis* and also can cause tick paralysis. The female (*right*) has a characteristic whitish, silver spot on the apex of the dorsal scutum. The females generally are significantly larger than the males (*left*).

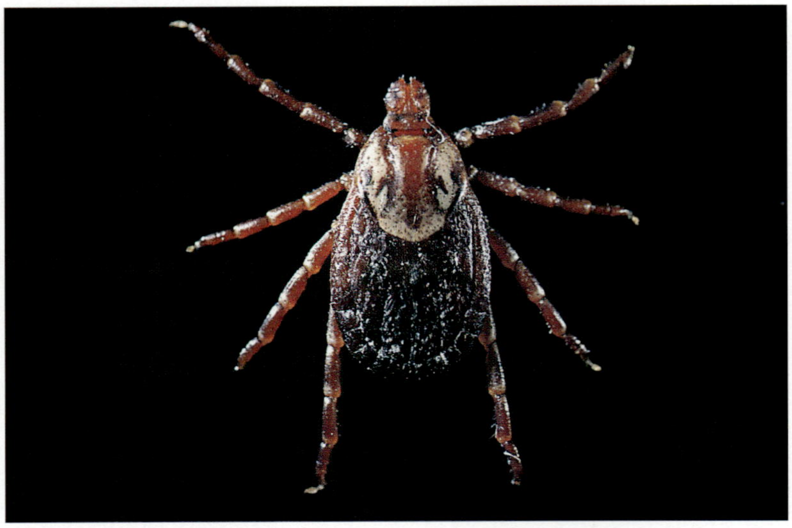

FIGURE 14-6 *Dermacentor variabilis* (adult female). *Dermacentor* ticks (or dog ticks) have an appearance distinct from ixodid ticks, as shown by this adult *D. variabilis* female. Adult dermacentor ticks are significantly larger than ixodid ticks, and have both a white dorsal scutum (ixodid ticks have a black scutum) and a black leathery sac distal to the dorsal scutum (ixodids have a tan–brown sac). Two major species of dermacentor ticks cause human tick-borne diseases in the United States: *D. variabilis* ticks and *Dermacentor andersoni* (wood ticks). *D. variabilis* ticks are predominantly clustered in the eastern states, whereas *D. andersoni* are predominantly found in western and Rocky Mountain states. Dermacentor ticks are the main vector for *Rickettsia rickettsii*. (*From* Spach *et al.* [4]; with permission.)

EHRLICHIOSIS

Characteristics of human monocytic and human granulocytic ehrlichiosis

	Human monocytic ehrlichiosis	Human granulocytic ehrlichiosis
Organism	*Ehrlichia chaffeensis*	*Ehrlichia equi*–like agent
Vector	*Amblyomma americanum*	*Ixodes scapularis*
Distribution	South central, Southeast	Northeast, upper Midwest

FIGURE 14-7 Characteristics of human monocytic and human granulocytic ehrlichiosis. In the United States, two distinct *Ehrlichia* species cause two types of ehrlichiosis: human monocytic ehrlichiosis and human granulocytic ehrlichiosis. In 1986, Maeda *et al.* [5] first described human monocytic ehrlichiosis, and in 1991 investigators isolated the causative agent (*Ehrlichia chaffeensis*). This organism subsequently has been isolated from amblyomma and dermacentor ticks, but most available data suggest that the amblyomma ticks probably are the predominant vector. More recently, Bakken *et al.* [6] described human granulocytic ehrlichiosis caused by an *Ehrlichia equi*–like agent. In 1996, Goodman *et al.* [7] cultivated this organism in cell culture. Ixodid ticks serve as the predominant vector for this *E. equi*–like agent. For both *Ehrlichia* species, the reservoirs probably include deer, dogs, and possibly small rodents.

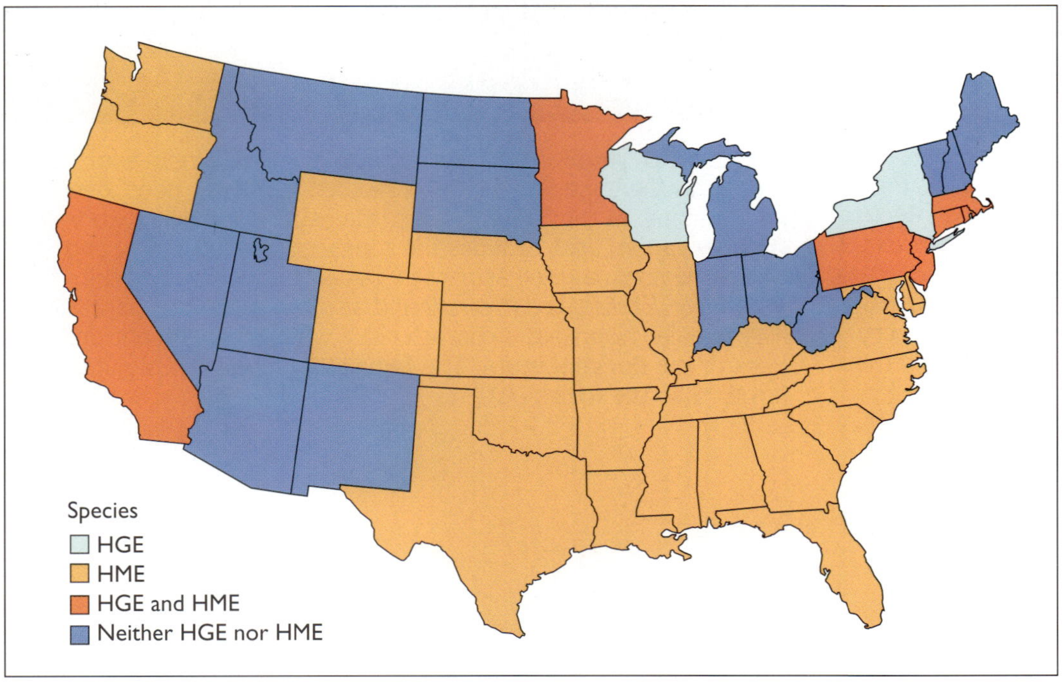

FIGURE 14-8 Distribution of ehrlichiosis in the United States between 1986 and 1996. More than 400 cases of human monocytic ehrlichiosis (HME) have been documented in more than 30 states. The regions with the highest number of cases correspond with the distribution of *Amblyomma americanum* ticks. Human granulocytic ehrlichiosis (HGE) predominantly occurs in the northeastern states and in the upper Midwest. Most investigators believe that the number of reported cases far underestimates the true incidence of ehrlichiosis. In part, this underestimation of true cases results from no systematic reporting system for cases of ehrlichiosis. Most cases of ehrlichiosis occur between April and August and involve rural residence or exposure [8].

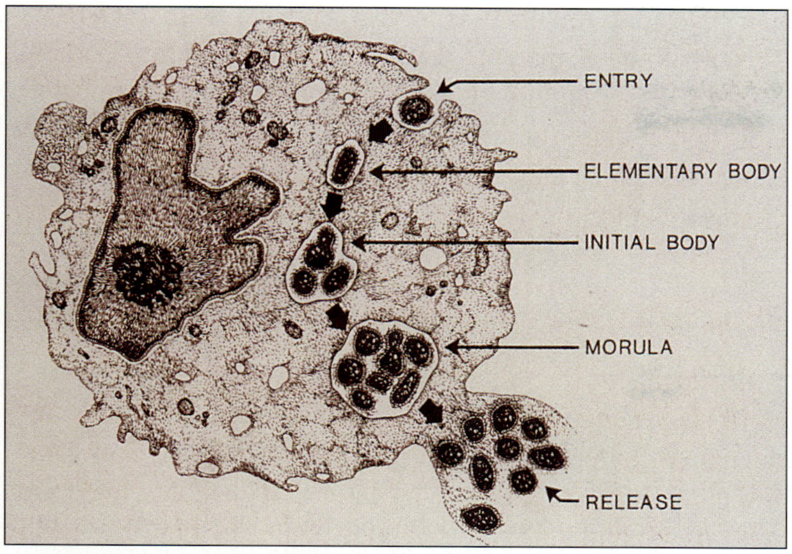

FIGURE 14-9 *Ehrlichia chaffeensis* growth cycle in an infected cell. Similar to *Chlamydia* organisms, *Ehrlichia* organisms pass through three developmental stages: elementary bodies, initial bodies, and morula. The elementary body represents a single, pleomorphic, 0.5-µm in diameter *Ehrlichia* organism (the stage of the organism that first enters a cell). These elementary bodies replicate by binary fission; within 3 to 5 days after infection they become initial bodies, a 1.0 to 2.5 µm in diameter cluster of *Ehrlichia* organisms. Subsequently during the next 7 to 12 days, further replication takes place and these clusters mature into a morula; the morula has a characteristic mulberry-like configuration. At this stage, the morula may be evident on a peripheral blood smear as an inclusion body. Most infected cells have several morula, each of which has multiple organisms within. (*Adapted from* McDade [9]; with permission.)

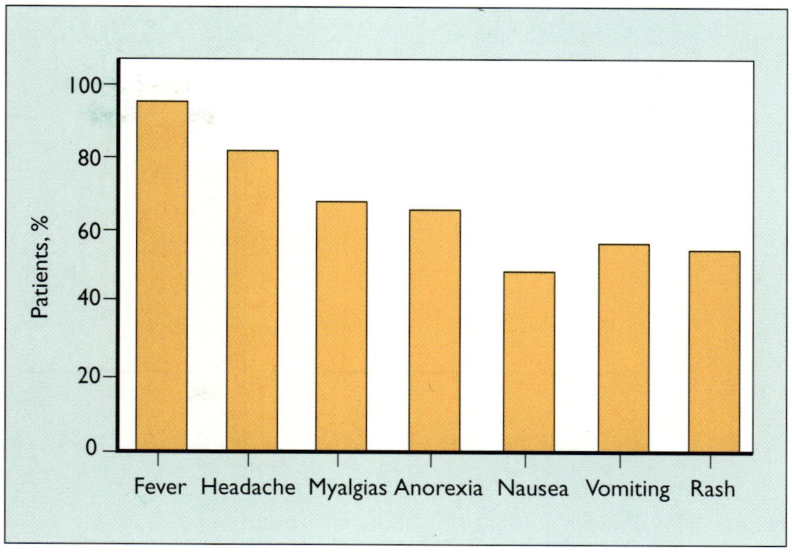

FIGURE 14-10 Clinical manifestations of patients with human monocytic ehrlichiosis. The incubation period for human monocytic ehrlichiosis is generally 7 to 10 days, and approximately 70% of patients have a history of a tick bite. The data shown in this figure reflect rates that include patients from all age groups. In general, rash occurs more frequently in children than in adults, with reported rates in children as high as 50% to 65%. At the time of initial presentation, the proportion of patients with rash is significantly lower, regardless of age. The rash typically appears as macular or petechial lesions located on the trunk or extremities. The most common symptoms (fever, headache, myalgias, and anorexia) can resemble more common illnesses such as influenza. Severe complications include severe neurologic involvement, respiratory failure, renal failure, and a toxic shock–like illness.

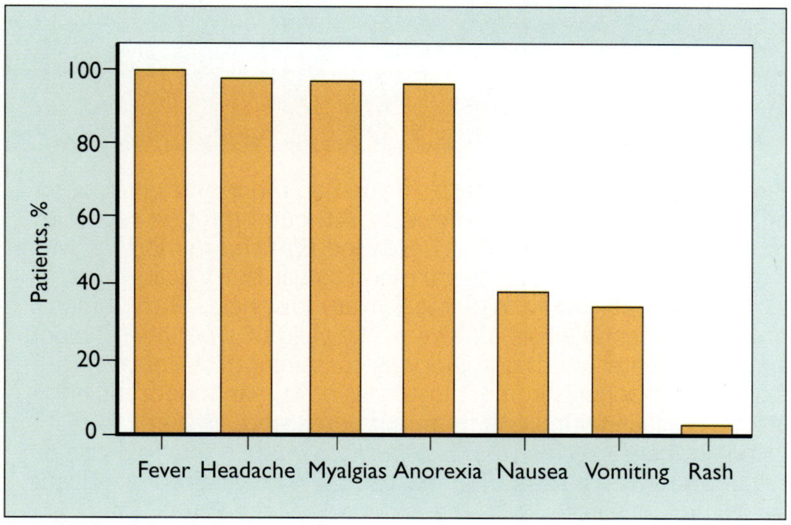

FIGURE 14-11 Clinical manifestations of patients with human granulocytic ehrlichiosis. Similar to human monocytic ehrlichiosis, the incubation period for human granulocytic ehrlichiosis is typically 7 to 10 days. Patients with human granulocytic ehrlichiosis also present with a flu-like illness. Rash, however, occurs much less frequently with human granulocytic ehrlichiosis than with human monocytic ehrlichiosis. Serious complications include involvement of the respiratory tract, central nervous system, liver, and renal system.

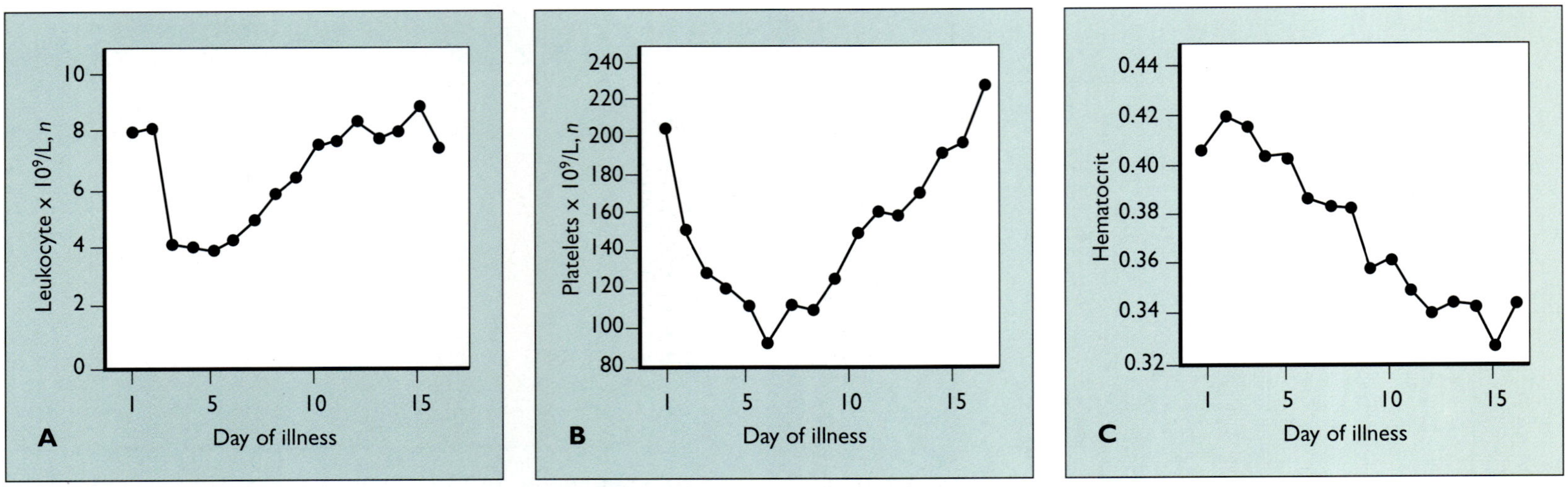

FIGURE 14-12 Hematologic alterations in patients with human monocytic ehrlichiosis. Data presented were obtained from 237 more seriously ill patients with human monocytic ehrlichiosis. During the first several days of illness, laboratory studies are generally normal or near normal. By day 3, however, the baseline leukocyte count (**A**) decreases by approximately 50%, with a leukocyte nadir occurring on days 3 through 7. Subsequently, the leukocyte count gradually returns to normal. Approximately 4% of patients develop atypical lymphocytosis beginning in the second week of the illness. Thrombocytopenia develops in approximately two thirds of patients (**B**), with the nadir occurring during days 5 through 8, followed by a gradual recovery with a return to baseline values by approximately 2 weeks. The course of hematocrit change differs significantly from leukocyte and platelet changes. The hematocrit begins to decline by approximately day 6 (**C**), but continues to steadily decrease until approximately day 12. The nadir appears to occur during days 12 through 16. The mechanism for the pancytopenia remains poorly characterized, but may relate to sequestration or destruction of various blood elements (the so-called hemophagocytic syndrome). (*Adapted from* Fishbein *et al.* [10]; with permission.)

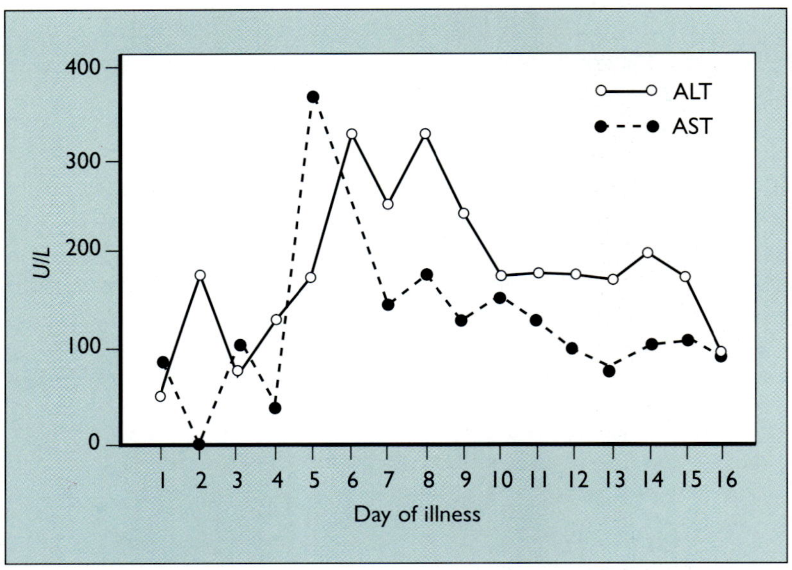

FIGURE 14-13 Liver function test alterations in patients with human monocytic ehrlichiosis. This figure shows the time course of the changes in liver function tests, representing data obtained from 237 more seriously ill patients with human monocytic ehrlichiosis. A significant increase in either aspartate aminotransferase (AST) or alanine aminotransferase (ALT) occurs in approximately 80% to 85% of these patients. During the first week of illness, liver function tests show a sharp rise, peaking on days 5 through 9 and returning to near baseline by approximately day 16. Jaundice, however, generally does not occur. (*Adapted from* Fishbein *et al.* [10]; with permission.)

Laboratory diagnosis of human monocytic ehrlichiosis and human granulocytic ehrlichiosis
Peripheral blood smear
Indirect immunofluorescence assay
Polymerase chain reaction

FIGURE 14-14 Diagnostic tests for human monocytic ehrlichiosis and human granulocytic ehrlichiosis. Although the first report of human monocytic ehrlichiosis described *Ehrlichieae morulae* within leukocytes visible on peripheral blood smear buffy coat, most experts consider buffy coat smears very low yield. With human granulocytic ehrlichiosis, however, the yield of a peripheral blood smear is greater, with granulocytes containing *Ehrlichieae* inclusions. The diagnosis in most instances of human monocytic ehrlichiosis is made by indirect immunofluorescence assay (IFA) testing using antigens specific to *Ehrlichia chaffeensis*; a fourfold rise or fall in titer, with a peak of at least 1:64, is considered diagnostic. Titers typically increase by the 3rd week of the illness. Diagnostic IFA titers for human granulocytic ehrlichiosis, using *Ehrlichia equi* antigen, are considered as 1:80 or greater; these diagnostic titers generally do not develop until the patient enters the convalescent phase. For both types of ehrlichiosis, polymerase chain reaction testing shows promise as an improved method to diagnose patients in the acute phase of the illness.

Treatment of ehrlichiosis

Therapy	Route	Pediatric dosage	Adult dosage	Duration, *d*
Doxycycline	Orally or intravenous	4.4 mg/kg/d divided in two doses on day 1, then 2.2 mg/kg/d divided in two doses	100 mg twice daily	5–10
Chloramphenicol	Orally or intravenous	50–75 mg/kg/d divided in four doses	500 mg four times daily	5–10

FIGURE 14-15 Therapy for human monocytic ehrlichiosis and human granulocytic ehrlichiosis. In general, the treatment of ehrlichiosis is similar to the treatment of Rocky Mountain spotted fever and is the same for human granulocytic ehrlichiosis and human monocytic ehrlichiosis. Available data suggest that doxycycline (or tetracycline) is the most effective drug for the treatment of ehrlichiosis. Doxycycline and tetracycline, however, are contraindicated in pregnancy. In addition, with children younger than 8 years of age, doxycycline (or tetracycline) can cause significant permanent staining of the teeth (available data suggest the development of tooth enamel occurs up to 8 y of age). The degree of darkening of the teeth is related to the cumulative dose of tetracycline or doxycycline, and the effect is more pronounced on primary teeth than on the larger, thicker permanent teeth. Because of this adverse effect, some consider doxycycline (or tetracycline) contraindicated in children younger than 8 years of age. Although *in vitro* studies suggest that *Ehrlichia* species are resistant to chloramphenicol, several reports have described patients with ehrlichiosis who were successfully treated with chloramphenicol. In children younger than 8 years of age, recommendations vary on whether to use doxycycline or chloramphenicol; factors to consider include the safety issues of doxycycline (teeth staining), the concerns for failures based on *in vitro* chloramphenicol data, and the remote (one in 25,000 to 40,000) possibility of aplastic anemia occurring from chloramphenicol. Overall, given that ehrlichiosis is a potentially fatal disease, most experts would consider it reasonable to treat suspected ehrlichiosis with doxycycline or tetracycline in a child younger than 8 years of age, especially if only a single course is used. Moreover, because doxycycline binds less readily with calcium than does tetracycline, doxycycline is less likely to cause staining of teeth and is, therefore, the preferred treatment.

BABESIOSIS

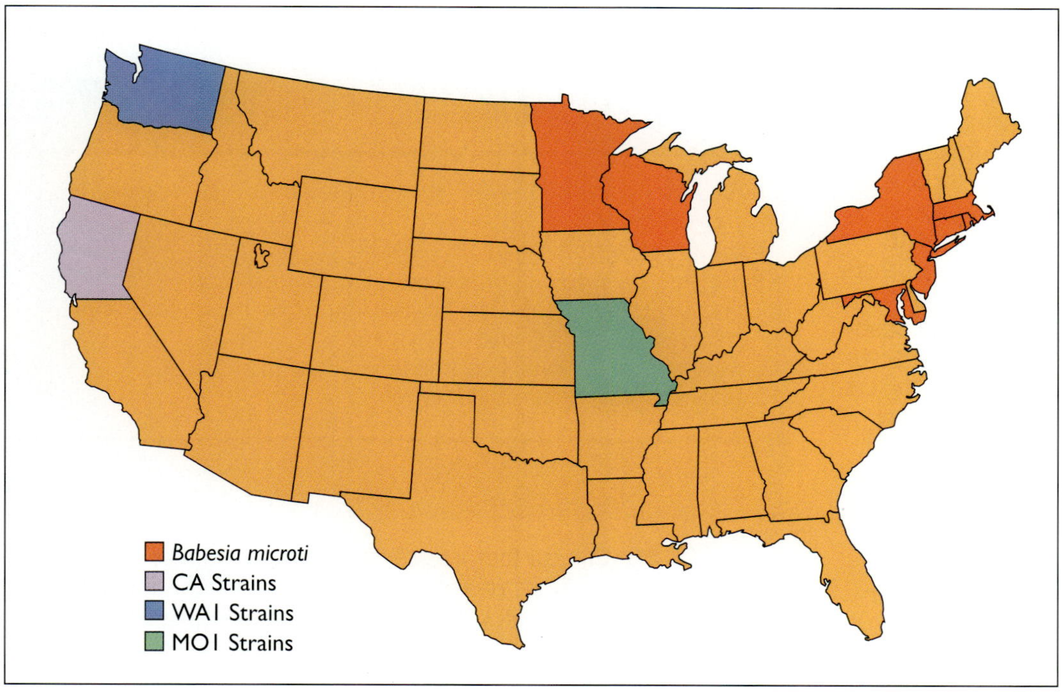

FIGURE 14-16 Babesiosis incidence in the United States. The highest prevalence of *Babesia microti* infection occurs in densely populated northeastern coastal regions and corresponds with the distribution of *Ixodes scapularis* ticks and their hosts. Three states (Washington, California, and Missouri) have reported cases of babesiosis that have involved *Babesia* species distinct from *B. microti*. The vector or vectors for *Babesia* in these states remains unknown, but presumably *Ixodes pacificus* is the vector in Washington and California. Most cases of babesiosis occur in the mid- to late summer. Overall, the number of cases is poorly defined, mainly because most persons who become infected with *Babesia* species do not develop significant clinical symptoms. Several reports have described rare cases of transfusion-associated babesiosis, and one report described maternal-fetal transmission of babesiosis.

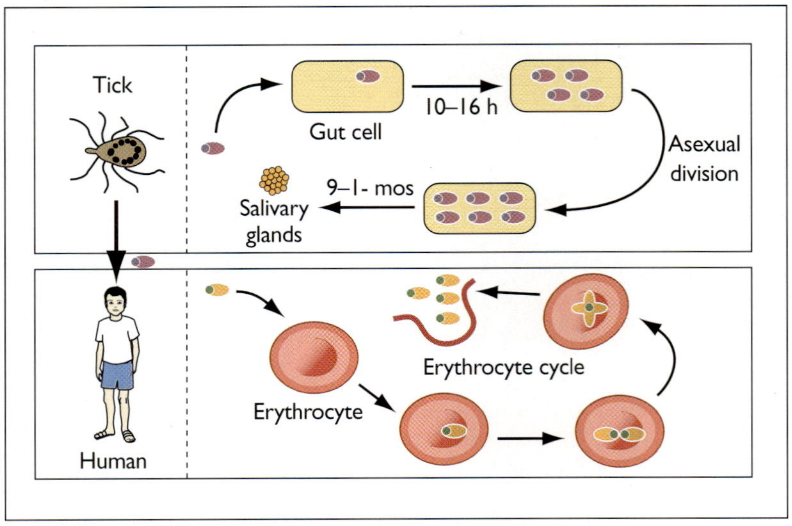

FIGURE 14-17 *Babesia* life cycle. Within a tick, *Babesia* parasites infect gut cells, undergo asexual division, and eventually migrate to the salivary glands. The organism is introduced into a human when the infected tick takes in a blood meal. Transmission usually involves the nymphal tick, but the duration of attachment required for transmission of *Babesia* species is not known. Once inside the human host, the *Babesia* parasites penetrate erythrocytes, undergo division, and eventually burst forth to infect other erythrocytes. Available data clearly suggest that *Babesia* species can be transmitted to humans concomitantly with *Borrelia burgdorferi*. (*Adapted from* Boustani and Gelfand [11]; with permission.)

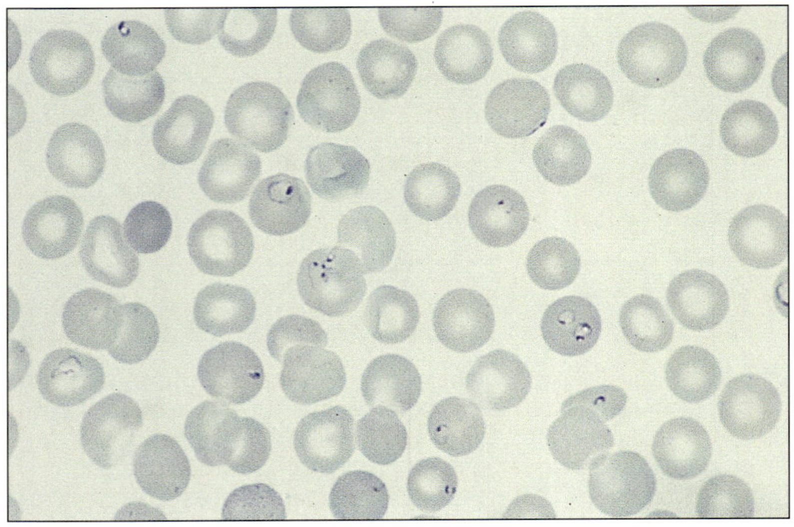

FIGURE 14-18 Peripheral blood smear of intraerythrocytic *Babesia* organisms. The diagnosis of babesiosis is usually made by viewing a Wright- or Giemsa-stained peripheral blood smear. The early forms of the intraerythrocytic babesia infection appear as cytoplasmic vacuoles with a single chromatin dot or several chromatin masses. Rarely, one may see the tetrad or "Maltese cross" forms; these are formed as the babesia cytoplasm coalesces into four compact masses. The predominant early form of babesia within erythrocytes closely resembles the appearance of *Plasmodium falciparum* ring forms, mainly because of the similar ring configuration and peripheral location of the organisms within the erythrocytes. *Plasmodium falciparum*, however, may have features not seen with *Babesia* species, including schizonts and gametocytes, as well as the presence of brownish pigment deposits (hemazoin) in older stages. Similar to diagnosing malaria, performing a thick blood smear increases the sensitivity of diagnosing babesiosis on a peripheral blood smear. (*From* Spach *et al.* [4]; with permission.)

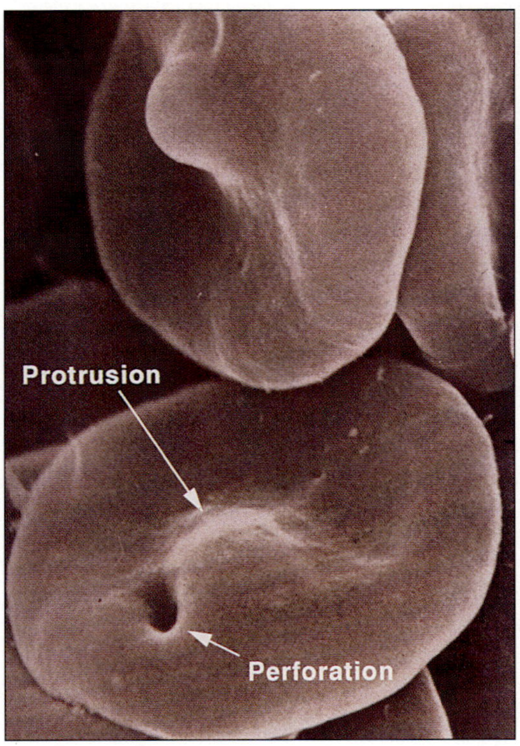

FIGURE 14-19 Electron microscopic image of intraerythrocytic *Babesia* organism. As the parasite leaves the erythrocyte, it causes significant damage to the erythrocyte membrane, including perforations, protrusions, and inclusions. The exact mechanism for hemolysis, however, remains poorly characterized. (*From* Sun *et al.* [12]; with permission.)

Clinical features of babesiosis
Subclinical or mild disease: epidemiologic studies suggest high incidence
Incubation period: typically 1–3 wk
Symptomatic illness: gradual onset and symptoms characterized by malaise, fatigue, anorexia, headache, myalgias, vomiting, and dark urine
Severe complications: hypotension, acute respiratory distress syndrome, renal failure

FIGURE 14-20 Clinical features of babesiosis. Available serologic data suggest that most *Babesia* species infections do not result in significant clinical symptoms. Although most European reports have described babesiosis among individuals who had previously undergone splenectomy, fewer than one third of the cases reported in the United States have involved persons without a spleen. The incubation period for *Babesia* species is typically 1 to 3 weeks, but may extend up to 6 weeks. The initial symptoms of babesiosis are nonspecific, often resembling influenza. The hallmark of the disease is the presence of hemolytic anemia. Characteristic laboratory abnormalities result from hemolysis and include anemia, thrombocytopenia, increased bilirubin, and increased lactic dehydrogenase. Severe complications include hypotension, acute respiratory distress syndrome, renal failure, and death. The presence of an erythema migrans skin rash strongly suggests concomitant infection with *Borrelia burgdorferi*.

Laboratory Diagnosis of Babesiosis
Peripheral blood smear
Indirect immunofluorescence assay
Polymerase chain reaction
Intraperitoneal inoculation of hamsters

FIGURE 14-21 Diagnosis of babesiosis. Microscopic examination of Giemsa- or Wright-stained blood smear may show *Babesia* organism ring forms that resemble *Plasmodium falciparum* ring forms; the presence of a tetrad of merozoites, or so-called "Maltese cross," is diagnostic for babesia infection. An indirect immunofluorescence assay titer of 1:64 or greater is considered positive, with titers or 1:256 or greater generally indicating acute babesia infection and titers of 1:64 or greater, but less than 1:256, usually indicating prior infection. Recently, investigators have developed a polymerase chain reaction–based assay for detection of *Babesia* organisms that appears to be promising. Intraperitoneal inoculation of hamsters is not a practical diagnostic method, but is occasionally used for research purposes.

Treatment of babesiosis

Therapy	Route	Pediatric dosage	Adult dosage	Duration, *d*
Clindamycin	Orally or intravenously	20–30 mg/kg/day divided in three doses	600 mg three times daily	7–10
Quinine (in addition to clindamycin)	Orally	25 mg/kg/d divided in three doses	650 mg three times daily	7–10
Exchange transfusion	Intravenously	2–3 blood volumes	2–3 blood volumes	—

FIGURE 14-22 Therapy for babesiosis. Clindamycin plus quinine is the regimen of choice for treating babesiosis. Chloroquine is ineffective and thus should not be substituted for quinine. In severe cases that require intravenous therapy, intravenous quinidine can substitute for oral quinine; in this circumstance, the patient should also receive intravenous clindamycin. One case report described a good response to the regimen of azithromycin (500 mg/d orally for 10 d) plus quinine. Another case report described a splenectomized adult man successfully treated with intravenous pentamidine (240 mg/d for 18 d) plus oral trimethoprim-sulfamethoxazole (3 g/d for 28 d). *In vitro* data suggest that atovaquone has excellent activity against *Babesia* species. Exchange transfusion is generally reserved for extremely ill patients who have a parasite burden greater than 10% and clinically significant hemolysis; exchange transfusion should be used in conjunction with antibiotic therapy.

Rocky Mountain Spotted Fever

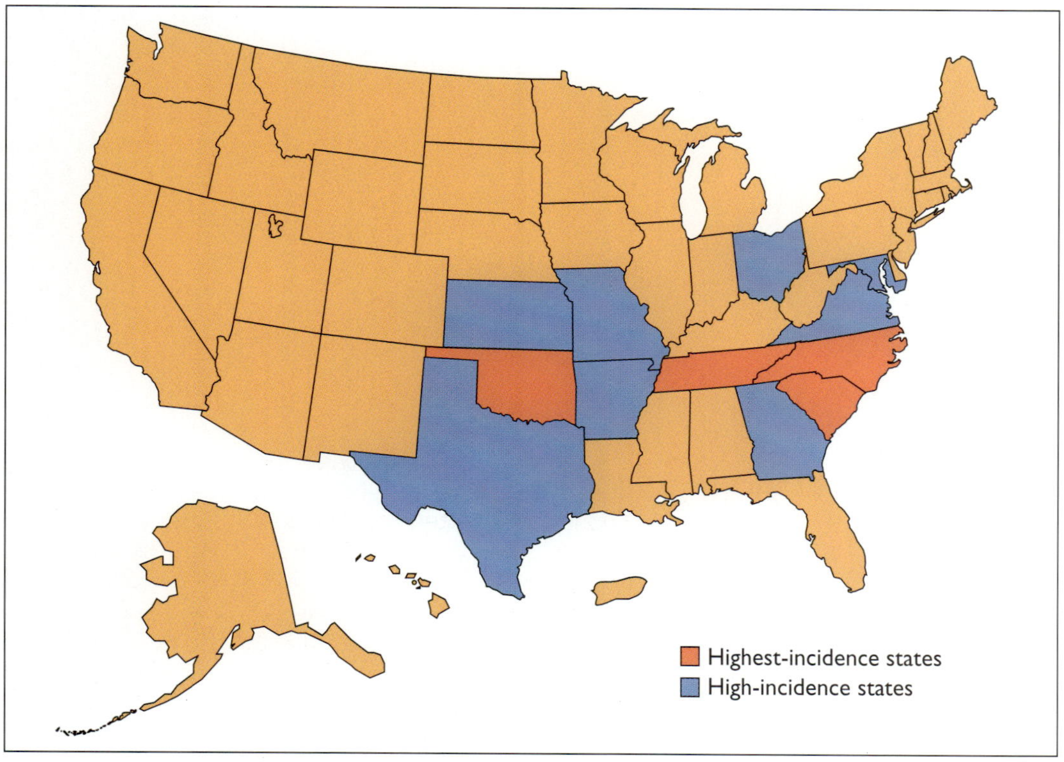

FIGURE 14-23 High and medium incidence rates of Rocky Mountain spotted fever (RMSF) in the United States. In 1906, Howard Taylor Ricketts first discovered RMSF among residents of the Bitter Root valleys of Montana and Idaho. These valleys, however, are no longer considered high incidence areas. Although RMSF has now been reported in almost every state, four states (North Carolina, South Carolina, Tennessee, and Oklahoma) have reported the highest number of cases in recent years. Other high incidence states in recent years include Maryland, Virginia, Georgia, Tennessee, Ohio, Missouri, Arkansas, Texas, and Kansas. Certain focal regions, such as Cowan and Rowan counties in North Carolina, are considered hyperendemic.

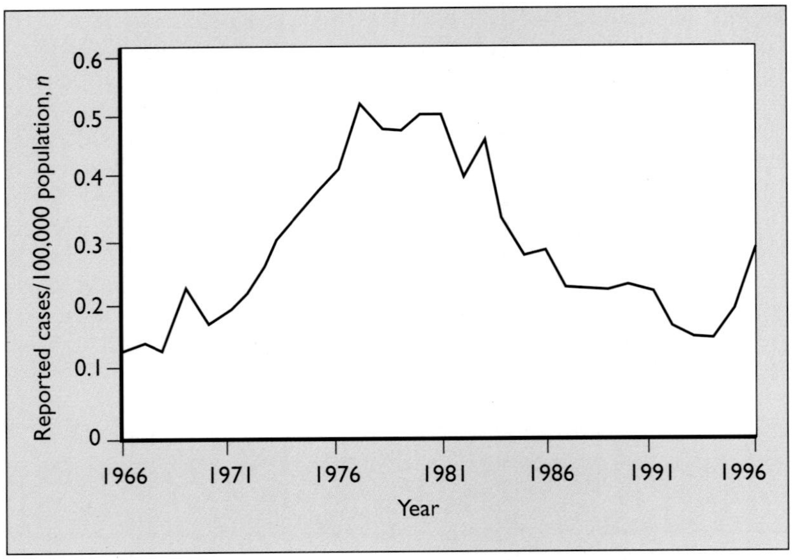

FIGURE 14-24 Rocky Mountain spotted fever (RMSF) incidence by year in the United States between 1966 and 1996. Surveillance data from the Centers for Disease Control and Prevention show significant fluctuations in the number of reported cases in the United States. The annual incidence rate generally fluctuates between 0.24 and 0.32 cases per 100,000 persons. The causative agent is *Rickettsia rickettsii.* Dermacentor ticks are the major vector for the transmission of *R. rickettsii* to humans, specifically *Dermacentor variabilis* in the eastern and southern regions and *Dermacentor andersoni* in the western regions. Approximately one in 20 dermacentor ticks harbor *R. rickettsii.* More than 95% of cases of RMSF occur between April 1 and September 30, corresponding with the seasonal feeding pattern of dermacentor ticks. In general, cases in the eastern and southern regions tend to peak in the spring and early summer; those cases in the west most often occur in the mid to late summer. Approximately 50% of persons with RMSF recall a tick bite within 14 days of their symptom onset [8].

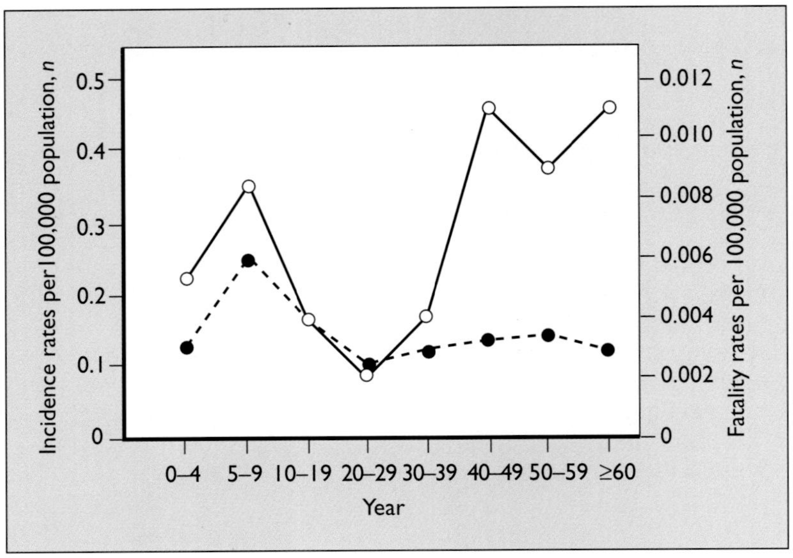

FIGURE 14-25 Age-specific incidence rates and age-specific fatality rates of Rocky Mountain spotted fever (RMSF) in the United States between 1981 and 1990. Centers for Disease Control and Prevention surveillance data from 1981 to 1990 show the highest incidence for laboratory-confirmed cases of RMSF among persons 5 to 9 years of age (*dashed line*). Persons aged 20 to 29 had the lowest incidence rates. Persons aged 40 years or older had the highest case-fatality rates: 8.2 % versus 2.3% for persons younger than 40 years of age (*solid line*). Those individuals who began therapy after the first 3 days of the onset of symptoms also had a higher case-fatality rate [13].

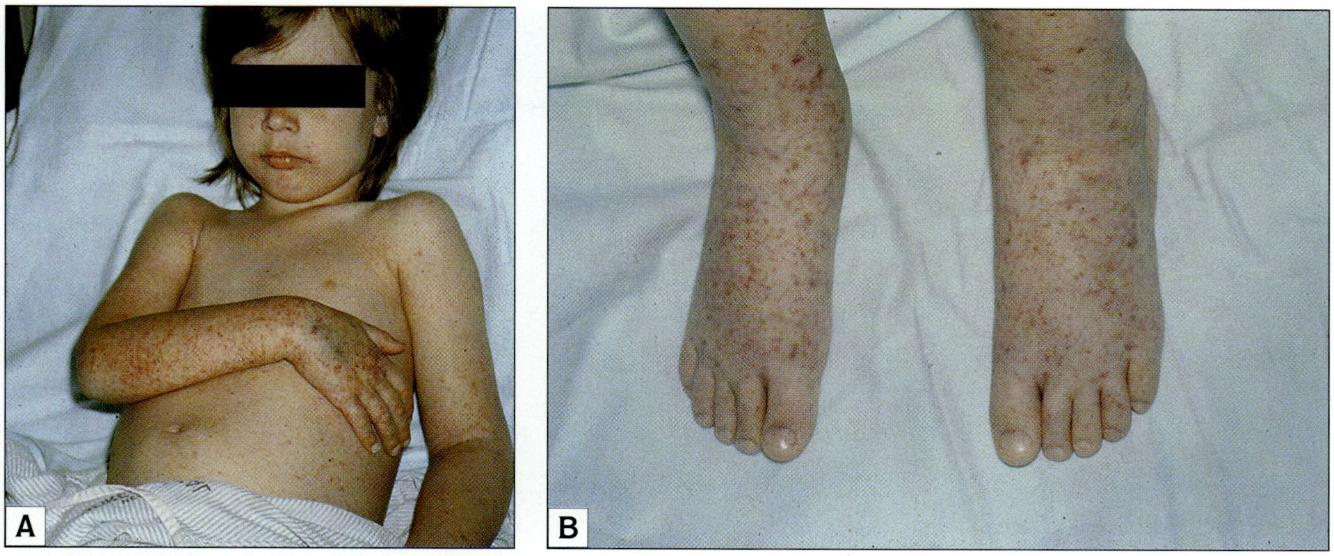

FIGURE 14-26 Skin rash in patient with Rocky Mountain spotted fever. Rash, which develops at some point in the illness in approximately 85% to 90% of persons infected with *Rickettsia rickettsii*, typically appears between days 3 and 5 of the clinical illness. Approximately 20% of patients, however, develop a rash on day 6 or later. In a significant proportion of patients, the rash does not appear petechial and does not involve the palms or soles. Early in the course of the illness, the rash typically appears maculopapular, but generally petechiae become evident. Classically, the rash begins on the extremities and gradually spreads more centrally to the trunk. The rash generally involves the palms and soles. **A,** A child with prominent rash involving the hands that has started to spread to the trunk. **B,** Edema in the patient's extremities. The presence of edema indicates significant capillary leak, suggesting the diagnosis of RMSF. (*Courtesy* of C.M. Wilfert, MD.)

Laboratory features of Rocky Mountain spotted fever
Normal leukocyte count with left shift, toxic granulations, and Döhle's bodies
Thrombocytopenia
Hyponatremia
Cerebrospinal fluid pleocytosis
Increased serum transaminases
Increased serum creatinine kinase

FIGURE 14-27 Laboratory features of Rocky Mountain spotted fever (RMSF). Although laboratory studies, *eg*, leukocyte count, platelet count, sodium level, and cerebrospinal fluid analysis can support the diagnosis of RMSF, they are not diagnostic. Although most patients with RMSF have a normal leukocyte count, there may be evidence of a shift to more immature band forms. Indeed, a normal leukocyte count with a marked left shift may help to distinguish RMSF from meningococcal disease. Although 30% to 50% of patients with RMSF will have mild thrombocytopenia (platelet count <150,000 cells/mL), only approximately 10% have severe thrombocytopenia (platelet count <10,000 cells/mL). Thrombocytopenia results from a consumption coagulopathy. Approximately 20% of patients develop hyponatremia. Typically, cerebrospinal fluid studies show mild pleocytosis (generally <100 cells/mL) and an elevated protein level. Low cerebrospinal fluid glucose occurs in less than 10% of patients. Other nonspecific findings include increased serum transaminase and serum creatine kinase levels.

Laboratory diagnosis of Rocky Mountain spotted fever
Serology
Indirect immunofluorescence assay
Latex agglutination assay
Skin biopsy
Direct immunofluorescence antibody staining
Immunoperoxidase staining
Polymerase chain reaction

FIGURE 14-28 Laboratory diagnosis of Rocky Mountain spotted fever (RMSF). An indirect immunofluorescence assay (IFA) titer to *Rickettsia rickettsii* of 1:64 or greater is considered diagnostic. Similarly, a latex agglutination assay of 1:128 or greater is considered diagnostic. The IFA and latex agglutination antibody titers typically become detectable 7 to 10 days into the illness. In general, most experts no longer recommend using the Weil-Felix proteus agglutination assay, mainly because of the poor sensitivity and specificity. A diagnosis of RMSF in the acute setting can be made by detecting *R. rickettsii* in a skin biopsy sample using either direct immunofluorescence antibody staining or immunoperoxidase staining; with either test, the organisms appear in the vascular endothelium and smooth muscle. These tests have similar sensitivity (approximately 75% to 80%) and specificity (>95%). In general, the immunofluorescent technique is more rapid, but immunoperoxidase staining provides easier antigen localization and concomitant viewing of the background histopathology. These tests are generally available only via research or reference laboratories. Polymerase chain reaction testing of a skin biopsy sample shows promise, but has not been standardized, nor is it widely available.

Treatment of Rocky Mountain spotted fever				
Therapy	**Route**	**Pediatric dosage**	**Adult dosage**	**Duration, *d***
Doxycycline	Orally or intravenously	4.4 mg/kg/d divided in two doses on day 1, then 2.2 mg/kg/d divided in two doses	100 mg twice daily	5–10
Chloramphenicol	Orally or intravenously	50–75 mg/kg/d divided in four doses	500 mg four times daily	5–10

FIGURE 14-29 Treatment of Rocky Mountain spotted fever (RMSF). Doxycycline (or tetracycline) is the most effective drug for the treatment of RMSF. These drugs, however, are contraindicated in pregnancy. In addition, with children younger than 8 years of age, doxycycline (or tetracycline) can cause significant permanent staining of the teeth (available data suggest the development of tooth enamel occurs up 8 y of age). The degree of darkening of the teeth is related to the cumulative dose of tetracycline or doxycycline, and the effect is more pronounced on primary teeth than on the larger, thicker permanent teeth. Because of this adverse effect, some consider doxycycline (or tetracycline) to be contraindicated in children younger than 8 years of age. This issue is complex and controversial: the clinician must balance the potential for teeth staining with the possible life-threatening consequences of RMSF, as well as the remote (one in 25,000 to 40,000) but real possibility of aplastic anemia occurring from chloramphenicol, the alternative drug. Overall, given that RMSF is a potentially fatal disease, most experts would consider it reasonable to treat suspected RMSF with doxycycline or tetracycline in a child younger than 8 years of age, especially if only a single course is used. Moreover, because doxycycline binds less readily with calcium than does tetracycline, doxycycline is less likely to cause staining of teeth and is, therefore, the preferred treatment. The mortality of inappropriately treated RMSF is approximately 15% to 20% compared with mortality rates of 3% to 6% when treated with doxycycline, tetracycline, or chloramphenicol.

Lyme Disease

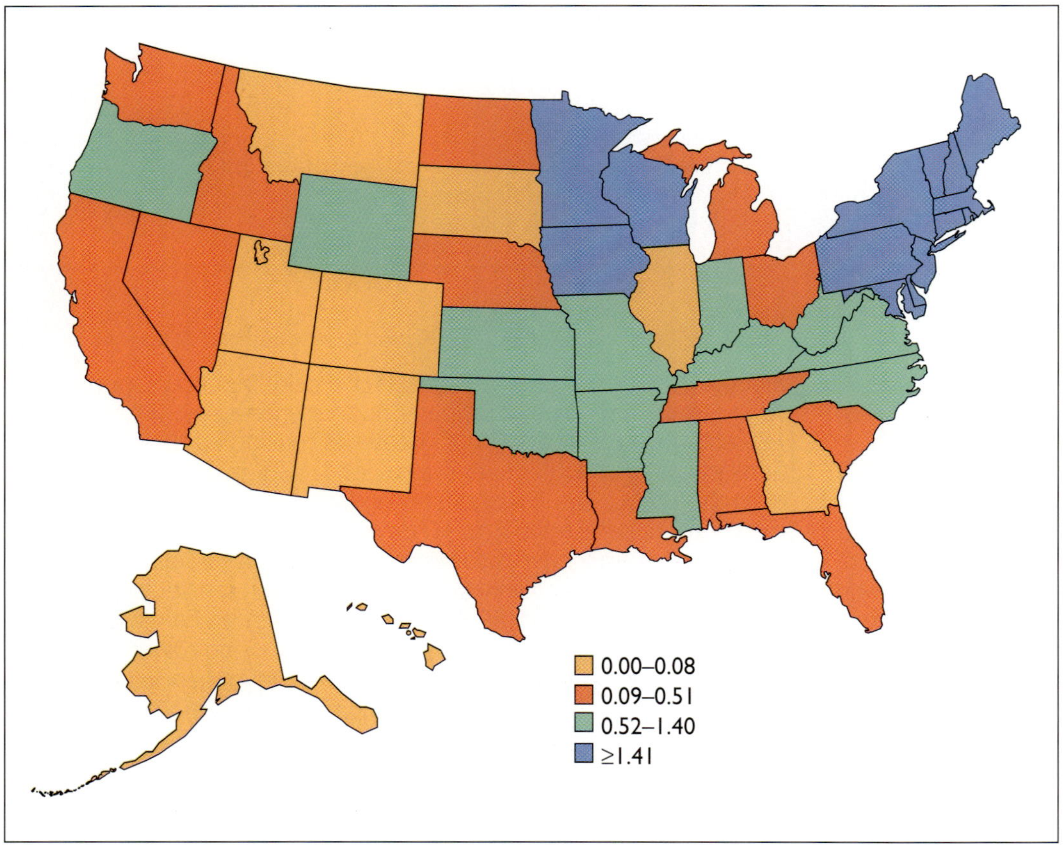

FIGURE 14-30 Lyme disease in United States in 1996. In 1996, a total of 16,455 cases of Lyme disease were reported to the Centers for Disease Control and Prevention, including cases from 45 states and Washington, DC. Most of the cases came from the Northeast, Mid-Atlantic, and North Central regions. Eight states (Connecticut, Rhode Island, New York, New Jersey, Delaware, Pennsylvania, Maryland, and Wisconsin) accounted for 91% of all reported cases of Lyme disease. Nantucket County had the highest incidence, with 1247 cases of Lyme disease per 100,000 persons. Five states (Alaska, Arizona, Colorado, Montana, and South Dakota) did not report any cases of Lyme disease in 1996. Cases had an almost equal male and female distribution.

The Centers for Disease Control and Prevention (CDC) initiated surveillance for Lyme disease in 1982, and in 1991 Lyme disease became a reportable disease. Lyme disease is the most common vector-borne disease in the United States. The CDC case definition consists of 1) erythema migrans rash of at least 5 cm, or 2) a positive serology result combined with at least one compatible manifestation of musculoskeletal, neurologic, or cardiovascular disease. Most states now require two-step serologic testing (enzyme immunoassay and Western immunoblot) for a serologic diagnosis of Lyme disease. Between 1982 and 1997, the overall trend is clearly an increase in the number of reported cases of Lyme disease.

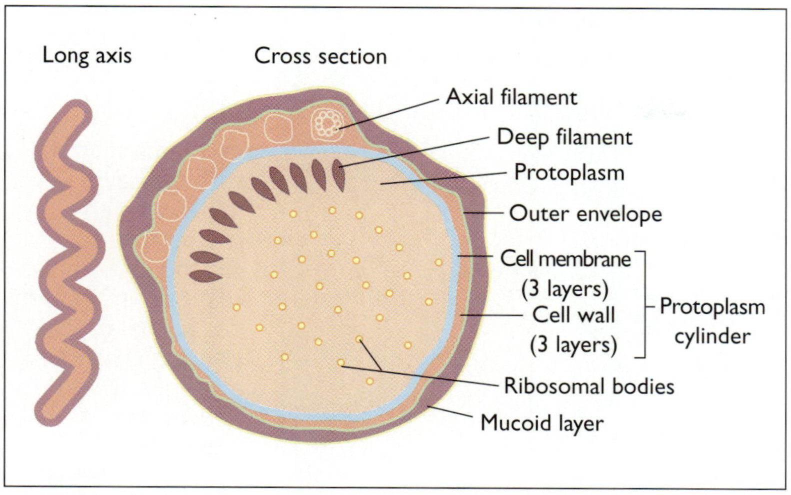

FIGURE 14-31 Structure of *Borrelia burgdorferi* spirochete. *B. burgdorferi*, the causative agent of Lyme disease, is a unicellular spirochete approximately 25 µm by 0.2 µm in size. The organism possesses many typical features of a spirochete, namely a loosely coiled spiral shape and a central protoplasmic cylinder surrounded by an outer envelope and mucoid layer. The axial filaments have a structure similar to flagella of other bacteria and probably are responsible for most of the organism's movement. Three spirochete genera (*Borrelia, Treponema*, and *Leptospira*) contain organisms within their genera that cause disease in humans. *Borrelia* can cause two types of tick-borne human disease: Lyme disease and relapsing fever. Recently, *B. burgdorferi* sensu lato has been subclassified into four species: 1) *B. burgdorferi* sensu stricto, 2) *Borrelia garinii*, 3) *Borrelia afzelii*, and *Borrelia japonica*. Each of these species has a predominant location in certain regions of the world; in North America, all isolates, to date, have been *B. burgdorferi* sensu stricto, whereas in Europe, most isolates have been *B. garinii* or *B. afzelii*. (*Adapted from* Schmid [14]; with permission.)

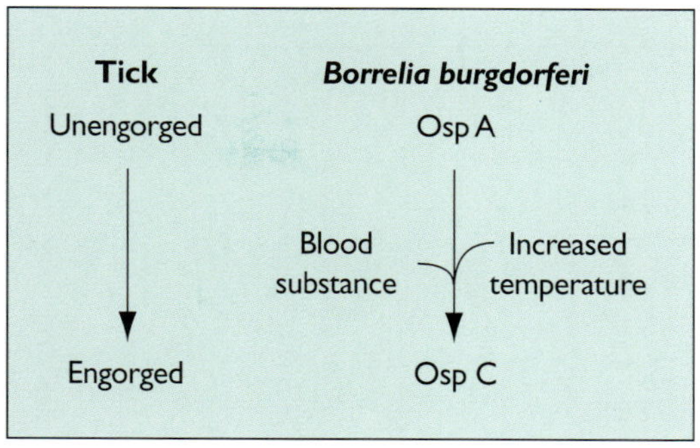

FIGURE 14-32 Changes in outer surface protein. Recent studies by Schwann *et al.* [15] have shown that the *Borrelia burgdorferi* organism in unfed ticks is predominantly covered by outer surface protein (Osp) A, but that after feeding for several days, OspC replaces OspA. Two environmental cues cause the change from OspA to OspC: 1) an increase in temperature in the tick that occurs during feeding as a result of close attachment to a mammal, and 2) an unidentified biochemical substance taken in with the mammal's blood. The spirochete makes the change by turning off the gene that codes for OspA and turning on the *OspC* gene. The spirochete's change from OspA to OspC occurs in the tick's gut, and only after this change has taken place will the spirochetes leave the gut and travel to the tick's salivary glands. It appears that *Borrelia burgdorferi* is not infectious in humans until the change to OspC takes place. Although the function of the outer surface proteins A and C remain poorly characterized, they probably play distinct roles in specific environments.

Stages of Lyme disease

Early		Late
Stage 1	**Stage 2**	**Stage 3**
Localized	Disseminated	Chronic

FIGURE 14-33 Stages of Lyme disease. Following inoculation of *Borrelia burgdorferi* from an ixodid tick, patients with *B. burgdorferi* infection can present with protean manifestations, and many investigators have likened Lyme disease to syphilis—another spirochete disease often referred to as "the great imitator". Similar to the three stages of syphilis, manifestations of untreated Lyme disease can be considered a three-stage disease. Stage 1 (localized disease) and 2 (disseminated disease) are often grouped together as representing early Lyme disease, with stage 3 representing late Lyme disease. Stage 1 usually represents localized erythema migrans, although patients in this phase often have systemic influenza–like symptoms. Stage 2 disease includes the appearance of multiple annular skin lesions, central nervous system involvement (acute meningitis, cranial nerve abnormalities, and peripheral neuropathy), cardiac involvement (conduction disturbances), and musculoskeletal involvement (migratory joint pains and brief attacks of arthritis). Stage 3 (chronic disease) most often affects the joints (arthritis) or the nervous system (encephalopathy, polyneuropathy, or leukoencephalitis).

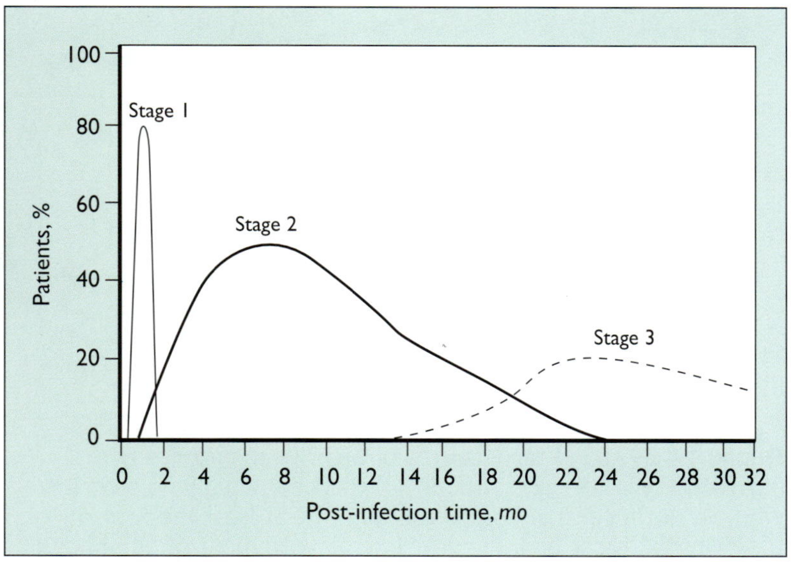

FIGURE 14-34 Time course and frequency of symptoms. Approximately 50% of persons with Lyme disease report a recent tick bite. Following the tick bite, the typical incubation period is 7 to 10 days (range, 3 to 31 d) prior to the onset of symptoms. The initial stage 1 symptoms occur in approximately 70% to 80% of infected individuals. Weeks after the initial tick bite, the skin, nervous system, and joints are the regions of the body that are most commonly involved as the spirochete spreads hematogenously. Stage 2 symptoms typically begin 4 to 10 weeks after the initial infection and they occur in approximately 50% of untreated patients. Stage 3 Lyme disease typically starts much later, often 1.5 to 2 years later; rarely, patients have the onset of stage 3 symptoms more than 5 years after their initial infection. (*Adapted from* Schmid [14]; with permission.)

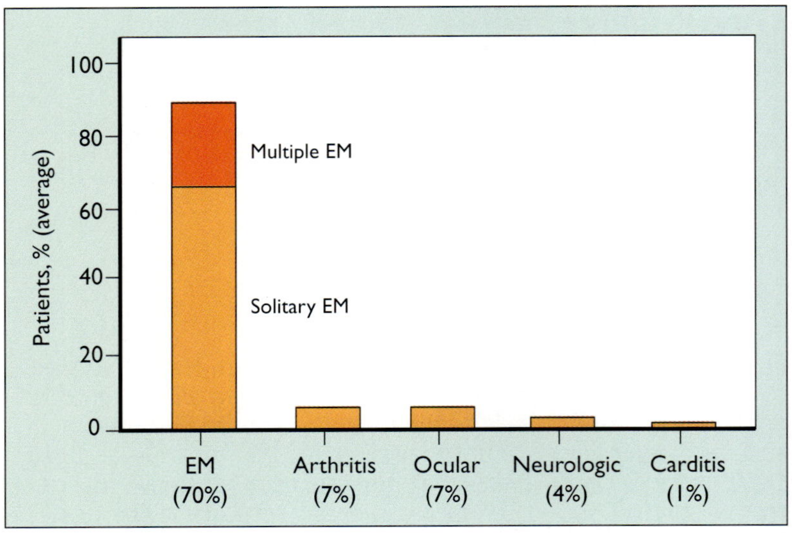

FIGURE 14-35 Frequency of specific clinical manifestations in children with Lyme disease. This figure depicts the most common clinical manifestations of Lyme disease in children. An erythema migrans rash occurs in approximately 90% of children, with 70% having a solitary erythema migrans rash and 20% having multiple erythema migrans lesions. Most studies suggest that arthritic, ocular, neurologic, and cardiac involvement generally occur in less than 10% of children with Lyme disease. Some studies, however, have suggested a higher rate of arthritis. Available data suggest that congenital Lyme disease occurs only rarely. In addition, transmission of *Borrelia burgdorferi* via breast milk has been documented [16].

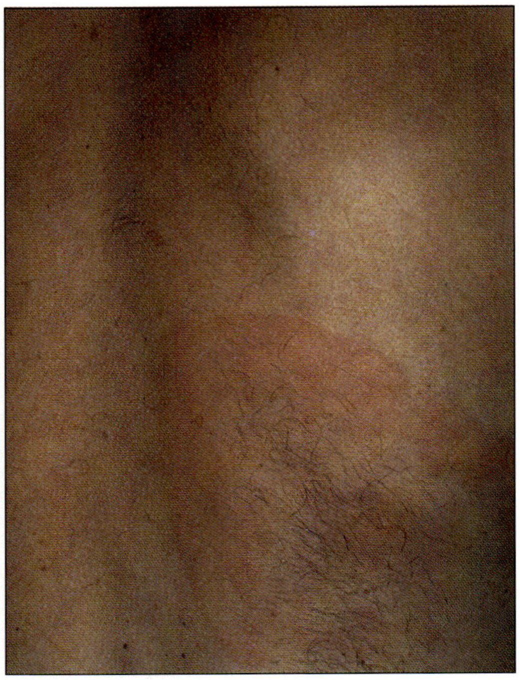

FIGURE 14-36 Erythema migrans rash in a patient with Lyme disease. This photograph shows a patient with Lyme disease who developed an erythema migrans rash on the right side of his back and flank. Erythema migrans typically develops 7 to 10 days after a tick bite and is present in 60% to 80% of patients. The erythema migrans rash typically appears as an erythematous, expanding, annular rash that frequently has partial central clearing. The rash averages 15 cm in diameter; if untreated, it persists for several weeks before gradually fading. Although the rash first appears at the site of the tick bite, multiple erythema migrans lesions can develop at sites away from the primary lesion. (*From* Spach and Liles [17]; with permission.)

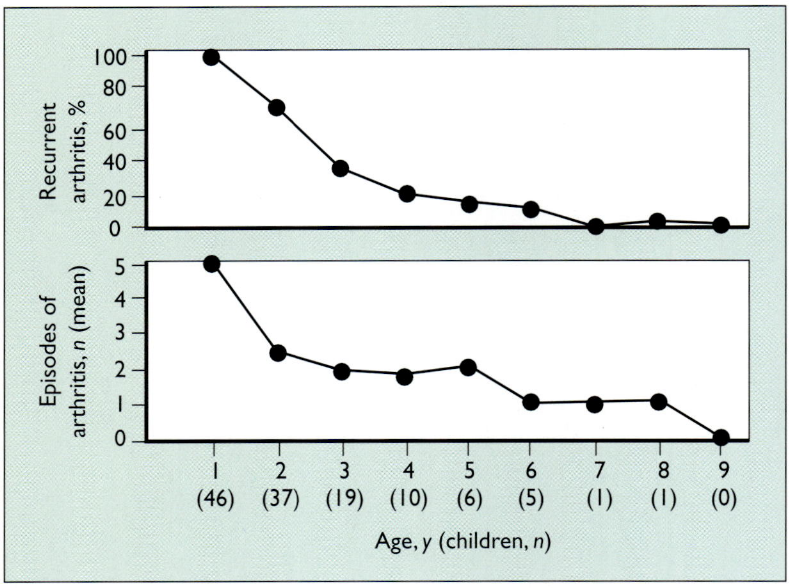

FIGURE 14-37 Long-term course of arthritis in children with untreated Lyme disease. Among 46 children with Lyme arthritis who did not receive antibiotic therapy (for at least the first 4 y of their illness), most typically developed involvement of one or two large joints. The knee was the joint most often affected. The children had a mean of five episodes of joint swelling in the first year of arthritis. As each year passed, the percentage of children with recurrent arthritis gradually decreased, as did the number of episodes per year for each child. By year 7, arthritis attacks were rare and when they did occur they involved only one episode per year. (*Adapted from* Szer *et al.* [18]; with permission.)

Laboratory diagnosis of Lyme disease
Serology
Enzyme immunoassay
Immunofluorescence antibody assay
Western immunoblotting
Cultures
Skin Biopsy
Polymerase chain reaction

FIGURE 14-38 Diagnostic tests for Lyme disease. In general, the diagnosis of Lyme disease depends on an accurate and detailed clinical assessment, and laboratory results should be viewed as supplemental information. Serologic testing should be considered as playing a secondary or supportive role; two-step serologic testing is recommended as outlined in Figure 14-45. Serologic tests have a high percentage of false-negative results during the initial 4 to 6 weeks of the patient's illness; false-positives can result from oral treponemes, syphilis, relapsing fever, Epstein-Barr viral infections, and rheumatoid arthritis. In addition, the lack of standardization of serologic testing has played a large role in the poor reliability of serologic testing. Investigators have cultured *Borrelia burgdorferi* from blood, cerebrospinal fluid, skin lesions, and a single synovial fluid specimen using a specialized culture medium referred to as Barbour–Stoenner–Kelly (BSK) medium. For routine clinical purposes, however, performing cultures has a low yield and is not practical; thus, it is generally not recommended. Although several case reports have described making a diagnosis of Lyme disease by taking a skin biopsy sample, this procedure is generally not done on a routine basis. Polymerase chain reaction (PCR)–based tests show some promise, but these tests have not become widely standardized. In addition, this test does not differentiate live from dead organisms. Most often, the PCR test has been used for cerebrospinal fluid or joint fluid analysis.

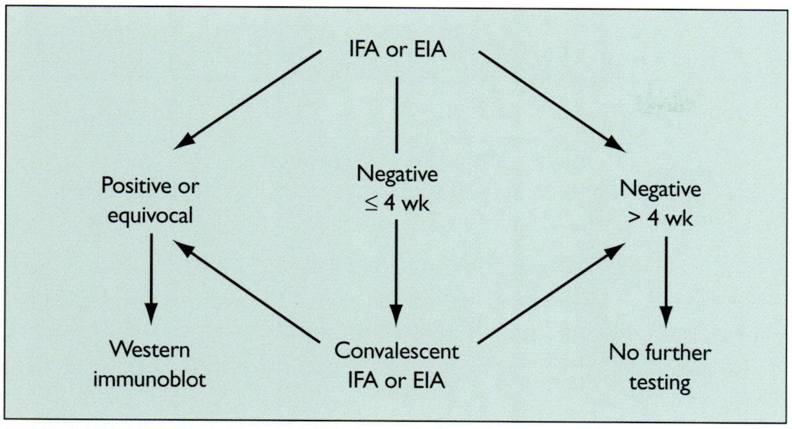

FIGURE 14-39 The current recommended approach to serologic testing of patients with suspected Lyme disease. These recommendations were made by expert groups that convened at the Second National Conference on Serologic Diagnosis of Lyme Disease in 1994. These groups included the Centers for Disease Control and Prevention, the Association of State and Territorial Public Health Laboratory Directors, the Food and Drug Administration, and the National Institutes of Health. In general, these groups recommended using a two-step diagnostic process, beginning with screening of suspected cases using either an enzyme immunoassay (EIA) or an immunofluorescent antibody (IFA) test. All positive or equivocal specimens should undergo "confirmatory" testing using a standardized Western immunoblot. Patients with a positive Western immunoblot result (see Fig. 14-46) are considered to have a positive serology test for Lyme disease. Patients who are more than 4 weeks into their illness and have a negative screening test do not need further testing. Patients who have a negative screening test, but are less than 4 weeks into their illness, should have a follow-up convalescent repeat screening test, and, if positive, subsequent Western immunoblot testing. If Western immunoblot testing is used for testing in the first 4 weeks of disease onset, then both IgM and IgG should be used. (*Adapted from* Centers for Disease Control and Prevention [19]; with permission.)

Criteria for a positive Western immunoblot serology test for Lyme disease

IgM (≥two bands), *kD*	21/24, 39, 41
IgG (≥five bands), *kD*	18, 21/24, 28, 30, 39, 41, 45, 58, 66, 93

FIGURE 14-40 Criteria for positive Western immunoblot test for Lyme disease. The recommendations from the expert groups that convened at the Second National Conference on Serologic Diagnosis of Lyme Disease in 1994 also standardized the criteria for a positive Western immunoblot serology test. The Western immunoblot IgM should be considered positive if at least two of the listed bands are present; the Western immunoblot IgG should be considered positive if at least five of the 10 bands listed are present. (*Adapted from* Centers for Disease Control and Prevention [20]; with permission.)

Treatment of Lyme disease in adults

Manifestation	Therapy	Route	Dosage	Duration, *d*
Early (erythema migrans)	Doxycycline	Orally	100 mg twice daily	14–21
	Amoxicillin	Orally	500 mg three times daily	14–21
	Cefuroxime axetil	Orally	500 mg twice daily	14–21
	Azithromycin	Orally	500 mg/dL, 250 mg once daily	7
Arthritis	Doxycycline	Orally	100 mg twice daily	30
	Amoxicillin	Orally	500 mg three times daily	30
	Ceftriaxone	Intravenously	2 g/d	14–21
Cardiac				
Mild (AV block with PR ≤0.3 s)	Doxycycline	Orally	100 mg twice daily	14–21
Serious	Ceftriaxone	Intravenously	2 g/d	14–21
Neurologic				
Mild (facial palsy)	Doxycycline	Orally	100 mg twice daily	21–30
	Amoxicillin	Orally	500 mg three times daily	21–30
Serious	Ceftriaxone	Intravenously	2 g/d intravenously	14–21

AV—atrioventricular; PR—pulse rate.

FIGURE 14-41 Treatment of Lyme disease in adults. The optimal dose and duration have not been well established for any therapy. Most experts recommend adjusting the duration of therapy based on the severity of the disease and the rapidity of response. In general, oral tetracycline (500 mg four times daily) can be substituted for oral doxycycline. Neither doxycycline nor tetracycline should be given to pregnant women, lactating women, or children younger than 8 years of age. The rationale for treating stage 1 Lyme disease is twofold: 1) to decrease the duration of the erythema migrans rash, and 2) reduce the probability that patients will develop later sequelae of Lyme disease. Success rates treating erythema migrans are high (>90%). The success in treating Lyme arthritis, however, has been variable, with approximately 50% of patients having a complete resolution of their arthritis within several weeks of completing antibiotic therapy. Patients who previously received intra-articular steroids have a lower response rate when treated with antibiotics. Approximately 60% of patients with neurologic involvement have a significant improvement after antibiotic treatment, although it may take months before a response is noted. Following therapy, some patients develop a fibromyalgia-like illness that does not respond to further antibiotic therapy. Prophylactic administration of antibiotics to patients who are bitten by a tick is controversial; some recommend prophylactic therapy only when the tick bite occurs in endemic areas.

Treatment of Lyme disease in children

Manifestation	Therapy	Route	Dose	Duration, *d*
Early (erythema migrans)	Amoxicillin	Orally	25–50 mg/kg/d divided in three doses	14–21
	Cefuroxime axetil	Orally	250 mg in three doses	14–21
	Erythromycin	Orally	30 mg/kg/d divided in four doses	14–21
Arthritis	Amoxicillin	Orally	50 mg/kg/d divided in three doses	30
	Ceftriaxone	Intravenously	75–100 mg/kg/d	14–21
	Penicillin G	Intravenously	300,000 U/kg/d divided in six doses (every 4 h)	14–21
Cardiac				
Mild (AV block with PR ≤0.3 s)	Amoxicillin	Orally	50 mg/kg/d divided in three doses	14–21
Serious	Ceftriaxone	Intravenously	2 g/d	14–21
	Penicillin G	Intravenously	300,000 U/kg/d divided in six doses (every 4 h)	14–21
Neurologic				
Mild (facial palsy)	Amoxicillin	Orally	50 mg/kg/d divided in three doses	21–30
Serious	Ceftriaxone	Intravenously	75–100 mg/kg/d	14–21
	Penicillin G	Intravenously	300,000 U/kg/d divided in six doses (every 4 h)	14–21

AV—atrioventricular.

FIGURE 14-42 Treatment of Lyme disease in children. Because large-scale treatment studies in children have not been performed, recommendations for children have been extrapolated from the adult data. Treatment of children younger than 8 years of age, however, does not include doxycycline or tetracycline because these antibiotics can cause permanent teeth staining. Children older than 8 years of age can receive doxycycline or tetracycline at a dose equivalent to the adult dose. Available data suggest that the long-term prognosis is excellent for children who have received therapy for Lyme disease. Indeed, several small studies suggest that children with arthritis have better response rates than adults do.

REFERENCES

1. Habicht GS, Beck G, Benach JL: Lyme Disease. *Sci Am* 1987, 257:78–83.
2. Brown RN and Lane RS: Lyme disease in California: a novel enzootic transmission cycle of *Borrelia burgdorferi*. *Science* 1992, 256:1439–1442.
3. Barinaga M: California rides its own bi-cycle. *Science* 1992, 256:1385.
4. Spach DH, Liles WC, Campbell GL, *et al.*: Tick-borne diseases in the United States. *N Engl J Med* 1993, 329:936–947.
5. Maeda K, Markowitz N, Hawley RC, *et al.*: Human infection with *Ehrlichia canis*, a leukocytic rickettsia. *N Engl J Med* 1987, 316:853–856.
6. Bakken JS, Dumler JS, Chen S-M, *et al.*: Human granulocytic ehrlichiosis in the upper Midwest United States: a new species emerging. *JAMA* 1994, 272:212–218.
7. Goodman JL, Nelson C, Vitale B, *et al.*: Direct cultivation of the causative agent of human granulocytic ehrlichiosis. *N Engl J Med* 1996, 334:209–215.
8. National Center for Infectious Disease Electronic Publications. Centers for Disease Control and Prevention website. Available at: http://www.cdc.gov/ncidod/publications. Accessed on May 20, 1998.
9. McDade JE: Ehrlichiosis: a disease of animals and humans. *J Infect Dis* 1990, 161:609–617.
10. Fishbein DB, Dawson JE, Robinson LE: Human ehrlichiosis in the United States, 1985 to 1990. *Ann Intern Med* 1994, 120:736–743.
11. Boustani MR, Gelfand JA: Babesiosis. *Clin Infect Dis* 1996, 22:611–605.
12. Sun T, Tenenbaum J, Greenspan J, *et al.* Morphologic and clinical observations in human infection with *Babesia microti*. *J Infect Dis* 1983, 148:239–248.
13. Centers for Disease Control and Prevention: *MMWR Morbidity Mortality Weekly Rep* 1991, 40:451–459.
14. Schmid GP: Epidemiology and clinical similarities of human spirochetal diseases. *Rev Infect Dis* 1989, 11(suppl 6):S1460–S1469.
15. Schwann TG, Piesman J, Golde WT, *et al.*: Induction of an outer surface protein on *Borrelia burgdorferi* during tick feeding. *Proc Natl Acad Sci USA* 1995, 92:2909–2913.
16. Shapiro ED: Lyme disease in children. *Am J Med* 1995, 98 (suppl):69S–73S.
17. Spach DH, Liles WC: Tick-borne diseases: an illustrated update. *Hosp Med* 1994, 30:25–36.
18. Szer IS, Taylor E, Steere AC: The long-term course of Lyme arthritis in children. *N Engl J Med* 1991, 325:159–163.
19. Centers for Disease Control and Prevention: Recommendations for test performance and interpretation from the Second National Conference on Serologic Diagnosis of Lyme Disease. *MMWR Morbidity Mortality Weekly Rep* 1995, 44:590–591.

CHAPTER 15

Infections in Immunocompromised Hosts

Patricia Flynn
Elaine Tuomanen

WITH THE INCREASINGLY LONG-TERM SURVIVAL of children with hematologic malignancies, solid tumors, and bone marrow or organ transplantation, the control of infectious diseases in the immunocompromised patient has become a major determinant of outcome. Loss of neutrophil function places the patient at particularly increased risk of bacterial and fungal infection. In contrast, loss of T- and B-cell functions increases the risk of all classes of infection. In addition, patients are susceptible to infections based on therapy involving infusions or in-dwelling lines and catheters. This broad range of diagnostic possibilities makes empiric therapy both necessary and challenging.

Classic syndromes that arise in immunocompromised patients include lesions of the mucosa and skin, pneumonitis, diarrhea, cystitis, and catheter-related infections. These syndromes arise from direct effect of chemotherapeutic agents on rapidly growing epithelial cells as well as loss of defenses against endogenous bacterial flora. Generalized sepsis can involve bacteria, fungi, or viruses. In these groups, the agents common in normal children remain prominent, but disease is often more severe. Equally common, however, are rarer and emerging pathogens. First-line anti-infectives are available for many of these classes of infection. However, because these patients usually undergo multiple rounds of therapy, resistance to anti-infectives is a persistent and real complication. This problem has prompted trials of adjunctive therapies such as cytokines, growth factors, gammaglobulin, and other investigational agents. The success of interferon in the treatment of chronic granulomatous disease raises hopes that reconstitution of the immunocompromised host's defense will be increasingly possible. Further, more attention has been directed to antimicrobial prophylaxis and administration of vaccines to control the risk of infection before the onset of disease. In this context, the remarkable success of trimethoprim-sulfamethoxazole in controlling disease due to *Pneumocystic carinii* stands as a stellar example.

This chapter presents an overview of the broad spectrum of disease in these patients and a general diagnostic and therapeutic approach. Syndromes are illustrated to demonstrate the diversity of causes of infections in these patients. Finally, the individual classes of infectious agents—bacteria, fungi, viruses, and others—are depicted with particular attention to the contrast between the classic localized disease of normal children and the severe, disseminated disease of immunocompromised patients.

PATHOGENS AND RISK PERIODS

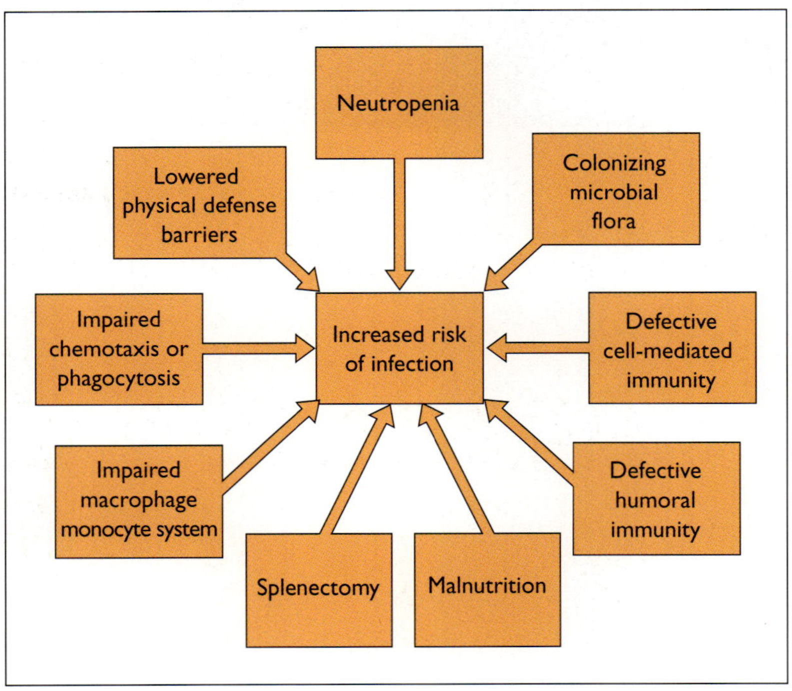

FIGURE 15-1 Contributors to the increased risk of infection in the immunocompromised host. Patients undergoing chemotherapy or immunoablative intervention are at increased risk of infection from both exogenous and endogenous infectious agents. Chemotherapy compromises physical barriers at mucous membranes and skin, increasing the risk of pathogen entry, both in terms of commensals and new agents. Loss of defenses further promotes overwhelming infection.

Classes of defects in host defense

Immune defect	Examples	Bacteria	Fungi	Parasites	Viruses
Interrupted integument	Intravenous needles Catheters Mucositis	*S. pyogenes* *S. aureus* Enterobacteriaceae *P. aeruginosa* Coagulase-negative staphylococci *Corynebacterium* Viridans streptococci	*Candida* *Mucoraceae* *Aspergillus* *Fusarium*		
Infusion infections	Blood products Intravenous fluids	*Salmonella* *Enterobacter* *Serratia*	*Candida*	*Plasmodium* *Toxoplama* *Babesia* *Trypanosoma*	Hepatitis B, C, E CMV EBV HIV HTLV
Neutrophil	Acute leukemia Chemotherapy	*S. pyogenes* *S. aureus* Enterobacteriaceae *P. aeruginosa* Enterococci	*Candida* *Aspergillus* *Mucoraceae* *Trichosporon* *Fusarium* *Pseudallescheria*		
T helper lymphocyte	Hodgkin's disease Chemotherapy Marrow transplant AIDS	*Listeria* *Salmonella* *Serratia* *Nocardia* *Mycobacterium* *Legionella* *Rhodococcus*	*Cryptococcus* *Candida* *Histoplasma* *Coccidoides* *Penicillium* *Pneumocystis*	*T. gondii* *Strongyloides* *Cryptosporidium* *Leishmania* *Isopora belli*	Measles HSV VZV CMV Adenovirus JC virus BK virus Echovirus
Gamma globulin	Multiple myeloma Chronic lymphocytic leukemia Chemotherapy Marrow transplant AIDS	*S. pneumoniae* *H. influenzae* *N. meningitidis*	*Pneumocystis*	*Giardia lamblia*	
Complement	Congenital defects	*Neisseria*			
Splenectomy	Posttrauma Sickle cell	*S. pneumoniae* *H. influenzae* *N. meningitidis*		*Babesia* *Plasmodium*	

CMV—cytomegalovirus; EBV—Epstein-Barr virus; HTLV—human T-cell leukemia virus; HSV—herpes simplex virus; VZV—varicella-zoster virus.

FIGURE 15-2 Classes of defects in host defense. These classes create different risk patterns for infecting organisms. Bacteria and fungi are the most prominent infectious agents in all classes of compromised defense, but specific causes differ depending on the class of immune defect. Viruses and parasites add to the picture regarding defects in T-cell function and infections from infusion of blood products or intravenous fluids. (*Adapted from* Armstrong [1]; with permission.)

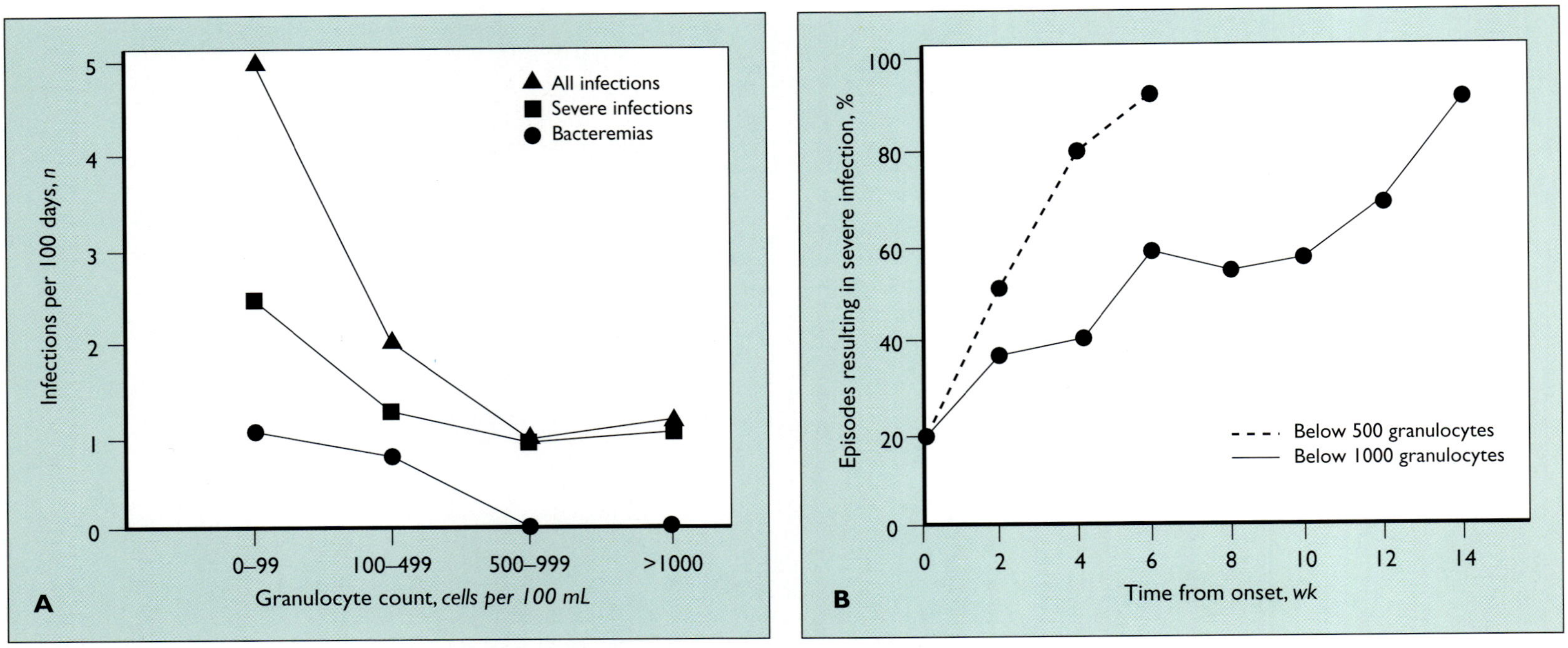

FIGURE 15-3 Risk of infection as a function of depth and length of neutropenia. **A,** Severe neutropenia, particularly at a level below 500 leukocytes per 100 µL, is associated with nearly universal infection, most often severe. **B,** When this level of neutropenia persists, virtually all patients become infected. These data have stood the test of time and are the foundation for the guidelines for immediate and aggressive management of fever in the neutropenic patient. (*Adapted from* Bodey *et al* [2]; with permission.)

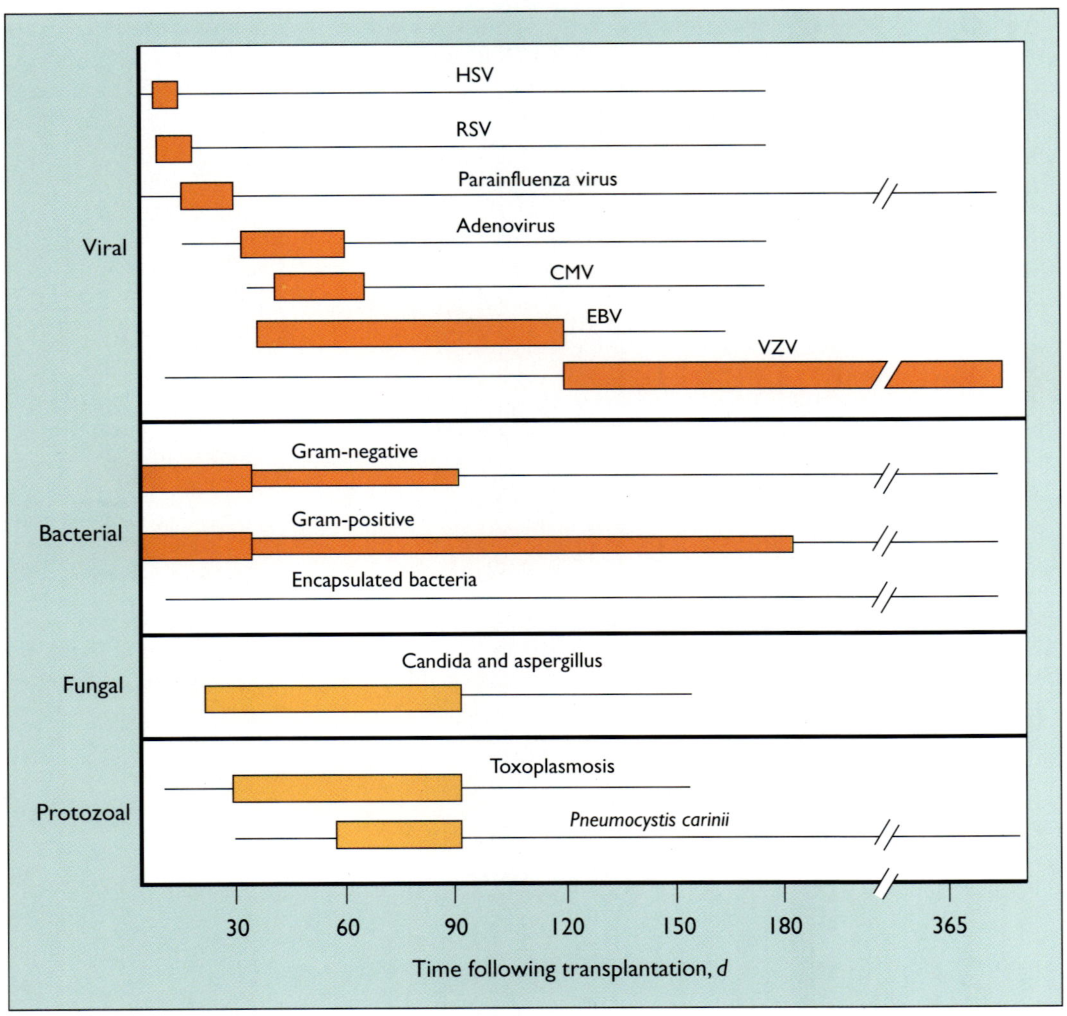

FIGURE 15-4 Timing of infections as a function of transplantation. During the first 4 weeks following immunoablative therapy, patients are at very high risk for bacterial sepsis or herpes simplex virus (HSV) and respiratory syncitial virus (RSV) infections. Thereafter, Epstein-Barr virus (EBV), cytomegalovirus (CMV), and other viruses are coupled with fungi, particularly *Candida* and *Aspergillus* spp. Late complications include varicella-zoster virus (VZV) and sepsis due to encapsulated bacteria. *Heavy bars* indicate period of highest risk. (*Adapted from* Patrick [3]; with permission.)

General Therapeutic Approach

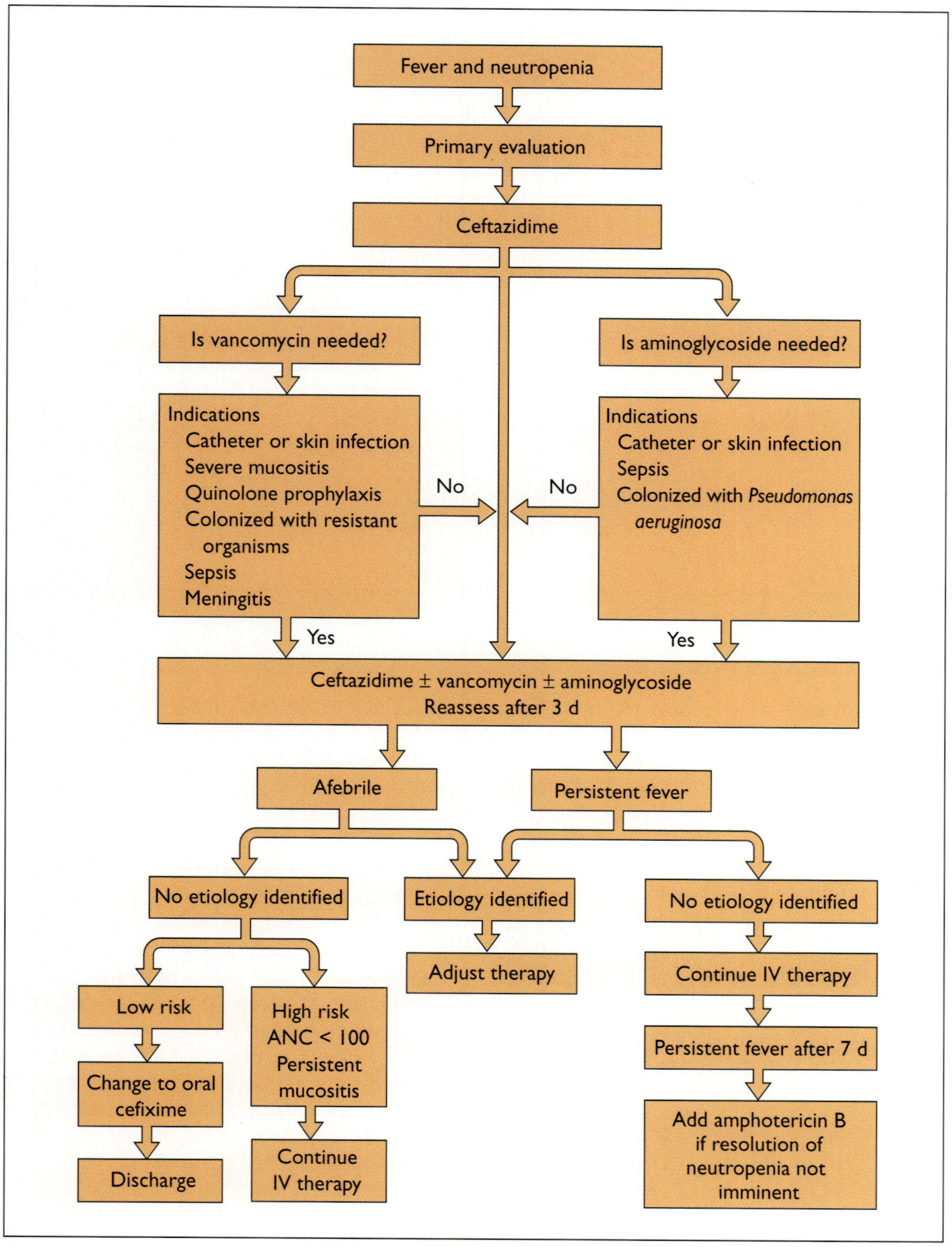

Figure 15-5 Treatment algorithm for fever and neutropenia. This algorithm is used at St. Jude Children's Research Hospital, Memphis, and serves as an example of the decisions to be made in the management of the immunocompromised patient with suspected infection based on fever with or without localizing signs. The first decision is whether there is a need to broaden monotherapy ceftazidime to include vancomycin for staphylococci or *Streptococcus viridans* or an aminoglycoside for pseudomonas infection. After 7 days, if fever persists, the decision to add antifungal therapy must be made. In contrast, if the fever resolves and the patient does not have any high-risk criteria, treatment can be switched to oral cefixime with discharge from the hospital.

Cytokine therapies for immunocompromised patients

Factor	Target diseases	Major function
GM-CSF	Bone marrow transplant neutropenia	Stimulates proliferation of neutrophil, monocyte, and eosinophil progenitors; enhances function of mature corresponding cells
G-CSF	Bone marrow transplant neutropenia	Stimulates proliferation of neutrophil progenitors; enhances function of mature neutrophils
IFN γ	Chronic granulomatous disease	Enhances function of neutrophils and monocytes/macrophages; increase expression of MHC class II antigens; enhances production of IgG subclasses
Erythropoietin	Anemia	Stimulates proliferation of erythrocytes
IVIG	Hypogammaglobulinemia HIV	Passive antibody replacement
M-CSF	Investigational	Stimulates proliferation of monocyte progenitors; enhances function of monocytes
IL-1 (α and β)	Investigational	Stimulation, proliferation, and differentiation of T, B, and other cells; induces fever, catabolism, and acute-phase proteins; induces proliferation of bone marrow cells; activates neutrophils and monocytes
IL-3	Investigational	Promotes growth of stem cells erythroid and myeloid progenitors
IL-6	Investigational	Promotes differentiation of B cells; induces production of immunoglobulins; induces acute-phase proteins
Stem cell factor	Investigational	Promotes multilineage differentiation
PIXY 321	Investigational	GM-CSF/IL-3 fusion protein promotes multilineage differentiation of stem cells

G-CSF—granulocyte colony-stimulating factor; GM-CSF—granulocyte–macrophage colony-stimulating factor; IFN—interferon; IL—interleukin; IVIG—intravenous immunoglobulin; M-CSF—macrophage colony-stimulating factor; MHC—major histocompatibility complex.

FIGURE 15-6 Cytokine therapies for immunocompromised patients. Reconstitution of the immune defects of immunocompromised patients has moved forward the availability of recombinant growth factors and cytokines. Neutropenia, lymphopenia, and anemia can be shortened with the application of growth factors. Cytokines are largely investigational but show promise for a wide variety of defects. Interferon is particularly beneficial to patients with chronic granulomatous disease. Gammaglobulin is used not only for hypogammaglobulinemia, but increasingly also for in many settings to provide passive antibody. (*Adapted from* Roilides and Pizzo [4]; with permission.)

Immunization after bone marrow transplantation

Vaccine	Allogenic BMT	Autologous BMT	Recommended time, *mo*
Tetanus toxoid	++	++	12
Diphtheria toxoid	++	++	12
Inactivated poliovirus	++	++	12
Measles (attenuated)	+/–	+/–	Individual
Rubella (attenuated)	+/–	+/–	Individual
Mumps (attenuated)	+/–	+/–	Individual
Influenza	+	+	6
Haemophilus influenzae	++	+	4–6
Streptococcus pneumoniae	++	+	4–6
Hepatitis B	+	+	

FIGURE 15-7 Schedule for immunizations after bone marrow transplantation (BMT). Following immunoablative therapy, engraftment of donor cells allows initiation of a schedule of reimmunization of the host. Nonliving vaccines are administered first. Live attenuated vaccines (measles, mumps, rubella) are delayed until demonstration of an adequate response to nonliving vaccine antigens (*eg*, tetanus). (*Adapted from* Ljungman *et al.* [5]; with permission.)

Syndromes with Multiple Causes

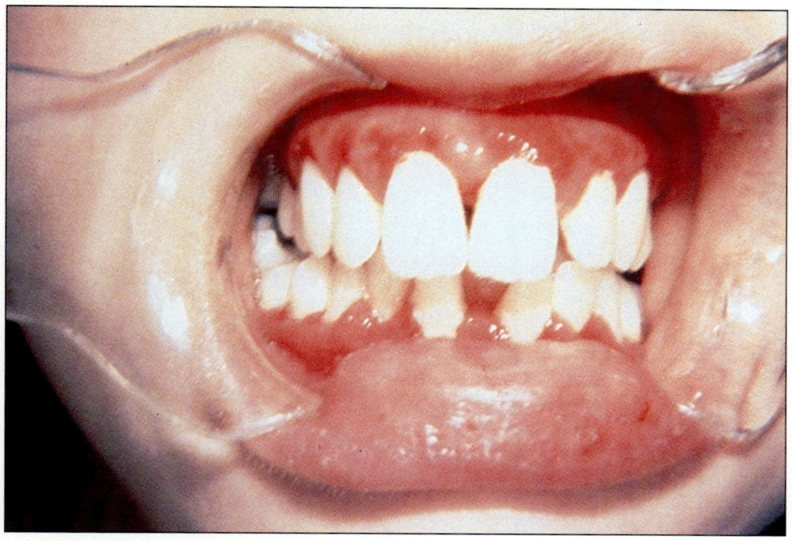

Figure 15-8 Mucositis. Chemotherapy, particularly cytosine arabinoside, directly destroys rapidly growing mucosal cells of the gastrointestinal, pulmonary, and urogenital tracts. This destruction promotes overgrowth of endogenous flora leading to mucositis. The most common cause is *Candida* spp, but overgrowth of oral bacterial flora is also common. Oral hygiene and topical application of antifungals provides palliative treatment until the epithelium regenerates.

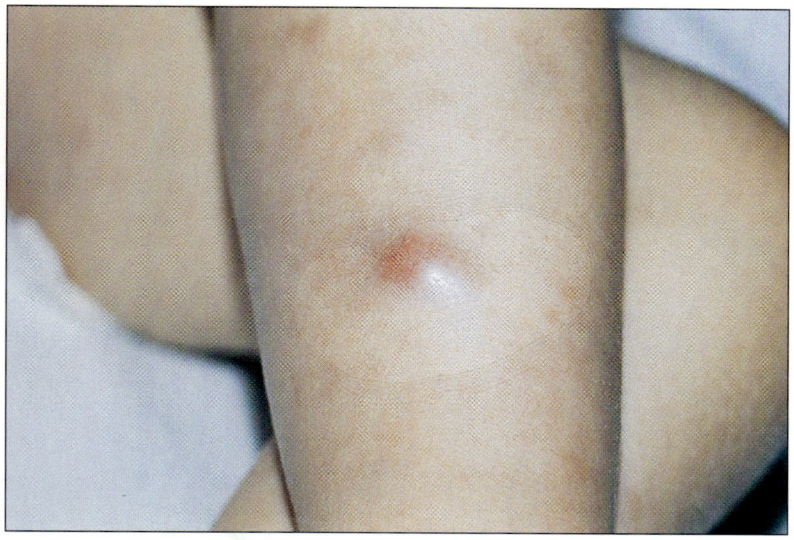

Figure 15-9 Cutaneous lesion. Virtually every infectious pathogen can produce cutaneous manifestations in the immunocompromised host. The differential diagnosis of such lesions can be inferred from Figure 15-2. However, the clinician must also differentiate infectious from noninfectious causes. The lesion shown is a cutaneous infiltration of leukemic cells.

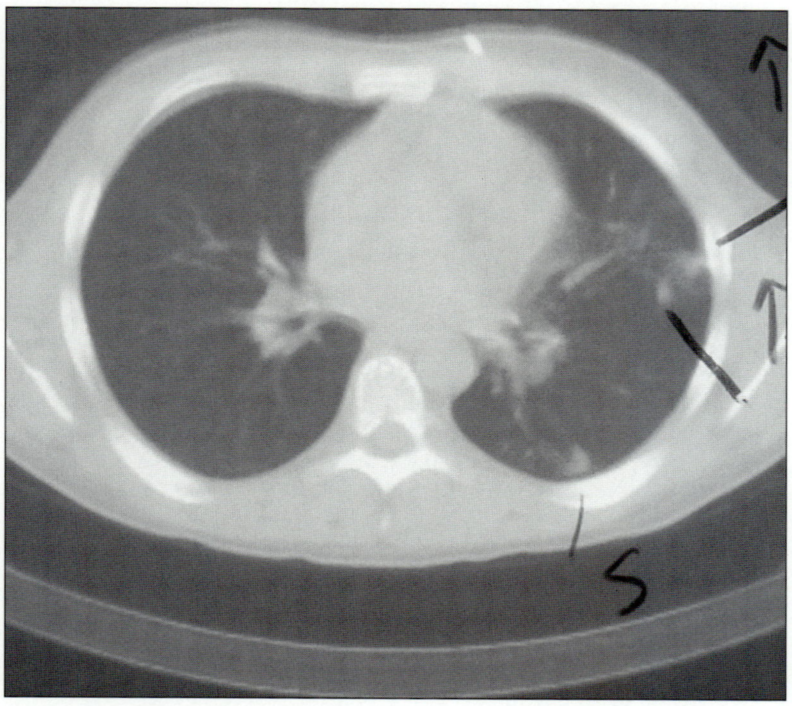

Figure 15-10 Bronchiolitis obliterans organizing pneumonia (BOOP). Virtually every infectious pathogen can produce pulmonary manifestations in the immunocompromised host. The wide differential diagnosis of such lesions is listed in Figure 15-11. Dyspnea and cough are associated with radiographic evidence of hyperaeration and consolidation (indicated by *bars*). Corticosteroids can be helpful. In addition to infectious causes, myeloproliferative disorders can be associated with widespread pulmonary infiltrates.

Infectious and noninfectious cases of pneumonitis in patients receiving a bone marrow transplant

Infectious	Noninfectious
Bacterial	Pulmonary damage by radiation
Enterobacteriaceae sp.	Pulmonary damage by chemotherapy (*eg,* bleomycin)
Staphylococcus aureus	Underlying malignancy
Legionella sp.	Pulmonary edema
Fungal	Alveolar hemorrhage
Aspergillus sp.	Idiopathic interstitial pneumonia
Mucor sp.	Pulmonary vascular disease
Candida sp.	Pneumomediastinum
Viral	
Cytomegalovirus	
Adenovirus	
Respiratory syncytial virus	
Parainfluenzae virus	
Influenzae virus	
Human herpesvirus 6	
Protozoan	
Pneumocystis carinii	

Figure 15-11 Infectious (*left*) and noninfectious (*right*) causes of pneumonitis in transplant recipients. Pneumonitis is perhaps the most common, serious manifestation of infection in this group of patients. The use of trimethoprim-sulfamethoxazole prophylaxis for *Pneumocystis* spp infections has greatly diminished the incidence of pneumonitis. Although bacterial causes are common soon after transplantation, fungal and viral causes are prominent, particularly after the first few weeks (see Figure 15-4).

Differential diagnosis of hemorrhagic cystitis

- Noninfectious
  - Chemotherapy (*eg*, cyclophosphamide)
  - Graft-versus-host disease
  - Mechanical trauma from Foley catheter
- Infectious
  - Viral
    - Adenovirus
    - Cytomegalovirus
    - Papovavirus (*eg*, BK virus)
    - Herpes simplex virus
  - Bacterial
    - Urinary tract infection, mainly gram-negative enteric organisms
  - Fungal
    - Urinary tract infection
    - Fungal ball

FIGURE 15-12 Differential diagnosis of hemorrhagic cystitis. The generalized mucositis associated with chemotherapy includes the bladder epithelium. Such hemorrhagic cystitis can be controlled with bladder irrigation. However, each case should be examined for viral causes, particularly adenovirus. Less common causes include bacterial and fungal urinary tract infections.

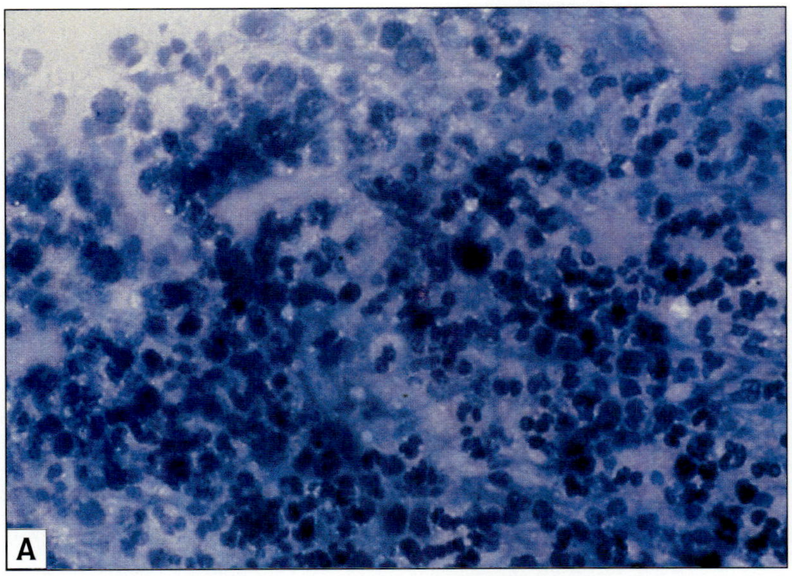

A

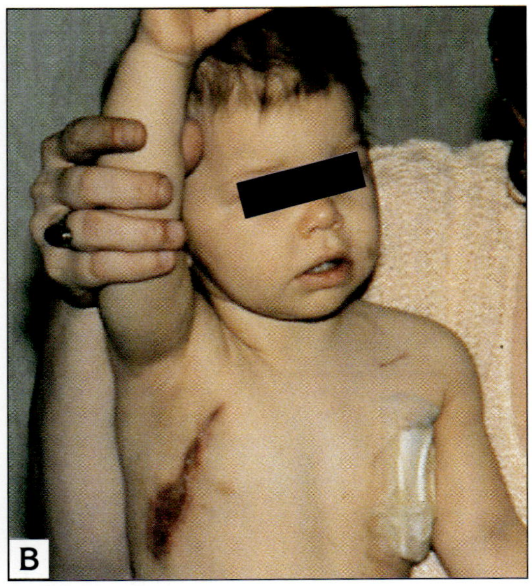

B

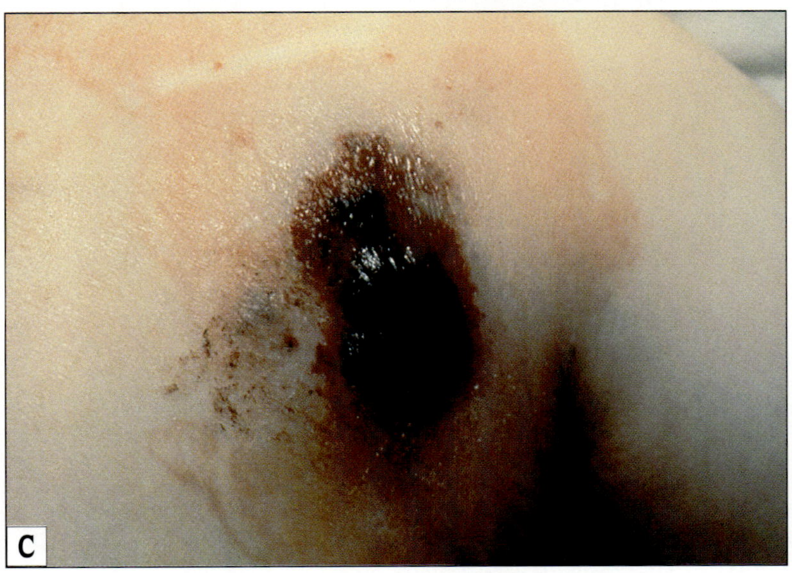

C

FIGURE 15-13 Catheter-related infections. In-dwelling catheters can become colonized with pathogens from contiguous skin, such as staphylococci, or agents causing bacteremia, such as *Candida* spp. Diagnosis involves differentiating infection only of the catheter from accompanying systemic or local infection. A bacterial count in fluid drawn from the catheter that is five- to tenfold higher than in peripheral blood indicates catheter-related infection, which can be managed with simple removal of the catheter if no longer needed. If continued use of a long-term catheter (*eg*, a Hickman or subcutaneous portal) is necessary, antimicrobial therapy may be successful in two thirds to three quarters of infections. In contrast, local inflammation of the tunnel tract indicates the need for both removal of the catheter and systemic anti-infective therapy. A particularly aggressive infection of a catheter site is associated with atypical mycobacteria, which requires wide surgical excision of the site to avoid chronic, persistent infection. **A** and **B**, Atypical mycobacteria: acid-fast bacilli in a Hickman catheter exudate *(panel A)*, and recurrent infection after suboptimal surgical debridement of an infected catheter tunnel tract *(panel B)*. **C**, Pseudomonas infection–induced necrotic lesion at exit site.

(continued on next page)

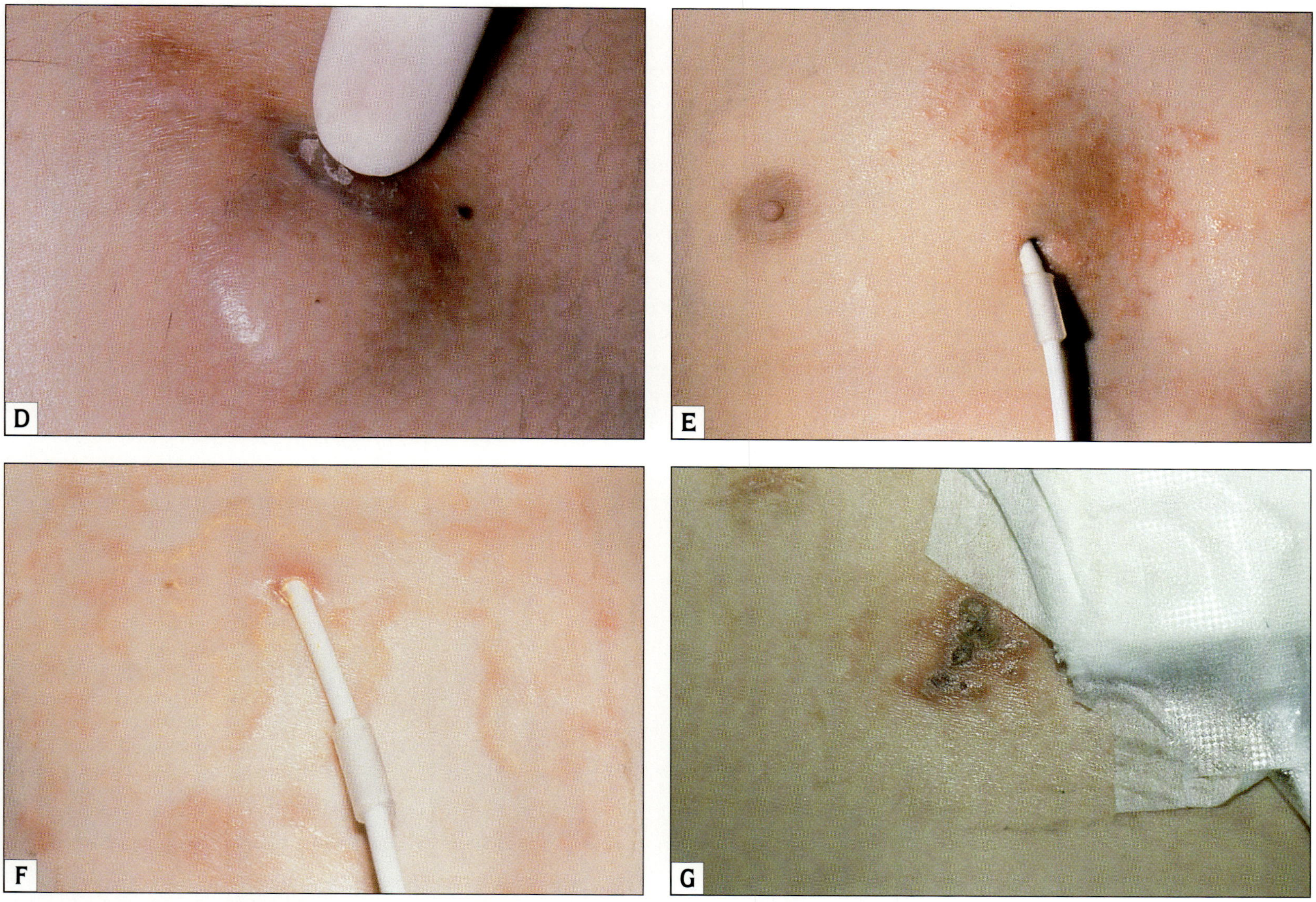

Figure 15-13 *(continued)* **D**, Culture-negative inflammation and tissue breakdown over a subcutaneous portal. **E**, *Candida albicans*–induced erythematous papular rash at exit site. **F**, *Microsporum canis* and *Candida parapsilosis*–induced serpentigenous lesion underlying plastic film dressing. **G**, Herpes simplex virus–induced vesicular and crusted lesions at exit site. This patient also had oral herpetic lesions. (*Panels A and F from* Ryan-Poirier [6]; with permission.)

Bacterial Infections

Common bacterial causes of fever in neutropenic patients
Gram-positive
Staphylococcus aureus
Coagulase-negative staphylococci
S. pneumonia
S. pyrogenes
Viridans streptococci
Enterococcus sp.
Corynebacterium sp.
Gram-negative
Escherichia coli
Klebsiella sp.
Pseudomonas aeruginosa
Enterobacter sp.

Figure 15-14 Common bacterial causes of fever in neutropenic patients. The incidence of bacteremia in neutropenic patients with fever is high enough to warrant empiric, aggressive antibiotic therapy. Endogenous flora account for many infections, and increased risk for these infections can be indicated by surveillance culture of the nose and rectum.

Emerging resistance to antibiotics in bacteria

Antibacterial agent	Resistant organisms
New cephalosporins	Gram-negative bacilli
Carbapenems	*Pseudomonas* sp., *Stenotrophomonas* sp., Enterobacteriaceae, staphylococci, enterococci, *Bacteroides* sp.
Semisynthetic penicillins, cephalosporins	Staphylococci, pneumococci
Aminoglycosides	Enterococci, gram-negative bacilli
Penicillins	Enterococci, pneumococci
Glycopeptides (vancomycin, teicoplanin)	Enterococci, staphylococci
Fluoroquinolones	Staphylococci, gram-negative bacilli

Figure 15-15 Emerging resistance to antibiotics in bacteria. As patients with neutropenia undergo multiple rounds of antibiotic therapy, development of antibiotic resistance is a common occurrence. Such resistant pathogens are also acquired nosocomially, particularly in the intensive care unit, where these patients commonly are cared for. (*Adapted from* Shlaes *et al.* [7]; with permission.)

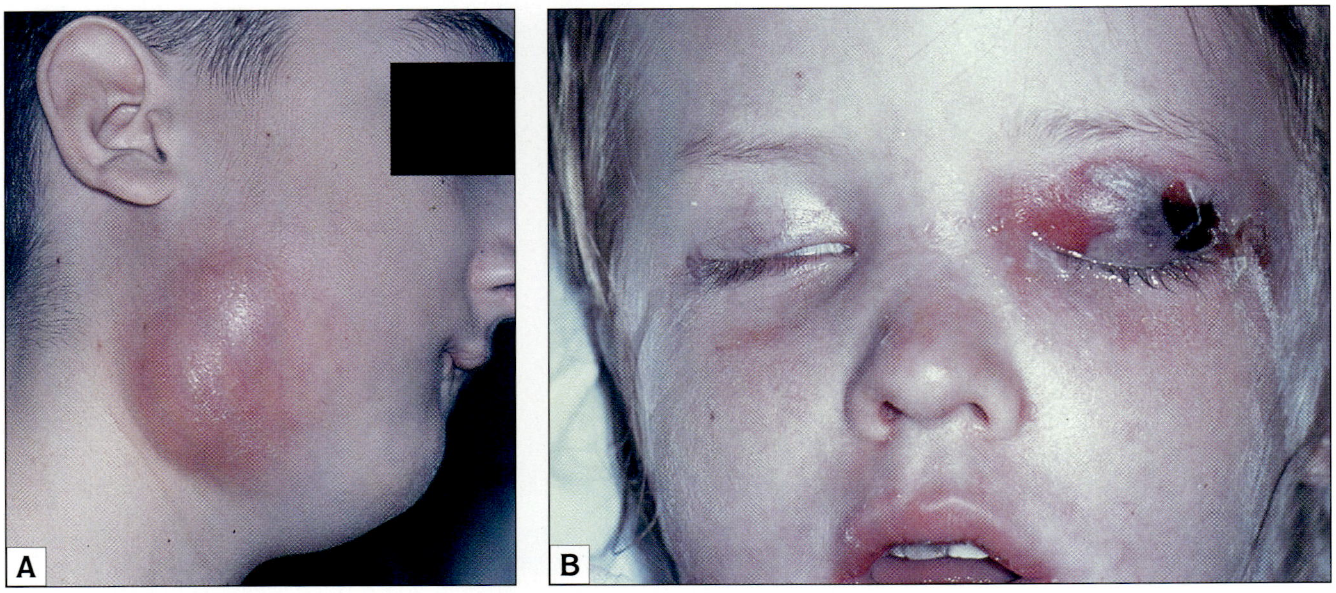

Figure 15-16 Abscesses caused by *Staphylococcus aureus*. Superficial infections of the skin and draining lymph nodes are characteristic of *S. aureus*. Although most infections respond to common antibiotics, a high local prevalence of methicillin-resistant strains may require the use of vancomycin. **A,** Abscess formation in a cervical lymph node. **B,** Periorbital cellulitis.

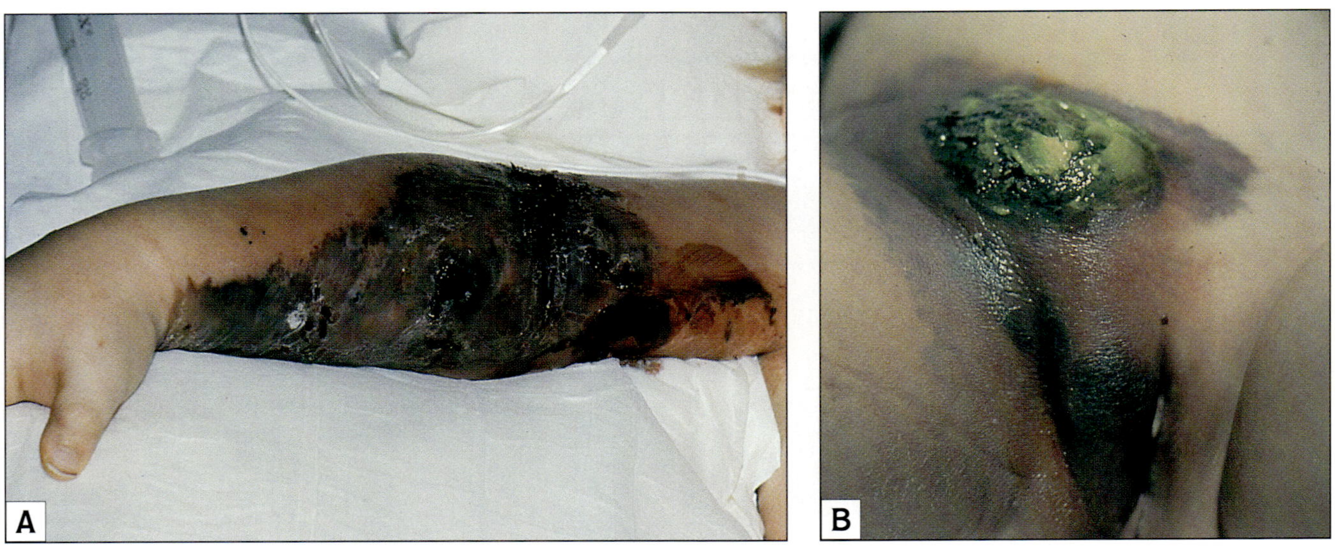

Figure 15-17 Gram-negative cellulitis. Although most cutaneous infections are caused by staphylococci, immunosuppressed patients develop necrotic skin lesions with gram-negative flora (*eg, Klebsiella* and *Pseudomonas* spp. and *Escherichia coli*). These lesions commonly are rapidly progressive, deep, and necrotic. **A,** Lesions of the arm. **B,** Lesions of the abdominal wall.

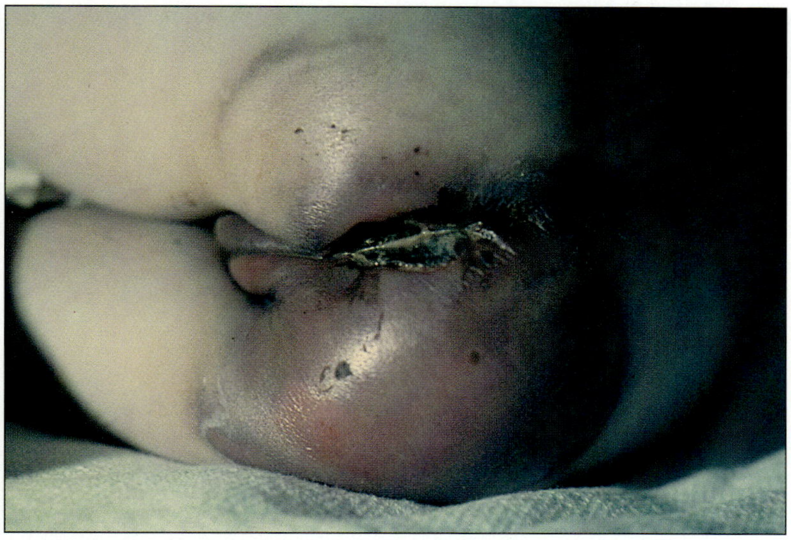

FIGURE 15-18 Perirectal cellulitis. Generalized mucositis, especially during chemotherapy, enhances the incidence of infection with endogenous flora. Gut colonization with *Pseudomonas* spp can indicate increased risk for perirectal cellulitis, which is particularly aggressive in this patient infected with *Pseudomonas aeruginosa*.

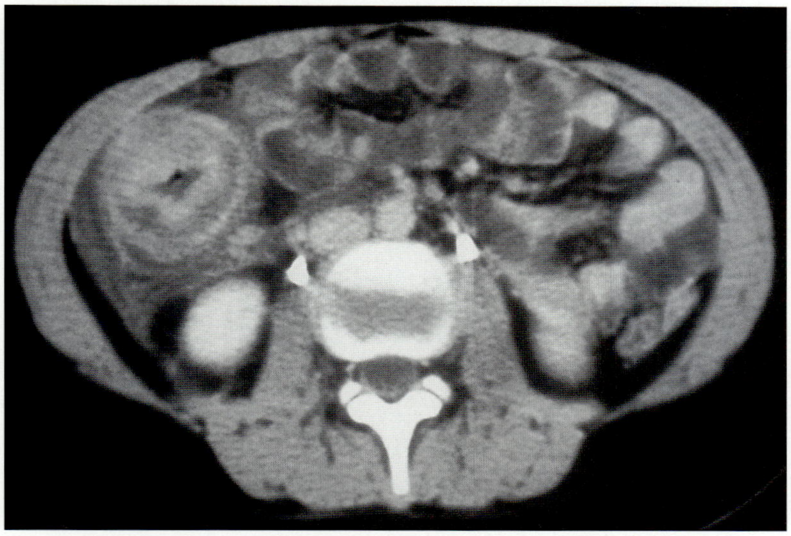

FIGURE 15-19 Typhilitis. Neutropenic patients can develop a necrotizing infection of the cecum and terminal ileum that mimics appendicitis. Causative organisms include *Pseudomonas*, Enterobacteriaceae, anaerobes, *Candida*, and *Aspergillus* (for which medical management usually is sufficient), and *Clostridium septicum*, which produces a fulminant, toxin-mediated myonecrosis.

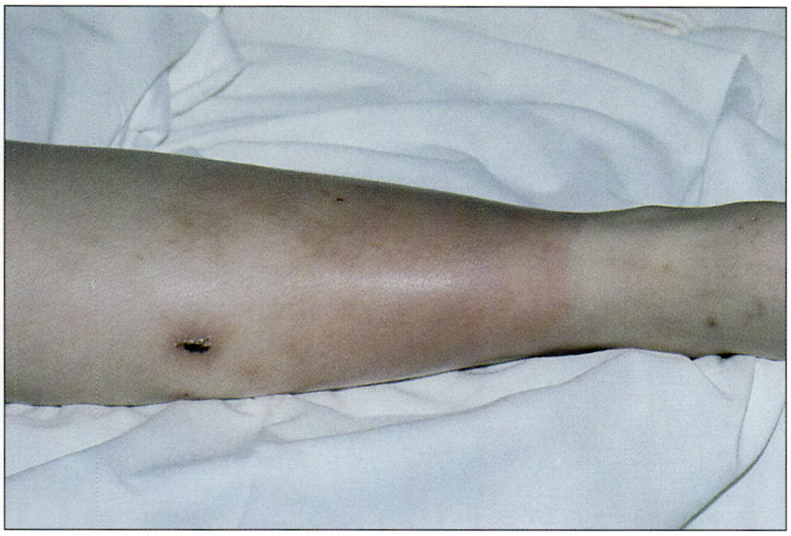

FIGURE 15-20 Erysipelas. Following a break in the skin, infection with *Streptococcus pyogenes* can cause this symptom complex of local painful induration and lymphatic spread. Distinction from the more intensive necrotizing soft tissue infections is important (see Fig. 15-22).

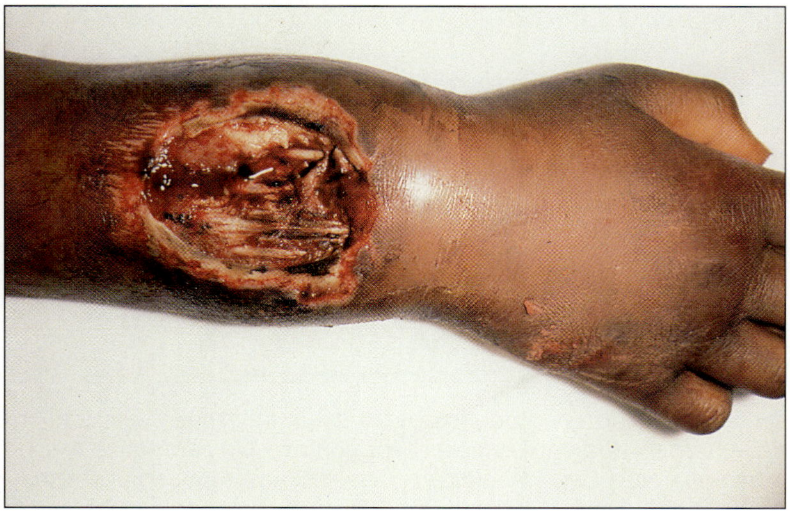

FIGURE 15-21 Necrotizing soft tissue infection. Several bacteria and fungi can produce this syndrome, including *Streptococcus pyogenes*, *Clostridium perfringens* (shown), mycobacteria, *Staphylococcus aureus*, *Vibrio*, *Aspergillus*, and *Mucor*. These infections can also be polymicrobial. The recent emergence of more aggressive forms of group A streptococcal infection, such as necrotizing fasciitis, require very aggressive therapy, including repeated surgical debridement and combination of antibiotherapy with β-lactams and clindamycin.

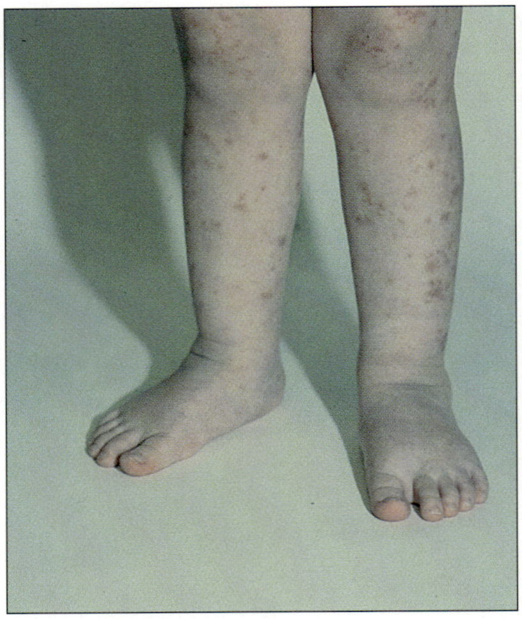

Figure 15-22 Aeromonas soft tissue infection. A recognized cause of watery diarrhea, *Aeromonas* organisms also cause sepsis in addition to skin and soft tissue infections. Sepsis caused by *Aeromonas* is similar to that caused by other gram-negative bacteria and may be polymicrobial, particularly in immunocompromised patients or those with hepatobiliary disease.

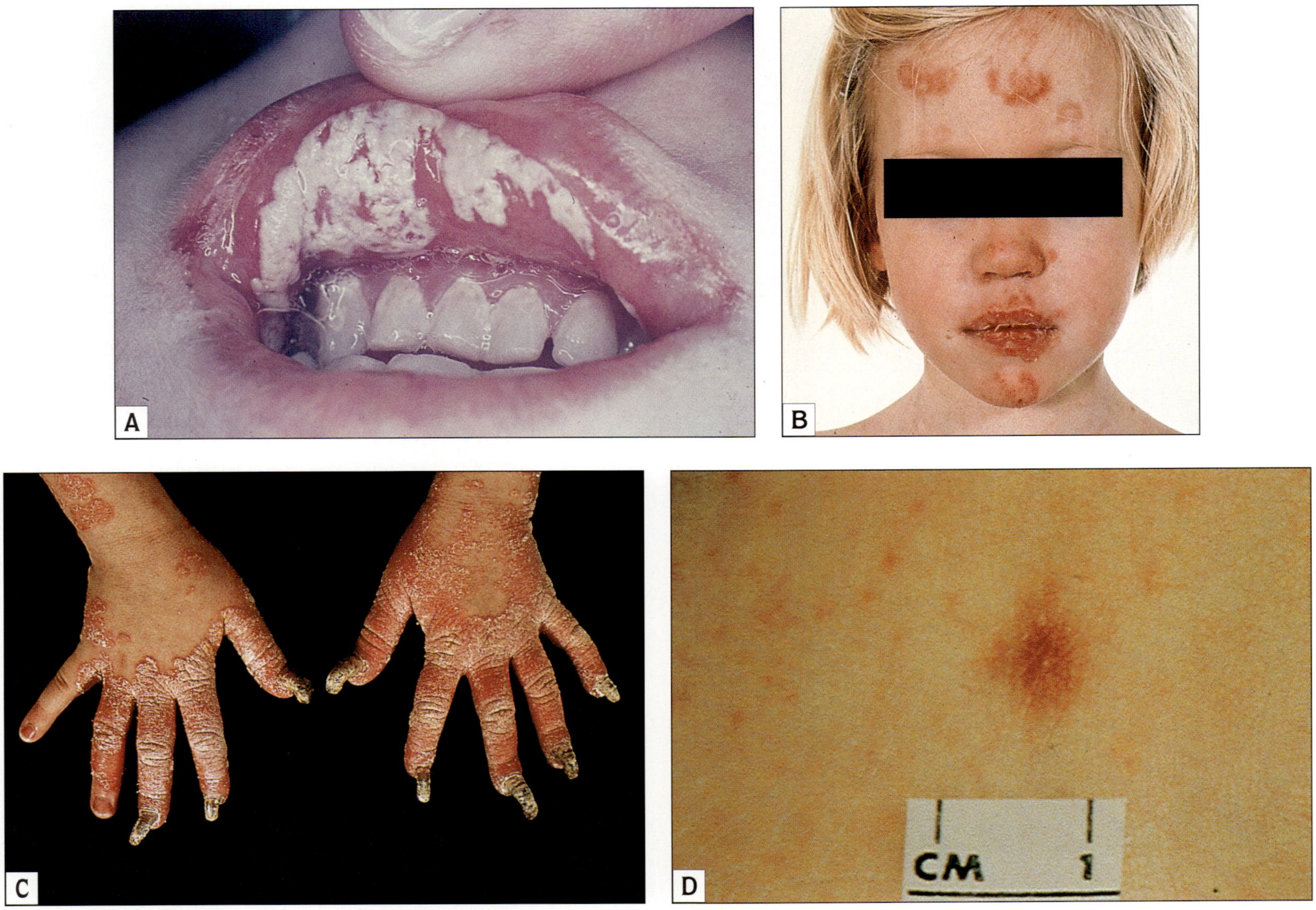

Figure 15-23 Various infections caused by *Candida* spp. *Candida albicans* or *Candida tropicalis* are major pathogens of immunocompromised patients, whereas *Candida krusei*, *Candida glabrata*, and *Candida parapsilosis* are increasing in frequency. **A,** Oral thrush. Most immunodeficient patients experience mild mucositis. **B** and **C,** Chronic mucocutaneous candidiasis. This condition is caused by an inherited T-cell defect associated with widespread, noninvasive cutaneous infections with *Candida albicans*. Severely immunocompromised patients can develop disseminated disease involving lesions of any organ. **D** through **G,** Manifestations of disseminated *C. tropicalis*: skin *(panel D)*,

(continued on next page)

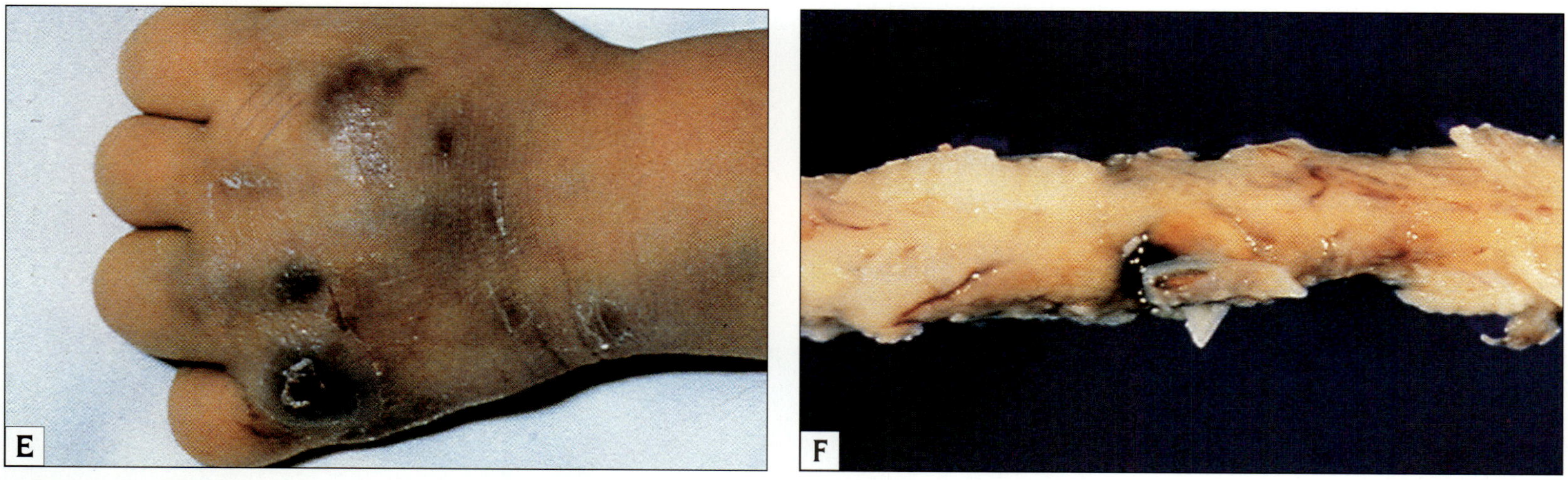

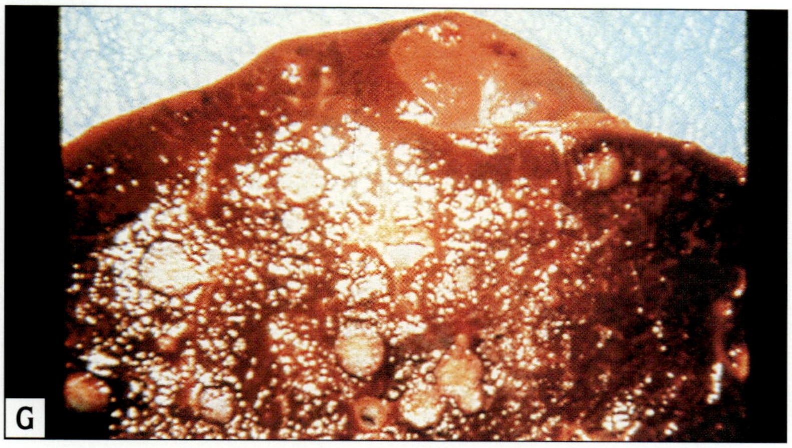

Figure 15-23 *(continued)* hand *(panel E)*, spinal cord *(panel F)*, and spleen *(panel G)*.

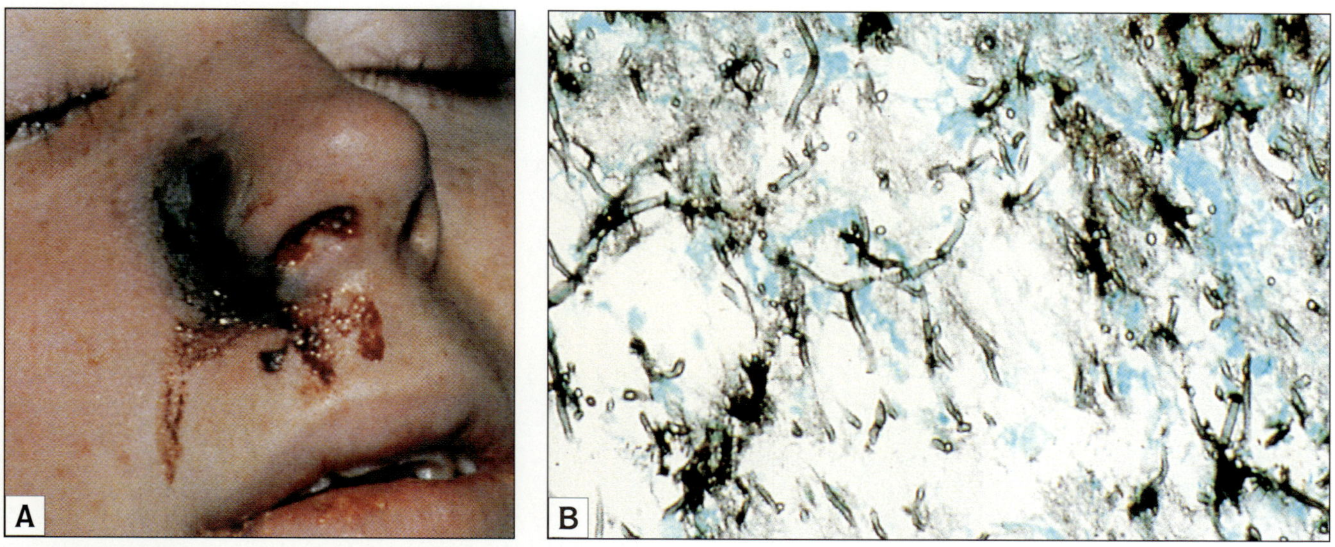

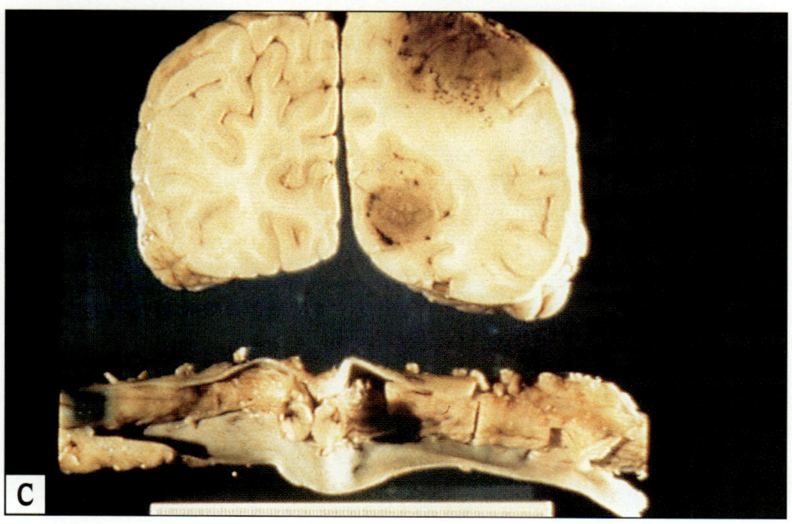

Figure 15-24 Invasive aspergillosis. *Aspergillus fumigatus* or *Aspergillus flavus* are generally acquired by the respiratory route and represent a major cause of infection in neutropenic patients, particularly after bone marrow transplantation. Disease is primarily cutaneous, sinus, pulmonary (often with a characteristic halo sign on computed tomography), or cerebral. **A,** Necrotic skin lesions from direction extension of sinus infection. **B,** Bronchoalveolar lavage (silver stain of hyphae). **C,** Focal brain lesions of cortex and deep structures. Aggressive therapy with amphotericin B and itraconazole can control the infection until the return of circulating neutrophils.

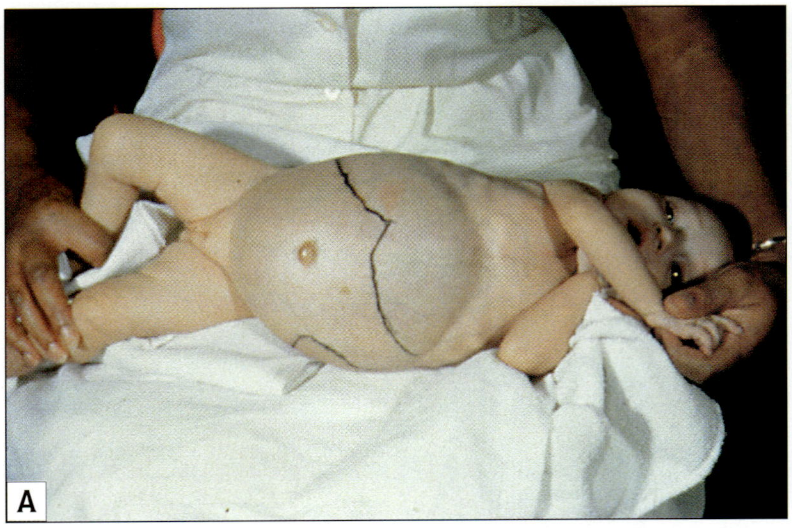

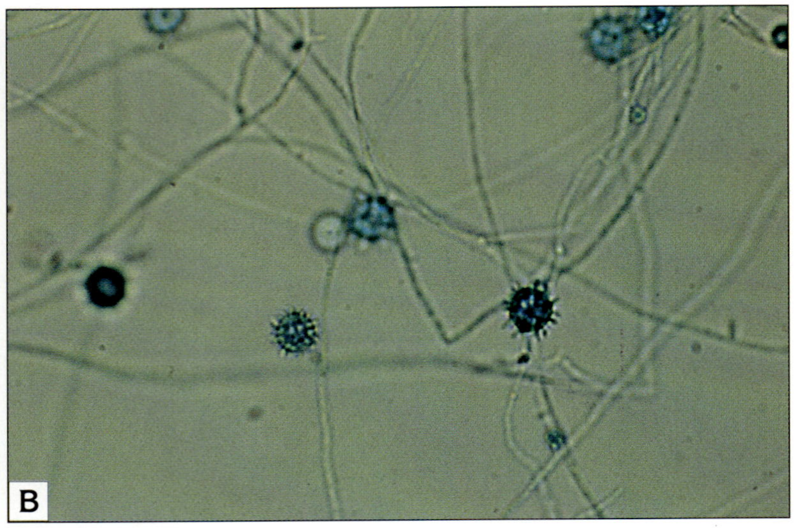

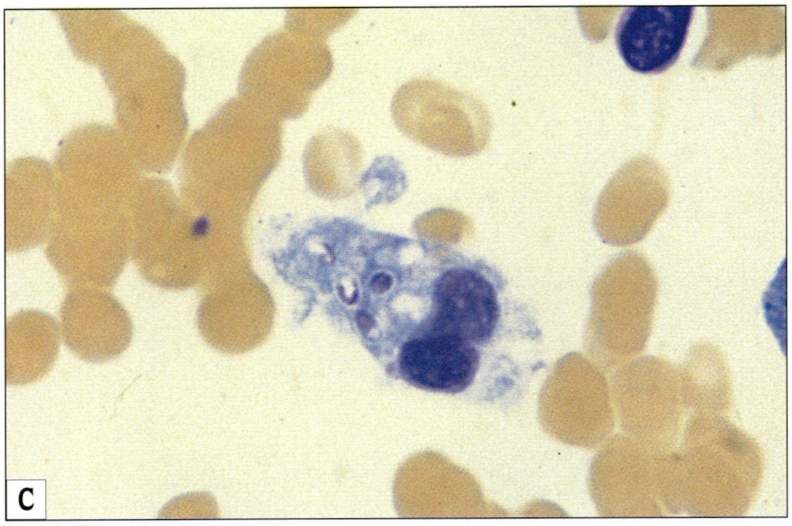

Figure 15-25 Progressive disseminated histoplasmosis. The most common primary systemic mycosis, histoplasmosis is endemic in the Ohio and Mississippi river valleys in the United States. **A,** The characteristic symptom complex of pulmonary infiltrates with hepatosplenomegaly caused by inhalation of microconidia and dissemination to the lymphoreticular system. **B,** Culture yields tuberculate macroconidia of the mold form (lactophenol cotton blue stain). **C,** In progressive disseminated disease in immunocompromised patients, bone marrow aspirate can demonstrate yeast forms in histiocytes (Giemsa stain).

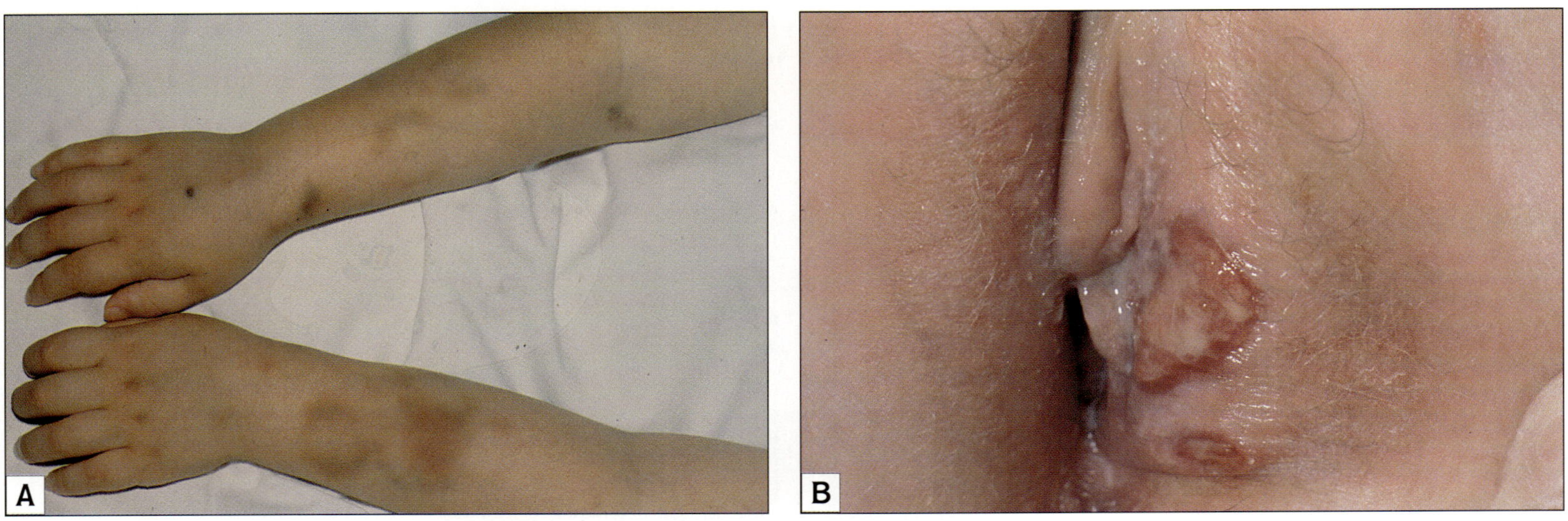

Figure 15-26 Blastomycosis. Infection with *Blastomyces dermatitidis* is rare and manifests as a primary pulmonary lesion followed by lymphohematogenous spread and granuloma formation. Pulmonary disease in immunocompromised hosts, particularly those with AIDS, can be primary or reactivation. **A** and **B**, Extrapulmonary disease is commonly cutaneous, with painless papular lesions (*panel A*) progressing through verrucous and ulcerative stages (*panel B*).

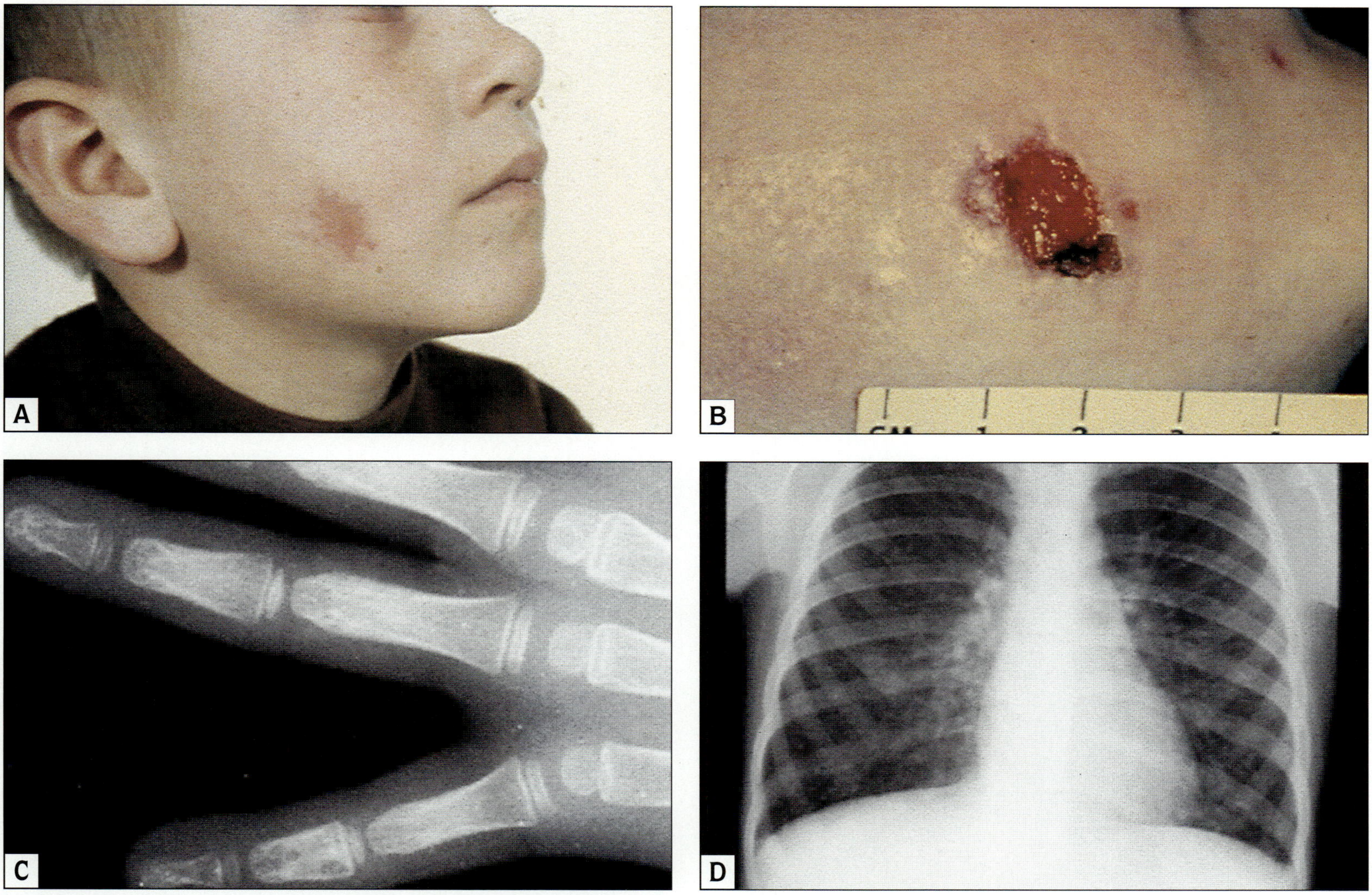

Figure 15-27 Manifestations of cryptococcosis. *Cryptococcus neoformans* is an encapsulated yeast that infects a wide range of immunosuppressed patients. Disseminated disease most commonly involves the brain following either an indolent course with a mass lesion or fulminant meningitis. **A** and **B**, Skin lesions (papules and ulcer, respectively). **C,** Osteolytic lesions. Immunosuppressed patients are rarely cured of infection and require maintenance therapy for the duration of immunocompromise. **D,** Nodular or diffuse infiltrates. Although primary pulmonary disease is most often self-limiting, such manifestations can occur.

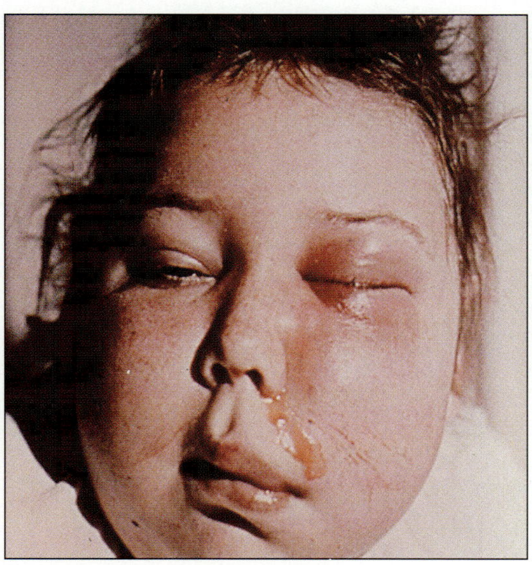

Figure 15-28 Rhinocerebral mucormycosis caused by *Rhizopus* spp. Inhalation into the sinuses of conidia of any of several genera of Mucorales can lead to highly fatal infection. Pulmonary, cutaneous, and disseminated forms of infection also occur.

A. Emerging fungal pathogens
Yeast
Trichosporon sp.
Malassezia sp.
Rhodotorula sp.
Phaeohyphomycosis
Curvularia sp.
Exserohilum sp.
Alternaria sp.
Hyalohyphomycosis
Fusarium sp.
Penicillium sp.
Pseudallescheria sp.

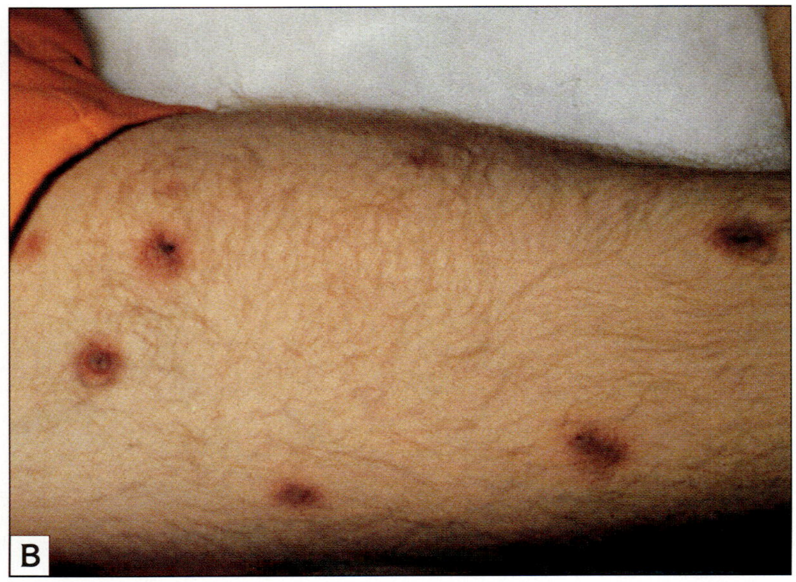

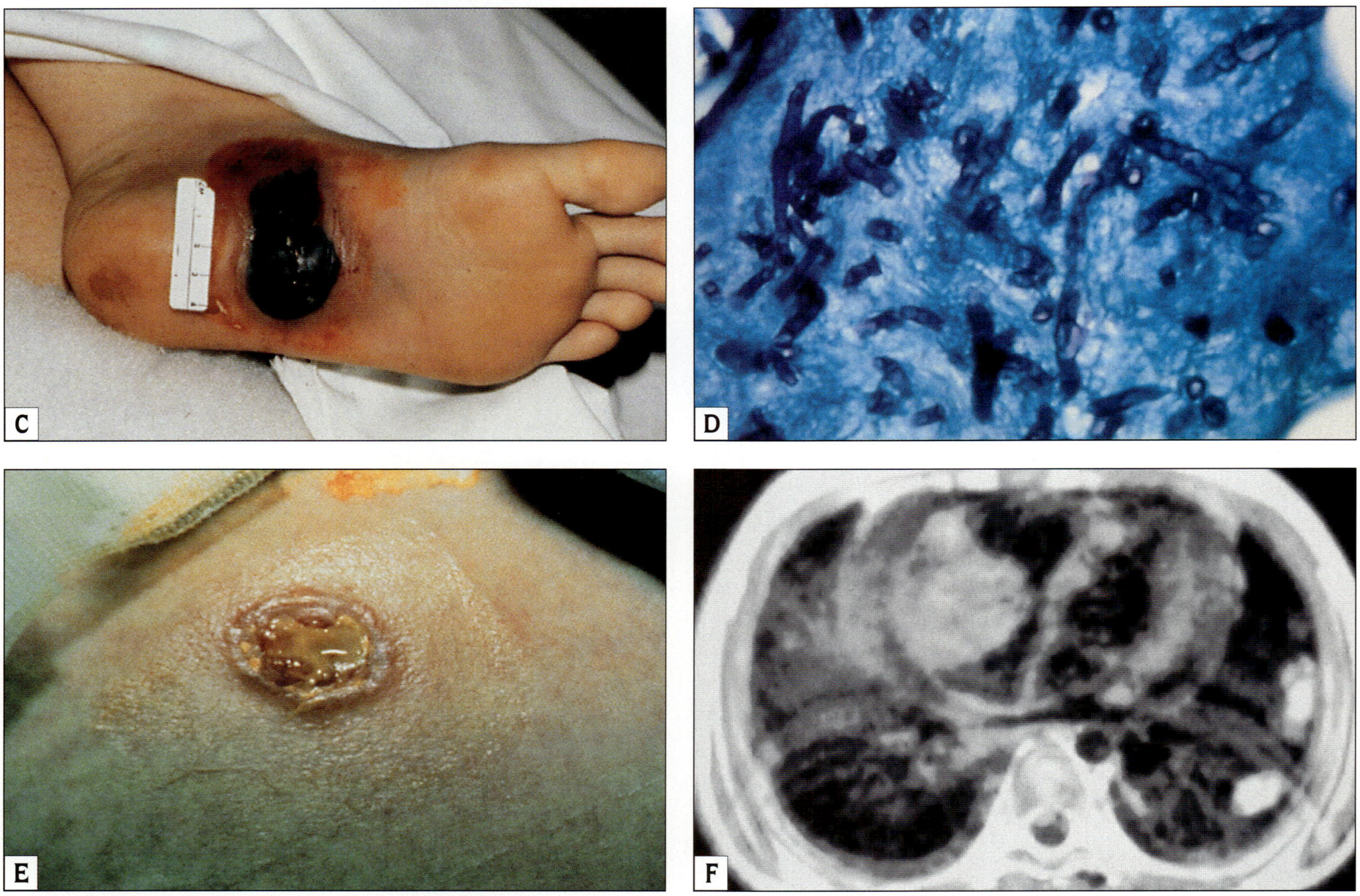

FIGURE 15-29 Emerging fungal infections. In the setting of severe immunosuppression, unusual fungi that are not pathogenic to the normal host can become problematic. **A**, Fungal pathogens. **B** through **G**, Necrotic lesions of the skin in disseminated disease caused by *Fusarium (panel B)*; local infection of the foot caused by *Fusarium (panel C)*; *Exserohilum* (silver stain of exudate) *(panel D)*; three manifestations of *Pseudallescheria boydii*, including cutaneous ulcerative lesion *(panel E)*, right atrial mass (magnetic resonance imaging) *(panel F)*,

(continued on next page)

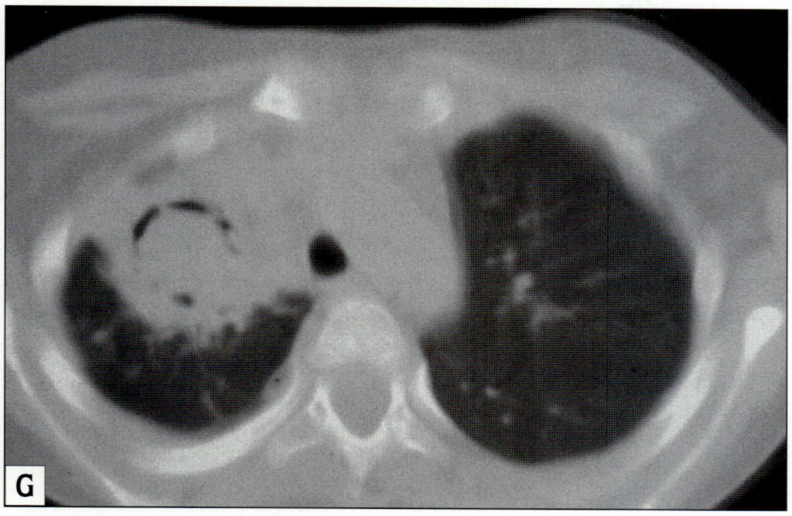

Figure 15-29 *(continued)* and classic mycetomata of the right lung (computed tomography) *(panel G)*. Many of these pathogens respond poorly to conventional antifungal therapy.

Viral Infections

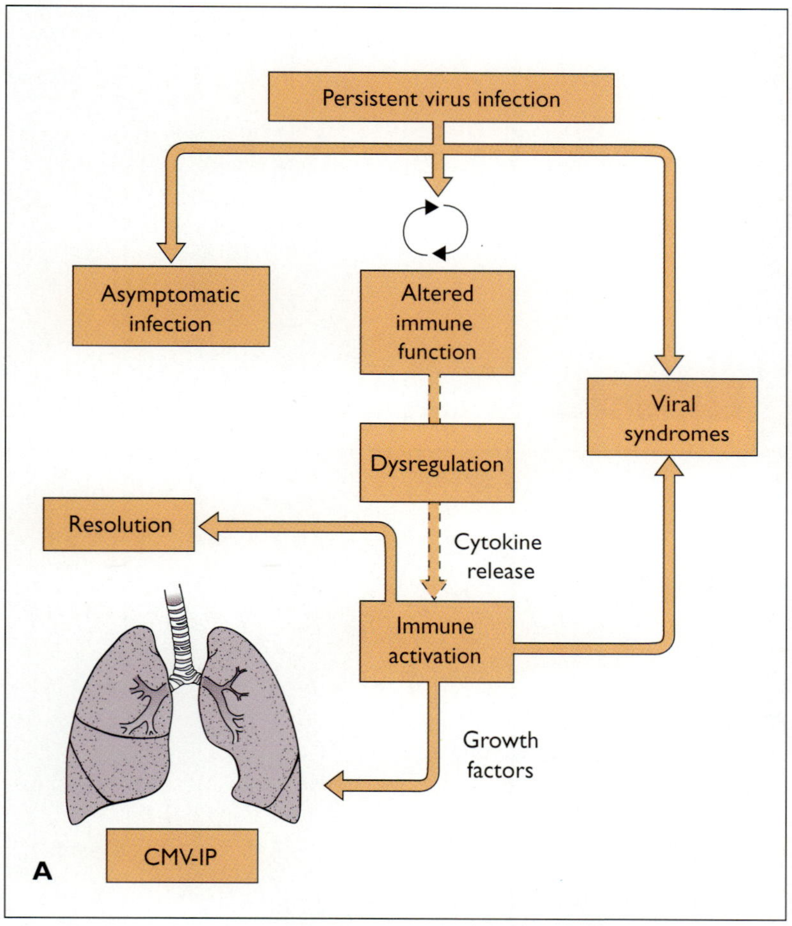

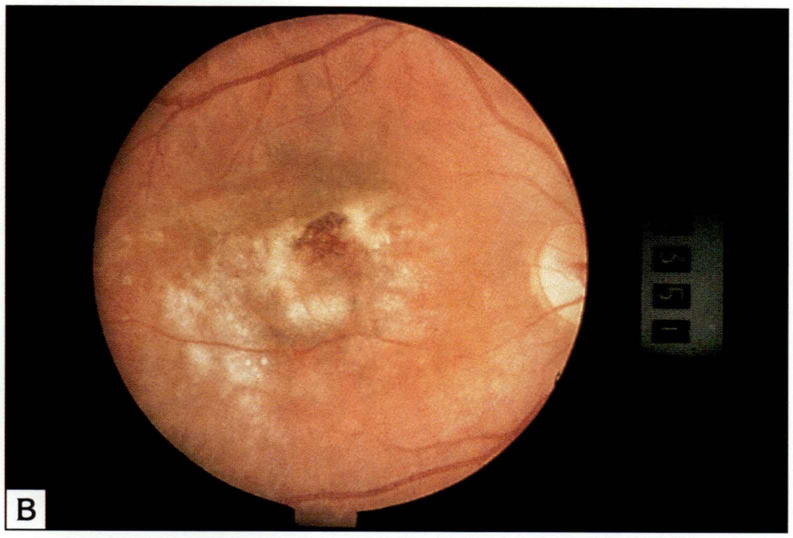

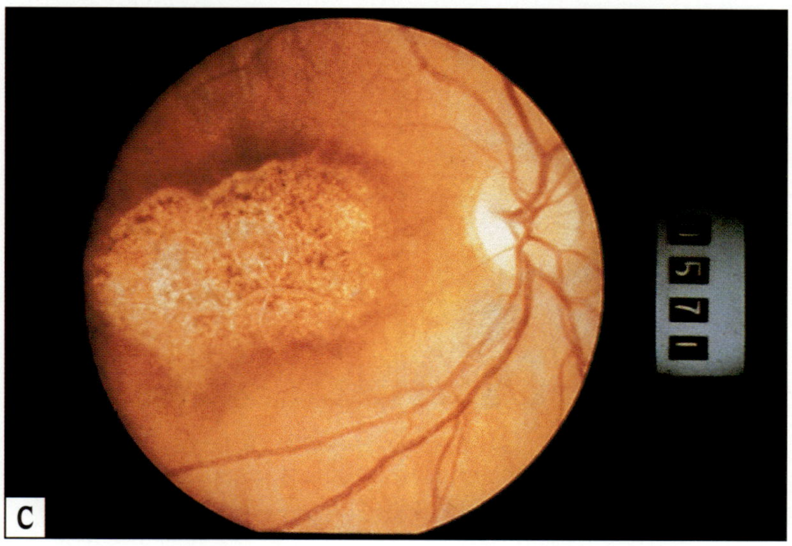

Figure 15-30 Cytomegalovirus (CMV) viremia. Patients with defects in cell-mediated immunity, particularly posttransplantation or with AIDS, develop persistent CMV viremia due to reactivation of endogenous disease or acquisition of new virus from blood or organ transplant. **A,** Infection cycle. **B** and **C,** Two examples of retinal lesions. Syndromes associated with disseminated disease commonly 4 to 12 weeks after transplantation include interstitial pneumonitis and hepatitis in addition to retinitis. The exceptionally high rate of infection in seronegative transplant recipients who receive tissue from a seropositive donor warrants prophylaxis with ganciclovir. (*Panel A adapted from* Zaia [8]; with permission.)

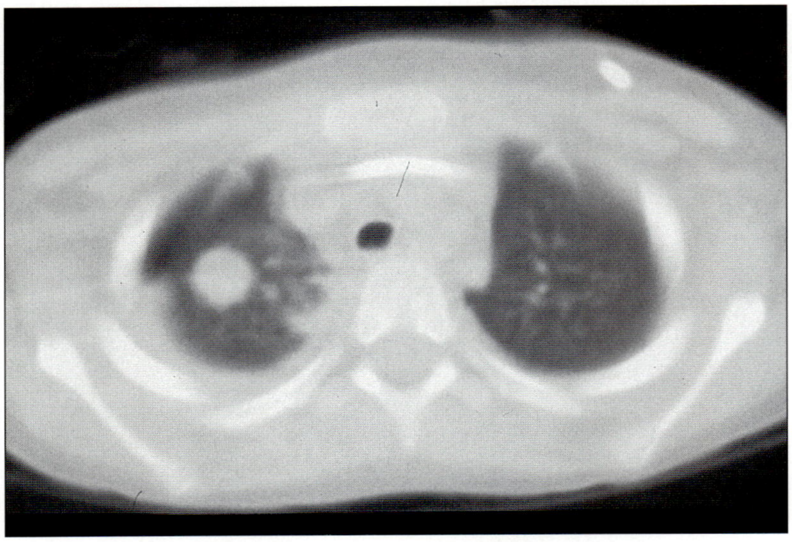

FIGURE 15-31 Lung computed tomographic image of a left pulmonary mass lesion caused by Epstein-Barr virus (EBV). Reactivation of latent EBV in transplant recipients is associated with systemic lymphoproliferative disease characterized by B-lymphocytic localized tumor masses. Pediatric patients with AIDS develop lymphocytic interstitial pneumonitis.

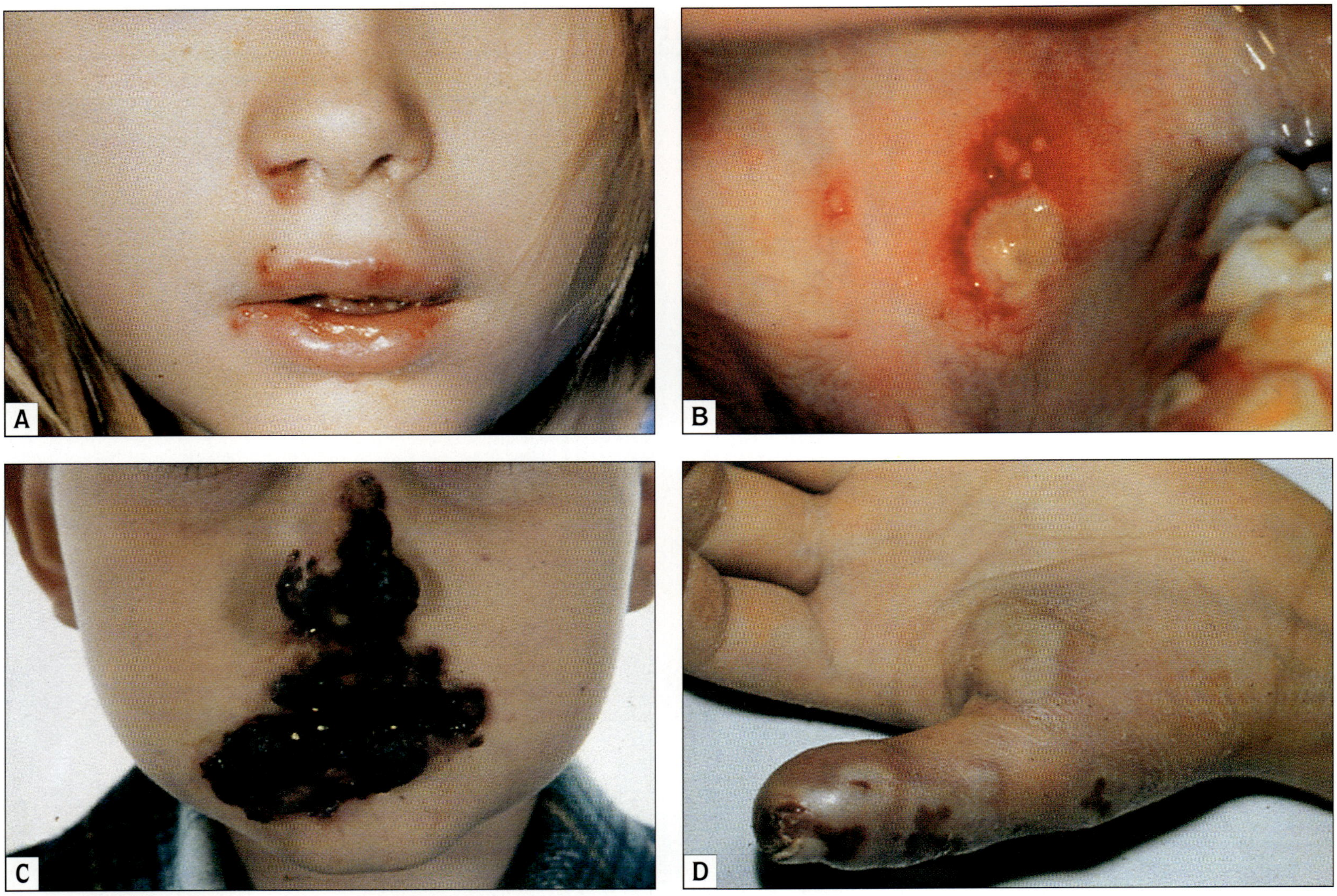

FIGURE 15-32 Herpes simplex virus (HSV). **A** through **E**, HSV infection in the immunocompromised host most commonly takes the form of protracted mucocutaneous lesions: orolabial vesicular lesions *(panel A)*, ulcerated lesion of the buccal mucosa *(panel B)*, advanced necrotic orolabial infection *(panel C)*, herpetic whitlow *(panel D)*,

(continued on next page)

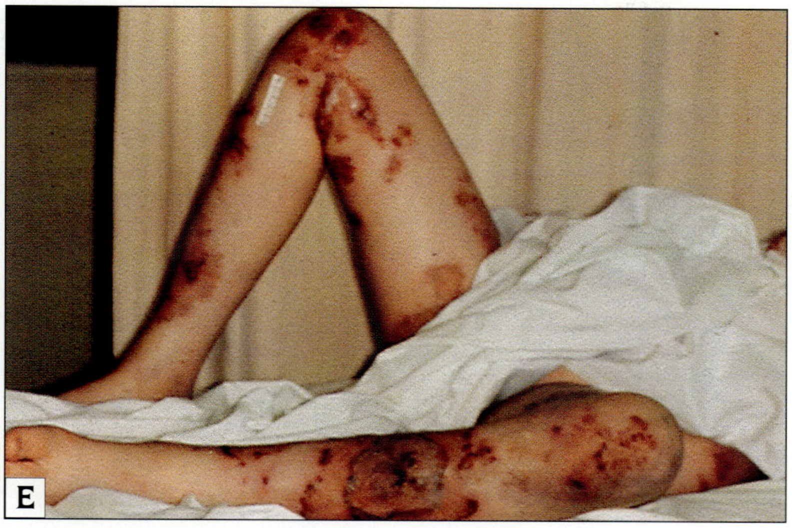
E

Figure 15-32 *(continued)* and severe disseminated cutaneous lesions *(panel E)*.

Acknowledgments

The authors thank Drs. W. Hughes, C. Patrick, and J. Shenep of St. Jude Children's Research Hospital, Memphis, TN for contributing illustrations. This work was supported in part by the National Cancer Institutes Core Grant P30 CA 21765 and the American Lebanese Syrian Associated Charities.

References

1. Armstrong D: History of opportunistic infection in the immunocompromised host. *Clin Infect Dis* 1993, 17 (suppl 2):S318–S321.
2. Bodey GP, Buckley M, Sathe YS, *et al.*: Quantitative relationship between circulating leukocytes and infection in patients with acute leukemia. *Ann Intern Med* 1966, 64:328–340.
3. Patrick C: Infections in bone marrow transplant recipients. In *Pediatric Infectious Diseases.* Edited by Long SS, Pickering LK, Prober G. New York: Churchill-Livingstone; 1992:634–639.
4. Roilides E, Pizzo PA: Perspectives on the use of cytokines in the management of infectious complications of cancer. *Clin Infect Dis* 1993, 17 (suppl 2):S385–S389.
5. Ljungman P, Johannson N, Aschan J, *et al.*: Immunizations after bone marry transplantation. *Bone Marrow Transplantation* 1995, 15:445–446.
6. Ryan-Poirier KA: Dermatologic findings with infections. In *Infections in Immunocompromised Infants and Children.* Edited by Patrick C. New York: Churchill-Livingstone; 1992.
7. Shlaes DM, Binczewski B, Rice LB: Emerging antimicrobial resistance and the immunocompromised host. *Clin Infect Dis* 1993, 17 (suppl 2):S527–S536.
8. Zaia JA: Viral infections associated with bone marrow transplantation. *Hematol Clin North Am* 1990, 4:603–623.

Chapter 16

Infections in Naturally Immunodeficient Hosts

Robert L. Roberts

MOST KNOWLEDGE ABOUT the primary immunodeficiency diseases has been acquired in the past three decades because most of these patients died in early childhood prior to 1960. Recognition of primary immunodeficiency diseases has expanded the understanding of immune system and how it works to fight invasive pathogens. The studies on children born with severe T-cell deficiencies such as DiGeorge syndrome helped physicians to understand how the human immunodeficiency virus (HIV), by destruction of CD4 cells, makes the patient susceptible to opportunistic infections.

The clinical features of specific immunodeficiencies are listed in this chapter but many share similar presentations. Recurrent or persistent respiratory infections are a common finding in many immunodeficient patients. The infections do not respond to antibiotics, or recur as soon as antibiotics are discontinued. There is often a history of persistent otitis media in infancy and of chronic sinusitis and bronchitis as the child matures. By adolescence, permanent lung damage may have occurred in the form of bronchiectasis or pneumatoceles. Respiratory infection must be distinguished from respiratory allergy, which is usually associated with a clear, nonpurulent discharge and is not usually associated with fever.

Careful analysis of the infections acquired by the immunodeficient patient may allow the physician to predict which branch of the immune system is defective. Cellular (T-cell) defects with or without antibody (B-cell) defects are usually more severe, becoming manifest as viral, fungal, and gram-negative encapsulated bacterial infections in the first months of life. A child with such a defect would be unlikely to survive to puberty without intensive medial intervention. Defects in antibody production alone are not usually apparent until the transplacentally acquired maternal antibodies are depleted (6–8 mo), at which time infections with gram-positive encapsulated bacteria may start to occur. However, children with a partial or subclass antibody defect have a more benign course, and may escape diagnosis until adolescence. Phagocytic cell defects may lead to bacterial infections of the respiratory tract, skin and mucous membranes. Patients are usually symptomatic in infancy, although milder cases may not be recognized until adolescence. Disorders of complement are rare, but may make the patient susceptible to recurrent bacterial infections, particularly neisserial infections such as *Neisseria gonorrhoeae* or *Neisseria meningitidis*, if the later components (C5–C9) are missing.

When an immunodeficiency is suspected in a patient, initial screening tests performed by most hospital laboratories may be used to gauge the patient's immune status. A complete blood count and differential can determine whether there are adequate numbers of white blood cells, and also allow for examination of their morphology. Antibody function may be measured quantitatively by immunoglobulin levels (IgG, IgA, IgM) and qualitatively by titers of specific antibody to antigens to which the patient has been immunized. Intradermal skin tests to agents such as mumps virus or tetanus toxoid test are used T-cell function. An elevated IgE level may suggest hyperimmunoglobulin E syndrome, which is associated with neutrophil chemotactic defects. The IgE level may also help distinguish an allergic from an infectious disease process. Total complement activity may be checked and specific components determined if this value is low.

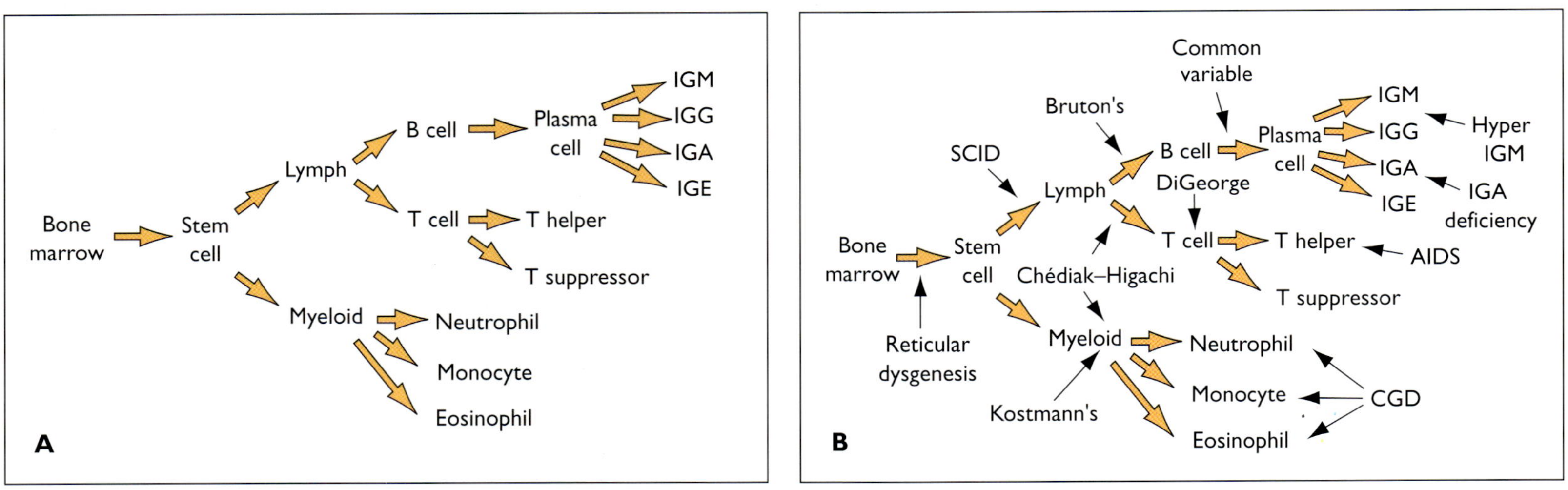

FIGURE 16-1 The immune system and its disorders. **A,** The normal immune system, with all hematopoietic cells proceeding from the bone marrow stem cell. The lymphoid and myeloid precursor cells differentiate to mature lymphocytes, granulocytes, and monocytes found in the peripheral blood. **B,** Some of the disorders or primary deficiencies of the immune system. Those specific disease entities will be discussed later in this chapter. The earlier the defect occurs in the differentiation process, the more severe the immunodeficiency tends to be. CGD—chronic granulomatous disease; SCID—severe combined immunodeficiency.

Primary phagocytic cell disorders

Disorder	Clinical features	Laboratory findings	Incidence*
Leukocyte adhesion deficiency	Delayed umbilical cord separation, gingivitis, bacterial infections; infections usually begin in infancy, particularly with more severe form	Leukocytosis, lack of surface adhesion receptors, decreased neutrophil chemotaxis, decreased natural killer cell activity	Approximately 60 cases of LAD-I and two cases of LAD-II reported (both in Israel)
Hyper-IgE syndrome (Jobs)	Eczema, respiratory infections, coarse facial features, osteoporosis; skin rash noted in infancy, but infections may start later	IgE very high, eosinophilia, decreased neutrophil chemotaxis	Approximately 50 cases in literature, but disease is probably underreported due to lack of specific diagnostic test
Chédiak–Higashi syndrome	Oculocutaneous albinisms, neuropathy, infections, tendency to develop malignancies; albinism and infections in infancy	Abnormal leukocyte granules, poor neutrophil chemotaxis, decreased natural killer cell activity	Approximately 200 cases reported
Specific-granule deficiency (lactoferrin deficiency)	Recurrent bacterial infections, extensive soft tissue infections; infections start in infancy	Lack specific granules in granulocytes, lactoferrin deficiency, poor neutrophil chemotaxis and killing	Five reported cases in 1993
Chronic granulomatous disease	Recurrent bacterial infections, granulomas that may obstruct genitourinary tract; most patients (70%) are diagnosed <12 mo of age, but a few are not diagnosed until adolescence	Lack of oxygen radical production, poor bacterial killing	Estimated incidence of 1:500,000 with ~66% X-linked and the rest autosomal recessive
Myeloperoxidase deficiency	Recurrent fungal or bacterial infections, but most are asymptomatic	Lack myeloperoxidase activity in neutrophils and monocytes	Estimated 1:2000 of partial defect and 1:4000 complete defect

* All numbers are approximations because not every reported case can be verified, and the more recent cases are not included.

FIGURE 16-2 Clinical and laboratory features of primary phagocytic cell disorders. Defective functioning of all phagocytic cells (neutrophils, eosinophils, and monocytes) occurs in leukocyte adhesions deficiency, chronic granulomatous disease, and Chédiak–Higashi syndrome. Myeloperoxidase deficiency only affects neutrophils and monocytes, and it has relatively high incidence of 1 in 2000 to 4000 individuals in the US general population. Patients with chronic granulomatous disease are at risk for acquiring infections with both common and unusual bacteria and fungi due to the decreased ability to kill catalase-positive organisms. Natural killer cells are defective in killing in leukocyte adhesion deficiency (LAD) due to lack of surface adhesion receptors and also in Chédiak–Higashi syndrome due to defects in microtubule assembly. (*Data from* Nathan and Oski [1].)

Common pathogens in patients with phagocytic cell disorders

Disorder	Pathogens
Congenital or cyclic neutropenia and leukocyte adhesion deficiency	Bacteria, gram-positive *Staphylococcus aureus* *Staphylococcus epidermidis* Streptococci, group A Bacteria, gram-negative *Pseudomonas* Enterobacteriaceae Fungus *Candida* species *Aspergillus fumigatus*
Chédiak–Higashi syndrome	*S. aureus* is predominant pathogen with increased susceptibility to other bacteria and fungi as in neutropenia
Hyper-IgE syndrome	*S. aureus* is predominant pathogen *Candida albicans, Haemophilus influenzae, Pseudomonas aeruginosa,* Group A streptococci, group A; *A. fumigatus*
Chronic granulomatous disease	Bacteria, catalase-positive *S. aureus* *Burkholdia cepacia* *Nocardia* Other gram-negative bacteria Fungus *A. fumigatus* *C. albicans*
Myeloperoxidase deficiency	*C. albicans*

FIGURE 16-3 Common pathogens in patients with phagocytic cell disorders. Patients with chronic granulomatous disease phagocytic cell disorders are very susceptible to common bacterial and fungal pathogens. Patients are also susceptible to a variety of catalase-positive organisms that are unusual pathogens for normal hosts. A positive culture for one of these organisms, such as *Serratia*, should alert the physician to consider the diagnosis of chronic granulomatous disease in a new patient. Patients with neutropenia and low bone marrow reserves are at great risk for overwhelming sepsis, although most patients with phagocytic disorders have a more indolent course.

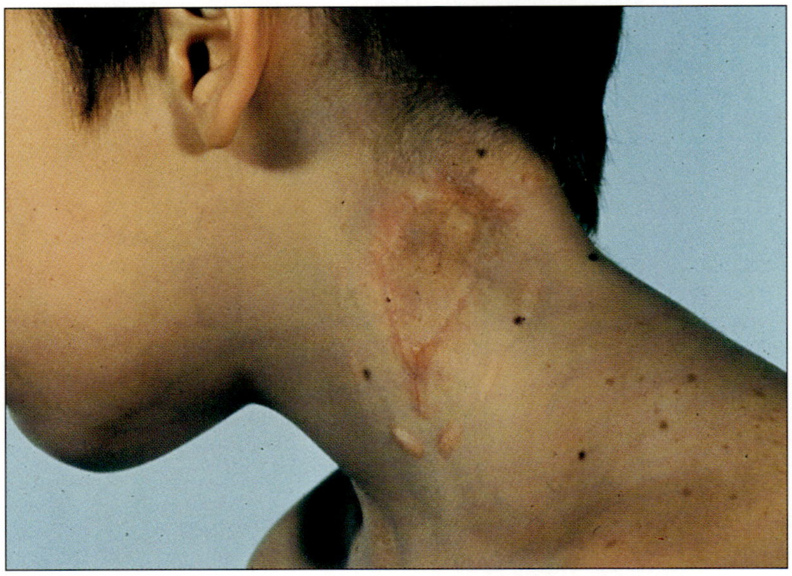

FIGURE 16-4 Suppurative lymphadenitis in chronic granulomatous disease (CGD). Suppurative lymphadenitis is a common feature of CGD, and often requires treatment with surgical drainage and intravenous antibiotics, as was the case for this boy with the X-linked form of the disease. The basic defect in both the autosomal and X-linked forms of CGD is the inability of the oxidase system, composed of both membrane and cytosolic proteins, to convert atmospheric oxygen to superoxide anion. Normally, the superoxide anion is converted to other reactive oxygen intermediates (ROI), such as hydrogen peroxide and hypochlorous acid (which kill intracellular catalase-positive bacteria and fungi, including *Staphylococcus aureus, Salmonella, Serratia, Pseudomonas,* and *Aspergillus)*. Catalase-negative bacteria, such as *Streptococcus*, are usually not a major pathogen for CGD patients because these organisms generate small amounts of hydrogen peroxide themselves, which contributes to their own demise. Catalase-positive organisms can destroy the hydrogen peroxide they produce, but they cannot adequately scavenge the much larger amounts of ROI generated by normal neutrophils.

CGD patients are prone to develop soft-tissue abscesses, pneumonia, hepatic abscesses, lung abscesses, and osteomyelitis (*see* Fig. 16-6). Perirectal abscesses are a common presentation of CGD in infancy. As a result of chronic inflammation, granulomas may also develop in the gastrointestinal or urinary tracts, leading to obstruction. The diagnosis of CGD can be made using various assays of ROI production, such as the nitroblue tetrazolium dye test (*see* Fig. 16-33), superoxide production by cytochrome-*c* reduction, and more recently, by flow cytometry. The routine care of CGD patients would include antibiotic prophylaxis, usually with daily trimethoprim-sulfamethoxazole, which concentrates in neutrophils and greatly increases the ability of neutrophils from CGD patients to kill bacteria. Other medications include interferon γ injections to non-specifically enhance host defenses, and itraconazole to prevent aspergillus and other fungal infections. Treatment of any significant infections should include intravenous antibiotics with empiric coverage of *S. aureus*, which is most common, and *Burkholdia cepacia*, which is most lethal. Treatment with amphotericin should be started if the patient is not responding to antibiotics. Cultures, including direct biopsy specimens, are often initially negative in CGD because of the neutrophils are able to bacteria within a small area but not to kill them. Thus, the infection may slowly progress over several weeks in a CGD patient before a positive culture is obtained. Trials of gene therapy have begun in CGD, and stem cell transplantation (from either bone marrow or cord blood) to cure CGD is gaining more acceptance.

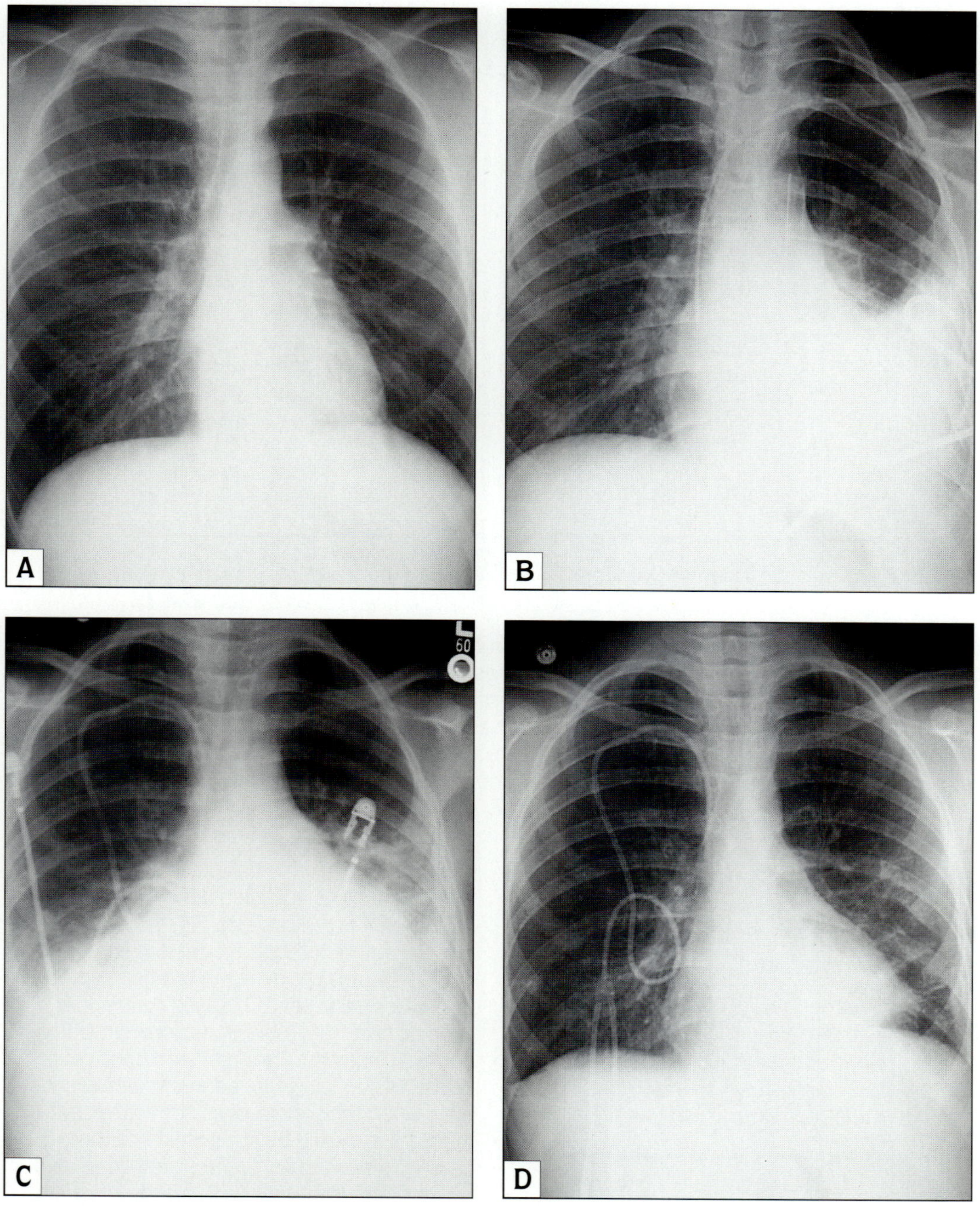

Figure 16-5 Chronic granulomatous disease (CGD). These four chest radiographs were made over a 5-month period in a 16-year-old boy with CGD. **A,** Initial photograph taken to investigate chest pain and fever occurring over 2 weeks. The image appears relatively normal, but a computed tomography scan revealed a consolidated lesion behind the cardiac shadow. A biopsy of the lesion grew *Aspergillus fumigatus*. **B,** An image taken approximately 2 months later. The infection spread to involve a large portion of the left lung despite amphotericin treatment and surgical excision of the initial lesions. The patient then started receiving granulocyte transfusions, and oral itraconazole was added to his amphotericin infusions. He was also receiving injections of interferon γ, which were increased to daily injections to further enhance his host defenses; granulocyte colony-stimulating factor was administered to increase both the number and function of his neutrophils. The patient began to improve clinically, and chest radiography showed some clearing of his lung lesions. **C,** Large pericardial and pleural effusions (negative for bacteria and fungi on culture) that appeared approximately 3 weeks after starting the granulocyte transfusions. The granulocyte transfusions were suspected of provoking an inflammatory response that caused the effusions and new lung infiltrates. **D,** The effusions gradually resolved after the transfusions were stopped. Itraconazole may prevent aspergillus infections in patients with CGD and should be considered in addition to other prophylactic medications, including antibiotics (usually Co-trimoxazole) and interferon γ injections [2,3].

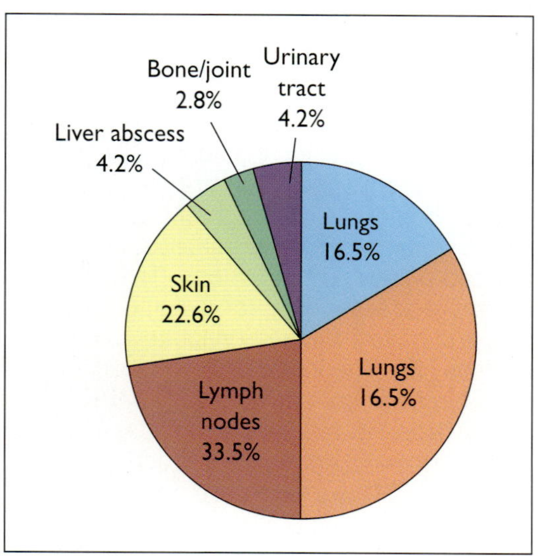

Figure 16-6 Sites of infection in chronic granulomatous disease. This graph represents the proportional distribution of infectious episodes by body site in 48 patients with chronic granulomatous disease followed up for 15 years [4]. The lymph nodes were the most common site of infection, and lymphadenopathy often accompanies infection of other sites, such as skin or lungs. Infections in the gastrointestinal or urinary tracts may lead to obstruction, which should be treated with steroids in addition to antibiotics. The percentage of liver infections was only 4.2%, which may reflect the fact that it may take several months to treat only one episode of liver abscesses. Obtaining a positive culture for an unusual organism such as *Serratia* from an infant should make the physician consider the diagnosis of CGD.

Surface receptors absent/reduced in leukocyte adhesion deficiency

Type	Receptors	Tissue distribution	Ligand
LAD-I	CD11a/CD18 (LFA-1)	Leukocytes	ICAM-1, ICAM-2
	CD11b/CD18 (CR3, Mac-1, Mo-1)	Granulocytes Monocytes Macrophages Natural killer cells B cells (activated)	ICAM-1, C3bi, fibrinogen
	CD11c/CD18 (p150, 95; CR4)	Granulocytes Monocytes Macrophages Lymphocytes (activated)	C3bi
LAD-II	CD62E (P selection, PADGEM, GMP-140)	Platelets Endothelium	sLewis-X, L-selectin (CD 15s)

ICAM—intracellular adhesion molecule; LFA—leukocyte function-associated antigen; GMP—guanosine monophosphate.

Figure 16-7 Absent or reduced surface receptors in leukocyte adhesion deficiency (LAD). The basic defect in LAD-I is a mutation in the gene for CD18, the β-chain of the CD11/CD18 complex. The three different α-chains (CD11a, CD 11b, CD 11c) account for three different receptors that are all missing in LAD-I because CD18 is necessary for expression on the surface. Neutrophils, monocytes, and lymphocytes are all lacking those receptors and are prevented from attaching to other cells that are essential for chemotaxis (*see* Fig. 16-8) LAD-II, which is much more rare than LAD-I, involves absence of another adhesion receptor.

Defects in leukocyte function in leukocyte adhesion deficiency

Phagocytic cells	Lymphocytes
Adherence and spreading to glass or plastic	Blastogenic response of T cells
Oxidative burst activity to particulate stimuli	Cytotoxicity of T cells
Degranulation in response to particulate stimuli	Cytotoxicity of natural killer cells
Antibody-dependent cytotoxicity	Interferon production
Cell aggregation	Cell aggregation

Figure 16-8 In vitro defects in leukocyte function in leukocyte adhesion deficiency. The lack of adhesion receptors (*see* Fig. 16-9) on leukocytes prevents the cells from attaching to other cells. Clinically, the defect in the neutrophils is of greater significance because neutrophils normally act very rapidly to contain invading bacteria. The high absolute neutrophil count (≥20,000) in leukocyte adhesion deficiency, even when the patient does not appear to be infected, is caused by the inability of the neutrophils to attach to the endothelium and migrate into the tissues [5]. All these patients had skin abscesses and approximately half had periodontitis. Over one third had omphalitis, which is often associated with delayed umbilical cord separation in newborns.

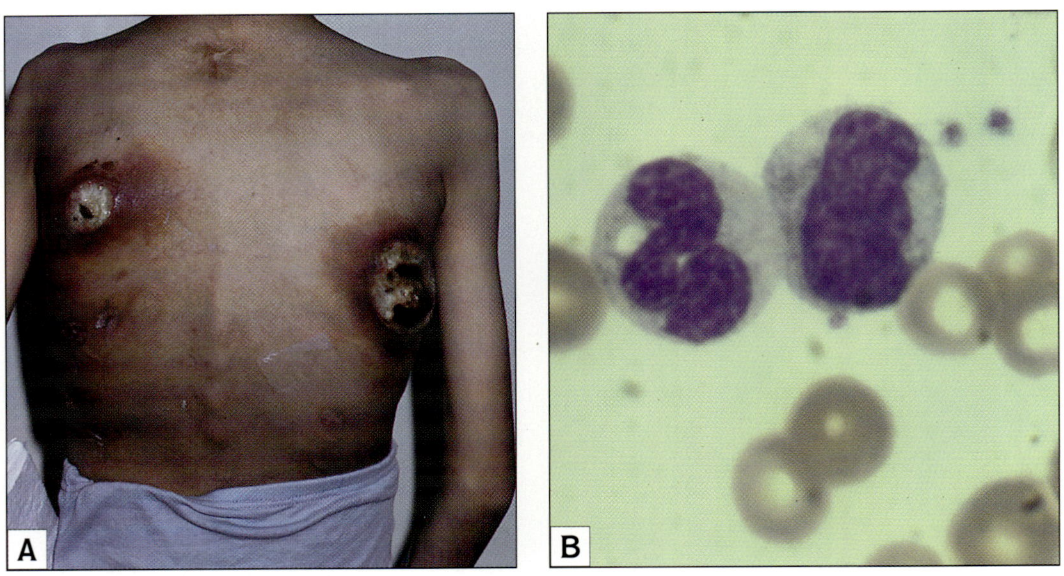

Figure 16-9 Specific-granule deficiency (SGD). Patients with SGD are very susceptible to bacterial and fungal infections, resulting in recurrent skin abscesses (**A**) and pulmonary infections. Their granulocytes lack secondary (or specific) granules and have a bilobed or kidney-shaped nucleus (**B**). The in vitro abnormalities found in their cells include very defective chemotaxis, decreased bactericidal activity, and abnormal oxidative burst activity. Although SGD is a very rare disorder (with fewer than 20 cases reported since it was first recognized in 1974), it does highlight the importance of specific granules to neutrophil function. This disease has also been referred to as lactoferrin deficiency because lactoferrin is found within the neutrophil specific granules.

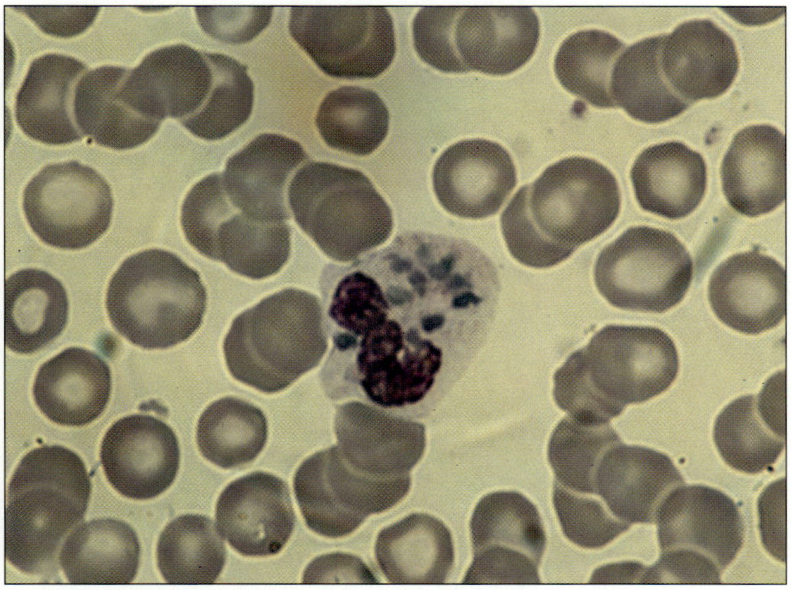

FIGURE 16-10 Peripheral blood neutrophil from patient with Chédiak–Higashi syndrome (CHS). Note the large granules within the neutrophils that may also be found in other peripheral blood leukocytes. Most patients will eventually develop an "accelerated" phase that is characterized by fever, jaundice, hepatosplenomegaly, and diffuse mononuclear cell infiltrates; this may lead to death. Other pertinent clinical features include partial oculocutaneous albinism and a progressive neuropathy. Neutropenia is common in CHS, and the neutrophils themselves display very slow chemotaxis owing to abnormal microtubule assembly. Natural killer activity is also decreased in CHS, which may increase their susceptibility to malignancies. At least 10 CHS patients have been treated with allogeneic bone marrow transplantations, which appeared to correct their hematologic abnormalities [6].

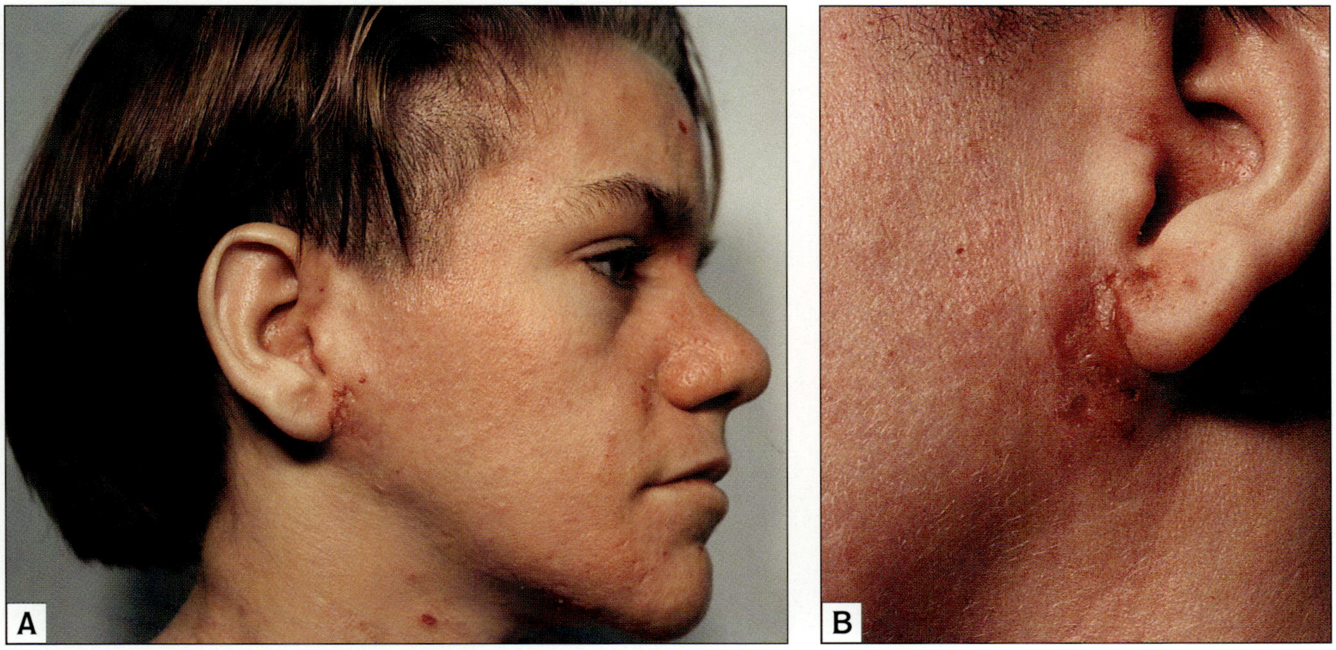

FIGURE 16-11 Hyper-IgE syndrome. **A,** This profile of a patient with hyper-IgE syndrome demonstrating the coarse facial features typical of this syndrome that become more prominent as the patient gets older. **B,** The impetiginized skin is also typical of the rash associated with hyper-IgE that usually begins as an eczematous eruption in early infancy. The most debilitating aspect of hyper-IgE is the pulmonary disease, typically manifest by pneumatoceles and progressive lung scarring. *Staphylococcus aureus* and candida are the most common lung pathogens. Cold abscesses (those lacking external signs of inflammation) are also characteristic of this disease—which accounts for the initial name for this disease, "Job's syndrome." Sinusitis and otitis are also very common in HIE, and gingivitis may occur. Laboratory studies reveal very high levels of IgE (usually between 10,000 and 20,000 U/mL) and eosinophilia. These patients have impaired ability to make specific antibodies, are often anergic in delayed skin testing, and have defective neutrophil chemotaxis, thus affecting all components of the immune system. The underlying defect is not known, although hyper-IgE has developed in some HIV-positive patients, implicating lack of T-cell control. Management of hyper-IgE consists primarily of antibiotics for treatment and prophylaxis, skin care including steroids and antifungal drugs, and pulmonary therapy to prevent further loss of lung function. Other treatments have included intravenous gamma globulin and interferon γ, both with limited success in some patients.

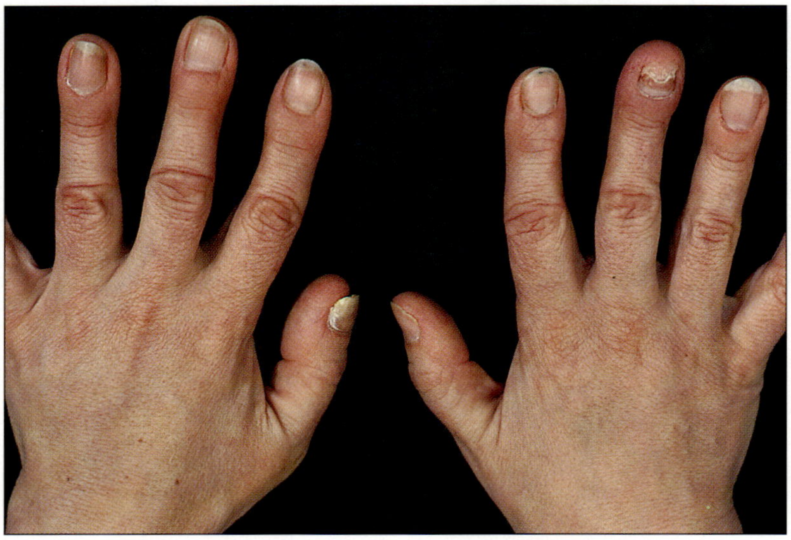

FIGURE 16-12 Hands of a woman aged 40 years with hyper-IgE syndrome. Clubbing of the fingers is very apparent due to the patient's recurrent pulmonary infections. The thumb nail on the left hand is discolored and infected with a fungus. The middle finger on the right hand is obviously swollen and red. Bone scan of the finger showed the infection in the finger had spread to underlying bone, thus resulting in osteomyelitis. Patients with hyper-IgE syndrome are also prone to develop osteoporosis, with a greater susceptibility to fractures.

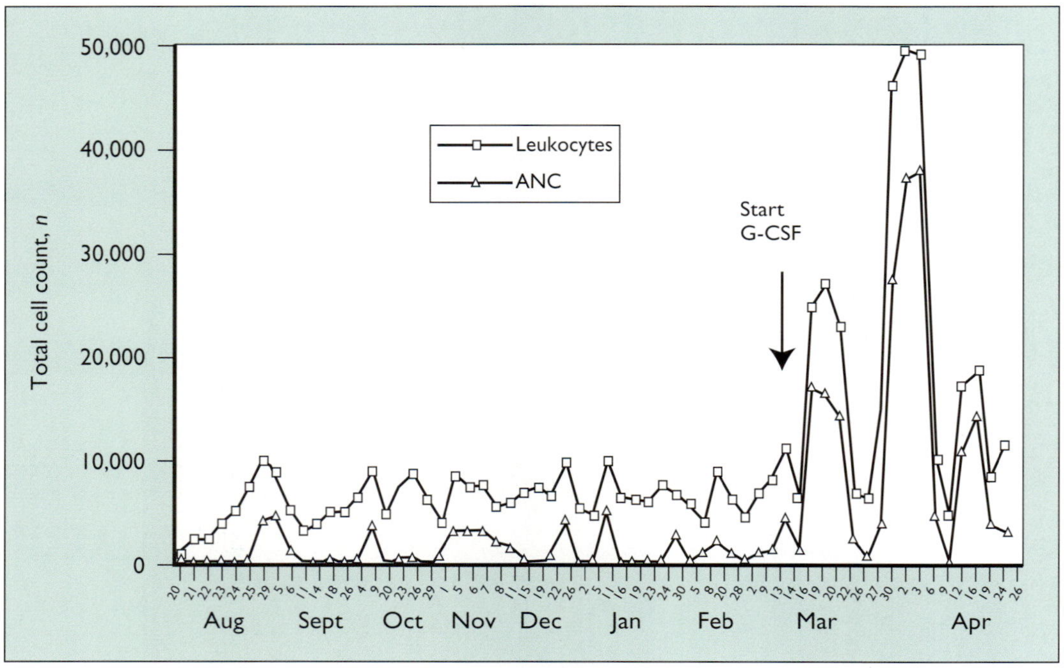

FIGURE 16-13 Cyclic neutropenia in a patient with hyper-IgM syndrome and the effects of granulocyte colony-stimulating factor. This patient had been diagnosed with hyper-IgM syndrome in infancy and had developed cyclic neutropenia with a 21-day cycle. The neutropenia period lasted 3 to 4 days and the absolute neutrophil count (ANC) dropped to less than 100. Administration of granulocyte colony-stimulating factor (5 μg/kg) induced an immediate increase:by the next day, the ANC was over 10,000. The patient's ANC eventually increased to greater than 40,000, but the level did decrease to under 500 for 1 to 2 days during the neutropenic phase. The cycle also decreased in length to approximately every 2 weeks. Therefore, although the patient continued to have cycles of neutropenia, his ANC remained high enough to protect him from major infections.

Clinical and laboratory features of primary B-cell or antibody-deficient syndromes

Disorder	Clinical features	Laboratory findings
X-linked agammaglobulinemia (Bruton's syndrome)	Recurrent pyogenic infections*	Absent immunoglobulins, absent B cells, normal T cells
Hyper-IgM syndrome	Recurrent bacterial and fungal infections, diarrhea	Low IgG, IgA, IgE; normal or high IgM; neutropenia; lack CD40 ligand on T cells
IgA deficiency	Recurrent respiratory infections, usually mild	Low or absent IgA, low IgG_2 subclass in symptomatic patients
Common variable immunodeficiency	Recurrent respiratory infections, autoimmune disease, lymphadenopathy*	Low immunoglobulins, B cells present
Transient hypogammaglobulinemia of infancy	Recurrent respiratory infections	Delayed immunoglobulin production until 3–4 y of age

* May sustain chronic meningoencephalitis due to enteroviruses.

FIGURE 16-14 Clinical and laboratory features of primary B cell or antibody-deficient syndromes. The recurrent infections usually do not begin until 5 to 6 months of age (when the maternal antibodies are depleted). Hyper-IgM syndrome is usually diagnosed by immunoglobulin levels, but it is actually the T cell that is defective, lacking the CD40 ligand necessary for immunoglobulin class switching. Patients with the more severe disorders may be treated with immunoglobulin preparations, with the exception of those with IgA deficiency, in which exogenous immunoglobulin may induce anaphylaxis due to anti-IgA antibodies.

Common pathogens in patients with primary B-cell or antibody-deficient disorders

Disorder	Pathogens
X-linked agammaglobulinemia (Bruton's syndrome)	Bacteria *Streptococcus pneumonia* *Haemophilus influenzae* *Staphylococcus aureus* *Pseudomonas aeruginosa* *Mycoplasma* *Salmonella, Shigella* *Campylobacter* Viruses (particulary enteroviruses) Parasites (*Giardia*)
Common variable immunodeficiency	Similar to Bruton's syndrome plus *Cryptosporidium*
Hyper-IgM syndrome	Similar to Bruton's syndrome plus: *Cryptosporidium* *Pneumocystis carinii* *Cryptococcus neoformans* Cytomegalovirus
IgA deficiency	Common viral and bacterial respiratory pathogens plus *Giardia*
Transient hypogammaglobulinemia of infancy	Common bacterial respiratory pathogens

Figure 16-15 Common pathogens in patients with primary B-cell or antibody-deficient disorders. Patients with Bruton's agammaglobulinemia are susceptible to a wide range of pathogens and will die soon after maternal antibodies are depleted unless immunoglobulin is replaced. Patients with common variable immunodeficiency and hyper-IgM syndrome are susceptible to opportunistic organisms, such as cryptosporidium, due to defects in their T-cell immunity as well as to the bacteria and viruses that act as pathogens in patients with Bruton's agammaglobulinemia.

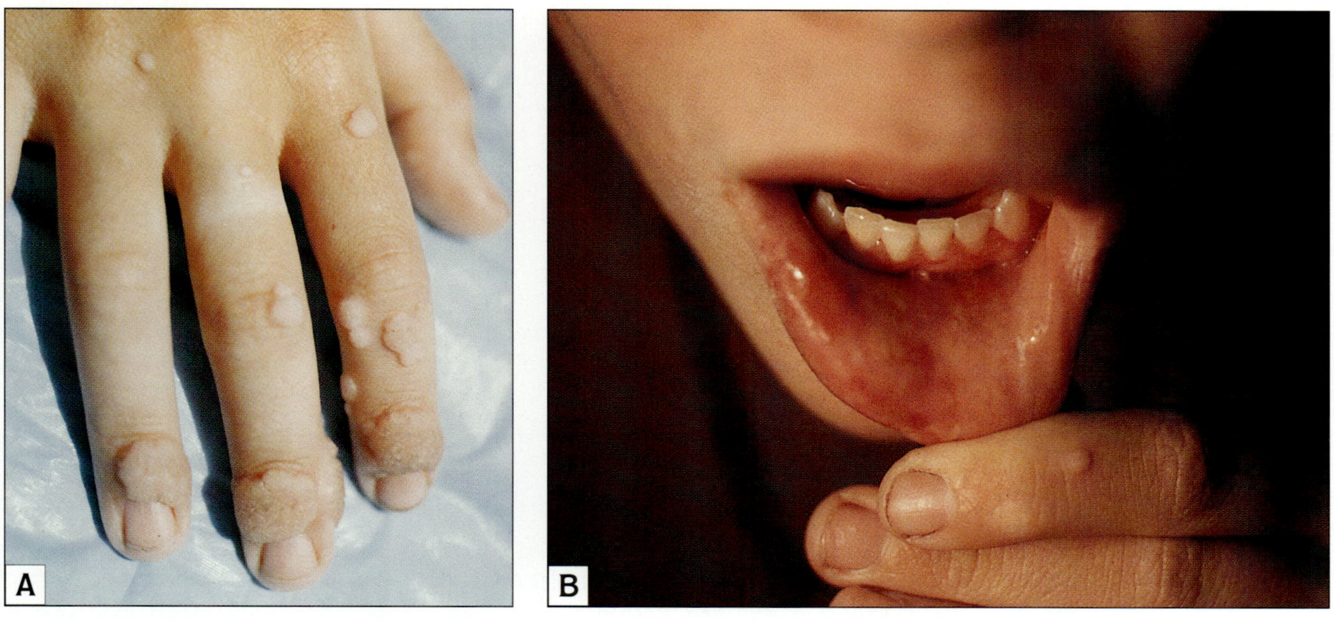

Figure 16-16 Common variable immunodeficiency. **A,** The verruca vulgaris began to appear on this patient's fingers at approximately 10 years of age when he also began to experience recurrent pneumonias with pleural effusions requiring chest tube drainage. At 12 years of age, laboratory evaluations found IgA (previously normal) below detectable levels, very decreased IgG_2 and IgG_4 subclasses, and an inability to respond to pneumococcal vaccine. **B,** Other problems included recurrent aphthous ulcers and 2 episodes of varicella-zoster. T-cell studies showed a decreased proliferative response to phytohemagglutinin and candida antigen. This patient was also of interest because he had been previously diagnosed with chronic mucocutaneous candidiasis (CMC) at 2 years of age. His disease had been under good control with ketoconazole until his pneumonias developed. Patients with CMC are at greater risk for bacterial, viral, and other fungal infections, and there are reported cases of patients with CMC developing common variable immunodeficiency [7].

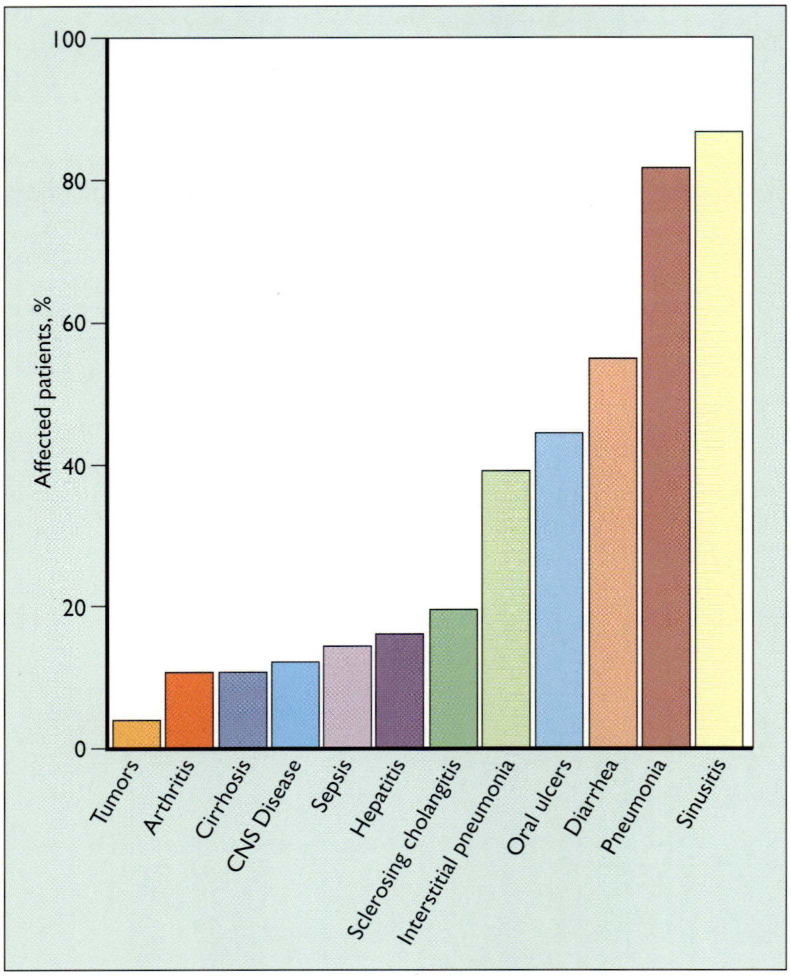

FIGURE 16-17 The clinical features of hyper-IgM syndrome as shown by the percentage of patients affected. This study was based on 56 patients documented to have hyper-IgM syndrome. Almost all of these disorders are directly related to an infectious agent except for the tumors. Over 80% had had sinusitis or pneumonia as might be expected with antibody deficiency, but almost 40% had *Pneumocystis carinii* pneumonia (interstitial pneumonia), which is associated with T-cell deficiency. They also have a number of gastrointestinal problems including sclerosing cholangitis, which often leads to liver failure. The basic defect in hyper-IgM syndrome is the lack of the CD40 ligand on T cells. However, many patients also have neutropenia, which further decreases their host defenses [8]. CNS—central nervous system.

Clinical and laboratory features of primary T-cell or cellular disorders

Disorder	Clinical features	Laboratory findings
Di George syndrome	Congenital heart disease, tetany, odd facies with low-set ears and small mouth, thrush	Hypocalcemia; low T cells, deletion in chromosome 22, absence of thymus
Nezelof syndrome	Recurrent bacterial, viral, and fungal infections; poor growth	Low T-cell number and function, high IgE, poor antibody response to specific antigens
Chronic mucocutaneous candidiasis	Recurrent skin and mucous membrane fungal infections, increased susceptibility to bacterial and viral infections	Low T-cell response to candida infection, endocrine abnormalities

FIGURE 16-18 Clinical and laboratory features of T-cell or cellular disorders. The immunologic defects in DiGeorge syndrome are extremely variable—from essentially normal to very poor T-cell function. The T-cell number and function in most patients with DiGeorge syndrome gradually improve as the patients get older. Nezelof syndrome is actually a combined disorder that also involves abnormal antibody production and is associated with thymic dysplasia. Most chronic combined mucocutaneous cases can be controlled ketoconazole, but these patients are very susceptible to bacterial and viral infections; this susceptibility becomes more apparent as they age.

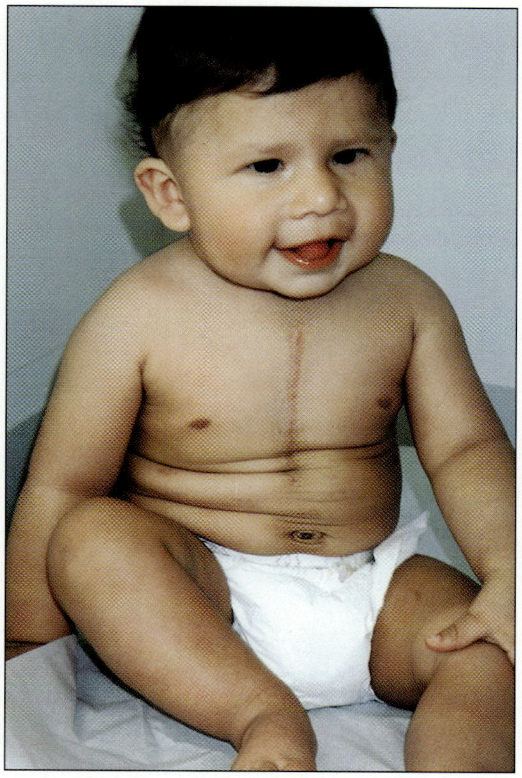

FIGURE 16-19 DiGeorge syndrome. The major features that comprise DiGeorge syndrome include congenital heart disease, hypocalcemia secondary to hypoparathyroidism, and defective T-cell immunity. The surgical scar on the chest of this infant indicates repair of heart disease caused by truncus arteriosus or interrupted aortic arch, which are common in this syndrome. This patient also has some of the facial features characteristic of DiGeorge:low-set ears, microstomia, and hypertelorism. All of these defects are caused by aberrant embryologic development of the third and fourth brachial arches and their derivatives, which includes the parathyroid glands, aortic arch, and thymus gland. There is a great variability in the penetrance of this syndrome, particularly the T-cell defect, with some infants having relatively normal T-cell number and function, whereas others have very decreased numbers of T cells and, subsequently, are much more susceptible to infections. Infants with very low T-cell functions are at risk for common pathogens including candida and viruses, such as herpes, and opportunistic infections, such as *Pneumocystis carinii*. The diagnosis of DiGeorge syndrome can be best confirmed by absence of thymus as detected by chest radiography or by direct inspection during surgery to correct their congenital heart defect. The detection of a deletion in chromosome 22 by a special fluorescent technique will be present in approximately 90% of DiGeorge patients, confirming the diagnosis. The T-cell number and function may improve if the infant does not die from the heart disease, although prophylaxis against *P. carinii* is recommended until T-cell function approaches normal. Bone marrow and thymic transplantation has been performed in severely immunocompromised patients.

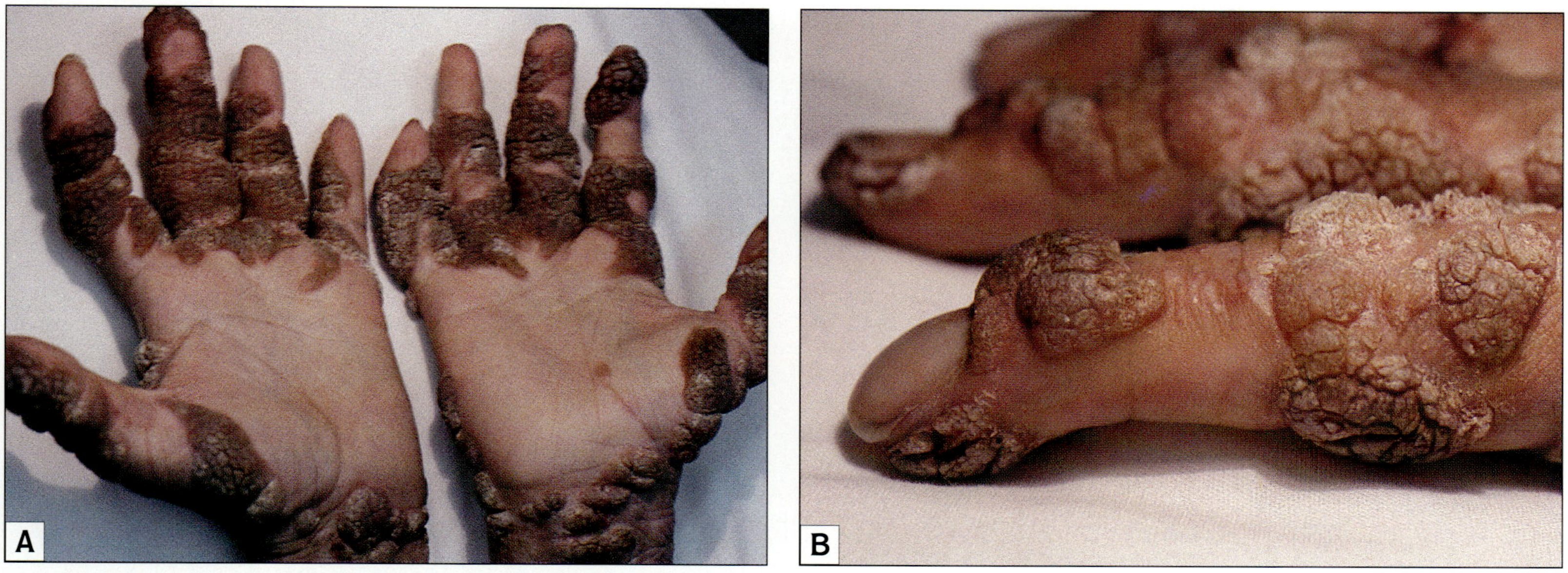

FIGURE 16-20 Nezelof syndrome. Nezelof syndrome is also known as cellular immunodeficiency with immunoglobulins. **A,** The fingers and a large portion of the hands of this 18-year-old man are covered with massive growths of verruca vulgaris (warts) that began in infancy. **B,** Close-up image of fingers. Warts are usually caused by the papovavirus and often occur in patients with defective cellular immunity. This patient had decreased numbers of the T cells that responded poorly in mitogen-stimulation assays. Patients with Nezelof syndrome are susceptible to both common and opportunistic microorganisms, similar to those encountered in DiGeorge syndrome. Immunoglobulins can be produced, but the ability to make specific antibody to pathogens is impaired. The patient shown initially had high serum levels of IgE (>30,000 U/mL) that declined to less than 1000 U/mL after starting infusions of intravenous gamma globulin. Bone marrow transplantation was not available for this patient; infusions of interleukin-2 were started to enhance his T-cell function but had to be stopped due to serious complications. The patient died at 20 years of age from his chronic pulmonary disease, with heavy growth of *Pseudomonas aeruginosa* in the lungs. This syndrome is now considered a variant of combined immunodeficiency with thymic dysplasia and aberrant immunoglobulin production.

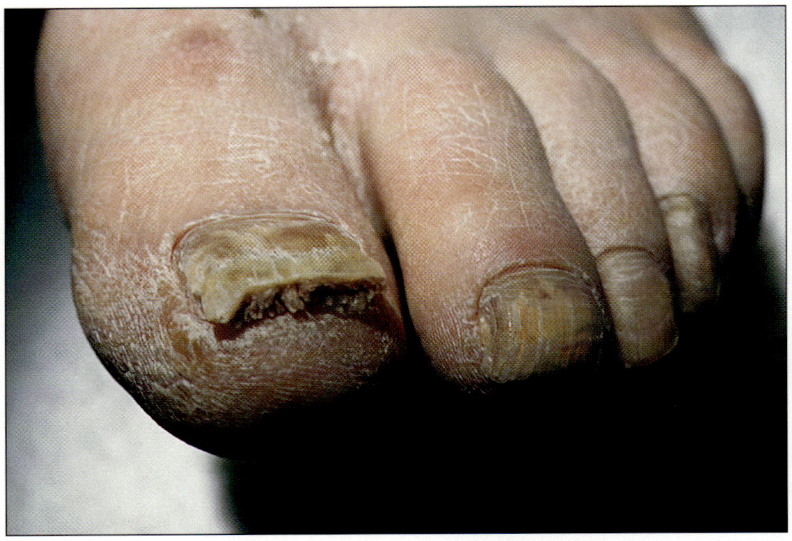

Figure 16-21 Chronic mucocutaneous candidiasis. Chronic mucocutaneous candidiasis is characterized by recurrent and chronic candidal infection of the mucous membranes, skin, and nails. These patients are also at risk for endocrinopathies and autoimmune disease. Treatment with oral ketoconazole is very effective in controlling the candidal infections, but it is now apparent that these patients are also susceptible to a number of bacterial and viral infections as they age. One of our patients with chronic mucocutaneous candidiasis later developed common variable immunodeficiency (*see* Fig. 16-16).

Disorders associated with chronic mucocutaneous candidiasis

Infections: dermatophytosis, viral, bacterial
Skin: vitiglio, alopecia, enamel dysplasia
Gastrointestinal: malabsorption, iron deficiency, hepatitis
Hematologic: aplastic anemia, hemolytic anemia, thrombocytopenia, neutropenia
Cancer: oropharynx, thymomas

Figure 16-22 Disorders associated with chronic mucocutaneous candidiasis (CMC). The disorders associated with CMC vary greatly among different patients and may be more significant that the candidiasis. More than 50% of patients are likely to suffer from severe bacterial or viral infections, and a number of deaths have been reported. All components of the immune system (*eg*, T cells, B cells, phagocytic cells) may be defective in CMC, and skin and gastrointestinal disorders also occur.

Clinical and laboratory features of primary combined T- and B-cell disorders

Disorder	Clinical features	Laboratory findings
Severe combined immunodeficiency Enzyme deficiencies X-linked (IL-2 receptor deficiency) Other	Recurrent bacterial, viral, and fungal infections; diarrhea; poor growth	Low T or B cells; enzyme deficiency as in adenosine deaminase deficiency
Reticular dysgenesis	Severe infections, diarrhea	Lymphopenia and granulocytopenia
Ataxia telangiectasia	Ataxia, telangiectasia, infections; symptoms appear at age 2 to 4 years	Low IgE and IgA; elevated α-fetoglobulin
Wiskott–Aldrich syndrome	Eczema, bleeding tendency, infections; high risk for malignancy	Thrombocytopenia, high IgA and IgE, low IgM; small platelet volume
Bare lymphocyte syndrome	Recurrent infections, diarrhea	Lack histocompatibility antigens
Short-limbed dwarfism	Dwarfism, sparse hair, infections	Skeletal deformities, leukopenia, hypogammaglobulinemia

Figure 16-23 Clinical and laboratory features of primary combined T- and B-cell disorders. Severe combined immunodeficiency tends to be the most severe disorder and is usually manifested early by failure to thrive, recurrent common childhood infections, and opportunistic infections. Ataxia telangiectasia and Wiskott–Aldrich syndrome may not be evident at birth, but the genes responsible for these disorders have been identified and can be used 1) for diagnosis in patients suspected of having these disorders, and 2) to detect the carrier state in siblings of these patients. Stem cell transplantation is the usual definitive treatment for these disorders although gene therapy is being attempted when the specific gene defect is identified.

Common pathogens in patients with primary T-cell and combined B- and T-cell disorders

Disorder	Pathogens
Di George syndrome (highly variable with regard to degree of immunodeficiency) and Severe combined immune deficiency (often more severe than Di George)	*Candida* sp (thrush common) Bacteria, common and opportunistic *Streptococcus pneumoniae* *Pseudomonas aeruginosa* *Mycobacterium* sp Viruses Herpes simplex virus Cytomegalovirus Varicella-zoster virus Protozoa *Pneumocystis carinii* *Crytosporidium*
Wiskott–Aldrich syndrome	Bacteria (encapsulated) *Haemophilus influenzae* *S. pneumoniae* *Candida* sp Viruses Herpes species Molluscum contagiosum Protozoa (*P. carinii*)
Ataxia telangiectasia	Bacteria (more common pathogens)
Chronic mucocutaneous candidiasis	Fungal *Candida albicans* (100%) Histoplasma Bacteria *Staphylococcus aureus* *S. pneumoniae* *H. influenzae* *Nocardia* Viruses (herpes species) Protozoa (*Giardia*)

FIGURE 16-24 Common pathogens in patients with primary T-cell and combined B- and T-cell disorders. Patients with combined T- and B-cell disorders are initially likely to become infected with common pathogens such as candida and streptococci, which usually will respond to conventional antimicrobial treatments. If the diagnosis of severe combined immunodeficiency is not made at an early age, however, these patients are at risk for acquiring opportunistic infections such as pneumocystis, which are more difficult to treat and more lethal. Patients with Wiskott–Aldrich syndrome may be treated for several years with immunoglobulin replacement and prophylactic antibiotics without developing life-threatening infections. Because patients with chronic mucocutaneous candidiasis live longer due to better antimicrobial drugs, they are highly susceptible to many bacteria and viruses.

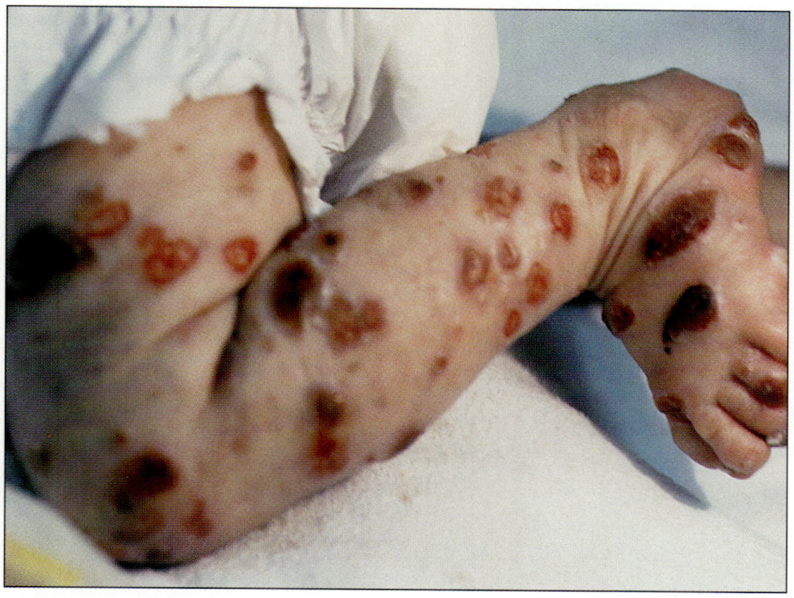

FIGURE 16-25 Severe combined immunodeficiency (SCID). This infant with SCID developed disseminated varicella infection resulting in massive skin lesions that persisted until he died several days later from invasion of the virus into the brain. A bone marrow transplantation had been planned, but the infection was too advanced (despite acyclovir therapy) for it to be effective. Infants with SCID typically present in the first few months of life with recurrent pneumonias, oral and cutaneous candidiasis, diarrhea, and failure to thrive. They are very susceptible to encapsulated bacteria (*Streptococcus pneumoniae*, *Haemophilus influenzae*) and also to opportunistic infections, such as *Pneumocystis carinii*. Several forms of SCID vary regarding the populations of T and B cells that may be present or absent and their function. There are both autosomal and X-linked forms of SCID, and the immunoglobulin levels may be decreased, normal, or elevated. SCID patients with deficiency of the adenosine deaminase enzyme may be treated with infusions of the enzyme, and gene therapy has been attempted to correct the defect in enzyme synthesis. However, stem cell transplantation (bone marrow or cord blood) is still the most effective means of treating this disorder.

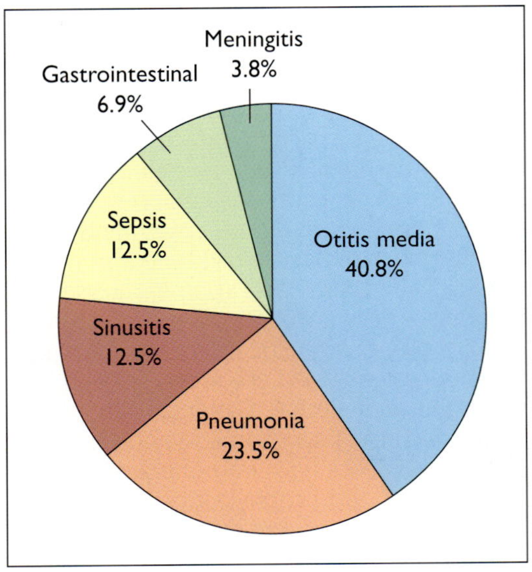

FIGURE 16-26 Relative frequencies of severe combined immunodeficiency (SCID) genotypes based on 108 SCID patients. Almost half of SCID cases were caused by mutations in the common cytokine receptor γ-chain, which is X-linked. Patients with adenosine deaminase (ADA) deficiency made up approximately 15% of the cases, and eight patients had Janus kinase 3 (JAK3) deficiency. One patient had reticular dysgenesis, and one had cartilage hair hypoplasia, but a specific mutation could not be identified in the remainder of the patients. However, 21 of these patients were found to have an autosomal recessive pattern of inheritance [9].

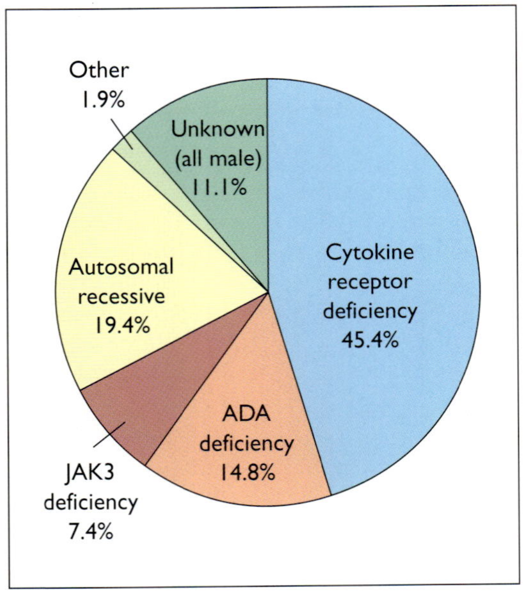

FIGURE 16-27 Sites of infections in Wiskott-Aldrich syndrome. Sites of reported infections in a large group of patients (*n* = 154) with Wiskott-Aldrich syndrome (WAS) with 289 episodes of infection during the observation period. This study included a large number of patients diagnosed with WAS prior to the availability of treatment modalities such as intravenous gamma globulin and, subsequently, many of these patients died at an early age. In an older group of WAS patients, sinusitis would be reported more often than otitis media. Infection was the leading cause of death in patients under 6 years of age followed by bleeding due to thrombocytopenia. Death due to malignancy was more common in older patients. Varicella and herpes simplex were the most common viruses identified as causing infections in these patients, and 9% developed *Pneumocystis carinii* pneumonia [10].

Clinical and laboratory features and pathogens of primary complement deficiency disorders

Deficiency	Clinical features	Laboratory findings	Pathogens
C1–C4	Infectious and autoimmune disorders	Decreased complement activity; absent specific component	Bacteria (encapsulated) *Streptococcus pneumoniae* *Haemophilus influenzae*
C5–C9	Severe *Neisseria* infections	Absent specific components; decreased complement activity	*Neisseria meningitidis* (meningitis) Disseminated gonococcal infection
Properdin	Meningococcal meningitis	Abnormal alternative pathway	*N. meningitidis*

FIGURE 16-28 Clinical features and laboratory findings in primary complement deficiency disorders. Complement deficiency disorders are very rare, and almost all (except C9) will result in decreased total complement activity (CH50 or CH100). The early component deficiencies (C1 through C4) are often associated with increased infections and autoimmune disease, whereas late component deficiency (C5 through C9) is usually associated only with neisserial infections. Those lacking C5 through C9 or properdin have increased susceptibility to neisserial infection and are candidates for meningococcal as well as pneumococcal vaccines because an increase in anticapsular antibody can enhance opsonization and phagocytic clearance through Fc receptors.

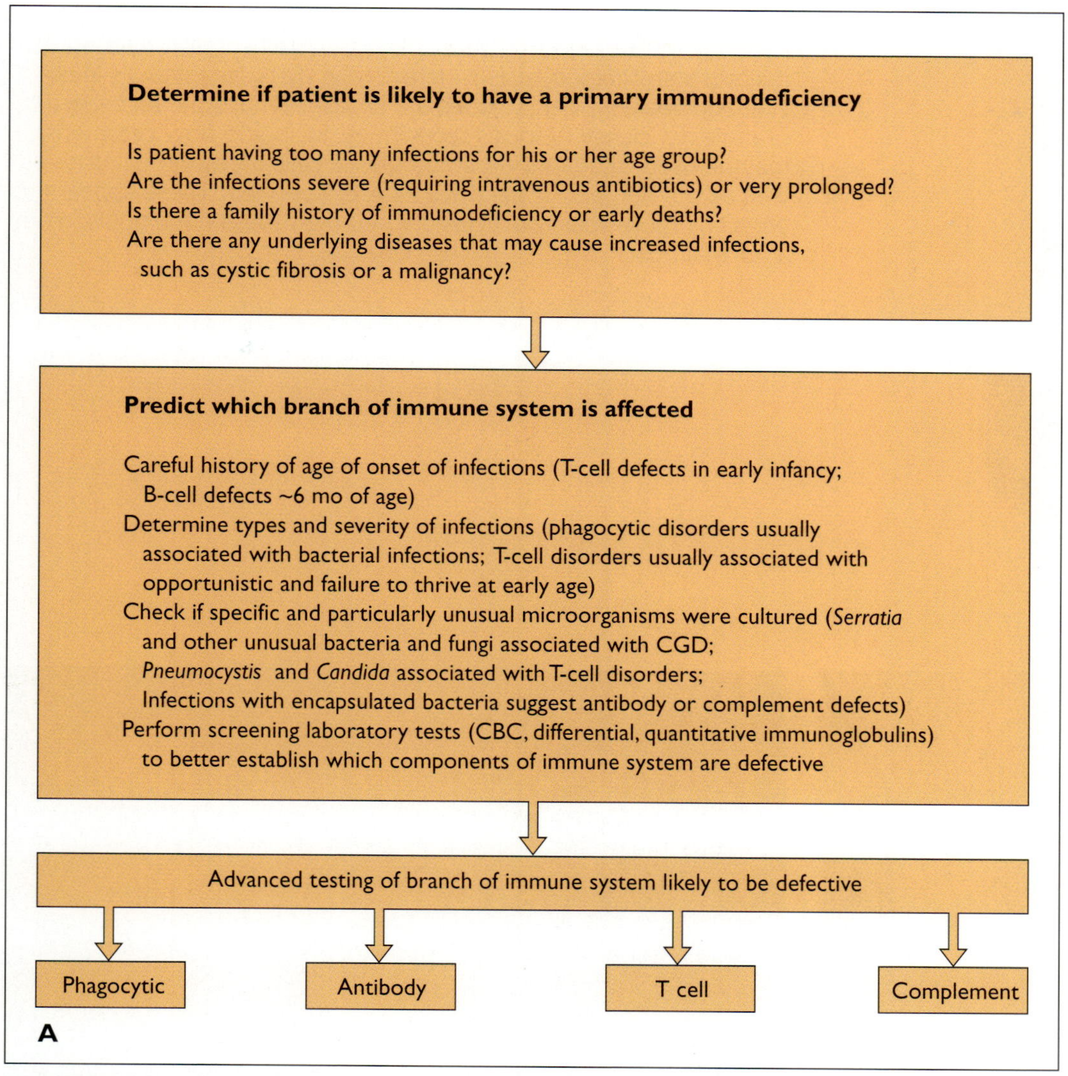

Figure 16-29 Laboratory testing for immunodeficiency. Screening tests, such as complete blood count and differential, should first be performed when immunodeficiency is suspected. **A,** The physician should also attempt to establish which branch of the immune system (phagocytic or T or B cell) is defective based on history and initial laboratory studies. **B,** Physicians should then proceed to the more complex and costly tests within that branch should be performed to establish a specific diagnosis. Complement deficiency, although not listed, can be screened for by testing complement hemolytic activity (CH50 or CH100). CBC—complete blood count; CGD—chronic granulomatous disease.

B. Laboratory testing for immunodeficiency

Phagocytic cell function	T-lymphocyte function	B-lymphocyte function
Complete blood count with differential	Complete blood count with differential	Immunoglobulin levels (IgG, IgA, IgM, IgE)
Nitroblue tetrazolium, superoxide production	Delayed hypersensitivity skin tests	Specific antibody titers to immunizations
Chemotactic and shape change assays	Proliferative response to mitogens, specific antigens	Isohemagglutinins (anti-A and anti-B)
Bactericidal and phagocytic activity	Enzyme assays (adenosine deaminase, purine nucleoside phosphorylase)	Flow cytometry for B-cell enumeration (CD19–CD21, surface immunoglobulin)
Cytotoxicity assays (antibody dependent)	Cytokine production (IL-2, interferon, IL-4, IL-6)	Immunoglobulin subclasses (IgG_1, IgG_2, IgG_3, IgG_4)
Flow cytometry (CD11/CD18, upregulation of Fc receptors)	Mixed lymphocyte culture (with allogenic cells)	Antibody responses to vaccines (primary and secondary)
		In vitro antibody production

IL–interleukin.

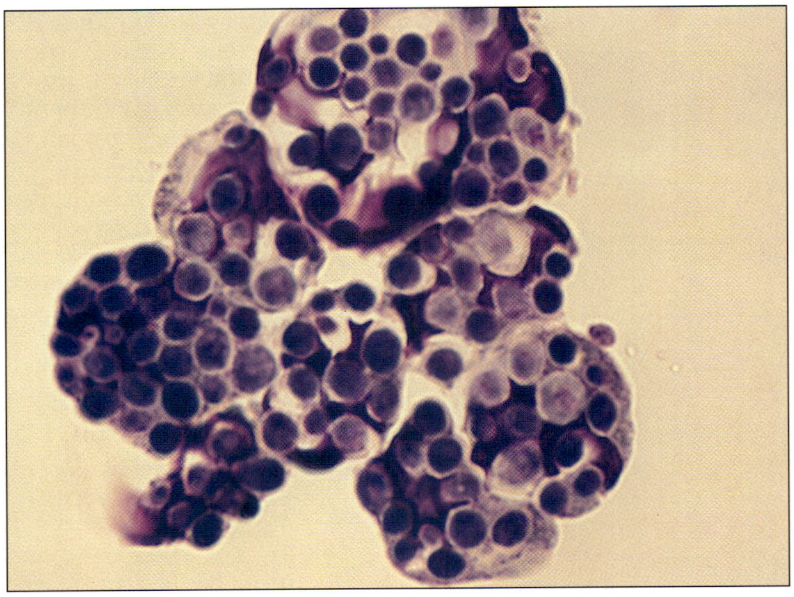

Figure 16-30 Laboratory evaluation of phagocytosis. Several neutrophils are ingesting yeast particles (stained dark blue) in this micrograph. Phagocytosis is defective in disorders such as leukocyte adhesion deficiency, Chédiak–Higashi syndrome, and specific granule deficiency. Various techniques, including flow cytometry, may be used to quantify the number of cells ingesting particles as well as the number of particles ingested per cell. There appears to be 10 or more yeast particles per cell with these neutrophils from a normal host.

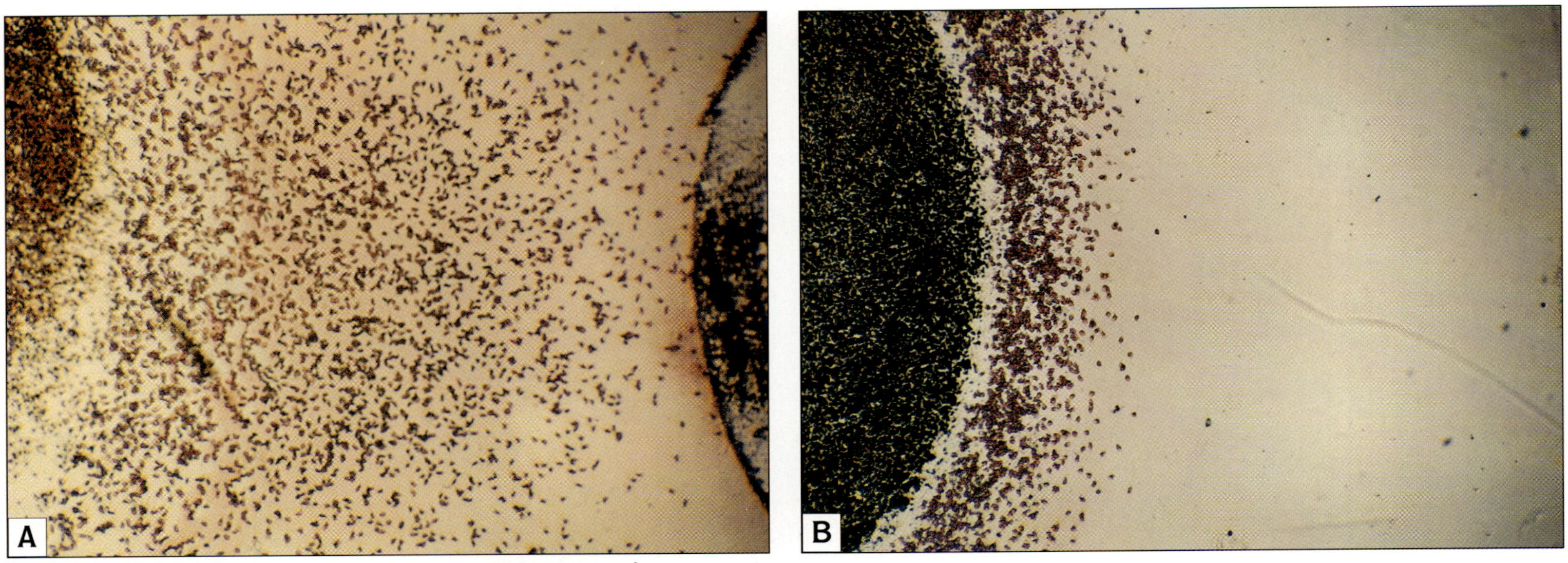

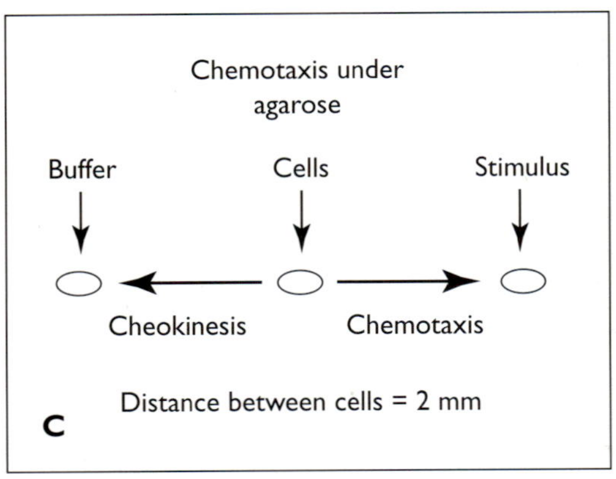

Figure 16-31 Laboratory evaluation of chemotaxis. The cells are first placed in the center well of an agarose gel and are allowed to migrate for 3 hours in a 37°C incubator. Then the cells are fixed and counted to determine how many cells migrate out and how far they migrate. **A**, Normal cells responding to zymosan-activated serum, with many actually traveling the whole distance (2 mm). **B**, Cells with a chemotactic defect, such as those with Chédiak–Higashi syndrome, hyper-IgE syndrome, or leukocyte adhesion deficiency migrate in fewer numbers and go a shorter distance. **C**, Graphic demonstration of chemotaxis-under-agarose technique. "Chemokinesis" refers to the random movement of leukocytes in the absence of a chemoattractant gradient.

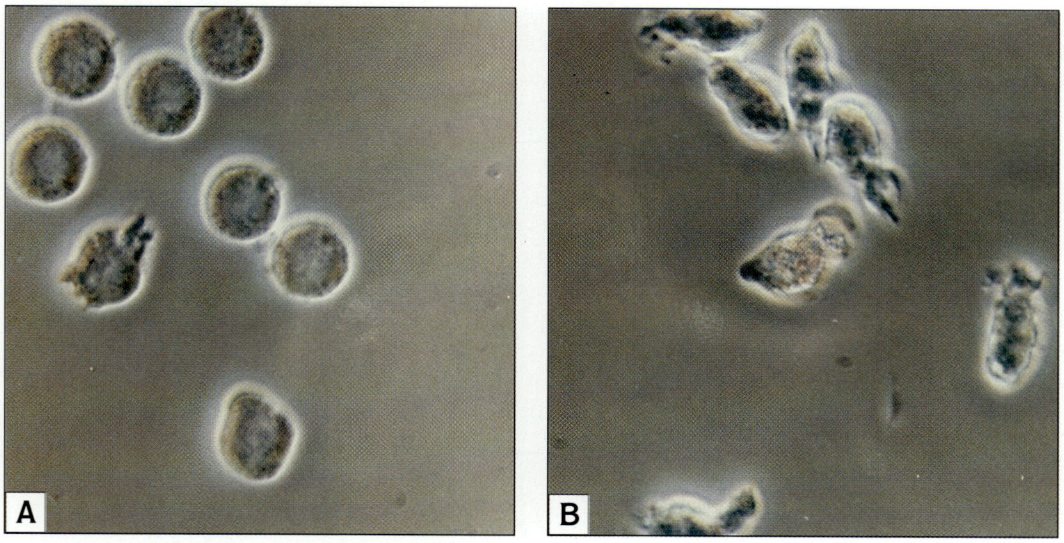

Figure 16-32 Laboratory evaluation of shape change and neutrophil aggregation. **A,** Neutrophils from a normal individual in their resting state are round without pseudopods, as usually seen in the peripheral blood. **B,** Following stimulation with complement-activated serum, the cells rapidly (within 60–120 s) acquire a more elongated shape, with pseudopods at one end and a knob-like uropod at the other end. The cells also begin to stick together and form aggregates. Shape change, which correlates with chemotaxis, can be assayed visually or by flow cytometry, and aggregation can be assayed by adapting a platelet aggregometer. Neutrophils from patients with Chédiak–Higashi syndrome or specific granule deficiency are more resistant to changing shape after stimulation, and neutrophils from patients with leukocyte adhesion deficiency do not aggregate as readily as cells from normal control subjects.

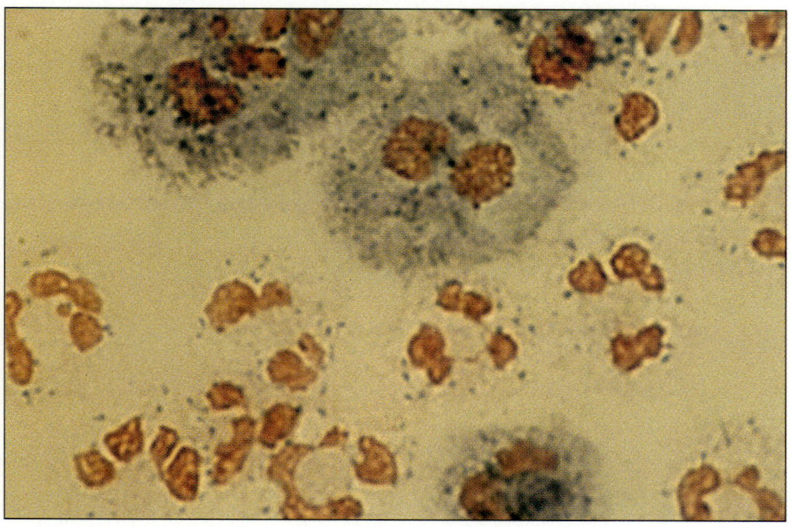

Figure 16-33 Nitroblue tetrazolium test for chronic granulomatous disease (CGD). These neutrophils from the mother of a patient with X-linked CGD have been exposed to nitroblue tetrazolium and phorbol myristate acetate to stimulate the oxidative burst. Blue staining of cytoplasmic granules indicates oxidation and production of oxygen radicals. The cells without blue granules are of the CGD phenotype. Approximately 50% of neutrophils from mothers of X-linked CGD patients are of normal phenotype, and 50% are of CGD phenotype due to random inactivation of the X chromosome in female patients. (*Courtesy of* E.S. Buescher, MD.)

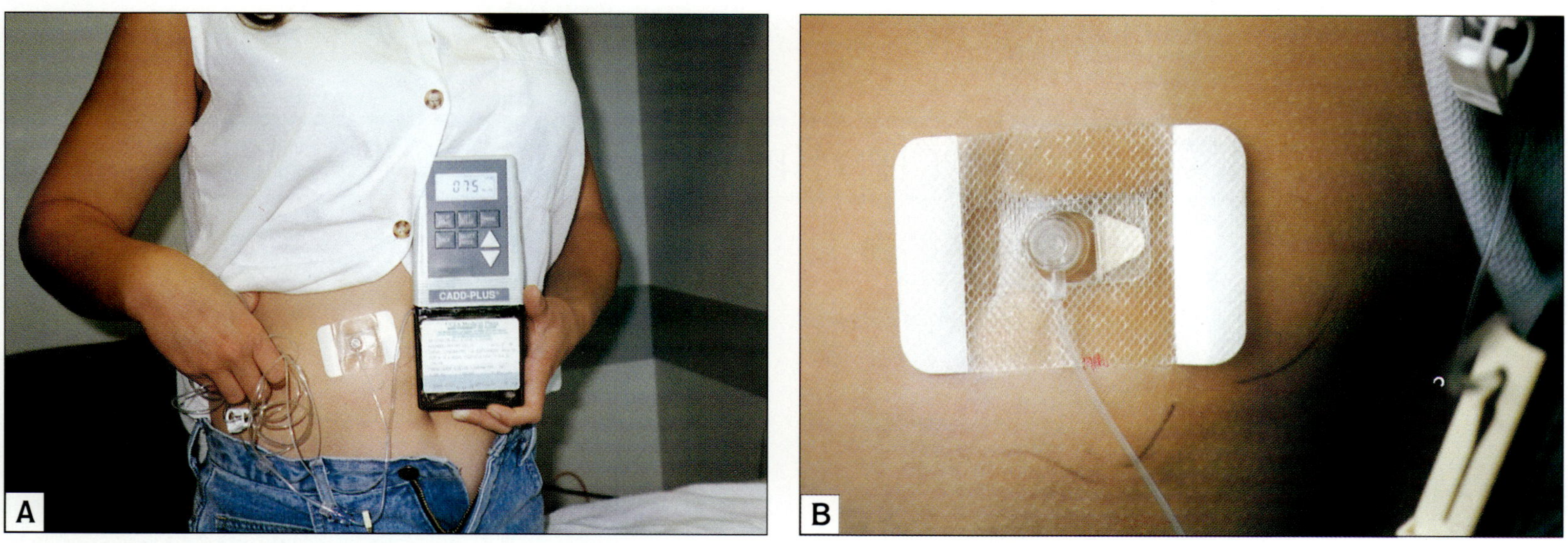

Figure 16-34 Administration of immunoglobulin therapy. Patients with severe antibody deficiency (Bruton's, hyper-IgM, and common variable syndromes) greatly benefit from immunoglobulin replacement therapy. Intramuscular injections of immunoglobulin are very painful and require frequent doses. Most patients tolerate intravenous immunoglobulin (IVIG) quite well, and high serum levels can be easily obtained by increasing the volume given. **A,** Subcutaneous infusion of IVIG. **B,** A small-bore needle implanted in the skin. Subcutaneous infusion can be used for patients with poor venous access or adverse reactions to intravenous administration.

Genetics of primary immunodeficiencies	
X-linked	**Autosomal recessive (chromosome number)**
Wiskott–Aldrich syndrome	Adenosine deaminase deficiency (20)
Chronic granulomatous disease*	Purine nucleoside phosphorylase deficiency (14)
Severe combined immunodeficiency*	Ataxia telangiectasia (11)
Hyper-IgM syndrome	Chronic granulomatous disease
Bruton's agammaglobulinemia	Different components of oxidase on chromosomes 1,7,16
X-linked lymphoproliferative syndrome	Leukocyte adhesion deficiency I (21)
Properdin deficiency	Di George syndrome (22)
	Chédiak–Higashi syndrome (1)
	Complement, classical pathway

* Also have autosomal recessive forms.

FIGURE 16-35 The genetics of primary immunodeficiency. The discovery of the genes responsible for several of the primary immunodeficiencies has greatly facilitated diagnosis in patients suspected of having a primary immunodeficiency; it also may be used for prenatal diagnosis if the parents already have an affected child. Unaffected carriers of the gene may also be identified. The recognition of the responsible gene also opens the possibility of gene therapy for these disorders as well as other treatment modalities if the gene product is also known.

REFERENCES

1. Nathan DG, Oski FA (eds): *Hematology of Infancy and Childhood*, ed 4. Philadelphia:WB Saunders; 1993.
2. Mouy R, Veber F, Blanche S, *et al.*: Long-term itraconazole prophylaxis against Aspergillus infections in thirty-two patients with chronic granulomatous disease. *J Pediatr* 1994, 125:998–1003.
3. Margolis D, Melnick D, Alling D, Gallin J: Trimethoprim-sulfamethoxazole prophylaxis in the management of chronic granulomatous disease. *J Infect Dis* 1990, 162:723–726.
4. Mouy R, Fischer A, Vilmer E, *et al.*: Incidence, severity, and prevention of infections in chronic granulomatous disease. *J Pediatr* 1989, 114:555–560.
5. Schmalstieg F: Leukocyte adherence defect. *Pediatr Infect Dis J* 1988, 7:867–872.
6. Haddad E, Le Deist F, Blanche S, *et al.*: Treatment of Chédiak-Higashi syndrome by allogenic bone marrow transplantation:report of 10 cases. *Blood* 1995, 85:3328–3333.
7. Herrod H: Chronic mucocutaneous candidiasis in childhood and complications of non-Candida infection:a report of the Pediatric Immunodeficiency Collaborative Study Group. *J Pediatr* 1990, 116:377–382.
8. Levy J, Espanol-Boren T, Thomas C, *et al.*: Clinical spectrum of X-linked hyper-IgM syndrome. *J Pediatr* 1997, 131:47–54.
9. Buckley R, Schiff R, Schiff S, *et al.*: Human severe combined immunodeficiency:genetic, phenotypic, and functional diversity in one hundred eight infants. *J Pediatr* 1997, 130:378–387.
10. Sullivan K, Mullen C, Blaese M, Winkelstein J: A multiinstitutional survey of the Wiskott-Aldrich syndrome. *J Pediatr* 1994, 125:876–885.

SELECTED BIBLIOGRAPHY

Habbal MHE, Strobel S: Leucocyte adhesion deficiency. *Arch Dis Child* 1993, 69:463–466.

Rich RR (ed):*Clinical Immunology:Principles and Practice*. Chicago:Mosby; 1996.

Steihm ER (ed): *Immunologic Disorders in Infants and Children*, ed 4. Philadelphia:WB Saunders; 1996.

INDEX

I

T